ALLERGIES AND INFECTIOUS DISEASES

MALARIA

ETIOLOGY, PATHOGENESIS AND TREATMENTS

ALLERGIES AND INFECTIOUS DISEASES

Additional books in this series can be found on Nova's website under the Series tab.

Additional e-books in this series can be found on Nova's website under the e-book tab.

ALLERGIES AND INFECTIOUS DISEASES

MALARIA

ETIOLOGY, PATHOGENESIS AND TREATMENTS

ANNA MARGRÉT PETERSON
AND
GERALD E. CALAMANDREI
EDITORS

Nova Science Publishers, Inc.
New York

For permission to use material from this book please contact us:
Telephone 631-231-7269; Fax 631-231-8175
Web Site: http://www.novapublishers.com

Library of Congress Cataloging-in-Publication Data

Malaria : etiology, pathogenesis, and treatments / editors, Anna Margrit Peterson and Gerald E. Calamandrei.
p. ; cm.
Includes bibliographical references and index.
ISBN 978-1-62100-363-2 (hardcover)
I. Peterson, Anna Margrit. II. Calamandrei, Gerald E.
[DNLM: 1. Malaria. WC 750]
LC classification not assigned
616.9'362--dc23

2011033

Published by Nova Science Publishers, Inc. † New York

Contents

Preface

Malaria remains one of the most overwhelming communicable diseases threatening the human race, disproportionately affecting populations of tropical and subtropical regions in the world. It is caused by five different species of *Plasmodium* parasite transmitted by female *Anopheles* mosquito. In this book, the authors present topical research in the etiology, pathogenesis and treatments of malaria. Some of the topics discussed include progress with RTS,S; global malaria eradication; malaria in the archaic Greek world; the role of human matrix metalloproteinases in malaria pathogenesis; artemisinin combination therapy for the treatment of childhood malaria; climate variations and malaria in China and natural acquired anti-plasmodium falciparum IgG antibody responses.

Chapter 1 - Malaria remains one of the most overwhelming communicable diseases threatening the human race, disproportionately affecting population of tropical and subtropical regions of the world. It is caused by five different species of Plasmodium parasite transmitted by female Anopheles mosquito. The etiological agents have remarkably complex way of target cells invasion and complication of the disease. The pathogenesis of malaria is multifaceted, and its degree of causing life threatening severe malaria depends on the *Plasmodium* species that cause infection, endemicity of the disease, age and the immune status of the infected host. It is certain that majority of deaths due to malaria is caused by *P. falciparum* which is known to be associated with several severe syndromes. Recent reports, mainly from Asia, indicated that *P.vivax* is also causing severe malaria. The basic pathological mechanisms behind these disorders, which are vital in designing protective vaccine and effective anti-malarial drug, are not completely understood yet and some are still debatable. Moreover, the earlier believe that some segments of the human population are naturally resistant to malaria due to polymorphism is also partly refuted. To the advantage of readers and for common understanding among scholars, it is necessary to review recent progresses on malaria research. To this effect, this chapter discusses an overview of recent findings related to malaria parasite, cellular and molecular means of target cell recognition, invasion, and mechanisms leading to complication of the disease, possible promising target areas of anti-malarial drug design, and the global trends of drug resistant strains of Plasmodium parasite.

Chapter 2 - Malaria has afflicted humans for aeons, being responsible for more deaths throughout history than any other disease. Today, infection with protozoan parasites of the genus *Plasmodium* still claims the lives of at least one million people each year, mainly children, in addition to the significant debilitation it causes to hundreds of millions more. Consequently, malaria has a drastic socioeconomic impact on endemic countries and therefore it has been the focus of global health initiatives for decades. Early attempts to eradicate malaria through targeting the mosquito vector failed; however, increased investment in existing control measures, such as the use of insecticide-impregnated bed nets, has been matched by renewed efforts to develop an efficacious vaccine. Sequencing of the genome of *P. falciparum*, which causes the most severe form of the disease, has improved knowledge of the malaria parasite's complex lifecycle, which, combined with a greater understanding of the human immune response to infection, has produced a number of novel candidate vaccines over the last two decades. Most notable among these is RTS,S which has shown much promise throughout a long development process, recently becoming the first candidate vaccine against human malaria to progress into phase III clinical trials. There is optimism, therefore, that in the foreseeable future RTS,S may become the first licensed antimalarial vaccine. Nevertheless, there are unresolved issues surrounding the lack of understanding of its mechanism of protection and doubt cast over its therapeutic potential. While the future success of RTS,S as a commercially available product is not certain, it is still likely to play a significant role in our ongoing fight against malaria, if only as a forerunner to a more refined second generation vaccine.

Chapter 3 - Nearly six decades ago, the Global Malaria Eradication Programme (GMEP) (1955–1969) launched resulted with spectacular successes in terms of reduction/interruption of malaria transmission and substantially minimized the malaria burden too. Malaria eradication (malERA) and the sharp reduction of malaria incidence to zero has been achieved in a few countries by employing the world's cheapest "silver bullet", the so called DDT (Dichloro-Diphenyl-Trichloroethane) as well as by administering the low-cost antimalarial, chloroquine. However, due to several compounding factors such as emergence of insecticide resistance, drug resistance, inadequate fund, lack of political willingness, fragile healthcare system, inappropriate planning, lack of logistical support and poor infrastructures, the over-promised and under-delivered GMEP has been abandoned in 1969; subsequently in 1970s the strategy has been modified from eradication to control. Thereafter, even today malaria kills a poor African *child for every 30 seconds and continues to be a* major public health problem *in* the resource-constrained countries of Africa, Asia, Latin amerce, and beyond.

At the moment there is a worldwide renewed interest on malERA giving rise to the global agenda, which is purely due to countrywide global partnership and adequate support of international donors. There is a ray of hope as the malaria map shrinks and malaria incidence falls and some countries may consider attacking remaining foci with an elimination agenda by employing frontline vector control tools like insecticide-treated nets (ITNs), indoor residual spraying (IRS) and by supplementing with active case-management of potent antimalarial like artemisinin-based combination therapy (ACT).

However, in the present day scenario, malERA seems to be an over-ambitious and unrealistic target. In this perspective, this chapter describes briefly on the global public health and socio-economic impacts of malaria and also explains how to provide a comprehensive insight on the global malERA through campaigns and how efforts could to be taken to create a malaria free world. Furthermore, it also outlines some of the current potential obstacles and barriers, and how we can address the issues and challenges with the existing tools and how we can improve and exploit them effectively to attain the meaningful global malaria eradication. Indeed, shaping a better planet, suitable to every individual and in particular for children are a matter of grave concern as well as a mission and it is one of our foremost senses of duty too.

Chapter 4 - Malaria is a major public health problem in developing countries and is the top ranked priority tropical disease of the World Health Organization. It is a leading cause of disease and death among children under five years, pregnant women and non-immune travellers/immigrants. Every year, there are about 500 million clinical attacks of malaria. Of these, 2-3 million are severe and about 1 million people die (about 3000 deaths every day). Malaria in pregnancy accounts for about 25% of cases of severe maternal anemia and 10-20% of low birth weight. About 40% of the world's population is at risk of malaria. According to the World Malaria Report, malaria is prevalent in 108 countries of the tropical and semitropical world (Africa; Amazon, central and southern America; central, south and southeast Asia; Pacific). The economic burden of malaria is huge, estimated to be $12 billion a year in Africa alone. Known since millennia, malaria continues to upsurge in incidence till date due to a variety of factors including but not limited to drug resistance, global climate change, changing agricultural practices, insecticide resistance mosquitoes, population movements and poverty, and political instability.

Malaria is caused by the protozoa *Plasmodium* (P) and transmitted by the bite of an infected female anopheline mosquito. There are five species known to cause infection namely, P. *falciparum*, P. *vivax*, P. *ovale*, P. *malariae*, and P. *knowlesi*. Infection due to P species other than P. *falciparum* is called non-*falciparum* malaria. P. *falciparum* causes the most severe disease and patients with this form of malaria may progress to life-threatening illness within hours. The P life cycle consists of an exoerythrocytic (asymptomatic) stage and erythrocytic (symptomatic) stage. Several human genetic polymorphisms and mutations have been observed to influence either clinical attack or severity of the disease, particularly hemoglobin and red cell antigens. Individuals living in endemic areas appear to develop partial immunity to malaria following repeated infections. Although malaria classically presents as a febrile paroxysm with headache, myalgia, nausea, vomiting, malaise, splenomegaly, anemia and thrombocytopenia, it is a great imitator and trickster with varied and dramatic manifestations especially in endemic regions. Malaria diagnostic tools include clinical criteria, light microscopy, rapid diagnostic tests (RDTs), and molecular diagnostic techniques. Light microscopy remains the gold standard for diagnosis of malaria; it permits determination of the infecting species as well as quantification of parasitemia, facilitating monitoring the response to therapy. Malarial target antigen for RDTs includes histidine-rich protein 2 of P. *falciparum*, a pan-malarial *Plasmodium* aldolase, and the parasite specific lactate dehydrogenase. Molecular technologies have been developed to improve the diagnosis of malaria, although these methods are limited by a number of factors including specialized equipment, continuing supplies, operator expertise, turnaround time and cost. Treatment of chloroquine sensitive non-falciparum malaria comprises administration of chloroquine followed by standard course of primaquine for radical cure. Therapeutic options for chloroquine resistance non-*falciparum* malaria include mefloquine, atovaquone-proguanil or a combination of quinine and tetracycline or doxycycline. Parenteral antimalarial is often required for falciparum malaria and includes artmisinin derivative or qunine/quinidine along with doxycycline or clindamycin. Artesunate is the preferred therapy for treatment of severe falciparum malaria in adults and children wherever intravenous artesunate is available. Strategies for malaria control include mosquito vector control, personal protection from mosquito bites and chemoprophylaxis. Malaria vaccine is still under trial.

Although mortality is rare with non-falciparum malaria, for patients with complicated falciparum malaria the mortality approaches 10-20%. Medico-legal autopsies in cases of sudden unexpected natural deaths have revealed malaria as the cause of death in a few cases. In a study conducted at Government Wenlock District Hospital in Mangalore, a malaria endemic area in South India, autopsy files revealed 5 cases of sudden death due to malaria diagnosed by histopathology between September 2004 and August 2008. Cerebral malaria, acute renal insufficiency, acute pulmonary edema and acute respiratory distress syndrome are possible mechanisms of sudden death due to malaria.

Chapter 5 - Malaria influenced human natural selection and, in particular, Plasmodium Falciparum exerted a major impact on human genome in comparison with every other pathogen. Different and discussed opinions exist, concerning the period in which Plasmodium Falciparum infection appeared in Hellenic peninsula, although it was stated that this protozoan came from central Africa and reached Mediterranean and Egyptian coasts through Nile Valley. Paleopathology is providing some convincing responses, by means of the biomolecular analysis on bone remains, a methodology introduced with increasing frequency in the last ten years. Unfortunately some limits, such as the very ancient age of the remains, cannot be overcome and in addition the state of preservation of samples may influence the sensibility of laboratory methodologies. It is also to remember that previously only the macroscopic study of skeleton was performed. On the ground of a largely shared valuation that the myths may be the remote mirror of really occurred historical events and that the mythical tails, arising from the archaic history as well as from the pre-historic age, are frequently represented in the ancient artistic manifactures [Corinthian and Athenian ceramics], the Authors endeavoured to establish a link between some archeological remains of Hellenic origin and mythical events concerning Hercules. In particular it was considered the tale recording the second labour of the Hero, when the Hydra of Lerna was defeated and killed.

In accordance with some theories, the fight of Hercules against monster endowed with multiple-heads, which both were reproducing and doubling after their excision, would be the clear memory of the attempt to reclaim the marshes in malarial district of Lerna. This area in Argolis, during the Neolithic age, would be an healthy place and some communities of fishers probably settled here, since fresh water from a coast lake were available. Subterrean rivers, coming from mountains in Argolis, supplied this lake. Nevertheless, an environmental change caused the lake to be covered with sand and the apperance of a marsh with subsequent likely disappearance of human settlements, approximately in 1250 b.C. This decline would have been caused by the appearance of Plasmodium Falciparum malaria. The study of epidemics, from an historical point of view, might benefit by archeological contribution and, in addition, by works of the crafstmen and artists, who depicted, in their manufactures, remarkable mythical events for ancient people.

However, paleopathological study possibly along with the integration of biomolecular analysis remain not replaceable approaches.

Chapter 6 - Human matrix metalloproteinases (MMPs) are a family of proteolytic enzymes able to destroy endothelial tight junctions, disrupt the subendothelial basement membrane, and modulate the activity of pro-inflammatory molecules and other MMPs. The regulation of balances between MMPs and their endogenous inhibitors (tissue inhibitors of metalloproteinases, TIMPs) plays a key role in either physiological processes, such as wound repair; or pathological, including tumor angiogenesis and neuroinflammation. Interestingly, in the last decade, growing evidence, in vivo and in vitro, on the involvement of MMPs and TIMPs in severe and complicated malaria has been emerging. In the present chapter, the data on altered levels MMPs and TIMPs available from human and murine models of malaria will be reviewed; and the well-established relationship between the host MMP-9 and parasite haemozoin (HZ), the lipid-enriched ferriprotoporphyrin IX crystal produced by Plasmodium parasite after haemoglobin catabolism, will be analyzed. Therefore, the functional role of deregulated balances between MMPs and TIMPs in the clinical progress towards complicated malaria (cerebral, lung and placental malaria), as well as the potential use of MMP inhibitors as an adjuvant treatment, will be discussed.

Chapter 7 - Malaria remains the most severe public health challenge facing most of the countries of the tropical and sub-tropical regions of the world. The disease is known to be associated with underdevelopment, poverty and ignorance. The World Health Organization has described malaria as a major contributor to high rate of the global infectious disease–related mortality and morbidity particularly in sub-Saharan Africa. Almost all of the malaria deaths in sub-Saharan Africa occur in children below five years of age and this translates to the child mortality of nearly 1 million each year. Early and effective treatment of childhood malaria is imperative because the majority of children who die from malaria do so within 48 hours of onset of illness. In addition, to the high malaria transmission intensity in sub-Saharan Africa, limited access to adequate treatment, increasing parasite resistance to affordable and safe medicines (chloroquine, sulphadoxine-pyrimethamine and amodiaquine); and inappropriate treatment at home or at community level, aggravate the malaria burden. The relentless increase in malaria parasites resistance to many conventional antimalarial drugs necessitated the introduction of artemisinin-based combination therapy (ACT). There is a growing international consensus that wide-scale, systematic implementation of ACT is one of the few effective measures that will enable malaria-endemic countries to achieve the ambitious goals set in Abuja in 2000 to 'roll back malaria'. The derivatives of artemisinin plant, Artemisia annua (Qinghao, Asteraceae) are currently considered the cornerstone of Plasmodium falciparum malaria treatment due to their potency and rapid action. Numerous evidence abound indicating that ACTs were very efficacious in the treatment of uncomplicated malaria among children in sub-Saharan Africa. These ACTs include; artemether-lumefantrine, artesunate-mefloquine, artesunate-amodiaquine, artesunate-sulphadoxine-pyrimethamine, artesunate-chlorproguanil-dapsone, and dihydroartemisinin-piperaquine. Most of the studies however acknowledged that more investigations are required for continuous safety monitoring and on the pharmacokinetics of these ACT varieties to provide more scientific information on the profiles of the drugs. There is need for continuous research to evaluate the tolerability, efficacy, effectiveness and cost of various combination therapy strategies, particularly relating to their potential use in Africa south of the Sahara, is imperative.

Chapter 8 - The incidence of malaria has decreased dramatically in 20th century China. However, there has been an evident re-emergence of malaria since 2000. The transmission of malaria is complicated, and climate variability may be one of the risk factors associated with the re-emergence of malaria. The relationship between malaria and climatic variables has been assessed in many regions, such as Africa and South America. However, limited studies have been conducted in China, and little is known about the impact of climate variations on malaria in that country. This chapter has systematically reviewed previous studies that examine the association between climatic variables and malaria in China; including research methods, findings, and limitations. Evidence has also been provided by a scenario-based study, projecting the future health burdens of malaria due to rising temperatures. Recommendations are presented at the end of the chapter for policy makers, public health practitioners, as well as clinicians to prevent and control malaria in a warming climate, not only in China but also in other developing countries.

Chapter 9 - Malaria is estimated to cause between 300 and 500 million clinical cases with about 700,000 to 1.6 million deaths every year, most (about 90%) of these deaths occur in sub-Sahara Africa. Thus, malaria remains a major cause of morbidity and mortality in sub-Sahara Africa. In Ghana malaria accounts for about 32.5% of all Out Patient attendances and about 24.6% of deaths in children under 5 years. The World Health Organization recommended the use of artemisinin based combination therapy (ACT) for the treatment of uncomplicated malaria to provide effective treatment against *P. falciparum* malaria and slow down the spread of drug resistance. Ghana has adopted the use of artesunate + amodiaquine for the treatment of uncomplicated malaria in the country since 2005. Malaria control in Ghana, like elsewhere in sub-Sahara Africa, relies on early diagnosis and prompt treatment of suspected cases and the home is where early recognition and in most cases prompt treatment is initiated. However, the current combination therapy is not widely available for home management as a result of the fear that making these drugs available may lead to abuse and therefore lead to the emergence of Plasmodium falciparum resistance to these drugs. Intermittent preventive treatment (IPT) has now been accepted as an important component of the malaria control strategy but has not been implemented in combination with timely home management to measure their impact on malaria prevalence in a target population. Findings reported in this chapter are from a two year implementation of a combined intermittent preventive treatment for children (IPTc) and timely home management of malaria using artesunate + amodiaquine. All children aged six to 60 months received home-based delivery of intermittent preventive treatment using amodiaquine + artesunate, delivered at home by community assistants every four months (six times in 24 months). Malaria parasite prevalence surveys were conducted before the first IPTc and four months after the third and sixth IPTc rounds. Results showed a significant reduction in malaria prevalence from 25% at baseline to 1% at year-two evaluation. At baseline, 13.8% of the children were febrile (axilary temperature of ≥37.50C) compared to 2.0% at year-two-evaluation. The improved access to ACT drugs for the treatment of suspected malaria in children aged six to 60 months could be one of the ways to achieve the Abuja target of getting 60% of under five suspected malaria cases into treatment within 24 hours of symptom onset, which was not achieved by 2005 as was targeted. If policy makers are bold enough to initiate policy to allow adults to participate in IPT at least once or twice in a year, this could further accelerate the reduction in malaria prevalence to a level that will reduce the public health burden of malaria.

Chapter 10 - Immunity to malaria has a major role in controlling the disease and its pathogenesis. Naturally acquired antibodies play a crucial role in developing immunity to malaria. Over the past two decades, anti-*Plasmodium falciparum* antibody prevalence to different malaria candidate antigens has been conducted in sera from individuals living in Thailand where malaria is endemic. They were village residents, occupational exposed soldiers, and patients with severe and uncomplicated malaria. Partial seroactivity was observed for anti-immunoglobulin (Ig) G antibodies to ring-infected erythrocyte surface antigens (erythrocyte membrane immunofluorescence [EMIF] whole parasite), Pf332, Pf155/Ring infected erythrocyte surface antigens (RESA), and the repeat region of the circumsporozoite (CS) protein (R32tet32). Prospective studies assessed only the anti-R32tet32 IgG antibody, unable to prevent malaria. Interestingly, all village residents, all occupational exposed soldiers, and all of those with acute falciparum malaria had IgG antibody responses to a late blood stage malaria antigen (whole). Furthermore, significant lowered levels of this antibody were seen in the patients who died, compared to those who recovered. Similar to whole sporozoite IgG antibody responses, significant lowered levels of sporozoite antibodies were observed in cerebral malaria compared to those with acute uncomplicated malaria. The exploration of naturally acquired anti-*P.falciparum* antibody prevalence, and its relation to the past's morbidity and mortality, may provide clue into malaria control strategies, especially vaccination.

Chapter 11 - Malaria is a classical tropical infection. This disease has been known for hundred years. However, it is still the public health problem worldwide. Basically, there are 4 well-known malaria parasite species that cause disease in human beings. However, within the past few years, the newest fifth species was reported. There are many reports on the fifth species of malaria in the present day. In this brief article, the author briefly reviews and presents details of the fifth species malaria.

Chapter 12 - Malaria fever, caused by four species of Plasmodium, is one of the commonest parasitic diseases plaguing mankind, particularly in the malaria-endemic regions of the world. The most widespread and virulent of the infection is caused by *Plasmodium falciparum*, which is known to affect millions of people annually.This write-up, a compilation of extracts of publications from especially, journals, and books, looks at how the infective protozoan has exploited the use of two hosts, mosquito and man, and while in man, the protozoan's ability to survive in different asexual forms; as hepatic sporozoites and erythrocyte merozoites. Exhibiting structural, biochemical and physiological features of typical Acomplexans, the sporozoites are able to attach to and breach membranes in their invasive journey through the insect-vertebrate hosts. The role of rhoptries and micronemes in the proper orientation of the sporozoite, as well as the further facilitation of the invasion by circumsporozoite protein (CSP) and thrombospondin-related anonymous protein (TRAP) is considered. Both CSP and TRAP are possible candidate proteins for the development of anti-malarial vaccines. While inside the erythrocytes (parasitized erythrocytes), the survival of the parasites depends on their utilization of the host's haemoglobin, which they need to hydrolyse, using a battery of proteases (plasmepsins, falcipain and metalloprotease, falcilysin), followed by detoxification to form haemozoin, the malarial pigment, a biocrystal. The formation of the haemozoin can be the target of attack of some anti-malarial therapies. The parasitisation of the erythrocytes is an adaptive survival strategy for the intruding protozoan, but to the host, it is the harbinger of various pathologies that culminate in a wide array of clinical features attributable to multi-organ failure and even death. Inside the parasitized erythrocytes, some parasite proteins or antigens are secreted to the surface of the erythrocyte membrane. The best characterized of these parasite proteins is PfEMP-1, a family of proteins encoded by the 'var' genes because each parasite contains many copies of the gene; and by switching expression between the copies, it is able to cause a remarkable degree of antigenic variation, a major ploy for survival. PfEMP-1 plays a key role in the parasite's ability to sequester in the microvasculature of the infected person, and to form rosettes with uninfected erythrocytes. The PfEMP-1 can also bind to a variety of host cell receptors, including CD 36, vCAM, P-selectin, etc. The severity of falciparum infection depends largely on the ability of parasitized erythrocytes to adhere to endothelial cells (ECs) and thus getting sequestered in the capillary network of vital organs such as brain, kidney, lungs and liver. Additionally, adhesion of the parasitised red cells to the ECs causes the activation of ECs, resulting in the over-expression of adhesive molecules and pro-inflammatory cytokines. The pathology of the infection could be ascribed to 'hyperadhesion', and could also be explained based on either the 'mechanical hypothesis', due to hypofusion of tissues, or 'cytokine hypothesis.' The most common complication of falciparum infection is anaemia, in which there could be ineffective erythropoiesis and dyserythropoiesis. Other clinical features are hepatic, renal and pulmonary dysfunctions and cerebral malaria. Attempts at using drugs to break the blood-stage life cycle target some important metabolic processes required for the survival of the parasite. The author and colleagues have shown that in sickle cell anaemia patients with falciparum parasites, the distribution of the reticulocytes is exponential, but in the non-parasitaemic, the distribution is polynomial.

Chapter 13 - This study attempts the reconstruction of the most characteristic clinical picture of the acute phase of malaria, the malarial paroxysm, describing the elements that participate on the part of the parasite and the host, the way they become integrated, and how they function to produce the classical clinical manifestations of what we call malaria.

Chapter 14 - Malaria continues to exert a strong selective pressure on humans resulting in genetic adaptations, such as haemoglobin structural variants (HbS, HbC, and HbE) and haemoglobin production disorders (α and β thalassaemias), which have reached high frequencies in populations exposed to malaria. Epidemiological studies have confirmed and expanded the hypothesis, originally formulated by Haldane on the basis of the geographical distribution of thalassaemia, that these adaptive traits have been maintained at such high frequency despite their fitness cost due to a selective advantage offered by protection against *Plasmodium falciparum* malaria. Moreover, there is evidence that this protection may vary according to the *P. falciparum* transmission intensity, which modulates the level of selective pressure, thus of the advantage conferred, and ultimately the frequency and dynamics of these adaptive traits in human populations. However, the mechanisms by which protection against malaria infection and disease is achieved in carriers of these traits remain elusive. In addition, clinical epidemiological studies have indicated that homozygote carriers of HbS may paradoxically be at a higher risk of severe malaria when infected with *P. falciparum*, thus emphasizing the importance of prompt and adequate treatment.

We aim to evaluate the current state of the art in relation to malaria pathogenesis with a particular focus on new insights into the biological mechanisms underlying the protection exerted by such genetic adaptations. Understanding these mechanisms in individuals carrying adaptive traits may unravel important clues as to what is necessary to induce protection against malaria, and may thus be of relevance for future vaccine design.

Chapter 15 - Malaria pathogenesis results from a complex interplay of pro-inflammatory and anti-inflammatory mediators produced as a result of innate responses following *Plasmodium* infection. These mediators interact with host tissues and organs resulting in damage and destruction that characterizes specific syndromes associated with red blood cell destruction, vascular endothelial disturbances, microvascular obstruction, respiratory distress, retinopathy, inflammatory responses to toxins and other parasite metabolites and placental tissue destruction. The malaria syndromes define uncomplicated malaria (UM), cerebral malaria (CM), placental malaria (PM), severe malarial anemia (SA), and severe malaria (SM). Approximately 515 million cases of malaria are reported annually with 1-3 million deaths occurring in children. Five *Plasmodium* species infect humans: *P. falciparum, P. vivax P.*

malariae P. ovale and P. knowlesi. Plasmodium falciparum is the agent most associated with severe and fatal malaria. Pregnant women and children make up the most vulnerable groups to develop severe pathogenesis from malaria infection. Cytokines, chemokines, vascular endothelial proteins, angiogenic factors, and other host mediators make up important mediators of pathogenesis in the host. In addition, other non-immunologic host molecules, parasite proteins, metabolites and toxins may contribute to severe pathogenesis in the host. Determining which of the mediators enhance adverse outcomes for disease progression and poor disease prognosis as well as identifying those mediators with protective effects is an area of intense investigation in malaria research. The cytokines tumor necrosis factor alpha (TNFα), interleukin (IL)-12, IL-1β, IL-10 and interferon gamma (IFNγ) are associated with the pathogenesis of cerebral malaria and severe anemia, with TNFα being strongly implicated with this form of malaria. Treatment of patients with neutralizing anti-TNFα antibodies was effective in resolving clinical symptoms. Low ratios of IL-10 to TNFα in serum correlate with severe anemia in contrast to high IL-10 to TNFα ratios seen in children with uncomplicated malaria. Levels of soluble ICAM-1, IL-1Ra, IL-2R, IL-4, IL-6, IL-6R, neopterin, angiopoeitin (ANG) 2 and TNFα are found to be highly elevated in patients with cerebral malaria, with TNFα being highly elevated in patients who died from cerebral malaria compared to patients with uncomplicated malaria. TNFα and ANG2 levels can predict poor prognosis with fatal outcomes in cases of cerebral malaria. A diagnostic test that is prognostic and capable of discriminating among the different malaria syndromes as well as distinguishing infections caused by non malaria pathogens will improve disease management of malaria and disease surveillance. A diagnostic test that incorporates host mediators of disease as well as parasite products and toxins would detect biomarkers of disease progression, diseases severity and development of cerebral malaria and will also be useful in determining the effectiveness of parasite clearance following drug treatment. In this chapter we examine studies performed to evaluate host mediators associated with malaria pathogenesis; uncomplicated malaria (UM), cerebral malaria (CM), placental malaria (PM), severe malarial anemia (SA), and severe malaria (SM) to determine the effectiveness of the mediators as biomarkers for malaria diagnosis.

Contributor List

Tsige Ketema
James W. L. Denny
Andrew W. Taylor-Robinson
Kaliyaperumal Karunamoorthi
Ritesh G. Menezes
Sadip Pant
Tanuj Kanchan
S. Senthilkumaran
Magdy A. Kharoshah
Ramadas Naik
Y. P. Raghavendra Babu
P. P. Jagadish Rao
Abul Fazil
Sergio Sabbatani
Sirio Fiorino
Mauro Prato
C. J. Uneke
Ying Zhang
Peng Bi
Janet Hiller
Yuwei Sun
Baofa Jiang
Collins K. Ahorlu
Piyatida Tangteerawatana
Srisin Khusmith
Viroj Wiwanitkit
Filiberto Malagón
Kwabena Nsiah
Benno Kreuels
Federica Verra
Ivan T. Matthews
Tobili Y. Sam-Yellowe

In: Malaria: Etiology, Pathogenesis and Treatments
Editor: A. M. Peterson and G. E. Calamandrei
ISBN: 978-1-62100-363-2

Chapter I

Pathogenesis of Severe Malaria and Treatment

*Tsige Ketema**
Department of Biology, College of Natural Sciences,
Jimma University, Jimma, Ethiopia

Abstract

Malaria remains one of the most overwhelming communicable diseases threatening the human race, disproportionately affecting population of tropical and subtropical regions of the world. It is caused by five different species of Plasmodium parasite transmitted by female Anopheles mosquito. The etiological agents have remarkably complex way of target cells invasion and complication of the disease. The pathogenesis of malaria is multifaceted, and its degree of causing life threatening severe malaria depends on the Plasmodium species that cause infection, endemicity of the disease, age and the immune status of the infected host. It is certain that majority of deaths due to malaria is caused by *P. falciparum* which is known to be associated with several severe syndromes Recent reports, mainly from Asia, indicated that *P.vivax* is also causing severe malaria. The basic pathological mechanisms behind these disorders, which are vital in designing protective vaccine and effective anti-malarial drug, are not completely understood yet and some are still debatable. Moreover, the earlier believe that some segments of the human population are naturally resistant to malaria due to polymorphism is also partly refuted. To the advantage of readers and for common understanding among scholars, it is necessary to review recent progresses on malaria research. To this effect, this chapter discusses an overview of recent findings related to malaria parasite, cellular and molecular means of target cell recognition, invasion, and mechanisms leading to complication of the disease, possible promising target areas of anti-malarial drug design, and the global trends of drug resistant strains of *Plasmodium* parasite.

* Department of Biology, College of Natural Sciences, Jimma University, P. O. Box 378, Jimma, Ethiopia. Correspondence to: E-mail: tsigeketema@gmail.com.

Keywords: Malaria, Pathogenesis, antimalarial drugs, *Plasmodium* species

1. Introduction

Despite the effort made to control malaria for more than a century, still it is a leading cause of morbidity and mortality in least developed region of the world. Until recent time, only the four *Plasmodium* species (*Plasmodium falciparum, P. vivax, P. ovale and P. malariae*) were identified as the only etiological agents of human malaria. However, the current reports from Asia (White, 2008) revealed that *P. knowlesi, a* simian parasite, is also responsible for human malaria and included as the fifth human malaria parasite. *P. falciparum* and *P. vivax* cause the major complication, with *P. falciparum* being the more virulent. It is indicated that about 1-3million mortality per year, mainly in children and pregnant women, are due to severe malaria caused by *P. falciparum* (Snow et al., 2005). Some of these severe malaria syndromes are severe anemia, cerebral malaria and acute respiratory distress (Haldar et al., 2007). According to the report of WHO/UNICEF (2005), of all malaria cases in the world, 60% were occurring in Africa with 75% of global *P. falciparum* malaria cases, from which 80% mortality is documented. Even though the public health importance of *P. vivax* is overshadowed by *P. falciparium*, it is the most important parasite in Asia and South America, accounting for more than half of malaria cases with about 390 million clinical cases annually (Price et al., 2007). Besides, studies from Indonesia, New Guinea papua showed a strong association between *P. vivax* infection and severe disease and death (Tjitra et al., 2008; Genton et al., 2008).

For detailed understanding of the pathogenesis of malaria associated complications, knowledge on the parasite's life cycle, which involves invasion of multiple tissues of human and mosquitoes, is crucial. Briefly, the life cycle of human malaria illness initiated when infected *Anopheles* mosquito inject sporozoites into skin. These sporozoites reside for awhile in the skin and some of them actively move from skin to blood circulation (Amino et al., 2006; 2008). Those that remain in the skin could be probabily destroyed by local phagocytic cells (Amino et al., 2008). Few of them may enter to lymphatic system and eliminated by host immune system (Yamauchi et al., 2007). The sporozoites (~ 70% in *P. berghei*) could get chance to enter blood circulation and transported by the hepatic artery or portal vein to the hepatic sinusoids that contains both endothelial and Kupffer cells (Amino et al., 2006). Then, each sporozoite actively traverse numerous kuffer cells and hepatocytes before starting invasion of single hepatocyte (Amino et al., 2008), although the role of this migration is not known yet. Lastly, the sporozoites invade hepatocyte by formation of parasitophorous vacuole (PV). Following invasion of hepatocytes, sporozoites develop and multiply into thousands of merozoites. The duration of pre-erythrocytic stages of the different malaria parasites slightly differ: on average, the duration is 5-6 days (*P. falciparum)*, 8 days (P. *vivax)*, 8-9 days (*P. knowlesi),* 9 days *(P. ovale),* and 13 days (P. *malariae)* (Anon, http://www3.niaid.nih.gov/ topics/Malaria/lifecycle.htm). In human host, the conversion of sporozoite into merozoite usually takes place in hepatocytes. In rodent malaria, however, this process is known to occur in skin before the sporozoites travel to liver (Gueirarda et al., 2010).

After parasitophorous vacuole (PV) rupture, the merozoites circulate in blood stream immediately start invasion of RBCs using several receptor-ligand interactions (Cowman and Crab, 2006). Merozoites develop and multiply asexually in RBCs. Like in the case of liver stage, duration for parasite development in RBC varies for different species of *Plasmodium*. For example, *P. falciparum, P. ovale* and *P. vivax* develop over 48 hours, but 24 hours in case of *P. knowlesi* and 72 hours for *P. malariae*. On averge, about 8-32 merozoites are produced from each parasite, and are able to invade other new RBCs. A small proportion (~ < 1%) of asexual parasites could change into gametocytes, extracellular and nonpathogenic stage to be picked by vector (Eichner et al., 2001). Gametocyte formation in *P. vivax* takes place soon after merozoites are released from liver, while in *P. falciparum* it develop much later (Miller et al., 2002), with peak number occurring one week after peak asexual stage densities (Pukrittayakame et al., 2008). Inside the mid gut of the vector, the parasite undergoes sexual reproduction (sporogony), which will then develop into sporozoites and migrates to salivary gland of the vector and gets ready for transmission to other host (Knell, 1991).

2. Invasion of Host Tissues by *Plasmodium*

2.1. Sporozoites Invasion of Hepatocyte

In malaria infection, host-parasite interaction plays vital role in invasion and complication of the disease. Interaction of *Plasmodium* parasite and host tissue is intiated upon the entry of sporozoites into host's skin. The migration of sporozoites through host cells by damaging cells plasma membrane until it joins blood circulation and enters to hepatocyte is critical for intiation of host response (Frevert, 2004). Secretion from micronemes, adhesion proteins including TRAP, secreted by the apical region of the parasite body, and sporozoite-specific transmembrane protein (SLARP), S6, are recognized to participates in the movement of sporozoites (Yuda and Ishino, 2004; Steinbuechel and Matuschewski, 2009). Moreover, different parasite related proteins such as CSP, SPECT-1, SPECT-2, and Phospholipase are also known to involve in the process of cell transverse, host cells surface receptors recognition and invasion, and induction of protective immunity (Matuschewski et al., 2002; Ishino et al., 2004).

Liver invasion by sporozoites are acheived through interaction between surface protein of the parasite, recombinant circumsporozoite protein (CSP) and heparin sulfate proteoglycans (HSPGs) on hepatocytes (Ancsin and Kisilevsky, 2004). It is thought that sporozoites passing through a number of liver cells are a prerequisite for invasion of specific hepatocyte, because it helps the parasite to secrete micronemal proteins necessary for invasion of a final hepatocyte (Mota et al., 2002). Such transverse process across several liver cells is assisted by the thrombospondin-related anonymous protein (TRAP) family and actin–myosin motor (Baum et al., 2006; Munter et al., 2009). HSPGs are indicated to intiate invasion of hepatocyte (Coppi et al., 2007). The study made on animal model also revealed that, the sporozoite asparagine-rich protein (SLARP) expressed in sporozoites and liver stage contributes to the intiation of *Plasmodium* liver stage development, as it was confirmed indirectly through observation that SLARP deficient *P. berghei* sporozoites completely failed to cause infection (Silvie et al., 2008b). Also it was shown that sporozoites overcome immune response Kupffer cells that would normally lead to parasite destruction, by secretion of the sporozoite surface protein CSP (Klotz et al., 2007).

Ono et al (2008) and Kumar et al. (2007) further affirmed the contribution of intracellular environment such as K^+ and uracil for activation of sporozoite. The activated sporozoites secrete surface adhesive proteins which interact with receptors on hepatocytes surface, tetraspanin CD81 and Cholestrol enriched microdomain, to facilitate internalization of the sporozoite (Mota et al., 2002; Silvie et al., 2006). Once the sporozoite enters to hepatocyte, it is belived that the parasite CSP enhances its growth and down regulates the expression of inflammatory genes (Singh et al., 2006). Moreover, genes upregulated in infective sporozoite (*UIS*s): *UIS*-3, *UIS-4,* and *pb36P,* are described as vital for the parasite development (Singh et al., 2006). Further, the mechanism of contribution of one of these genes, *UIS-3,*was well studied *in vitro* and the result revealed that, *UIS-3* interact with the liver fatty acid binding protein (L-FABP), to deliver fatty acid to developing liver stage parasite (Mikolajczak et al., 2007).

Very recently, a detailed study was conducted on the host early cellular events and factors influencing parasite infectivity and sporozoite development. In the study, the gene expression profile of human liver cells, HepG2-A16, exposed to non- irradiated sporozoites of *P. falciparum* was critically analyzed under laboratory condition. The finding showed that within the first 30 minutes of infection, the expression of at least 742 genes, that regulate diverse biological functions including immune system, cell adhesion and communications, metabolism pathways, cell cycle regulation and signal transduction were altered. The finding also depicited that alteration of cellular events governed by these genes, including host defence response, and occurance of condition that favors sporozoite growth and survival in hepatocyte (Chattopadhyay et al., 2011).

2.2. Merozoites Invasion of Erythrocyte

The release of Merozoites from liver and their immediate invasion of RBCs are critical for complication of the disease. Merozoites egress is mainly assisted by aspartic proteases and cystein proteases, found in exoneme of the parasite (Silva et al., 1996; Blackman, 2008). For instance, subtilisin-like serine protease, PfSUB1, is confirmed to involve in merozoite release from parasitophorous vacuole (PV). As to the mechanism, just before the merozoites are released from PV, PfSUB1 is discharged from exonemes of the parasite into the PV space (Yeoh et al., 2007), where it mediate proteolytic maturation of abundantly expressed, papain-like cysteine proteases, called serine repeat antigens (SERA) (Aly and Matuschewski, 2005). Therefore, PfSUB1 might trigger egress of merozoites through activation of SERA enzymes (Koussis et al., 2009). However, other members of SERA activated by PfSUB1 remain to be identified.

It is clear that the quick invasion of RBCs by merozites reduces the exposure of parasites surface antigens to the host immune response and increase the probability of many RBCs invasion (Silvie et al., 2008a). The initial process of invasion of RBCs is the attachment of merozoites to the surface of RBC at any direction, which is mediated by merozoite surface protein (MSP1) with band 3 on the erythrocyte surface (Goel et al., 2003) and GPI-anchored surface proteins (Gilson et al., 2006). This is followed by reorientation of the apical end, a region containing specialized secretary organelles such as rhoptries, micronemes, and dense organelles of the merozoite towards the erythrocyte surface. The re-orientation phase is mediated by transmembrane protein apical membrane antigens (AMA-1) (Mitchell et al., 2004). Then, an erythrocyte binding antigen (EBAs) binds to glycophorine proteins of erythrocytes, which is responsible for formation of PV. Accordingly, the following antigens of the parasite: erythrocyte binding antigens (EBA)-140, EBA-175, sialic acid residue and EBA-181, bind to Glycophorine C, Glycophorine A, and unknown receptors on RBCs (reviewed in Silvie et al., 2008a), respectively. One of these parasite antigens, EBA-175, is well studied and defined as it is composed of 7 regions and 2 cysteine-rich segments (F1 and F2) located at the N-terminus in region II, which are responsible for glycophorin A binding to the erythrocyte membrane (Sim et al., 1994). Very recently, it was suggested that region II of EBA-175 is the possible candidate ligand-blocking malaria vaccine devlopment, due to its less vulnerability to polymorphism (Jianga et al., 2011).

There is also an assumption that proteins found in the apical organelles, including Duffy binding-like erythrocyte binding protein and *P. falciparum* reticulocyte binding-like homologue (PfRH4) have adhesive role to attach erythrocyte receptors (Triglia et al., 2005; Iyer et al., 2007). In consistant with this, *in vitro* study conducted on serum antibody collected from malaria exposed individual and purified rabbit immunoglobuline G (IgG), showed reactivity to the domain of PfRh4 and inhibit entry of *P. falciparum* into human erythrocytes, respectively (Tham et al., 2009). Recently, complement receptor-1, the host erythrocyte receptor is identified as receptor for PfRH4 *P. falciparum* invasion ligand (Thama et al., 2010). EBAs have analogous function in *P. vivax* and *P. knowlesi*, for invasion while the reticulocyte binding-like homologue, PfRH, proteins have homology to ligands of *P. vivax* and *P. yoelii* (Miller et al., 2002). Further more, from in vitro studies, it is confirmed that *P. falciparum* has multiple pathways of invasion of erythrocytes (Lobo et al., 2004; Deans et al., 2007). A new *P. falciparum* erythrocyte binding protein, named as GPI-anchored micronemal antigen (GAMA), is found in micronemes of the merozoite, sporozoites, and ookinate stage of the parasite; and membrane linked through a glycosylphosphatidylinositol (GPI) anchor is also identified (Hindi et al., 2009). The same protein is also described to be highly conserved in all species of *Plasmodium* (Hindi et al., 2009).

The interaction between parsite ligand and host cell receptor creates a complex process, termed parasite-host cell junction, which leads to invagination of RBCs plasma membrane and facilitate engulfment of the parasite and formation of PV (Amino et al., 2008). During invasion of erythrocytes, three proteins, MSP-1, AMA-1, and *Plasmodium* thrombospondin-related apical merozoite protein (PTRAMP), are removed from the surface of merozoites by the action of the parasite's subtilisin-like protease 2 (SUB2) (Green et al., 2006). The purpose of SUB2 clearance of these proteins is to facilitae erythrocyte invasion (Hindi et al., 2009).

Even though residing in cells that lack standard biosynthetic pathways and internal organelles provide immunological advantage to the parasite, it is an impediment for intracellular parasites to get all growth requirements to achieve maximum growth and replication. However, in order to overcome this difficulty, *Plasmodium* parasite restrict its feeding to hemoglobin (Hb), expand its surface area through the formation of a tubovesicular network, and export various proteins wastes, which are virulent metabolites, into the surface of RBCs (reviewed in Leiriao et al., 2004). Moreover, genomic and biochemical evidences showed that *Plasmodium* parasite has lost the ability to de novo biosynthesis of essential molecules such as the purine ring and amino acid as RBC lacks organelles used for these biosynthesis (Gardner et al., 2002; Olszewski et al., 2009). Therefore, the parasite is enforced to depend on hosts sources and limited to simple metabolic pathways. The energy production path way in *Plasmodium* parsite is also restricted to glycolysis followed by fermentation and little or no oxidative phosphorylation (Sherman, 1998). Few years back, study carry out on the genomic analysis of a parasite revealed that genes encoding all necessary enzymes to run TCA cycle are active and expressed during intraerythrocytic developmental cycle (Bozdech et al., 2003). However, Foth et al. (2005) confirmed that the acetyl-coA synthesized by pyruvate dehydrogenase, encoded by *P. falciparum* genome, are confined to the apicoplast (Bozdech et al., 2003), and mainly consumed for biosynthesis of fatty acid instead of running TCA cycle. Heme and isoprenoid biosynthesis are also carried out by apicoplast (Ralph et al., 2004).

Furthermore, *Plasmodium* parasite degrades about 75% of total Hb of RBC in digestive vacuole for acquisition of amino acid used for biosynthesis of protein (Liu et al., 2006). The byproduct released during Hb degradation, heme, is detoxified by heme polymerase into hemozoin, malaria pigment. Degradation of Hb elevates the level of some amino acids such as alanine, valine, and histidine inside and outside of RBC in trophozoite stage. Where as, other amino acids derived from arginine including ornithine and citrulline depleted as the level of arginine decrease to undetectable level (Olszewski et al., 2009).

As the parasite grows and multiplies in red blood cell, the membrane permeability and cytosolic composition of the host cell is altered, it become permeable for uptake of material and disposal of metabolic wastes (Kirk et al., 2005). Therefore, during the late erythrocyte stage parasite proteins are exported to surface of host RBC through sequence *Plasmodium* export element (PEXEL) (Marti et al., 2005). Some of these export proteins are responsible for adherence to the surface of non parasitized RBCs after their release into blood. There are proteins reported to be involved in intraerythrocytic parasite development. Membrane associated 592 and soluble proteins 644 in human and mouse, respectively, are required for the parasite development (Pasini et al., 2006; 2008). Moreover, an early transcribed membrane protein (ETRAMPs), which is abundant on membrane of PV are also known to involve in parasite development (Spielmann et al., 2006). As the number of merozoite in PV increase, the vacuole ruptures and different metabolic products, toxin, parasite antigen, and pigments are released into blood. These products are responsible for initiation of pathological events.

3. Malaria Complications and Their Pathogenesis

3.1. Cerebral Malaria (CM)

CM is a leading cause of malaria related death among non-immune cases and children (Molyneux et al., 1989). There are a number of assumptions regarding the pathogenesis of CM. The most recognized notion is the elevated release of proinflammatory cytokines such as tumor necrosis factor (TNF)-α potent inducer, interferon (IFN)-γ, lymphotoxin, NO, Interleukin (IL)-6 and IL-1β, due to activation of Toll-like receptor (TLR) (Lyke et al., 2004; Jaramillo et al., 2005; Franklin et al., 2009). The pathologic and protective roles of some of these cytokines are dependent on their concentration and induction time. For instance, early high IFN-γ production is associated with protection against malaria (D'Ombrain et al., 2008).

Pro-inflammatory cytokines are thought to be important in controlling cerebral malaria disease (Vreden et al., 1992), but their over production may contribute for the occurrence of cerebral malaria, characterized by loss of vascular cell integrity, tissue edema, and blockage of microvessels with parasitized RBCs (pRBCs) and/or mononuclear cells which end ups with complication of the disease (Medana et al., 2001). But still, the exact cellular and molecular pathogenesis is unknown. The mechanical blockage of blood vessels by pRBCs with late stage of *P. falciparum* (Miller et al., 2002), leukocytes and platelets (Armah et al., 2005), secretion of cytokines and chemokines (Hunt and Grau, 2003; Sarfo et al., 2005), angiogenic failure (Armah et al., 2005), immune status, genetic variation of the host, and parasite factors (Hunt and Grau, 2003; Gitau and Newton, 2005) are reported to involve in the pathogenesis of CM. Sequestration of pRBCs to endothelial tissue has advantages for the parasite to escape from spleen and immune clearance and create conducive microhabitat for parasite survival (Cranston et al., 1984). In vitro studies of *P. vivax* malaria also showed cytoadherance of pRBCs to chondroitin sulfate A, a receptor expressed in placental, pulmonary and cerebral microvasculature (Rogerson et al., 2007; Traore et al., 2000). However, the frequency of cytoadherence of *P. vivax* pRBCs is less widespread and lesser magnitude than due to *P. falciparum* (reviewed in Anstey et al., 2007), and *P. vivax* pRBCs are accumulated in lung like in non-human malaria infections (Anstey et al., 2007).

The pro-inflammatory cytokines mentioned above and glycosylphosphatidylinositol (GPI) play important role in adherence of pRBCs to endothelial cells of deep tissues by upregulating the expression of adhesion molecules, surface receptors that facilitate cell-cell interaction, such as CD36, ICAM-1, thrombospondin, E-selectin, VCAM-1, and chondoctrin sulphate (Schofield et al.,1996). The endothelium activation is achieved by the angiogenic factors, angiopoietin-2 (Ang -2) released from endothelial cells and vascular endothelial growth factor (VEGF) (Yeo et al., 2008). Study on animal model, *P. berghei* ANKA, revealed that the major adhesion molecule, CD36 for sequestration of pRBCs is analogous to that of human malaria, *P.falciparum* (Franke-Fayard et al., 2005) except that the way the pathology begin and develop in mice is not dependent of CD36 (Patel et al., 2008). Recently, it was concluded that since the pathology of rodent cerebral malaria shares many features with human, it is suggested that rodents are relevant model to study cerebral malaria pathogenesis (Baptista et al., 2010).

In addition to pRBC, leukocyte and platelates are also play important role in pathogenesis of CM. Some *in vitro* studies indicated that, they accumulate in brain microvessels of cerebral malaria cases to modulate the adherence of pRBCs to brain endothelium (Wassmer et al., 2004; Armah et al., 2005). Several *in vitro* studies were conducted to reveal the mechanism employed by platelates to induce CM. The result showed that platelates and thrombocytopenia induced clumping of *P. falciparum* parasitized RBCs are highly associated with CM (Wassmer et al., 2008). Mechanism of platelates inducted CM is, due to contact dependent proapoptotic effect of platelates on TNF-activted human brain microvascular endothelial cells (HBEC) (Wassmer et al., 2006a). The tumor growth factor (TGF)-β released from activated platelates induces the process of HBEC killing (Wassmer *et al.*, 2006a). Also platelates play great role in alteration of brain endothelium function (Wassmer *et al.*, 2006b).

During RBCs lysing, HZ are released and engulfed by phagocytic cells such as monocytes, neutrophils, and macrophages (Arese and Schwarzer, 1997). Hemozine-fed human monocytes secrete matrix metalloproteinase-9 (MMP-9) enzyme (Bergin et al., 2005) Specific lipoperoxide derivatives produced by HZ is thought to play a role in modulating production of MMP-9 and other cytokines (Prato et al., 2008). MMP-9 has ability to invade matrix proteins, disrupts basal lamina, and increase production of TNF-α from its precursors (Prato et al., 2005). The matrix protein degrading ability of MMP-9 is important in pathogenesis of cerebral malaria by destructing a blood brain barrier, leading to local hemorrhage and extravasation of phagocytic cells and parasitized RBCs into brain tissues, which is a hallmark of CM (Prato et al., 2008).

Nitric Oxide (NO), in mammalian cells elicited by macrophages in response to the effect, GPI and Hz (Riley et al., 2006), are proposed mediator of severe malaria (Maneerat et al., 2000). Despite contradictory results from different clinical studies (Dondorp et al., 1998), it is generally accepted that NO has protective role against severe malaria (Hobbs et al., 2002). Similarily *P. falciparum* GPIs can induce NO synthase expression in *Anopheles stephensi* midgut epithelium *in vivo* in a manner analogous to mammalian and also NO-mediated inactivation of malaria parasites in vector (Anstey et al., 1996). Its mechanism of protection is through endotoxin tolerance in animal model (Zingarelli et al., 1995) and down regulation of endotoxin-induced TNF-α in animal model and human monocytes (Iuvone et al., 1996). The other possible way of NO protection against malaria is through induction of heme-oxygenase-1 (HO-1), enzyme involve in degradation of heme into biliverdin, iron and CO (Gramaglia et al., 2006). The induced HO-1 and CO binds to Hb, and then prevents its oxidation and production of heme in animal model (Pamplona et al., 2007). Biliverdin is also play preventive role of oxidative changes leading to inflammatory reactions in patient's body (Vitek and Schwertner, 2007).

NO and arginine, the substrate for nitric oxide synthase, are usually low in severe malaria. Where as Hb and arginase, an enzyme that catalyzes arginine, is much higher in severe malaria (Janka et al., 2010). Even though, the exact mechanism for hypoarginiemia in human is not clearly known yet, the frequent lysing of RBC is proposed to cause it in sickle-cell disease patients (Morris et al., 2005). Explanation given by Morris et al. (2005) for the enhanced arginase activity in parasite infected cultures is that, during RBC lysis host arginase continuously degrades extracellular arginine pool. To prove this view, Olszewski et al. (2009) incubated a culture consisting of infected RBCs with uninfected RBCs under laboratory condition. The result, however, indicated that even intensive lysing of RBCs (100%) is insufficient to account for the high level of arginase activity. Thus, reason for reduction of arginine is not host related; rather the parasite's arginase is responsible for the arginine depletion as it is confirmed conversion of arginine into ornithine by the parasite leads to hypoargininemia in model animal (*P. berghe)* infection (Olszewski et al., 2009).

On the other hand, low level of NO in host body and hypoargininemia, leads to upregulation of ICAM-1 (intracellular adhesion molecule 1), which facilitate the process of sequestration of pRBCs to the vascular endothelium leading to CM (Gramaglia et al., 2006). It is also suggested that *Plasmodium* arginase is an important factor in cerebral malaria pathogenesis (Olszewski et al., 2009). Thus, different researchers recommended arginine supplementation for the treatment of malaria infection as it improve endothelial function, reduce adherence of pRBCs to endothelium, consequently reduce cerebral malaria, and increase exhaled NO levels for clinical malaria patients. Moreover, combination therapy that incorporates a parasite arginase inhibitor is suggested to reduce the pathologies (Weinberg et al., 2008; Olszewski et al., 2009).

3.2. Severe Anemia

Severe malarial anemia, a condition when hemoglobin level is < 5 g/dL, mainly caused by *P falciparum,* is responsible for most cause of mortality to children in endemic regions (Ekvall, 2003). *P.vivax* is a chief risk factor for severe anemia in vivax-endemic areas as well, particularly in young children (Tjitra et al., 2008; Genton et al., 2008); it is more severe in areas where chloroquine resistance is common (Price et al., 2007).

The mechanism of severe anemia due to malaria is appears multi-factorial that involve intensive hemolysis of circulating erythrocytes, both infected and non-infected, and dyserythropoiesis. Though it is certain that the fate of infected RBCs is lysing, it is higher in *P.vivax* pRBCs (Handayani *et al.*, 2009) and altered surface nature can be quickly cleaned, by the spleen leading to anemia. However, the mechanism behind hemolysis of non-infected RBCs was not clear for several years. Studies showed that for every infected RBC destroyed, the number of non pRBCs removed from circulation during *P. vivax* is much higher (~32) (Boutlis et al., 2006) than *P. falciparum* (~8) (Collins et al., 2003). The findings of some researches, however, revealed that glycosylphosphatidyl-inositol (GPI) of *P. falciparum,* toxin released when infected RBCs rupture, is inserted into non-parasitized RBCs membranes and results in recognition by circulating anti-GPI antibodies or complement binding and leads to subsequent elimination. This notion is confirmed and strongly supported by Brattig et al., (2008).

The other assumption of uninfected RBCs lysing is when a ligand such as RAP-2 (Sterkers et al., 2007) and MSP-7 (Tewari et al., 2005), of parasite aborted entry remain on the surface of non-infected RBCs initiate opsonization by specific antibodies which accelerate both complement mediated lysis and phagocytosis by macrophage (Haldar and Mohandas, 2009). Moreover, erythrocyte clearance may be associated to other changes such as oxidative damage (Griffiths et al., 2001), reduced deformability, (Dondorp et al., 2002) and phosphatidylserine (PS) externalization (Kiefer and Snyder, 2000). Erythrocytes signaling pathways and β2-AR-induced cAMP production are results in increasing adhesiveness of normal erythrocytes although it is severe in sickle erythrocytes (Hines et al., 2003).

Dyserythropoiesis, a condition when RBCs synthesis is affected in bone marrow due to the effect of cytokines and other inducer of inflammation such as hemozoin (Chitnis, 2001) also contributes for malaria related anemia. For instance, IL-6 induces hepcidin expression, which is a master regulator of iron trafficking, leading to decreased iron availability for erythropoiesis (Chasis and Mohandas, 2008). Other factors also known to affect erythrocyte synthesis through different mechanisms including, TGF (tumor growth factor) which inhibit erythroblast proliferation; TNF- α induces cleavage of major erythroid transcription factor, GATA-1; IFN-γ enhance macrophage production of TRAIL (TNF-related apoptosis-inducing ligand) which inhibits erythroblast differentiation (reviewed in Chasis and Mohandas, 2008). There is also a view that severe anemia is linked with Th1 cytokines. Decreased level of IL-12 is associated with severe anemia (Haldar and Mohandas, 2009). As suppression of IL-12 decreases production of IFN-γ and IFN-α, and induction of IL-10, this inturn is stimulated by infection (Ouma et al., 2008). Moreover, in children with severe anemia, the circulating level of TNF-α, IL-6, IL-1b, IL-1RA, MIP1a and MIP-1b are reported increased (Haldar and Mohandas, 2009). In fact, there is no conclusive evidence supporting the role of these cytokines in suppression of erythropoiesis. Furthermore, Th2 cytokines such as IL-4 play an important role in erythropoietic suppression. The study conducted on murine malaria parasite *P.chabausi* showed that, IL-4 increases iron uptake and storage in activated macrophages, and thus deviates iron to suppress erythropoiesis, which may occur by a STAT6- dependent mechanism, the development of hemoglobin producing erythroblasts (Thawani et al., 2009).

3.3. Acute Respiratory Distress (ARDS)

Among highly recognized malaria complications, acute respiratory distress syndrome (ARDS), characterized by epithelial apoptosis and interstitial and intra-alveolar edema, and fibrosis of lung (Schnapp et al., 2006), is known to cause high mortality rate, ~ 40% (Rubenfeld et al., 2005). Some severe clinical symptoms associated to ARDS are hypoxaema, dyspnea, airway obstruction, high level of parasitemia, and general respiratory insufficiency (Sharma and Mohan, 2007). Unlike other disorder related to malaria, this syndrome is common among adults than children (Taylor et al., 2006; Mohan et al., 2008). It is much associated with *P. falciparum* infection, even though fatal cases of ARDS are rarely reported from *P. vivax* infection (Taylor et al., 2006; Mohan et al., 2008). The mechanism of lung injury in malaria infection is not studied well. However, there is a hypothesis in which ARDS is initiated by high level of oxidative (Marthru et al., 1994) and nitrogen radicals (Ferrante et al., 1999). These radicals have potential to cause tissue damage and post translational modification of some host proteins in lung fluids leading to functional change *in vitro* (Bowler et al., 2004; Valko et al., 2007). Gole et al. (2000) also identified some modified plasma proteins by nitrogen oxidative radicals in patients with ARDS. There is also another veiw that IL-6 and IL-8, induced by pro inflammatory cytokines such as TNF-α and IL-1, are responsible for expression of endothelial ligand on vessel of lung to promote sequestration of pRBCs in lung but less massive than in brain (Taylor et al., 2006). Moreover, activated macrophages and neutrophils are also reported to involve in pulmonary lung sequestration (Duarte et al., 1985). In agreement with this, study made on PbANKA animal model showed that sequestration of pRBCs in lung is mediated by CD36 is important in pathogenesis of ARDS through inflammation and endothelial damage (Schofield et al., 2002; Lovegrove et al., 2008). But, in vivax malaria the mechanism is different. It is due to cytokine mediated alveolar alteration and permeability (Suratt and Parsons, 2006). Recently, in *P. berghei* ANKA-infected DBA/2 mice, circulating vascular permeability factor, VEGF, is found to cause lung vascular permeability in malaria-associated acute lung injury (Epiphanio et al., 2010). On the same model inhibition of circulating VEGF mediate protection against ARDS (Epiphanio et al., 2010).

Schnapp et al. (2006), critically analyze protein profile of patients with ARDS and able to identify novel proteins such as IGFBP-3 which involve in pathogenesis of ARDS. The IGFBP-3, highly produced during ARDS and mediates suppressive apoptosis of lung fibroblasts, play important role in lung injury. On the other hand cytochrome C initiator of apoptosis through activation of a cascade of biochemical reactions and subsequent cell death

(Jiang and Wang, 2004), is also pointed out to cause this apoptosis as its level is elevated in serum of LPS- induced acute lung injury in mice (Kuwano et al., 2006). In general proteins profile analysis showed that, proteins interaction during ARDS is very complex and redundant (Chang et al., 2008).

For the purpose of diagnosis some systemic proteins such as surfactant protein (SP)-D (Eisner et al., 2003), Clara cell protein (CC16) (Lesur et al., 2006), KL-6 (Ishizaka et al., 2004), lung inflammatory markers, S100 A8 and A9 proteins (De Torre et al., 2006), and soluble receptor for advanced glycation end-products (Uchida et al., 2006) have been reported as a biological marker of ARDS. Since the syndrome is manifested by endothelial damage and increased vascular permeability (Ware and Matthay, 2000), it is thought that through damaged membrane, lung epithelial proteins diffuse to circulation in patients with ARDS (Hermans and Bernard, 1999). Therefore, elevated level of these systemic proteins is an indicative of lung injury. Some of these proteins were further evaluated for their potential to serve as a biological marker in some ARDS patients. The result showed that SP-D and KL-6 level were significantly higher than in normal which depicited their potential to be used as markers for ARDS diagnosis (Determann et al., 2010).

3.4. Acute Renal Failure (ARF)

ARF, life threatening severe malaria complication is responsible for high mortality rate, frequently associated to *P. falciparum* infection (Parkash et al., 2003). It is common in non immune adult and older children (Manan et al., 2006). But some time dehydration caused due to vomiting in young children is associated to transient impairment of renal function (Barsoum, 2000). The trend of ARF prevalence in Asia for all *Plasmodium* species including *P. knowlesi* is increasing to about 60% (Cox-Singh et al., 2008) but in sub-Saharan Africa the incidence is very low (Wasiu and Kayode, 2004). The exact mechanism of ARF is also not known, but different studies indicated that pathogenesis of ARF is due to exaggerated induction of proinflammatory cytokines such as TNF-α, IFN-γ, IL-1α, IL-6, and IL-8, leading to vasoconstriction and increase vascular permeability (Das, 2008). Moreover, knob (PfEMP1) mediated sequestration of pRBCs and hemozoin-fed monocytes adherance to the vascular endothelial cells of kidney are also the major contributor of ARF (Baruch et al., 1995; Nguansangiam et al., 2007). Rosetting, mediated by binding of surface antigen, PfEMP1-DBLα of pRBCs to complement receptor 1, CD31, and heparan sulfate-like glycosaminoglycans of uninfected RBCs (Horata et al., 2009) cause aggregation of RBCs in capillary endothelium of all organs including kidney are also mediator of ARF (Baruch et al., 1995). Increased plasma viscosity, chemical mediators, catecholamine release, intravascular coagulation, hyprebilirubinaemia and hyperparasitaemia are indicated as contributor of ARF (Eiam-Ong and Sitprija, 1998; Sural et al., 2000).

Acute tubular necrosis, a condition characterized by an abrupt decline in renal function, acute elevation in plasma blood urea nitrogen (BUN) and serum creatinine are principal pathologic mechanism of malaria related ARF (Eiam-Ong and Sitprija, 1998; Parkash et al 2003). It is believed that acute tubular necrosis is caused by renal ischemia. The ischemia leads to decreased production of vasodilators such as, NO, and prostaglandin I_2, or PGI_2 by the tubular epithelial cells, leading to further vasoconstriction and hypoperfusion (Lameire and Vanholder, 2001).

3.5. Splenomegaly and Splenic Rupture

Naturally the spleen is a filter machine of altered cells including RBCs in human body. Rarely malara patients from endemic and higher antimalarial drug resistance regions develop splenomegaly and splenic rupture, life threatening clinical manifestation mainly due to *P .falciparum* malaria but not frequent in *P.vivax* (Baird, 2007). Except reports on incidence of splenomegaly and splenic rupture from different regions, detail studies on cause and pathogenesis are almost none. Among few reports on cause of splenomegaly, Bedu-addo and Bates (2002) reported that hyper-reactive malaria (41%), followed by B-lymphoproliferative disorder are the most common disorder associated with massive splenomegaly (22%). Other study suggested that severe anemia exhibited significant association with splenomegaly, longer fever duration, and lower parasitemia (Buffet *et al.*, 2009), which confirms the postulation of severe anemia is linked to a spleen-dependent mechanism.

4. Innate Resistance to Malaria

Some segement of population are naturally resistant to malaria for several reasons, including polymorphism. Thus, genetic variations influence the severity and ultimate out comes of the disease. For several decades, people with Duffy blood group negative or lack of receptor ligand glycophorin A on their erythrocytes (Miller et al., 1976) were considered naturally resistant to *P. vivax* malaria infection. The global prevalent allel for resistance was FY*A, while in across sub-Saharan Africa FY*B allel was identified (Howes et al., 2011). Polymorphism of human red blood cells such as sickle cell trait, heterozygote, (HbAS)) whose protective mechanism thought involve enhancement of innate and acquired immunity thalassemia, and glucose-6-phosphate-dehydrogenase deficiency were associated with innate protection against malaria infection (Pattanapanyasat et al., 1999; Aidoo et al., 2002; Williams et al., 2005). Other trait, heptoglobin (Hp), genotype that determine the efficacy of hemoglobin clearance after malaria induced hemolysis, and alter antioxidant and immune functions, is also associated with reduce incidence of malaria infection in Kenyan children (Atkinson et al., 2007). Similarly, pyruvate kinase deficiency, the second most common erythrocyte enzyme disorder in human, have protection against malaria and avoid multiplication of *P. falciparium* in human erythrocytes (Ayi et al., 2008). However, few years back, contradictory findings were reported on how RBC polymorphisms affect susceptibility to malaria infection. The finding from field and case studies showed the lack of consistency with the former thinking.

Regarding the protective role of heterozygous sickle cell hemoglobin (HBS), the study conducted by Aidoo et al., (2002) showed the variability of its protection among different age groups (protection was detected between the age of 2 and 15). Similarly, the case study conducted on five *P. falciparium* infected sibling of a family in the United States revealed that among two children having sickle cell anemia, one developed severe life threatening malaria and hemolysis. From the remaining three children who had sickle cell anemia, two of them had complicated malaria (Glikman et al., 2007). Although, sickle cell trait has some protection against malaria, there is also a possibility to expose patients to severe malaria, and hemolytic conditions. Likewise, the study conducted on mosquito vectors (*Anopheles gambiae* and *A. Funetus*), which were ELISA positive for the *P.vivax* circumsporozoite protein VK 247, revealed the possible transmission of *P.vivax* infection among duffy blood group-negative inhabitants of Kenya (Ryan et al., 2006). This is further evidenced by the study conducted on inhabitants of Brazil, Amazone region (Cavasini et al., 2007), which support the potential transmission of the *P.vivax* infection among Duffy blood group negative individuals.

5. Evolution of Antimalarial Drugs

Until the First World War, the population of the Western world had relied on quinine extracted from cinchona bark. With decrease in the supply of quinine during this time, it was enforced to develop the first synthetic antimalarial drugs acridines and the 8-aminoquinolines, including primaquine, the then pamaquine (reviewed in Grgerson and Plow, 2005). However, these synthetic drugs were highly toxic and failed to replace the quinine. Around 1934, chloroquine (CQ) was synthesized shortly followed by amodiaquine by incorporation of an aromatic structure to CQ side chain (Schlitzer, 2007). But the therapeutic efficacy of amodaquine significantly decline due to biotransformation of its p-aminophenol moiety into a quinonimine (ONeill et al., 1998). At the time of discovery CQ, it was felt to be too toxic for use. But, gradually it became the cornerstone of the malaria eradication campaign of the 1950s and 1960s (Gergerson and Plow, 2005). In 1962 high level of CQ resistance was reported from Asia (Peters, 1971) and then disseminated throughout the world except in few foci (WHO, 1996; 2010).

With time, the development of synthetic drugs focused on targeting different metabolic pathways unique to the parasite is popularized. As a result, derivatives of pyrimidine such as antifolate, biguanides, proguanil and chlorproguanil were synthesized and found effective against *Plasmodium* parasite (Gergerson and Plow, 2005). Shortly after proguanil, pyrimethamine (Daraprim), Dihydrofolate Reductase (DHFR) inhibitor was developed. Up on utilization, pyrimethamine showed outstanding efficacy both in prophylaxis and therapy (Delannoy and Hugon, 1954; Miller, 1957), even it was effective against CQ-resistant parasites (Powell et al., 1963). However, shortly after its introduction resistant strains were emerged (Petersen, 1987). This necessitates looking for other alternative antimalarial drugs such as sulfa drugs. Sulfonamides and sulfones, whose active component is sulfanilamide, were developed in 1932. Sulfadoxine also showed efficacy as a prophylactic and remedial against *P. falciparum* with single 1g dose, although it is slow schizontocidal agent (Gergerson and Plow, 2005). In 1959, sulfadoxine combination with pyrimethamine was used for treatment of human falciparum infections (Hurly, 1959). After the introduction of sulfadoxine-pyrmethamine into clinical practice, mefloquine and halofantrine, aryl amino alcohol derivatives of quinine were developed by the U.S. Army (Gergerson and Plow, 2005). Then, due to cross resistance between quinine and the aryl amino alcohol derivatives, resistance developed shortly to these drugs (Smithuis et al., 1993). Sulfadoxine-pyrmethamine combination is faster schizontocidal activity and improved clinical response was acheived and found logical drug to combat multidrug resistant infections. However, resistance to this drug also documented after successful effective periods. This enforces to look for other effective combination drugs, such as artemether-lumefantrine, artesunate-amodiaquine, and artesunate-mefloquine, which have been current in use in most malaria endemic regions (WHO, 2010).

6. Global Trends of Antimalarial Drug Resistant

According to the definition given by the World Health Organization (WHO), drug resistance in malaria parasite is the ability of *Plasmodium* strain to survive and/or multiply in the presence of anti-malarial drug with level greater than minimum effective concentration (MEC) despite proper administration and adequate absorption (WHO, 1973).

Since human exposure to anti-malaria drug, resistance has been reported for *P. falciparum* and *P. vivax* of the four species of human malaria parasites (Table-1). Factors facilitating the emergence of resistance strains are drug pressure due to exposure to sub-therapeutic level, drug elimination half-life, the immune status of infected cases, the number of parasites exposed to the drug; the coexisting of other antimalarial drugs in the blood to which the parasite is not resistant, the transmission intensity, and poor drug quality could be among the reasons (Shah and Ahmad, 1996; Basco, 2004; White and Pongtavornpinyo, 2003).

6.1. Drug Resistance in *Plasmodium* spp

P. falciparum surprisingly resistant to almost all antimalarial drugs in regimen for the past several decades, although the geographical expansion and prevalence rates of resistance to individual drugs were differ. The global history of anti-malarial drug resistance evidence showed that *P. falciparum* was highly resistant to CQ: the effective, cheapest and safest drug, Amodiaquine, and Sulfadoxine–pyrimethamine almost in all malaria endemic regions of the world (Wellems and Plowe, 2001; WHO, 2010). This is because of frequent point mutations such as *crt*, *mdr1*, *dhfr*/*dhps*, and others in malaria parasite genes which has association with resistance trait (Hayton and Su, 2004; Hyde, 2007). For instance chloroquine resistance in *P. falciparum* has been linked to mutation of digestive vacuole protein encoded by CQ resistance transporter, (*pfcrt*) gene particularily *pfcrt K*76T, located on chromosome 7, has central role in CQ resistance character both *in vitro*, and *in vivo* (Martin and Kirk, 2004; Mita et al., 2006).

However, mutation of CQ resistance transporter (*pfcrt*) gene homologous in *P.vivax* didnt shows CQ resistance trait (Nomura et al., 2001). Other *in vitro* study showed that *P. vivax* parasites carrying Tyr976Phe mutation of *Pvmdr1* showed reduced susceptibility to CQ (Barnadas et al., 2008), though it needs further analysis. Even though, the prevalence of CRPf became beyond tolerable level in most malaria endemic regions many decades ago, but still it is effective drug in some parts of Central America, where its efficacy was confirmed 100% (WHO, 2010).

Like wise *P. falciparum* resistance to SP is related to mutations of the dihydropteroate synthase, encoded by *pfdhps genes*, located on chromosome 8, and dihydrofolate reductase, encoded by *pfdhfr* genes, located on chromosome 4 (Wernsdorfer and Noedl, 2003). Also mutations at codons 58 and 117 of the *Pvdhfr* gene have been associated with treatment failure in *P.vivax* (Imwong et al., 2003). However, the association of the mutant allele pv-*dhps*/*pv-dhfr* with clinical resistance to SP in *P. vivax* is not clear (Mehlotra and Henry-Halldin, 2009). On the other hand in East Africa, the *pfdhfr*/*pfdhps* triple mutant *pfdhfr* N108-I51-R59 and double mutant *pfdhps* G437and E540 are confirmed to predictive trait for SP treatment failure, whereas in West Africa the *pfdhps* alleles didn't show any predictive value (Kublin et al., 2002; Mockenhaupt et al., 2005).

Table 1. Reports on frequently documented antimalarial drug resistant P. falciparum Parasite [Bloland, 1998; 2001; Abdel-Hameed, 2003; WHO, 1990; 2001, 2010]

Antimalarial drug	Countries from which resistance strains reported		
	Africa	Asia	S. America
Chloroquine	Somalia, Guinea , Burkina Faso, Kenya, Coted Ivoire, Ethiopia, Cameron, Gambia, Gabon, Nigeria, Zimbabwe, Zambia, Tanzania, Uganda, Malawi	Bangladesh, Iran, Afghanistan, Pakistan, Saudi Arabia, Vietnam India, Thailand, cambodia	Venezuela, Guyana, Panama Colombia, Thai-Cambodia
Amodiaquine	Burkina Faso, Cameroon, Congo, Gabon, Sierra Leone, Sudan Tanzania	Middle East	South America
Sulfadoxine–pyrimethamine	Malawi, Tanzania, Kenya, Botswana, Tanzania, Kenya, Ethiopia	Viet Nam, Indonesia, Malaysia, Philippines, Afghanistan, Iran, Pakistan, Tajikistan, Yemen, India, Nepal	Colombia Ecuador, Peru
Mefloquine	Benin, Nigeria Low TF	Cambodia–Thailand Myanmar, Viet Nam	Brazil, Guyana, Venezuela
artemether–lumefantrine [Coartem]	Efficacy > 85% , except in Tanzania – mainland [8-10%], Ghana and Burkina Faso	Indonesia, Philippines, Yemen, Bangladesh, India, Thailand, Nepal Myanmar, Cambodia	Brazil, Ecuador, Guyana, Suriname, Venezuela
artesunate–amodiaquine	Eritrea, Burkina Faso, Uganda, Rwanda, Kenya	Myanmar, Indonesia Afghanistan, Yemen	
artesunate–mefloquine	Cameroon and Nigeria	Cambodia, Myanmar Thailand, Bangladesh	Suriname

NB. TF= treatment failure.

Currently, in all malaria endemic regions where SP treatment failure was documented, artemisinin-based combination therapies (ACTs) are a frontline treatment (WHO, 2010). The rationale behind the use of a combination therapy is, highly potent and fast acting artemisinin derivatives combination with drug of long half-life can enhance rapid parasite clearance and elimination of symptom (WHO, 2006). Moreover, combination therapies have gametocidal activity which limits probability of transmission of the parasite (Grimberg and Mehlotra, 2011). ACTs antimalarial drugs, such as artemether-lumefantrine, artesunate-amodiaquine, and artesunate-mefloquine are being used in all malaria endemic regions of the world (Schlitzer, 2008; White, 2008). Since its introduction, artemether-lumefantrine is widely used in about 56 countries as first line drug. It is the most effective, easy to deliver and safe drug to patients (WHO, 2010). However, recently reports from different regions are showing the declining efficacy of the drug (Table 1), but in Africa the efficacy is still greater than 85% (WHO, 2010), except two studies from Ghana and Burkina Faso which were ≥10% treatment failure (Zongo et al., 2007; Kobbe et al., 2008). The genetic mechanism of treatment failure to artemether-lumefantrine is not known yet. However, there is an assumption that treatment failure to this drug could be due to inadequate absorption of the lumefantrine (Price et al., 2006; WHO, 2010), because its absorption is enhanced by the intake of fatty foods (Ezzet and Karbwang, 1998). Furthermore, recently the association between artemisinin resistance phenotype of *P. falciparum* strains and point mutation at *pfmdr1, pfatp6* (or *pfserca*), and *pfcrt*, *ubp-1* were investigated. But the finding showed lack of link between the mutations and resistance phenotype (Imwong et al., 2010).

Table 2. Some reports on frequently documented antimalarial drug resistant *P. vivax* parasite [WHO, 1990; 2001; 2010]

Antimalarial drug	Countries from which resistance strains were documented		
	Africa	*Asia*	*S. America*
Chloroquine	Madagascar, Ethiopia	Indonesia [Papua New Guinea, Irian Jaya, West Kalimantan, Papua, India, Vietnam, Dawei, south Myanmar	Peru, Brazil Colombia
Amodiaquine	Effective	Effective	Effective
Sulfadoxine–pyrimethamine	Effective	Effective	Effective
Mefloquine	Effective	Effective	Effective

Quinine (QN), a second line of treatment, is still effective and drug of choice for pregnant women and complicated malaria cases (WHO, 2010), except in Venezuela and South- East Asia where higher treatment failure (≥ 20%) is reported (Pukrittayakamee et al., 2000; WHO, 2010). Mechanism of QN resistance of *P. falciparum* is proved to be due to multifactorial bases resulted from different mutations, such as mutation of transporter genes *pfcrt*, and *pfmdr1* (Reed et al., 2000; Lakshmanan et al., 2005). Also polymorphism of *P. falciparum* sodium/hydrogen exchanger, (*pfnhe*1) gene (PF13_0019), microsatellite (ms4760) Dd2 harbors point mutations and a DNNND repeated unit polymorphism are indicated to have contribution to QN resistance *in vitro* (Ferdig et al., 2004). However, a recent study conducted on 83 isolates obtained from malaria patients' showed that, lack of significant association between point mutation to ms4760 and *in vitro* susceptibility to quinine (Andriantsoanirina et al., 2010). But still, QN remain effective drug against severe *P. falciparum* infection and resistant *P. vivax* strains.

The frequency of antimalarial drug resistance by *P. vivax* malaria is much lesser than *P. falciparum*. In most malaria endemic region of the world CQ is still used as first line drug for treatment of *P. vivax* infection, with recommended dose of 25mg base/Kg body weight for consecutive 3 days at 24hrs interval, since 1946 (WHO, 2001). However, chloroquine-resistant *P. vivax* (CRPv) has been emerging from different *P. vivax* malaria endemic regions after the first report documented from Indonesia, New Guinea Papua (Rieckman et al., 1989) (Table-2). Other drugs used for treatment of *P. vivax* malaria are still effective (WHO, 2010). Resistance of other *Plasmodium* species *P. ovale* and *P. malariae* to antimalarial drug is not well studied. Generally, it is belived that these parasites are sensitive to CQ except one CQ resistant *P. malariae* parasite reported from Indonesia (Maguire et al., 2002).

7. Potential Target Area of Anti-Malarial Drug Design

The tremendous increased emergence and dissemination of antimalarial drug resistant *P. falciparum*, adverse effect and high cost of some drugs has prompted the search for new and effective antimalarial drugs. It is obvious that increased antimalarial drug resistance, besides increasing the rate of morbidity and mortality (Mahomva et al., 1996), increases the cost of malaria control program (WHO, 1990).

Several approaches were undergoing to develop effective and noncostly antimalarial drugs. Among these efforts, use of combination chemotherapies, relatively older one, following re-optimization or re-formulation procedure is the most practiced anitmalaria drug design. Accordingly, different combination drugs such as Amodiaquine/sulfadoxine/ pyrimethamine (Dorsey et al., 2002; Schellenberg et al., 2002), Amodiaquine/artesunate (Adjuik et al., 2002), Artesunate/sulfadoxine/pyrimethamine (Dorsey et al., 2002), Artemether/lumefantrine (Lefevre et al., 2001), and Chlorproguanil/dapsone (Kublin et al., 2002) are developed to enhance the efficacy of available drugs. It is belived that a combination strategy provides synergetic effect and slow rate of parasite resistance to newly developed drugs (Rosenthal, 2003). In parallel to this, invention of analogous compound from exsisting antimalarial drugs in use by modification of certain structure is another potential approach under development to overcome the emerging resistant. This method is relatively easier to make as it doesn't require advanced knowledge on mechanism of action of the compound and target identification. This method is extensively used for development of 4-aminoquinolines compounds (Posner et al., 2003).

The third and promising approach is evaluation of drugs originally produced for other aliments as there are some shared biochemical pathways among organisms (Loyevsky and Gordeuk, 2001). Recently it is reported that some antiretroviral and anticancer drugs showed potential to inhibit of *Plasmodium* parasites. Among antiretroviral drugs assessed HIV -1 protease inhibitors, and other protease inhibitors including lopinavir, saquinavir, ritonavir, and indinavir, are proved as effective against *P. falciparum* in vitro (Peatey et al., 2010). The proposed mechanism of action of these antiretroviral drugs against *Plasmodium* parasite is, through inhibition of parasite's aspartic proteases, found on PV (Skinner-Adams et al., 2007). Similarily, non-nucleoside reverse transcriptase inhibitor, TMC-125, antiretroviral drug reported to have a potent activity against *P. falciparium* (Grimberg et al., 2009). This drug is hypothesized to inhibit parasite enzymes PfTERT, a catalytic reverse transcriptase component of telomerase involve in initiation of DNA synthesis (Figueiredo et al., 2005). This approach is thought to be helpful for further investigation on other potential reverse transcriptase inhibitors to develop novel antimalarial drugs (Grimberg and Mehlotra, 2011).

Drug resistance reverser is another innovative strategy used to retain some inexpensive and tolerable antimalarial agents in regimens (van Schalkwyk et al., 2001). The significant work of Martine et al., (1987), which showed a possibility of reversing CQR in *P. falciparum using* verapamil, creates a new prospective for reversal of CQ, which is novel class of drug that can kill the parasite and reverse resistance to the drug it self (Egan and Kaschula, 2007). Since then intensive efforts on co-adminstration of CQ with other drugs for *P. falciparum* treatment were undergoing (van Schalkwyk and Egan, 2006; Guantai and Chibale, 2010). Consequently, almost all drugs evaluated for co-adminstration with CQ showed successful result except one drug, chlorpheniramine (Egan and Kaschula, 2007). Moreover, Egan and Kaschula (2007) reported the co-admisteration of primaquine and antiretroviral protease inhibitors (PIs) such as saquinavir, ritonavir, and indinavir as effective CQR reversers. Furthermore, other antimicrobial agents and antidepressant were assessed and showed potential to reverse CQ and mefloquin resistance (Egan and Kaschula, 2007).

The noblest approach which will be a promising for antimalaria drug design is identification of new target for development of new antimalarial agents. This approach specifically focuses on unique nature of the parasite biology and biochemical pathways (Macreadie et al., 2000; Rosenthal, 2003). Accordingly, several targets were identified and even for most of them drugs are already design and commercialized. Some of these potential targets are; heme polymerization process (Chou and Fitch, 1993) and enzymes involved in heme degradation (Silva et al., 1996), the first enzyme involve in Isoprenoid synthesis by mevalonate/non–mevalonate pathway, 1–deoxy–D–xylulose–5–phosphate reductoisomerase (DXR) (Macreadie et al., 2000), PfPK5, cyclin-dependent kinase unique to *P. falciparum*, (Brinen et al., 2003), Plasmodium hexose transporter, PfHT (Parbhu et al., 2008) and Adenosine deaminase, involve in purine metabolism (Sriram et al., 2009). Recently, the advancement in high throughput screening methods, an approach used to screen a number of compounds within short time, create a promising progress in discovering new haem-targeting drugs (de Villiers and Egan, 2009). However, some drawbacks associated to target-based drug discovery such as difficulty in prediction and identification of targets crucial for the parasite growth and survival in host body, lack of noble classes of compound for all well identified and validated targets, and the possibility of frequent resistance emergence to a single cellular target, could be discouraging conditions of this approach (Dharia et al., 2010). Therefore, recently drug screening direction recommended is shifting to cell-based assays, yielding thousands of potent antimalarial compounds. But, the challenge here is knowledge of the mechanism of action of these compounds to facilitate medicinal chemistry (Dharia et al., 2010).

8. Antimalarial Drugs in Pipeline

Even though there is no drug for immediate use, some antimalarial drugs are at advanced stages of clinical trials of promising efficacy. For example some combination drugs such as Piperaquine/Dihydroartemisinin, Dapson/Chlorproguanil/Artesunate, and Pyronaridine/ Artesunate are found in clinical studies with good efficacy rate (Bathurst and Hentschel, 2006). Pyronaridine is a member of class 4-amonoquinoline whose quinoline heterocycle structure is replaced by an aza-acridine. The most significant quality of pyronaridine is, unlike other compound of the same class don't generate hazardious thio due to the presence of the second side chain (Biagini et al., 2008). Some years back reports on resistances to the Pyronaridine and cross resistance with other drugs in the same class was documented from *in vitro* test (Pradines et al., 1999). But, the combination of pyronaridine with artesunate showed higher efficacy (Ringwald et al., 1996) and currently it is in phase III clinical trial (http://www.mmv.org). There are also other antimalarial formulations mainly belongs to class 4-aminoquinolines already started clinical evaluation. AQ-13 is a CQ derivative with a shortened side chain tert-butyl-Isoquine produced by interchanging the hydroxyl and the diethylaminomethyl residue at the phenyl ring of amodiaquine to overcome toxic quinonimine production, showed potency against CQ resistance strains (ONeill et al., 2003).

The other drug in advanced stage of clinical trial is Tafenoquine, 8-aminoquinoline drug derivative of primaquine, with short life time, only two weeks (reviewed in Kiszewski et al., 2010). The basic structural difference from primaquine is the trifluoromethylphenyloxy substituent in Tafenoquine to increase sporontocidal activity of the drug (Schlitzer, 2008). But still Tafenoquine has some risk causing hemolysis in glucose-6-phosphate-dehydrogenase-deficient humans like primaquine (Shanks and Edstein, 2005). Several studies have shown very good protective efficacy of this drug (Mcintyre et al., 2003; Walsh et al., 2004). But, Tafenoquine resistance in *Leishmania major* due to increased glycolytic ATP synthesis was documented (Manzano et al., 2011). Tafenoquine is currently in its final stages of development and is going through Phase IIb/III clinical trials (reviewed in Kiszewski et al., 2010).

Fosmidomycin and Azithromycin, non combination formulations, are also at different level of clinical trials. A new target drug design Fosmidomycin is an inhibitor of 1-desoxy-Dxylulose- 5-phosphate reductoisomerase (DXR) (Jomaa et al., 1999), combination with antibiotic clindamycin twice a day for three consecutive days showed effective cure rate (Borrmann et al., 2006; Oyakhirome et al., 2007). Azithromycin, a new antibiotic, is also confirmed to have great efficacy as prophylactic against *P. vivax* infection (Heppner et al., 2005). The cure rates of Azithromycin are much increase with combination with quinine (Noedl et al., 2007).

Furamidine (DB75), a drug of choice for African trypanosomiasis and visceral leishmaniasis, is currently under evaluation to be formulated for malaria treatment (Schlitzer, 2008). It is now on phase-II clinical trial against *P. vivax* and uncomplicated *P. falciparum* infections (Ward et al., 2011). Pafuramidine (DB289), 2, 5-bis-(4-amidinophenyl) furan-bis-*O*-methylamidoxime, is also a promising new orally adminstared candidate active antiparasitic compound with clinical efficacy of 96% in *P. falciparum*-infected patients (Yeramian et al., 2005). The mechanism of action of Pafuramidine is hypothesized to interfer function of enzymes involve in DNA synthesis (Bell et al., 1991). However, phase I/II evaluation of the prophylactic activity of pafuramidine in healthy volunteers' didnt show significant clinical prophylactic efficacy (Nyunt et al., 2009). Moreover, attempt made to combine Pafuramidine with other antibiotics was not successful (Purfield et al., 2008).

On the other hand Ferroquine a compound contains a lipophilic ferrocenyl structure in the side chain of CQ, but designed to not fit to substrate binding site of CQ and don't affected by mutation of pfcrt gene (Biot et al., 1997) is become effective against CQ resistant strains (Delhaes et al., 2001). Currently it is in phase-I clinical trial and proved to be safe and tolerable up to 1,600 mg single dose and up to 800 mg in repeated dose among asymptomatic young male infected with *P. falciparum* (Mombo-Ngoma et al., 2011). Similarily, T3 antimalarial drug originally designed to inhibit phospholipid metabolism in intra-cellular stage of parasite is also in clinical trial for severe malaria (Margout et al., 2009). For T3 complete cure was achieved in *P. falciparum*-infected Aotus monkeys with a dose of 0.054 mmol (0.03 mg)/kg (Wengelnik et al., 2002).

8. Conclusion

Even though much progress has been made in malaria research, there is still a lot awaits further research in order to eradicate or at least significantly reduce the mortality and morbidity caused by malaria. Complete cellular and molecular mechanisms of parasite-host interaction, host cells invasion, and pathogenesis of the parasite, which could be a target for drug design and vaccine development, are not completely understood yet. However, the completed sequenced genome of *Plasmodium* parasite and advancement in drug target search methods such as in silico, and throughput screening methods, could create great hopes to the effort being made to identify novel drug target and development of new antimalarial drugs.

References

Abdel-Hameed, A.A. (2003). Antimalarial drug resistance in the Eastern Mediterranean Region. *Eastern Mediterranean Heal. J.,* 9 492-508.

Adjuik, M., Agnamey, P., Babiker, A., Borrmann, S., Brasseur, P., Cisse, M., Cobelens, F., Diallo, S., Faucher, J. F., Garner, P. Gikunda, S, Kremsner, P.G., Krishna, S., Lell, B., Loolpapit, M., Matsiegui, P.B., Missinou, M.A., Mwanza, J., Ntoumi, F., Olliaro, P., and Osimbo, P. (2002). Amodiaquine-artesunate versus amodiaquine for uncomplicated Plasmodium falciparum malaria in African children: a randomised, multicentre trial. *Lancet, 359,* 1365-1372.

Aidoo, M., Terlouw, D.J., Kolczak, M.S., McElroy, P.D., ter Kuile, F.O., Kariuki, S., Nahlen, B.L., Lal, A.A., and Udhayakumar, V. (2002). Protective effects of the sickle cell gene against malaria morbidity andmortality. *Lancet, 359,* 1311-1312.

Aly, A.S.I., and Matuschewski, K. (2005). A malarial cysteine protease is necessary for *Plasmodium* sporozoite egress from oocysts. *J. Exp. Med.*, *202*, 225-230.

Amino, R., Giovannini, D., Thiberge, S., Gueirard, P., Boisson, B., Dubremetz, J.F., Prevost, M.C., Ishino, T., Yade, M., and Menard, R., (2008). Host cell transversal is important for progression of the malaria parasite through the derms to the liver. *Cell Host Microbe, 3,* 88-96.

Amino, R., Thiberge, S., Martin, B., Celli, S., Shorte, S., Frischknecht, F., and Menard, R. (2006). Quantitative imaging of plasmodium transmission from mosquito to mammal. *Nat. Med., 12,* 220-224.

Ancsin, J. B., and Kisilevsky, R. (2004). A binding site for highly sulfated heparan sulfate is identified in the N terminus of the circumsporozoite protein: significance for malarial sporozoite attachment to hepatocytes. *J. Biol. Chem.*, 279, 21824–21832.

Andriantsoanirina, V., Menard, D., Rabearimanana, S., Hubert, V., Bouchier, C., Tichit, M, Le Bras, J., and Durand, R. (2010). Association of microsatellite variations of Plasmodium falciparum Na+/H+ exchanger (Pfnhe-1) gene with reduced in vitro susceptibility to quinine: lack of confirmation in clinical isolates from Africa. *Am. J. Trop. Med. And Hyg., 82*, 782-7.

Anon. Malaria: Life Cycle of the Malaria Parasite. http://www3.niaid.nih.gov/topics/Malaria/lifecycle.htm.

Anon. http://rbm.who.int/cmc_upload/0/000/014/923/am_toc.htm/ (accessed 23 November 2010).

Anstey, N. M., Weinberg, J. B. Hassanali, M. Y. Mwaikambo, E. D. Manyenga, D., Isukonis, M. A., Arnelle, D.R., Hollis, D., McDonald, M.I., and Granger, D.L. (1996). Nitric oxide in Tanzanian children with malaria: inverse relationship between malaria severity andnitric oxide production/nitric oxide synthase type 2 expression. *J. Exp. Med., 184,* 557–567.

Anstey, N.M., Handojo, T., Pain, M.C.F., Kenangalem, E., Tjitra, E., Price, R.N., and Maguire, GP. (2007). Lung injury in vivax malaria: pathophysiological evidence for pulmonary vascular sequestration andposttreatment alveolar-capillary inflammation. *J. Infect. Dis., 195,* 589–596.

Anstey, N.M., Russell1, B., Yeo, T.W., and Price1, R.N. (2009). The pathophysiology of vivax malaria. *Trends Parasitol, 25*, 220-226.

Arese, P. and Schwarzer, E. (1997). Malarial pigment (haemozoin): a very active 'inert' substance. *Ann. Trop. Med. Parasitol.,* 9, 1501–516.

Armah, H., Dodoo, A.K., Wiredu, E.K., Stiles, J.K., Adjei, A.A., Gyasi, R.K., Tettey, Y. (2005). High-level cerebellar expression of cytokines and adhesion molecules in fatal, paediatric, cerebral malaria. *Ann. Trop. Med. Parasitol.,* 99, 629-647.

Atkinson, S.H., Mwangi, T.W., Uyoga, S.M., Ogada, E., Macharia, A.W., Marsh, K., Prentice, A.M., Williams, T.N. (2007). The haptoglobin 2-2 genotype is associated with a reduced incidence of Plasmodium falciparum malaria in children on the coast of Kenya. *Clin. Infect. Dis. 44,* 802-809.

Ayi, K., Min-Oo, G., Serghides, L., Crockett, M., Kirby-Allen, M., Quirt, I., Gros, P., and Kain, K.C. (2008). Pyruvate kinase deficiency and malaria. *Engl. J. Med., 358*, 1805-10.

Baptista, F.G., Pamplona, A., Pena, A.C., Mota, M.M., Pied, S., and Vigario, A.M. (2010). Accumulation of Plasmodium berghei-Infected Red Blood Cells in the Brain Is Crucial for the Development of Cerebral Malaria in Mice. *Infect. Immunol., 78,* 4033-4039.

Barnadas, C., Ratsimbasoa, A., Tichit, M., Bouchier, C., Jahevitra, M. Picot, S., and Menard, D. (2009). *Plasmodium vivax* resistance to chloroquine in Madagascar: clinical efficacy andpolymorphisms in Pvmdr1 and Pvcrt-o genes. *Antimicr. Agents Chemother., 52,* 4233-4240.

Baruch, D.I., Pasloske, B.L., Singh, H.B., Xiahui, B., Ma, X.C., Feldman, M., and Taraschi, T.F., Howard, R.J. (1995). Cloning of the *P. falciparum* gene encoding PfEMP 1, a malarial variant antigen and adherence receptor on the surface of parasitized human erythrocyte. *Cell, 82,* 77–87.

Barsoum, R.S. (2000). Malaria acute renal failure. *J. Am. Soc. Nephrol., 11,* 2147–54.

Basco, L.K. (2004). Quality of anti-malarial drugs used for self-medication. *Am. J. Trop. Med. Hyg., 70,* 245-250.

Bathurst, I., and Hentschel, C. (2006). Medicines for venture: sustaining antimalarial drug development. *Trends Parasitol, 22*, 301– 307.

Bedu-Addo, G., and Bates, I. (2002). Causes of massive tropical splenomegaly in Ghana. *Lancet, 360,* 449-454.

Bell, C.A., Cory, M., Fairley, T.A., Hall, J.E., and Tidwell, R.R. (1991). Structure-activity relationships of pentamidine analogs against Giardia lamblia and correlation of antigiardial activity with DNA-binding affinity. *Antimicrob. Agents Chemother., 35,* 1099–1107.

Bergin, P.J., Sicheng, W., Qiang, P., andMarianne, Q. (2005). Secretion of matrix metalloproteinase-9 by macrophages, *in vitro*, in response to *Helicobacter pylori* FEMS *Immunol. Med. Microbiol., 45,* 159-169.

Biagini, G.A., O'Neill, P.M., Bray, P.G., and Ward, S.A. (2005). Current drug development portfolio for antimalarial therapies. *Curr. Opin. Pharmacol., 5,* 473–478.

Biot, C., Glorian, G., Maciejewski, L. A., and Brocard, J. S. (1997). Synthesis and antimalarial activity in vitro and in vivo of a new ferrocene-chloroquine analogue. *J. Med. Chem., 40*, 3715–3718.

Blackma, M. J. (2008). Malaria proteases and host cell egress an emerging cascade. *Cell Microbiol., 10*, 1925-1934.

Bloland, P.B. (2001). *Drug resistance in malaria* Geneva, World Health Organization, (WHO/CDS/CSR/DRS/2001/4).

Bloland, P.B., Kazembe, P.N., Oloo, A.J., Himonga, B., Barat, L.M., and Ruebush, T.K. (1998). Chloroquine in Africa: critical assessment and recommendations for monitoring and evaluating chloroquine therapy efficacy in Sub-Saharan Africa. *Trop. Med. Inter. Heal, 3*, 543–52.

Borrmann, S., Lundgren, I., Oyakhirome, S., Impouma, B., Matsiegui, P.B., Adegnika, A.A., Issifou, S., Kun, J. F., Hutchinson, D., Wiesner, J., Jomaa, H., and Kremsner, P.G. (2006). Fosmidomycin plus clindamycin for treatment of pediatric patients aged 1 to 14 years with Plasmodium falciparum malaria. *Antimicrob. Agents Chemother., 50*, 2713-2718.

Boutlis, C., Yeo, T.W., and Anstey, N.M. (2006). Malaria tolerance – for whom the cell tolls? *Trends Parasitol.*, *22*, 371–377.

Bowler, R.P., Duda, B., Chan, E.D., Enghild, J.J., Ware, L.B., Matthay, M.A., and Duncan, M.W. (2004). Proteomic analysis of pulmonary edema fluid and plasma in patients with acute lung injury. *Am. J. Physiol. Lung Cell Mol. Physiol., 286,* 1095–1104.

Bozdech, Z., Llinas, M., Pulliam, B.L., Wong, E.D., Zhu, J., andDeRisi, J.L. (2003). The transcriptome of the intraerythrocytic developmental cycle of *Plasmodium falciparum. PLoS Biol, 1*, E5.

Brattig, N.W., Kowalsky, K., Liu, X., Burchard, G.D., Kamena, F., and Seeberger, P.H. (2008). *Plasmodium falciparum* glycosylphosphatidylinositol toxin interacts with the membrane of non-parasitized red blood cells: a putative mechanism contributing to malaria anemia. *Microbes Infect. 10*, 885-891.

Brinen, L.S., andStout, T.J. (2003). Can Mosquitoes Be Bitten? A New Hope for Anti-Malarial Drug Design. *Structure*, *11,* 1309–1317.

Buffet, P.A., Safeukui, I., Milon, G., Mercereau-Puijalon, O., and David, P.H. (2009). Retention of erythrocytes in the spleen: a double-edged process in human malaria. *Curr. Opin. Hematol.*, *16,* 157-164.

Bullock, B. M. (1996). *Pathophysiology: Adaptations and alterations in function* (4th edn). Philadelphia: Lippincott.

Cavasini, C.E., Mattos, L.C., Couto, A.A., Bonini-Domingos, C.R., Valencia, S.H., Neiras, W.C., Alves, R.T., Rossit, A.R., Castilho, L., and Machado, R.L. (2007). *Plasmodium vivax* infection among Duffy antigen-negative individuals from the Brazilian Amazon region: an exception? *Trans. R. Soc. Trop. Med. Hyg., 101*,1042-1044.

Chang, D.W., Hayashi1, S., Gharib, S.A., Vaisar, T., King, S.T., Tsuchiya, M., Ruzinski, J.T., Park, D.R., Matute-Bello, G., Wurfel, M.M., Bumgarner, R., Heinecke, J.W., and Martin,

T. R. (2008). Proteomic andComputational Analysis of Bronchoalveolar Proteins during the Course of the Acute Respiratory Distress Syndrome. *Am. J. Respir. Crit. Care Med., 178*, 701–709,

Chasis, J.A., and Mohandas, N. (2008). Erythroblastic islands: niches for erythropoiesis. *Blood, 112,* 470-478.

Chattopadhyay, R., de la Vega, P., Paik, S.H., Murata, Y., Ferguson, E.W., Richie, T.L. and Ooi, G.T. (2011). Early transcriptional responses of HepG2-A16 liver cells to infection by *Plasmodium falciparum* sporozoites *J. Biol. Chem.,* Paper in Press.

Chitnis, C.E. (2001). Molecular insights into receptors used by malaria parasites for erythrocyte invasion. *Curr. Opin. Hematol., 8,* 85-91.

Chou, A. C. andFitch, C. D. (1993). Control of heme polymerase by chloroquine andother quinoline derivatives. *Biochem. Biophys. Res. Commun., 195*, 422- 427.

Colins, W., Jeffery, G.M., and Roberts, J.Q. (2003). A retrospective examination of anemia during infection of humans with Plasmodium vivax. *Am. J. Trop. Med. Hyg., 68*, 410–412.

Coppi, A., Tewari, R., Bishop, J.R., Bennett, B.L., Lawarence, R., Esko, J.D., Billker, O., and Sinnis, P. (2007). Heparan sulfate proteoglycans provide a signal to Plasmodium sporozoites to stop migrating and productively invade host cells. *Cell Host Microbe., 2*, 316-327.

Cowman, A.F. and Crab, B.S. (2006). Invasion of red blood cells by malaria parasites. *Cell, 124*, 755-766.

Cranston, H. A., C.W. Boylan, G. L. Carroll, S. Sutera, J. R. Williamson, I. Y. Gluzman, andD. J. Krogstad. *Plasmodium falciparum* maturation abolishes physiologic red cell deformability. *Sci., 223,* 400–402, 1984.

Das, B.S. (2008). Renal failure in malaria. *J. Vector Borne Dis., 45*, 83–97.

De Torre, C., Ying, S.X., Munson, P.J., Meduri, G.U., and Suffredini, A.F. (2006). Proteomic analysis of inflammatory biomarkers in bronchoalveolar lavage. *Proteomics, 6,* 3949–3957.

de Villiers, K.C. and Egan, T.J. (2009). Recent Advances in the Discovery of Haem-Targeting Drugs for Malaria and Schistosomiasis. *Molecules, 14,* 2868-2887.

Deans, A., Nery, S., Conway, D.J., Kai, O., Marsh, K., and Rowe, J.A. (2007). Invasion Pathways and Malaria Severity in Kenyan *Plasmodium falciparum Clinical Isolates. Infect. Immun., 75,* 3014–3020.

Delhaes, L., Abessolo, H., Biot, C., Berry, L., Delcourt, P., Maciejewski, L., Brocard, J., and Camus, D. (2001). Diven vitro and in vivo antimalarial activity of ferrochloroquine, a ferrocenyl analogue of chloroquine against chloroquine-resistant malaria parasites. *Parasitol. Res., 87,* 239–244.

Determann, R.M., Royakkers, A.A., Haitsma, J.J., HZhang, H., Slutsky, A.S., Ranieri, V.M., and Schultz, M.J. (2010). Plasma levels of surfactant protein D andKL-6 for evaluation of lung injury in critically ill mechanically ventilated patients. *BMC Pulmonary Medicine, 10:6.*

Dharia, N.V., Bright, A.T., Westenberger, S.J., Barnes, S.W., Batalov, S., Kuhen, K., Borboa, R., Federe, G.C., McClean, C.M., Vinetz, J.M., Neyra, V., Llanos-Cuentas, A., Barnwell, J.W., Walker, J.R., and Winzeler, E.A. (2010). Whole-genome sequencing andmicroarray analysis of *ex-vivo Plasmodium vivax* reveal selective pressure on putative drug resistance genes. *PNAS, 107,* 20045-20050.

D'Ombrain, M.C., Robinson, L.J., Stanisic, D.I., Taraika, J., Bernard, N., Michon, P., Mueller, I., and Schofield, L. (2008). Association of early interferon-gamma production with immunity to clinical malaria: a longitudinal study among Papua New Guinean children. *Clin. Infect. Dis., 47*, 1380-7.

Dondorp, A.M., Nyanoti. M., Kager, P.A., Mithwani, S., Vreeken, J., and Marsh, K. (2002). The role of reduced red cell deformability in the pathogenesis of severe falciparum malaria and its restoration by blood transfusion. *Trans. R. Soc. Trop. Med. Hyg., 96*, 282-286.

Dondorp, A.M., Planche, T., de Bel, E.E., Angus, B.M., Chotivanich, K., Silamut, K., Ruangveerayuth, R., Hoek, F., Romijn, J., Kager, P.A., Vreeken, J., and White, N. J. (1998). Nitric oxides in plasma, urine and cerebrospinal fluid in patients with severe falciparum malaria. *Am. J. Trop. Med. Hyg., 59,* 497-502.

Dorsey, G., Njama, D., Kamya, M. R., Cattamanchi, A., Kyabayinze, D.,Staedke, S. G., Gasasira, A. and Rosenthal, P. J. (2002). Sulfadoxine/pyrimethamine alone or with amodiaquine or artesunate for treatment of uncomplicated malaria: a longitudinal randomised trial. *Lancet 360,* 2031-2038.

Duarte, M.I., Corbett, C.E., Boulos, M., and Amato, N.V. (1985). Ultrastructure of the lung in falciparum malaria. *Am. J. Trop. Med. Hyg., 34,* 31–35.

Egan, T.J.; Kaschula, C.H. (2007) Strategies to reverse drug resistance in malaria. *Curr. Opin. Infect. Dis., 20*, 598-604.

Eiam-Ong, S., and Sitprija, V. (1998). Falciparum malaria and the kidney: a model of inflammation. *Am. J. Kidney Dis., 32*, 361-75.

Eichner, M., Diebner, H.H., Molineaux, L., Collins, W.E., Jeffery, G.M., and Dietz, K. (2001). Genesis, sequestration and survival of *Plasmodium falciparum* gametocytes: parameter estimates from fitting a model to malariatherapy data. *Trans. R. Soc. Trop. Med. Hyg., 95*, 497-501.

Eisner, M.D., Parsons, P., Matthay, M.A., Ware, L., Greene, K. (2003). Acute Respiratory Distress Syndrome Network. Plasma surfactant protein levels and clinical outcomes in patients with acute lung injury. *Thorax, 58*, 983-988.

Ekvall, H. (2003). Malaria andanemia. *Curr. Opin. Hematol., 10,* 108-114.

Epiphanio, S., Campos, M.G., Pamplona, A., Carapau, D., Pena, A.C., Ataíde, R., Monteiro, C.A.A., Félix, N., Costa-Silva, A., Marinho, C.R.F., Dias, S., and Mota, M.M. (2010).VEGF Promotes Malaria-Associated Acute Lung Injury in Mice Journal: *PLoS Pathog., 6,* e1000916.

Ezzet, F., Ezzet, R., and Karbwang, J. (1998). Population pharmacokinetics andtherapeutic response of CGP 56697 (artemether+benflumetol) in malaria patients. *British J. Clin. Pharmaco, 46*, 553–561.

Ferdig, M.T., Cooper, R.A., Mu, J., Deng, B., Joy, D.A., Su, X., and Wellems, T.E. (2004). Dissecting the loci of low-level quinine resistance in malaria parasites. *Mol. Microbiol.*, 52, 985–97.

Ferrante, R.J., Hantraye, P., Brouillet, E., and Beal, M.F. (1999). Increased nitrotyrosine immunoreactivity in substantia nigra neurons in MPTP-treated baboons is blocked by inhibition of neuronal nitric oxide synthase. *Brain Res., 823*, 177–182.

Figueiredo, L.M., Rocha, E.P., Mancio-Silva, L., Prevost, C., Hernandez-Verdun, D., Scherf, A. (2005). The unusually large *Plasmodium* telomerase reverse-transcriptase localizes in a discrete compartment associated with the nucleolus. *Nucl. Acid. Res., 33,* 1111-1122.

Foth, B.J., Stimmler, L.M., Handman, E., Crabb, B.S., Hodder, A.N., and McFadden, G.I. (2005). The malaria parasite *Plasmodium falciparum* has only one pyruvate dehydrogenase complex, which is located in the apicoplast. *Mol. Microbiol.,* 55, 39–53.

Franke-Fayard, B., Fonager, J., Braks, A., Khan, S.M., and Janse, C.J. (2010). Sequestration and Tissue Accumulation of Human Malaria Parasites: Can We Learn Anything from Rodent Models of Malaria? *PLoS Pathogens, 6,* e1001032.

Franklin, B.S., Parroche, P., Ataide, M.A., Lauw, F., Ropert, C., de Oliveira, R.B., Pereira, D., Tada, M.S., Nogueira, P., da Silva, L.H., Bjorkbacka, H., Golenbock, D.T., and Gazzinelli, R.T. (2009). Malaria primes the innate immune response due to interferongamma induced enhancement of toll-like receptor expression and function. *Proc. Natl. Acad. Sci. USA, 106,* 5789–5794.

Frevert, U. (2004). Sneaking in through the back entrance: the biology of malaria liver stages. *Trends Parasitol.,* 9, 417–424.

Gardner, M.J., Hall, N., Fung, E., White, O., Berriman, M., Hyman, R.W., Carlton, J.M., Pain, A., Nelson, K.E., Bowman, S., Paulsen, I.T., James, K., Eisen, J.A., Rutherford, K., Salzberg, S.L., Craig, A., Kyes, S., Chan, M.S., Nene, V., Shallom, S.J., Suh, B., Peterson, J., Angiuoli, S., Pertea, M., Allen, J., Selengut, J., Haft, D., Mather, M.W., Vaidya, A.B., Martin, D.M., Fairlamb, A.H., Fraunholz, M.J., Roos, D.S., Ralph, S.A., McFadden, G.I., Cummings, L.M., Subramanian, G.M., Mungall, C., Venter, J.C., Carucci, D.J., Hoffman, S.L., Newbold, C., Davis, R.W., Fraser, C.M., and Barrell, B. (2002). Genome sequence of the human malaria parasite *Plasmodium falciparum. Nature, 419*, 498–511.

Genton, B., D'Acremont, V., Rare, L., Baea, K, Reeder, J.C., Alpers, M.P., and Muller, I. (2008). *Plasmodium vivax* and mixed infections are associated with severe malaria in children: a prospective cohort study from Papua New Guinea. *PLoS Med, 5*, 127

Gilson, P.R., Nebl, T., Vukcevic, D., Moritz, R.L., Sargeant, T., Speed T.P., Schofield, L., Crabb, B.S. (2006). Identification and stoichiometry of glycosylphosphatidylinositol-anchored membrane proteins of the human malaria parasite *Plasmodium falciparum. Mol. Cell Proteomics, 5,* 1286–1299.

Gitau, E.N., and Newton, C.R. (2005). Review Article: blood-brain barrier in falciparum malaria. *Trop. Med. Int. Health, 10*, 285-292.

Glikman D, Nguyen-Dinh P, Roberts JM, Montgomery CP, Daum RS, andMarcinak JF (2007). Clinical malaria and sickle cell disease among multiple family members in Chicago, Illinois. *Pediatrics,* 120, 745-748.

Goel, V.K., Li, X., Chen, H., Liu, S.C., Chishti, A.H., Oh, S.S. (2003). Band3 is a host receptor bin ding merozoite surface protein 1 during the *Plasmodium falciparum* invasion of erythrocytes. *Proc. Nati. Acad. Sci. USA, 100*, 5164-5169.

Gole, M. D., Souza, J.M., Choi, I., Hertkorn, C., Malcolm, S., Foust, R.F., and Finkel, B. (2000). Plasma proteins modified by tyrosine nitration in acute respiratory distress syndrome. *Am. J. Physiol. Lung Cell Mol. Physiol., 278,* 961–967.

Gramaglia, I., Sobolewski, P., Meays, D., Contreras, R., Nolan, J.P., Frangos, J.A., Intaglietta, M., and van der Heyde, H.C. (2006). Low nitric oxide bioavailability contributes to the genesis of experimental cerebral malaria. *Nat. Med., 12,* 1417–1422.

Green, J.L., Hinds, L., Grainger, M., Knuepfer, E., and Holder, A.A. (2006). *Plasmodium* thrombospondin related apical merozoite protein (PTRAMP) is shed from the surface of merozoites by PfSUB2 upon invasion of erythrocytes. *Mol. Biochem. Parasitol., 150,*114–117.

Gregson, A. and Plowe, C.V. (2005). Mechanisms of Resistance of Malaria Parasites to Antifolates. *Pharmacol. Rev. 57,*117–145, 2005.

Griffiths, M. J., Ndungu, F., Baird, K.L., Ezzeter, D.P., Marsh, K., and Newton, C.R. (2001). Oxidative stress and erythrocyte damage in Kenyan children with severe *Plasmodium falciparum* malaria. *Br. J. Haematol., 113,* 486-491.

Grimberg, B.T. and Mehlotra, R.K. (2011). Expanding the Antimalarial Drug Arsenal—Now, But How? *Pharmaceuticals, 4,* 681-712.

Grimberg, B.T., Jaworska, M.M., Hough, L.B., Zimmerman, P.A., and Phillips, J.G. (2009,). Addressing the malaria drug resistance challenge using flow cytometry to discover new antimalarials. *Bioorg. Med. Chem. Lett., 19*, 5452-5457.

Guantai, E., and Chibale, K. (2010) Chloroquine resistance: Proposed mechanisms and counter measures. *Curr. Drug Deliv.*, *7*, 312-323.

Gueirarda, P., Tavaresa, J., Thibergea, S., Bernexb, F., Ishinoa, T., Milonc, G., Franke–Fayardd, B., Jansed, C.J., Menarda, R., andAminoa, R. (2010). Development of the malaria parasite in the skin of the mammalian host *PNAS, 107.*

Haldar, K., and Mohandas, N. (2009). Malaria, erythrocytic infection, and anemia. *American Society of Hematology*. PP, 88-93.

Haldar, K., Murphy, S.C., Milner, D.A., Taylor, T.E. (2007). Malaria: mechanism of Erythrocytic infection and pathological correlates of severe disease. *Annu. Rev. Pathol. Mech. Dis., 2,* 217-249.

Handayani, S., Chiu, D.T., Tjitra, E., Kuo, J.S., Lampah, D., Kenangalem, E., Renia, L., Snounou, G., Price, R.N., Anstey, N.M., and Russell, B. (2009). High deformability of Plasmodium vivax infected red blood cells undermicrofluidic conditions. *J. Infect. Dis., 199*, 445–450.

Hayton, K. andSu, X. Z. (2004). Genetic and biochemical aspects of drug resistance in malaria parasites. *Curr. Drug Targets Infect, Disorder, 4*, 1-10.

Heppner, D.G., Walsh, D.S., Uthaimongkol, N., Tang, D.B., Tulyayon, S., Permpanich, B., Wimonwattrawatee, T., Chuanak, N., Laoboonchai, A., Sookto, P., Brewer, T.G., McDaniel, P., Eamsila, C., Yongvanitchit, K., Uhl, K., Kyle, D.E., Keep, L.W., Miller, R.E., and Wongsrichanalai, C. (2005). Randomized, controlled, double-blind trial of daily oral azithromycin in adults for the prophylaxis of Plasmodium vivax malaria in Western Thailand.*Am. J. Trop. Med. Hyg., 73,* 842-849.

Hermans, C., and Bernard, A. (1999). Lung epithelium-specific proteins: characteristics and potential applications as markers. *Am. J. Respir. Crit. Care Med., 159*, 646-678.

Hindi, L., Green, J.L., Knuepfer, E., Grainger, M., and Holder, A.A. (2009). Novel Putative Glycosylphosphatidylinositol-Anchored Micronemal Antigen of *Plasmodium falciparum* That Binds to Erythrocytes. *Eukaryo. cell, 8,* 1869–1879.

Hines, P.C., Zen, Q., Burney, S.N., Shea, D.A., Ataga, K.I., Orringer, E.P., Telen, M.J., Parise, L.V. (2003). Novel epinephrine and cAMP-mediated activation of BCAM/Lu-dependent sickle (SS) RBC adhesion. *Blood, 101*, 3281–3287.

Hobbs, M. R., Udhayakumar, V., Levesque, M. C. , Booth, J., Roberts, J. M., Tkachuk, A. N., Pole, A., Coon, H., Kariuki, S., Nahlen, B. L., Mwaikambo, E. D., Lal, A. L., Granger, D. L., Anstey, N. M., and Weinberg. J. B. (2002). A new NOS2 promoter polymorphism associated with increased nitric oxide production andprotection from severe malaria in Tanzanian and Kenyan children. *Lancet, 360*, 1468–1475.

Horata, N., Kalambaheti, T., Craig, A., and Khusmith, S. (2009). Sequence variation of PfEMP1-DBLα in association with rosette formation in *Plasmodium falciparum* isolates causing severe and uncomplicated malaria. *Malar. J.*, 8, 184.

Howes, R.E., Patil, A.P., Piel, F.B., Nyangiri, O.A., Kabaria, C.W., Gething, P.W., Zimmerman, P.A., Barnadas, C., Beall, C.M., Gebremedhin, A., Ménard, D., Williams, T.N., Weatherall, D.J., and Hay, S.I. (2011). The global distribution of the Duffy blood group. *Nat. Comms., 2,* 266.

Hunt, N.H., and Grau, G.E. (2003). Cytokines: accelerators and brakes in the pathogenesis of cerebral malaria. *Trends Immunol., 24*, 491-499.

Hurly, M.G.D. (1959). Potentiation of pyrimethamine by sulphadiazine in human malaria. *Trans. R. Soc. Trop. Med. Hyg., 53,*412–413.

Hyde, J. E. (2007). Drug-resistant malaria - an insight. *The FEBS J.*, 274, 4688-4698.

Imwong, M., Pukrittakayamee, S., Renia, L., Letourneur, F., Charlieu, J.P., Leartsakulpanich, U., Looareesuwan, S., White, N.J., and Snounou, G. (2003). Novel point mutations in the dihydrofolate reductase gene of *Plasmodium vivax*: evidence for sequential selection by drug pressure. *Antimicrob. Agents Chemother., 47,* 1514–1521.

Imwong, M., Dondorp, A.M., Nosten, F., Yi, P., Mungthin, M., Hanchana, S., Das, D., Phyo, A.P., Lwin, K.M., Pukrittayakamee, S., Lee, S.L., Saisung, S., Koecharoen, K., Nguon, C., Day, N.P.J Socheat, D., andWhite, N.J. (2010). Exploring the contribution of candidate genes to artemisinin resistance in *Plasmodium falciparum. Antimicrob. Agents Chemother.*, *54*, 2886-2892.

Ishino, T., Yano, K., Chinzei, Y., andYuda, M. (2004). Cell-passage activity is required for the malaria parasite to cross the liver sinusoidal cell layer. *PLoS Biol.*, *2*, 77–84.

Ishizaka, A., Matsuda, T., Albertine, K.H., Koh, H., Tasaka, S., Hasegawa, N., Kohno, N., Kotani, T., Morisaki, H., Takeda, J., Nakamura, M., Fang, X., Martin, T.R., Matthay, M.A., and Hashimoto, S. (2004). Elevation of KL-6, a lung epithelial cell marker, in plasma and epithelial lining fluid in acute respiratory distress syndrome. *Am. J. Physiol. Lung Cell Mol. Physiol., 286*, 1088-1094.

Iuvone, T., Acquisto, F.D., Carnuccio, R., and Di Rosa, M. (1996). Nitric oxide inhibits LPS-induced tumor necrosis factor synthesis in vitro and *in vivo*. *Life Sci.*, *59*, 207–211.

Iyer, J., Grüner, A.C., Renia, L., Snounou, G., and Preiser, P.R. (2007). Invasion of host cells by malaria parasites: A tale of two protein families. *Mol. Microbiol., 65*, 231–249.

Janka, J.J., Koita, O.A., Traore, B., Traore, J.M., Mzayek, F., Sachdev, V., Wang, X., Sanogo, K., Sangare, L., Mendelsohn, L., Masur, H., Kato, G.J., Gladwin, M.T., and Krogstad, D.J. (2010). Increased pulmonary pressures andmyocardial wall stress in children with severe malaria. *J. Infect. Dis., 202,* 791-800.

Jaramillo, M., Godbout, M., and Olivier, M. (2005). Hemozoin induces macrophage chemokine expression through oxidative stress-dependent and–independent mechanisms. *J. Immunol., 174*, 475–484.

Jiang, X., and Wang, X. (2004). Cytochrome C-mediated apoptosis. *Annu. Rev. Biochem., 73*, 87-106.

Jianga, L., Gaura, D., Mua, J., Zhoua, H., Longa, C.A., andMillera, L.H. (2011). Evidence for erythrocyte-binding antigen 175 as a component of a ligand-blocking blood-stage malaria vaccine. *PNAS, 108,* 7553-7558.

Jomaa, J., Wiesner, S., Sanderbrand, B., Altincicek, C., Weidemeyer, M., Hintz, I., TSrbachova, M., Eberl, J., Zeidler, H. K., Lichtenthaler, D., Soldati, E. and Beck, H. (1999). Inhibitors of the nonmevalonta path way of isoprenoid synthesis as antimalarial drugs. *Sci., 285,* 1573 –1576.

Kiefer, C.R., and Snyder, L.M. (2000). Oxidation and erythrocyte senescence. *Curr. Opin. Hematol.*, 7, 113-116.

Kirk, K., Martin, R.E., Broer, S., Howitt, S.M., and Saliba, K.J. (2005). Plasmodium permeomics: membrane transport proteins in the malaria parasite. *Curr. Top. Microbiol. Immunol., 295*, 325–356.

Kiszewski, A.E. (2011). Blocking *Plasmodium falciparum* Malaria Transmission with Drugs: The Gametocytocidal and Sporontocidal Properties of Current and Prospective. *Antimalaria Pharmaceuticals, 4,* 44-68.

Klotz, U., and Frevert U. (2007). Malaria circumsporozoite protein inhibits the respiratory burst in Kupffer cells. *Cell Microbiol., 9*, 2610-2628.

Knell, A.J. (1991), *Malaria*. Oxford University Press.

Kobbe, R., Klein, P., Adjei, S., Amemasor, S., Thompson, W.N., Heidemann, H., Nielsen, M.V., Vohwinkel, J., Hogan, B., Kreuels, B., Bührlen, M., Loag, W., Ansong, D. and May, J. (2008). A randomized trial on effectiveness of artemether-lumefantrine *versus* artesunate plus amodiaquine for unsupervised treatment of uncomplicated *Plasmodium falciparum* malaria in Ghanaian children. *Malar. J., 7,* 261.

Koussis, K., Withers-Martinez, C., Yeoh, S., Child, M., Hackett, F., Knuepfer, E., Juliano, L., Woehlbier, U., Bujard, H., and Blackman, M.J. (2009). A multifunctional serine protease primes the malaria parasite for red blood cell invasion. *EMBO J., 28,* 725–735.

Kublin, J.G., Dzinjalamala, F.K., Kamwendo, D.D., Malkin, E.M., Cortese, J.F., Martino, L.M., Mukadam, R.A., Rogerson, S.J., Lescano, A.G., Molyneux, M.E., Winstanley, P.A., Chimpeni, P., Taylor, T.E., and Plowe, C.V. (2002). Molecular markers for failure of sulfadoxine-pyrimethamine and chlorproguanil-dapsone treatment of *Plasmodium falciparum* malaria. *J. Infect. Dis., 185,* 380–388.

Kumar, K.A., Garcia, C.R., Chandran, V.R., Van-Rooijen, N., Zhou, Y., Winzeler, E. and Nussenzweig V. (2007). Exposure of *Plasmodium* sporozoites to the intracellular concentration of potassium enhances infectivity andreduces cell passage activity. *Mol. Biochem. Parasitol., 156*, 32-40.

Kuwano, K., Hamada, N., Yamada, M., Fukumoto, J., Kaneko, Y., Maeyama, T., MichihiroYoshimi1, Aoyama, M., and Nakanishi, Y. (2006). Cytochrome c levels in serum and bronchoalveolar lavage fluid in lung injury. *Oral presentation.*

Lakshmanan, V., Bray, P.G., Verdier-Pinard, D., Johnson, D.J., Horrocks, P., Muhle, R.A., Alakpa, G.E., Hughes, R.H., Ward, S.A., Krogstad, D.J., Sidhu, A.B., and Fidock, D.A. (2005). A critical role for PfCRT K76T in *Plasmodium falciparum* verapamil-reversible chloroquine resistance. *EMBO J., 24*, 2294–305.

Lameire, N., and Vanholder, R. (2001). Pathophysiologic Features and Prevention of Human and Experimental Acute Tubular Necrosis. *J. Am. Soc. Nephrol., 12,* S20–S32, 2001

Lefevre, G., Looareesuwan, S., Treeprasertsuk, S., Krudsood, S., Silachamroon, U., Gathmann, I., Ezzet, R. andBakshi, R. (2001). A clinical andpharmacokinetic trial of six doses of artemether- lumefantrine for multidrug-resistant *Plasmodium falciparum* malaria in Thailand. *Am. J. Trop. Med. Hyg., 64*, 247-256.

Leiriao, P., Rodrigues, C.D., Albuquerque, S.S. and Mota, M.M. (2004). Survival of protozoan intracellular parasites in host cells. *EMBO reports, 5,* 1142-1147.

Lesur, O., Langevin, S., Berthiaume, Y., Legare, M., Skrobik, Y., Bellemare, J.F., Levy, B., Fortier, Y,. Lauzier, F., Bravo, G., Nickmilder, M., Rousseau, E., and Bernard, A. (2006). Critical Care Research Group of the Quebec Respiratory Health Network. Outcome value of Clara cell protein in serum of patients with acute respiratory distress syndrome. *Intensive Care Med., 32,* 1167-1174.

Liu, W., Kimball, E., andRabinowitz, J.D. (2006). A high-performance liquid chromatography-tandem mass spectrometry method for quantitation of nitrogen-containing intracellular metabolites. *J. Am. So.c Mass Spectrom.,* 17, 37–50.

Lobo C, de Frazao , K., Rodriguez, M., Reid, M., Zalis, M., and Lustigman, S. (2004). Invasion Profiles of Brazilian Field Isolates of *Plasmodium falciparum*: Phenotypic and Genotypic Analyses. *Infect. Immunol. 72*, 5886–5891.

Lovegrove, F. E., Gharib, S.A., Peña-Castillo, L., Patel, S.N., Ruzinski, J.T., Hughes, T.R., Liles, W.C., and Kain, K.C.(2008). Parasite Burden and CD36-Mediated Sequestration Are Determinants of Acute Lung Injury in an Experimental Malaria Model. *PLoS Pathog., 4, (5)*, e1000068.

Loyevsky, M. and Gordeuk, V. R. (2001). Iron chelators. In *Antimalarial Chemotherapy: Mechanisms of Action, Resistance, and New Directions in Drug Discovery* (ed. P. J. Rosenthal), pp. 307-324. Totowa, NJ: Humana Press.

Lyke, K.E., Burges, R., Cissoko, Y., Sangare, L., Dao, M., Diarra, I., Kone, A., Harley, R., Plowe, C.V., Doumbo, O.K., and Sztein, M.B. (2004). Serum levels of the proinflammatory cytokines interleukin-1 beta (IL-1beta), IL- 6, IL-8, IL-10, tumor necrosis factor alpha, and IL-12(p70) in Malian children with severe Plasmodium falciparum malaria and matched uncomplicated malaria or healthy controls. *Infect. Immunol., 72,* 5630-5637.

Macreadie, I., Ginsburg, H., Sirawaraporn, W., and Tilley, L. (2000). Antimalarial drug development and new targets. *Parasitol. Today, 16,* 438-444.

Maguire, J.D., Sumawinata, I.W., Masbar, S., Laksana, B., Prodjodipuro, P., Susanti, I., Sismadi, P., Mahmud, N., Bangs, M.J., and Baird, J.K. (2002). Chloroquine-resistant Plasmodium malariae in south Sumatra, Indonesia. *Lancet, 360,* 58-60.

Mahomva, A.I., Peterson, D.E., and Rakata, L. (1996). Chloroquine resistant *falciparum* malaria in Mutare District, eastern Zimbabwe. *Central African J. Med., 42,* 112–3.

Maneerat, Y., Viriyavejakul, P., Punpoowong, B., Jones, M., Wilairatana, P., Pongponratn, E., Turner, G.D., and Udomsangpetch, R. (2000). Inducible nitric oxide synthase expression is increased in the brain in fatal cerebral malaria. *Histopathology, 37*, 269-77.

Manan, J. A., Ali, H., and Manohar Lal, M. (2006). Acute renal failure associated with malaria. *J. Ayub. Med. Coll Abbottabad., 18.*

Manzano, J.I., Carvalho, L., Perez-Victoria, J.M., Castanys, S., and Gamarro. F. (2011). Increased Glycolytic ATP Synthesis Is Associated with Tafenoquine Resistance in *Leishmania major. Antimicrob. Agents Chemother., 55,* 1045-1052.

Margout, D., Wein, S., Gandon, H., Gattacceca, F., Vial, H.J., and Bressolle, F.M. (2009). Quantitation of SAR97276 in mouse tissues by rapid resolution liquid chromatography-mass spectrometry. *J. Sep. Sci., 32,* 1808-15.

Marthru, M., Rooney, M.W., Dries D.J., Hirsch, L.J., Barnes, L., and Tobin, M.H. (1994). Urine hydrogen peroxide during ARDS in patients with and without sepsis. *Chest, 105,* 232–236.

Marti, M., Baum, J., Rug, M., Tille, L., and Cowman, A.F. (2005). Signal mediated export of proteins from the malaria parasite to the host erythrocyte. *J. Cell Biol., 171*, 587-592.

Martin, R. E., and Kirk, K. (2004). The Malaria Parasite's Chloroquine Resistance Transporter is a Member of the Drug/Metabolite Transporter Superfamily. *Mol. Biol. Evol., 21,* 1938–1949.

Martin, S.K., Oduola, A.M., and Milhous, W.K. (1987). Reversal of chloroquine resistance in *Plasmodiumfalciparum* by verapamil. *Sci., 235*, 899-901.

Matuschewski, K., Nunes, A. C., Nussenzweig, V., and Menard, R. (2002). *Plasmodium* sporozoite invasion of insect and mammalian cells is directed by the same dual binding system. *EMBO J., 21,* 1597-1606.

Mcintyre, J.A., Castaner, J., and Bayes, M. (2003). Taf enoquine succinate. *Drugs Future, 28,*859–869.

Medana, I. M., Chaudhri, G., Chan-Ling, T., and Hunt, N.H. (2001). Central nervous system in cerebral malaria: "innocent bystander" or active participant in the induction of immunopathology? *Immunol. Cell Biol., 79,* 101–120.

Mehlotra, R. K., Henry-Halldin, C.N., and Zimmerman, P.A. (2009). Application of pharmacogenomics to malaria: A holistic approach for successful chemotherapy. *Pharmacogenomics 10*, 435-449.

Mikolajczak, S.A., Jacobs-Lorena, V., MacKellar, D.C., Camargo, N., and Kappe, S.H.I. (2007). L-FABP is a critical host factor for successful malaria liver stage development. *Inter. J. Parasito.,* 37, 483-489.

Miller, L.H., Baruch, D.I., Marsh, K., and Doumbo, O.K. (2002). The pathogenic basis of malaria. *Nature, 415*, 73–679.

Miller, L.H., Mason, S.J., Clyde, D.F., and McGinniss, M.H. (1976). The resistance factor to *Plasmodium vivax* in blacks. The Duffy-blood-group genotype, FyFy. *N. Engl. J. Med.,* 295.

Miller, M.J. (1957). Further studies on malaria suppression by monthly drug administration. *Am. J. Trop. Med. Hyg.,* 6, 625–637.

Mita, T., Kaneko, A., Hombhanje, F., Hwaihwanje, I., Takahashi, N., Osawa, H., Tsukahara, T., Masta, A., Lum, J.K., Kobayakawa, T., Ishizaki, T., and Bjorkman, A. (2006). Role of pfmdr1 mutations on chloroquine resistance in Plasmodium falciparum isolates with pfcrt K76T from Papua New Guinea. *Acta Trop., 98*, 137-144.

Mitchell, G.H., Thomas, A.W., Margos, G., Dluzewski, A.R., and Bannister, L.H. (2004). Apical membrane antigen1, a major malaria vaccine candidate, mediates the close attachment of invasion of merozoites to host red blood cells. *Infect. Immunol., 72,*154-158.

Mockenhaupt, F.P., Bousema, T.J., Eggelte, T.A., Schreiber, J., Ehrhardt, S., Wassilew, N., Otchwemah, R.N., Sauerwein, R.W., and Bienzle, U. (2005). *Plasmodium falciparum dhfr* but not *dhps* mutations associated with sulphadoxine-pyrimethamine treatment failure and gametocyte carriage in northern Ghana. *Trop. Med. Int. Health, 10,* 901–908.

Mohan, A., Sharma, S.K., and Bollineni, S. (2008). Acute lung injury andacute respiratory distress syndrome in malaria. *J. Vector Borne Dis., 45,*179–193.

Molyneux, M.E., Taylor, T.E., Wirima, J.J., and Borgstein, A. (1989). Effect of rate of infusion of quinine on insulin andglucose responses in Malawian children with falciparum malaria. *Q. J. Med., 71,* 441.

Morris, C. R., Kato, G.J., Poljakovic, M., Wang, X., Blackwelder, W.C., Sachdev, V., Hazen, S.L., Vichinsky, E.P., Morris, S.M., Jr., and Gladwin, M.T. (2005). Dysregulated arginine metabolism, hemolysis-associated pulmonary hypertension and mortality in sickle cell disease. *JAMA,* 294, 81–90.

Mota, M.M., Hafalla, J.C., and Rodriguez, A. (2002). Migration through host cells activates *Plasmodium* sporozoites for infection. *Nat. Med., 8*, 1318–1322.

Mombo-Ngoma, G., Supan, C., Dal-Bianco, M.P., Missinou1, M. A., Matsiegui, P., Salazar, C. L. O., Issifou1, S., Ter-Minassian, D., Ramharter, M., Kombila, M., Kremsner, P. G., and Lell, B. (2011). Phase I randomized dose-ascending placebo-controlled trials of ferroquine -a candidate anti-malarial drug- in adults with asymptomatic Plasmodium falciparum infection. *Malar. J., 10*, 53.

Munter, S., Sabass, B., Selhuber-Unke, C., Kudryashev, M., Hegge, S., Engel, U., Spatz, J.P., Matuschewski, K., Ulrich S. Schwarz, U.S. and Frischknecht, F. (2009). Plasmodium Sporozoite Motility Is Modulated by the Turnover of Discrete Adhesion Sites. *Cell Host Microbe*, 6, 551-562.

Nguansangiam, S., Day, N.P.J., Hien, T.T., Mai, N.T.H., Chaisri, U., and Riganti, M. (2007). A quantitative ultrastructural study of renal pathology in fatal *Plasmodium falciparum* malaria. *Trop. Med. Int. Heal, 12,* 1037–50.

Noedl, H., Krudsood, S., Leowattana, W., Tangpukdee, N., Thanachartwet, W., Looareesuwan, S., Miller, R.S., Fukuda, M., Jongsakul, K., Yingyuen, K., Sriwichai, S., Ohrt, C., and Knirsch, C. (2007). In Vitro Antimalarial Activity of Azithromycin, Artesunate, and Quinine in Combination and Correlation with Clinical Outcome. *Antimicrob. Agents Chemother*, 51, 651-656.

Nomura, T., Carlton, J.M.R., Baird, J.K., del Portillo, H.A., Fryauff, D.J., Rathore, D., Fidock, D.A., Su, X., Collins, W.E., McCutchan, T.F., Wootton, J.C., and Wellems, T.E. (2001). Evidence for Different Mechanisms of Chloroquine Resistance in 2 Plasmodium Species That Cause Human Malaria. *The J. Infec. Dis., 183*, 1653-1661.

Nyunt, M. M., Hendrix, C.W., Bakshi, R.P., Kumar, N., and Shapiro, T.A. (2009). Phase I/II evaluation of the prophylactic antimalarial activity of pafuramidine in healthy volunteers challenged with Plasmodium falciparum sporozoites. *Am. J. Trop. Med. Hyg., 80,* 528-35.

O'Neill, P.M., Bray, P.G., Hawley, S.R., Ward, S.A. B. K. andPark, B.K. (1998). 4-Aminoquinolines past, present andfuture: a chemical perspective. *Pharmacol. Ther., 77*, 29– 58.

Olszewski, K.L., Morrisey, J.M., Wilinski, D., Burns, J.M., Vaidya, A.B., Rabinowitz, J.D., and Llina′ s1, M. (2009). Host-Parasite Interactions Revealed by *Plasmodium falciparum* Metabolomics *Cell Host and Microbe, 5,* 191–199.

O'Neill, P.M., Mukhtar, A., Stocks, P.A., Randle, L.E., Hindley, S., Ward, S.A., Storr, R.C., Bickley, J.F., O'Neil, I.A., Maggs, J.L., Hughes, R.H., Winstanley, P.A., Bray, P.G., and Park, B.K. (2003). Isoquine and Related Amodiaquine Analogues: A New Generation of Improved 4-aminoquinoline Antimalarials, *J. Med. Chem., 46,* 4933-4945.

Ono, T., Cabrita-Santos, L., Leitao, R., Bettiol, E., Purcell, L.A., Diaz-Pulido, O., Andrews, L.B., Tadakuma, T., Bhanot, P., Mota, M.M., and Rodriguez, A. (2008). Adenylyl cyclase alpha and cAMP signaling mediate Plasmodium sporozoite apical regulated exocytosis and hepatocyte infection. *PLoS Pathog., 4*, e1000008.

Ouma, C., Davenport, G.C., Were, T., Otieno, M.F., Hittner, J.B., Vulule, J.M., Martinson J., Ong'echa, J.M., Ferrell, R.E. andPerkins, D.J. (2008). Haplotypes of IL-10 promoter variants are associated with susceptibility to severe malarial anemia andfunctional changes in IL-10 production. *Hum. Genetics, 124,* 515-524.

Oyakhirome, S., Issifou, S., Pongratz, P., Barondi, F., Ramharter, M., Kun, J. F., Missinou, M. A., Lell, B., and Kremsner, P. G. (2007). Randomized Controlled Trial of Fosmidomycin-Clindamycin versus Sulfadoxine-Pyrimethamine in the Treatment of Plasmodium falciparum Malaria. *Antimicrob. Agents Chemother, 51,* 1869-1871.

Pamplona, A., Ferreira, A., Balla, J., Jeney, V., Balla, G., Epiphanio, S, Chora, A., Rodrigues, C.D., Gregoire, I.P., Cunha-Rodrigues, M., Portugal, S., Soares, M.P.,and Mota, M.M. (2007). Heme oxygenase-1 andcarbon monoxide suppresses the pathogenesis of experimental cerebral malaria. *Nature Med., 13*, 703 – 710.

Parkash , J, Singh, A.K., Kumar, N.S., and Saxene, R.K. (2003). Acute renal failure in plasmodium vivax malaria. *J. Assoc. physicians India, 51*, 265-267.

Pasini, E. M., Kirkegaard, M., Salerno, D., Mortensen, P., Mann, M., and Thomas, A.W. (2008). Deep-coverage mouse red blood cell proteome: a first comparison with the human red blood cell. *Mol. Cell Prot., 7,* 1317-1330.

Pasini, E.M., Kirkegaard, M., Mortensen, P., Lutz, H.U., Thomas, A.W., and Mann, M. (2006). In-depth analysis of the membrane and cytosolic proteome of red blood cells. *Blood, 108*, 791-801.

Patel, A.P., Staines, H.M., andKrishna, S. (2008). New antimalarial targets: the example of glucose transport. *Travel Med. Infec. Dis, 6*, 58-66.

Pattanapanyasat, K., Yongvanitchit, K., Tongtawe, P., Tachavanich, K., Wanachiwanawin, W., Fucharoen, S., and Walsh, D.S. (1999). Impairment of *Plasmodium falciparum* growth in thalassemic red blood cells: further evidence by using biotin labeling and flow cytometry. *Blood*, *93*, 3116-3119.

Peatey, C.L., Andrews, K.T., Eickel, N., MacDonald, T., Butterworth, A.S., Trenholme, K.R., Gardiner, D.L., McCarthy, J.S., and Skinner-Adams, T.S. (2010). Antimalarial asexual stage-specific and gametocytocidal activities of HIV protease inhibitors. *Antimicrob. Agents Chemother.*, *54*, 1334-1337.

Peters, W. (1970). *Chemotherapy and Drug Resistance in Malaria.* London Academic Press.

Peters, W. (1971). Malaria. Chemoprophylaxis and chemotherapy. *BMC, 2,* 95-98.

Petersen, E. (1987). In vitro susceptibility of Plasmodium falciparum malaria to pyrimethamine, sulfadoxine, trimethoprim and sulfamethoxazole, singly and in combination. *Trans. R. Soc. Trop. Med. Hyg., 81,* 238–241.

Posner, G. H., Paik, I. H., Sur, S., McRiner, A. J., Borstnik, K., Xie, S. and Shapiro, T. A. (2003). Orally active, antimalarial, anticancer, artemisinin-derived trioxane dimers with high stability andefficacy. *J. Med. Chem., 46*, 1060-1065.

Powell, R. D., Brewer, G.J., and Alving, A.S. (1963). Studies on a strain of chloroquine-resistant Plasmodium falciparum from Colombia, South America. *Am. J. Trop. Med. Hyg., 12*, 509–512.

Prabhu, N., Joseph, P.I.D., and Chinnaswamy, P. (2008). *In vitro* antileptospiral activity of aqueous extract of *Eclipta alba* Linn. *Antiseptics*, *105*, 300- 302.

Pradines, B., Mamfoumbi, M. M., Parzy, D., Medang, M.O., Lebeau, C., J Mbina, J.R.M., Doury, J.C., and Kombila, M. (1999). In vitro susceptibility of African isolates of *Plasmodium falciparum* from Gabon to pyronaridine. *Am. J. Trop. Med. Hyg., 60,* 105-108.

Prato, M., Gallo, V., Giribaldi, G., and Arese, P. (2008). Phagocytosis of haemozoin (malarial pigment) enhances metalloproteinase-9 activity in human adherent monocytes: role of IL-1beta and15-HETE. *Malar. J., 7,* 157.

Prato, M., Giribaldi, G., Polimeni, M., Gallo, V., and Arese, P. (2005). Phagocytosis of hemozoin enhances matrix metalloproteinase-9 activity and TNF-alpha production in human monocytes: role of matrix metalloproteinases in the pathogenesis of falciparum malaria. *J. Immunol.*, *175,* 6436-6442.

Price, R. N., E. Tjitra, C. A. Guerra, S. Yeung, N. J. White, andN. M. Anstey (2007). Vivax malaria: neglected and not benign. *Am. J. Trop. Med. Hyg.*, *77*, 79–87.

Price, R.N., Uhlemann, A.C., van Vugt, M., Brockman, A., Hutagalung, R., Nair, S., Nash, D., Singhasivanon, P., Anderson, T.J., Krishna, S., White, N.J., andNosten, F. (2006). Molecular andpharmacological determinants of the therapeutic response to artemether-lumefantrine in multidrug-resistant *Plasmodium falciparum* malaria. *Clin. Infect. Dis., 42,* 1570–1577.

Pukrittayakamee, S., Chantra, A., Vanijanonta, S., Clemens, R., Looareesuwan, S., and White, N.J. (2000). Therapeutic responses to quinine and cBrinenmycin in multidrug-resistant falciparum malaria. *Antimicrob. Agents Chemother.*, *44*, 2395-2398.

Pukrittayakamee, S., Imwong, M., Singhasivanon, P., Stepniewska, K., Day, N.J., and White, N.J. (2008). Effects of Different Antimalarial Drugs on Gametocyte Carriage in P. vivax Malaria. *Am. J. Trop. Med. Hyg.*, *79,* 378-384.

Purfield, A.E., Tidwell., R.R., and Meshnick, S.R. (2008). Interactions of DB75, a Novel Antimalarial Agent, with Other Antimalarial Drugs *InVitro*. *Antimicrob. Agents Chemother., 52,* 2253-2255,

Ralph, S.A., van Dooren, G.G., Waller, R.F., Crawford, M.J., Fraunholz, M.J.,Foth, B.J., Tonkin, C.J., Roos, D.S., andMcFadden, G.I. (2004). Tropical infectious diseases: metabolic maps andfunctions of the Plasmodium falciparum apicoplast. *Nat. Rev. Microbiol., 2,* 203–216.

Reed, M. B., Saliba, K.L., Caruana, S.R., Kirk, K., and Cowman, A. F. (2000). Pgh1 modulates sensitivity and resistance to multiple antimalarials in *Plasmodium falciparum. Nature, 403*, 906–909.

Rieckman, K.H., Davis, D.R., and Hutton, D.C. (1989). *Plasmodium vivax* resistance to holoroquine? *Lancet, 2*, 1183-1184.

Riley, E. M., Wahl, S., Perkins, D.J., and Schofield, L. (2006). Regulating immunity to malaria. *Parasite Immunol., 28,* 35–49.

Ringwald, P., Bickii, J., and Basco, L. (1996). Randomised trial of pyronaridine versus chloroquine for acute uncomplicated falciparum malaria in Africa. *Lancet, 347,* 24–28.

Rogerson, S.J., Hviid, L., Duffy, P.E., G Leke, R.F., and Taylor, D. W. (2007). Malaria in pregnancy: pathogenesis andimmunity. *Lancet Infect. Dis.*, *7*, 105–117.

Rosenthal, P.J. (2003). Antimalarial drug discovery: old and new approaches. *The J. Exper. Biol., 206,* 3735-3744.

Rubenfeld, G.D., Caldwell, E., Peabody, E., Weaver, J., Martin, D.P., Neff, M., Stern, E.J., and Hudson, L.D. (2005). Incidence and outcomes of acute lung injury. *N. Engl. J. Med., 353,* 1685-1693.

Ryan, J.R., Stoute, J.A., Amon, J., Dunton, R.F., Mtalib, R., Koros, J., Owour, B., Luckhart, S., Wirtz, R, A., Barnwell, J.W., and Rosenberg, R. (2006). Evidence for transmission of Plasmodium vivax among a Duffy antigen negative population in Western Kenya. *Am. J. Trop. Med. Hyg., 75,* 575-581.

Saeed, S.A., Waqar, M.A., Zubairi, A.J., Bhurgri, H., Abdullah Khan, A., Gowani, S. A. S., Waqar, S.N., Choudhary, M.I., Jalil, S., Zaidi, A.H., and Ara, I. (2005). Myocardial ischaemia and reperfusion injury: Reactive oxygen species and the role of neutrophil. *JCPSP, 15,* 507-514.

Sarfo, B.Y., Armah, H.B., Irune, I., Adjei, A.A., Olver, C.S., Singh, S., Lillard, J.W., and Stiles, J.K. (2005). *Plasmodium yoelii* 17XL infection up-regulates RANTES, CCR1, CCR3 andCCR5 xpression, and induces ultrastructural changes in the cerebellum. *Malar. J., 4*, 63.

Schellenberg, D., Kahigwa, E., Drakeley, C., Malende, A., Wigayi, J., Msokame, C., Aponte, J. J., Tanner, M., Mshinda, H., Menendez, C. and Alonso, P.L. (2002). The safety and efficacy of sulfadoxine-pyrimethamine, amodiaquine, and their combination in the treatment of uncomplicated *Plasmodium falciparum* malaria. *Am. J. Trop. Med. Hyg.,* 67, 17-23.

Schlitzer, M. (2007). Malaria Chemotherapeutics Part I: History of Antimalarial Drug Development, Currently Used Therapeutics and Drugs in Clinical Development. *Chem. Med. Chem., 2*, 944 – 986.

Schlitzer, M. (2008). Antimalarial drugs—what is in use andwhat is in the pipeline? *Arch. Pharm., 341*, 149-163.

Schnapp, L.M., Donohoe, S., Chen, J., Sunde, D.A., Kelly, P.M., Ruzinski, J., Martin, T., and Goodlett, D.R. (2006). Mining the acute respiratory distress syndrome proteome: identification of the insulin-like growth factor (IGF)/IGF-binding protein-3 pathway in acute lung injury. *Am. J. Pathol., 169*, 86–95.

Schofield, L., Hewitt, M.C., Evans, K., Siomos, M.A., and Seeberger, P.H. (2002). Synthetic GPI as a candidate anti-toxic vaccine in a model of malaria. *Nature, 418*, 785–789.

Schofield, L., Novakovic, S., Gerold, P., Schwarz, R. T., McConville, M. J., andTachado, S. D. Tyrosine kinase dependent signal transduction in vascular endothelial cells by glycosylphosphatidylinositol toxin of plasmodium upregulates ICAM, VCAM and E-selectin expression andincrease leukocyte cytoadherence. (1996) *J. Immunol.,* 156, 1886–1896.

Shah, M.A., and Ahmad, Z. (1996). Malaria trends in general practice in Karachi, Pakistan. *Journal of the College of Physicians and Surgeons–Pakistan*, *6*, 62–4.

Shanks, G.D., and Edstein, M.D. (2005). Modern malaria chemophylaxis. *Drugs, 65*, 2091 – 2110.

Sharma, S.K., and Mohan, A. (2007). Acute respiratory distress syndrome. In: Grover A, Aggarwal V, Gera P, Gupta R, editors. *Manual of medical emergencies*. 3rd edn. Delhi, Pushpanjali Medical Publishers pp. 396–402.

Sherman, I.W. (1998). Carbohydrate Metabolism of Asexual Stages. In *Malaria, Parasite Biology, Pathogenesis and Protection,* (I.W. Sherman, Eds) pp. 135–143, Washington, D.C.: ASM Press.

Silva, A., Lee, A., Gulnik, S., Majer, P., Collins, J., Bhat, T., Collins, P., Cachau, R., Luker, K., Gluzman, I. Y., Francis, S. E., Oksman, A., Goldberg, D. E. and Erickson, J.W. (1996). Structure and inhibition of plasmepsin II, a hemoglobin-degrading enzyme from Plasmodium falciparum. *J. Proc. Natl. Acad. Sci. USA, 93,* 10034- 10039.

Silvie, O., Goetz, K., and Matuschewski, K. (2008b). A Sporozoite Asparagine-Rich Protein Controls Initiation of Plasmodium Liver Stage Development. *PLoS Pathog., 4,* e1000086.

Silvie, O., Mota, M.M., Matuschewski, K., and Prudencio, M. (2008a). Interactions of the malaria parasite and its mammalian host. *Current Opinion in Microbiol., 11*, 352–359.

Sim, B.K., Chitnis, C.E., Wasniowska, K., Hadley, T.J., and Miller, L.H. (1994). Receptor and ligand domains for invasion of erythrocytes by *Plasmodium falciparum. Sci, 264,* 1941-1944.

Singh, A.P., Buscaglia, C.A., Wang, Q., Levay, A., Nussenzweig, D.R., Walker, J.R., Wineler, E.A., Fujii, H., Fontoura, B.M.A., and Nussenzweig, V. (2006). *Plasmodium* circumsporozoite protein promotes the development of the liver stages of the parasite. *Cell, 131,* 492-504.

Skinner-Adams, T.S., Andrew, K.T., Melville, L., McCarthy, J., and Gardiner, D.L. (2007). Synergistic interactions of the antiretroviral protease inhibitors saquinavir and ritonavir with chloroquine and mefloquine against *Plasmodium falciparum in vitro. Antimicrob. Agents Chemother., 51*,759-762.

Smithuis, F.M., van Woensel, J.B., Nordlander, E., Vantha, W.S., andter Kuile, F.O. (1993) Comparison of two mefloquine regimens for treatment of Plasmodium falciparum malaria on the northeastern Thai-Cambodian border. *Antimicrob. Agents Chemother., 37*, 1977–1981.

Snow, R.W., Guerra, C.A., Noor, A.M., Myint, H.Y., and Hay, S.I. (2005). The global distribution of clinical episodes of *Plasmodium falciparum* malaria. *Nature, 434*, 214–217.

Spielmann, T., Gardiner, D.L., Beck, H.P., Trenholme, K.R., andKemp, D.J. (2006). Organization of ETRAMPs and EXP-1 at the parasite–host cell interface of malaria parasites. *Mol. Microbiol., 59,* 779-794.

Sriram, S., Srilakshmi, J.K., Meenaa, V., and Sasikumar, C. (2009). Adenosine deaminase from *Plasmodium falciparum* as a Potential Drug Target in Anti- Malarial Drug Designing: A Bioinformatic Approach. *Ethnobotanical Leaflets, 13,*639-647.

Steinbuechel, M., andMatuschewski, K. (2009), Role for the Plasmodium sporozoite-specific transmembrane protein S6 in parasite motility andefficient malaria transmission. *Cellular Microbiol., 11*, 279–288.

Sterkers, Y., Scheidig, C., da Rocha, M., Lepolard, C., Gysin, J., and Scherf, A. (2007). Members of the low-molecular-mass rhoptry protein complex of *Plasmodium falciparum* bind to the surface of normal erythrocytes. *J. Infect. Dis., 196,* 617-621.

Suratt, B.T., and Parsons, P.E. (2006). Mechanisms of acute lung injury/acute respiratory distress syndrome. *Clin. Chest Med.,* 27, 579–589.

Sural, S., Sharma, R.K., Gupta, A., Sharma, A.P., and Gulati, S. (2000). Acute renal failure associated with liver disease in India: etiology and outcome. *Ren. Fail, 22,* 623–34.

Taylor, W.R., Canon, V., and White, N.J. (2006). Pulmonary manifestations of malaria: recognition and management. *Treat. Respir. Med., 5,*419–428.

ter Kuile, F.O., Nosten, F., Thieren, M., Luxemburger, C., Edstein, M.D., Chongsuphajaisiddhi, T., Phaipun, L., Webster, H.K., and White, N.J. (1992). High-dose mefloquine in the treatment of multidrug-resistant falciparum malaria. *J. Infect. Dis., 166,* 1393–1400.

Tewari, R., Ogun, S.A., Gunaratne, R.S., Crisanti, A., and Holder, A.A. (2005). Disruption of *Plasmodium berghei* merozoite surface protein 7 gene modulates parasite growth in vivo. *Blood*, *105*, 394-396.

Tham, W., Wilson, D.W., Reiling, L., Chen, L., Beeson, J.G., and Cowman, A.F. (2009). Antibodies to Reticulocyte Binding Protein-Like Homologue 4 Inhibit Invasion of *Plasmodium falciparum* into Human Erythrocytes. *Infec andimmune, 77*, 2427–2435.

Thama, W., Wilsona, D.W., Lopatickia, S., Schmidtb, C.Q., Tetteh-Quarcoob, P.B., Barlowb, P.N., Richarda, D., Corbina, J.E., Beesona, J.G., and Cowmana, A.F. (2010). Complement receptor 1 is the host erythrocyte receptor for Plasmodium falciparum PfRh4 invasion ligand. *PNAS, 107,* 17327–17332.

Thawani, N., Kulkarni, M.A., and Sohani, S. (2009). Factors Associated with Coverage and Usage of Long-Lasting Insecticidal Nets in Madagascar. *J. Trop. Med., 451719.*

Tjitra, E., Anstey, N.M., Sugiarto, P., Warikar, N.E., Karyana, K.M., Lampah, D.A., and Price, R. N. (2008). Multidrug-resistant *Plasmodium vivax* associated with severe and fatal malaria: a prospective study in Papua, Indonesia. *PLoS Med, 5,* e128.

Traore, B., Muanza, K., Looareesuwan, S., Supavej, S., Khusmith, S., Danis, M., Viriyavejakul P., and Gay, F. (2000). Cytoadherence characteristics of Plasmodium falciparum isolates in Thailand using an in vitro human lung endothelial cells model. *Am. J. Trop. Med. Hyg.*, *62*, 38–44

Triglia, T., Duraisingh, M.T., Good, R.T., and Cowman, A. F. (2005). Reticulocyte-binding protein homologue 1 is required for sialic acid-dependent invasion into human erythrocytes by *Plasmodium falciparum*. *MoL. Microbiol.*, *55*, 162–174.

Uchida, T., Shirasawa, M., Ware, L.B., Kojima, K., Hata, Y., Makita, K., Mednick, G., Matthay, Z.A., and Matthay, M.A. (2006). Receptor for advanced glycation end-products is a marker of type I cell injury in acute lung injury. *Am. J. Respir. Crit. Care Med., 173*, 1008-1015.

Valko, M., Leibfritz, D., Moncol, J., Cronin, M.T., Mazur, M., and Telser, J. (2007). Free radicals and antioxidants in normal physiological functions and human disease. *Int. J. Biochem. Cell Biol., 39,* 44-84.

van Schalkwyk, D. A., Walden, J. C. and Smith, P. J. (2001). Reversal of chloroquine resistance in *Plasmodium falciparum* using combinations of chemosensitizers. *Antimicrob. Agents Chemother*, *45,* 3171-3174.

van Schalkwyk, D.A., and Egan, T.J. (2006). Quinoline-resistance reversing agents for the malaria parasite *Plasmodium falciparum*. *Drug Resist. Updat.*, *9*, 211-226.

Vitek, L., and Schwertner, H.A. (2007). The Heme Catabolic Pathway and its Protective Effects on Oxidative Stress-Mediated Diseases. *Advan. Clin. Chem., 43*, 1-57

Vreden, S.G., van den Broek, M.F., Oettinger, M.C., Verhave, J.P., Meuwissen, J.H., and Sauerwein, R.W. (1992). Cytokines inhibit the development of liver schizonts of the malaria parasite Plasmodium berghei in vivo. *Eur. J. Immunol., 22*, 2271-2275.

Walsh, D.S., Eamsila ,C., Sasiprapha, T., Sangkharomya, S., Khaewsathien, P., Supakalin, P., Tang, D.B., Jarasrumgsichol, P., Cherdchu, C., Edstein, M.D., Rieckmann, K.H., and Brewer, T.G.(2004). Efficacy of monthly tafenoquine for prophylaxis of Plasmodium vivax and multidrug-resistant P. falciparum malaria. *J. Infect. Dis., 190,* 1456-63.

Waller, D., Krishna, S., Crawley, J., Miller, K., Nosten, F., Chapman, D., ter Kuile, F.O., Craddock, C., Berry, C., Holloway,P.A.H., Brewster, D., Greenwood, B.M., and White, N.J. (1995). Clinical features and outcome of severe malaria in Gambian children. *Clin. Infect. Dis., 21,* 577–87.

Ward, C.P., Wong, P.E., Burchmore, R.J., de Koning, H.P., and Barrett, M.P. (2011). Trypanocidal furamidine analogues: influence of pyridine nitrogens on trypanocidal activity, transport kinetics, and resistance patterns. *Antimicrob. Agents Chemother., 55,* 2352-2361.

Ware, L.B., and Matthay, M.A. (2000). Acute respiratory distress syndrome. *N. Engl. J. Med., 342,* 1334-1349.

Wasiu, A.O., and Kayode, A.A. (2004). Pediatric acute renal failure in southwestern Nigeria. *Kidney Int., 66,* 1541–1548.

Wassmer, S.C., Combes, V., Candal, F.J., Juhan-Vague, I., and Grau, G.E. (2006b). Platelets potentiate brain endothelial alterations induced by *Plasmodium falciparum. Infect. Immun., 74*, 645-53.

Wassmer, S.C., de Souza, J.B., Frère, C., Candal, F.J., Juhan-Vague, I., and Grau, G.E. (2006a). TGF-beta1 released from activated platelets can induce TNF-stimulated human brain endothelium apoptosis: a new mechanism for microvascular lesion during cerebral malaria. *J. Immunol., 176,* 1180-4.

Wassmer, S.C., Taylor, T., Maclennan, C.A., Kanjala, M., Mukaka, M., Molyneux, M.E., and Grau, G.E. (2008). Platelet-induced clumping of *Plasmodium falciparum*-infected erythrocytes from Malawian patients with cerebral malaria-possible modulation in vivo by thrombocytopenia. *J. Infect. Dis., 197,* 72-8.

Weinberg, J.B., Lopansri, B.K., Mwaikambo, E., and Granger, D.L. (2008). Arginine, nitric oxide, carbon monoxide, andendothelial function in severe malaria. *Curr. Opin. Infect. Dis.,* 21, 468-475.

Wellems, T.E., and Plowe, C.V. (2001). Chloroquine-resistant malaria. *J. Infect. Dis., 184,* 770–776.

Wengelnik K, Vidal V, Ancelin ML, Cathiard AM, Morgat JL, Kocken CH, Calas M, Herrera S, Thomas AW, and Vial HJ. (2002). A class of potent antimalarials and their specific accumulation in infected erythrocytes. *Sci., 295,* 1311-4.

Wernsdorfer, W.H., and Noedl, H. (2003). Molecular markers for drug resistance in malaria: use in treatment, diagnosis andepidemiology. *Curr. Opin. Infect. Dis., 16*, 553–558.

White, N.J. (2008). *Plasmodium knowlesi*: the fifth human malaria parasite. Editorial Commentary. *Clin. Infect. Dis., 46*,172-173.

White, N.J., and Pongtavornpinyo. W. (2003). The *de novo* selection of drug-resistant malaria parasites. *Proceedings of the Royal Society of London. Series B: Biol. Scie.* 270:545–554.

WHO, (1973). *Chemotherapy of malaria and resistance to antimalarials*. Geneva, Technical Report Series, No. 529.

WHO, (1990). Practical chemotherapy of malaria. Report of a WHO Scientific Group. Geneva, World Health Organization, (WHO Technical Report Series, No. 805).

WHO, (1995). *Management of uncomplicated malaria and use of antimalarial drugs for the protection of travellers*. WHO/MAL 96.1075. Geneva: World Health Organization,

WHO, (2001). The use of antimalarial drugs: Report of an informal consultation (WHO/CDS/RBM/2001.33). *Geneva, Switzerland,* 2001.

WHO/UNICEF (2005). World malaria report, WHO, Geneva

WHO, (2006). *Guidelines for the treatment of malaria*. WHO/HTM/MAL/2006.1108.

WHO, (2010). *Global report on antimalarial efficacy and drug resistance*: 2000-2010 ISBN: 9789241500470.

Williams, T.N., Mwangi, T.W., Roberts, D.J., Alexander, N.D., Weatherall, D.J., Wambua, S., Kortok, M., Snow, R.W., and Marsh, K. (2005). An immune basis for malaria protection by the sickle cell trait. *PLoS Med., 2,* e128.

Yamauchi, L.M., Coppi, A., Snounou, G. and Sinnis, P. (2007). *Plasmodium* sporozoites trickle out of the injection site. *Cell Microbio., 9(5),* 1215-1222.

Yeo, T.W., Lampah, D.A., Gitawati, R., Tjitra, E., Kenangalem, E., Piera, K., Price, R.N., Duffull, S.B., Celermajer, D.S, Anstey, N.M. (2008). Angiopoietin-2 is associated with decreased endothelial nitric oxide and poor clinical outcome in severe falciparum malaria. *Proc. Natl. Acad. Sci. USA, 105*(44), 17097-102.

Yeo, T.W., Lampah, D.A., Gitawati, R., Tjitra, E., Kenangalem, E., McNeil, Y.R., Darcy, C.J., Granger, D.L., Weinberg, J.B., Lopansri, B.K., Price, R.N., Duffull, S. B., Celermajer, D. S., and Anstey, N.M. (2007). Impaired nitric oxide bioavailability and L-arginine reversible endothelial dysfunction in adults with falciparum malaria. *JEM, 204*, 2693-2700.

Yeoh, S., O'Donnell, R.A., Koussis, K., Dluzewski, A.R., Ansell, K.H., Osborne, S.A., Hackett, F., Withers-Martinez, C., Mitchell, G.H., Bannister, L.H., Bryans, J.S., Kettleborough, C.A., and Blackman, M.J. (2007). Subcellular discharge of a serine protease mediates release of invasive malaria parasites from host erythrocytes. *Cell 131*, 1072–1083.

Yeramian, P., Meshnick, S. R., Krudsood, S., Chalermrut, K., Silachamroon, U., Tangpukdee, N., Allen, J., Brun, R., Kwiek, J. J., Tidwell, R., and Looareesuwan, S. (2005). Efficacy of DB289 in Thai patients with *Plasmodium vivax* or acute, uncomplicated *Plasmodium falciparum* infections. *J. Infect. Dis., 192,* 319-322.

Yuda, M., and Ishino, T. (2004). Liver invasion by malarial parasites – how do malarial parasites break through the host barrier? *Cell Microbiol., 6,* 1119–1125.

Zingarelli, B., Halushka, P.V., Caputi, A.P., and Cook. J. A. (1995). Increased nitric oxide synthesis during the development of endotoxin tolerance. *Shock, 3*, 102–108.

Zongo, I., Dorsey, G., Rouamba, N., Tinto, H., Dokomajilar, C., Guiguemde, R.T, Rosenthal, P.J. and Ouedraogo, J.B. (2007). Artemether-lumefantrine versus amodiaquine plus sulfadoxine-pyrimethamine for uncomplicated falciparum malaria in Burkina Faso: a randomised non-inferiority trial. *The lancet, 369*, 491-498.

In: Malaria: Etiology, Pathogenesis and Treatments
Editors: A. M. Peterson and G. E Calamandrei
ISBN: 978-1-62100-363-2

Chapter II

Progress with RTS,S: The Most Advanced Candidate Vaccine Against Human Malaria

***James W. L. Denny*[1] *and Andrew W. Taylor-Robinson*[2*]**
School of Medicine[1] and Institute of Molecular and Cellular Biology[2],
University of Leeds, United Kingdom.

Abstract

Malaria has afflicted humans for aeons, being responsible for more deaths throughout history than any other disease. Today, infection with protozoan parasites of the genus *Plasmodium* still claims the lives of at least one million people each year, mainly children, in addition to the significant debilitation it causes to hundreds of millions more. Consequently, malaria has a drastic socioeconomic impact on endemic countries and therefore it has been the focus of global health initiatives for decades. Early attempts to eradicate malaria through targeting the mosquito vector failed; however, increased investment in existing control measures, such as the use of insecticide-impregnated bed nets, has been matched by renewed efforts to develop an efficacious vaccine. Sequencing of the genome of *P. falciparum*, which causes the most severe form of the disease, has improved knowledge of the malaria parasite's complex lifecycle, which, combined with a greater understanding of the human immune response to infection, has produced a number of novel candidate vaccines over the last two decades. Most notable among these is RTS,S which has shown much promise throughout a long development process, recently becoming the first candidate vaccine against human malaria to progress into phase III clinical trials. There is optimism, therefore, that in the foreseeable future RTS,S may become the first licensed antimalarial vaccine. Nevertheless, there are unresolved issues surrounding the lack of understanding of its mechanism of protection and doubt cast over its therapeutic potential. While the future

* Address correspondence to this author at the Institute of Molecular and Cellular Biology, University of Leeds, Clarendon Way, Leeds LS2 9JT, UK; Tel: 0044 113 343 2893; Fax: 0044 113 343 2882; E-mail: a.w.taylor-robinson@leeds.ac.uk.

success of RTS,S as a commercially available product is not certain, it is still likely to play a significant role in our ongoing fight against malaria, if only as a forerunner to a more refined second generation vaccine.

Keywords: Malaria, *Plasmodium falciparum*, immunity, vaccine, RTS,S

Introduction

Humans have been plagued for millennia by malaria, an infectious disease that is thought to have affected prehistoric man [1, 2]. Malaria in humans is caused by five species of protozoan parasite from the genus *Plasmodium* which are spread via the female *Anopheles* mosquito [3, 4]. *P. falciparum* is the most dangerous, accounting for more deaths worldwide than any of the other species.

Malaria is currently endemic in 109 countries and is found on every continent on Earth, bar Antarctica, but is confined to mainly tropical regions [5, 6]. The estimated global population is 6.9 billion people [7], of which 3.3-3.6 billion are at risk of contracting malaria [5, 8]. It is estimated that there are 300-500 million clinical cases worldwide annually [9]. The 1-3 million deaths that result equate to a death every 10-30 seconds [10, 11]. 90% of deaths are due to *P. falciparum* and occur principally in young children in sub-Saharan Africa.

The distribution of malaria is mainly among socioeconomically lower developed countries, further perpetuating their cycle of poverty. It is thought to cost these endemic nations approximately $12 billion a year, most of which Africa has to bear [12, 13]. Annual losses of 1.3% in economic growth may be attributed at least in part to lost person hours and therefore to reduced productivity [14]. Furthermore, children who miss school suffer from impaired education which ultimately affects their future employment prospects [14].

Over the past half century, many non-governmental organisations have been established to implement a variety of malaria initiatives. The first large-scale international effort was the Global Malaria Eradication Programme (GMEP), initiated by the World Health Organization (WHO) in 1955 and aimed to eradicate malaria [15]. This was abandoned in 1969 due to years of neglect; instead, control became the strategy of subsequent decades. Relatively recently, a resurgence of public awareness called for an increased effort in the use of control measures. This sparked The Bill and Melinda Gates Foundation (BAMGF) in 2007 to announce that eradication should be attempted again [15, 16]. Rapid support from the WHO led to the formation of the Malaria Elimination Group, which now works toward this. Another important organisation is the Program for Appropriate Technology in Health (PATH) which, in 2004, led to the formation of the Malaria Control and Evaluation Partnership in Africa [17]. This works with Africa's governments and the Roll Back Malaria (RBM) partnership to deliver control and prevention interventions across the continent [17]. Elimination, and ultimately eradication, is thought to be possible with current tools; however, large-scale attempts to control malaria have had a turbulent history, successful in some parts of the world but failing in many others, and practice of these methods continues to be neglected [15].

This has been a commonly held view for years and allowed vaccines to gain increasing attention, leading in 1999 to the formation of the PATH Malaria Vaccine Initiative (MVI) [17]. MVI helps accelerate malaria vaccine development, and, in 2001, formed a relationship with GlaxoSmithKline (GSK) based on a promising candidate vaccine known as RTS,S [18]. By 2006, an additional $207.6 million had been invested which has helped progress RTS,S to where it stands today [18].

MVI is currently looking at four vaccines, with RTS,S being the most advanced (Figure 1) [11]. Their drive for a vaccine has been perpetuated by 50 years of failures and inadequacies in alternative preventative measures [5, 19]. Negligence and poor implementation are ultimately responsible for the failure to eradicate malaria and not the control measures themselves. Consequently, a vaccine may be the only real shot at eradication; it was achieved with smallpox, which sets a precedent for all other infectious diseases, including malaria.

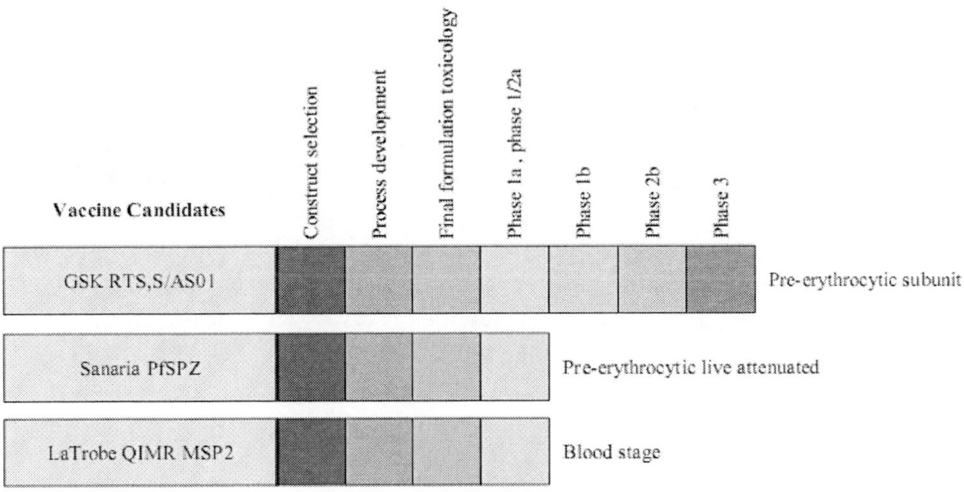

Figure 1. Diagram to show the relative advanced progress of RTS,S compared to other leading malaria candidate vaccines.

This chapter aims to introduce malaria as a disease, incorporating key areas of understanding including lifecycle, transmission, pathogenesis, pathophysiology and epidemiology. This is followed by assessment of existing control methods which provides a context for the subsequent sections that focus on immunology and vaccinology. The spotlight concentrates on *P. falciparum* and RTS,S throughout. Before concluding, problems with RTS,S and its potential future are discussed.

Lifecycle and Clinical Features

Malaria has a complex lifecycle which is broadly similar for all *Plasmodium* species that infect humans. Differences in the requirements for host cell invasion of each species lead to different aetiologies and therefore different clinical presentations. Malaria involves a number of clinical symptoms which are mainly associated with the blood stage of infection.

Lifecycle

A person becomes infected when, during the course of taking a blood meal, a female *Anopheles* mosquito inoculates them with *Plasmodium* sporozoites harboured in the mosquito's saliva. Once the sporozoites enter the bloodstream they proceed rapidly to the liver where they invade hepatocytes and undergo asexual reproduction (hepatic schizogony) to produce intracellular liver schizonts [20-22]. In the case of *P. vivax* and *P. ovale* hypnozoites may also be formed [2, 20]. These too grow within hepatocytes but remain quiescent and are responsible for persistence of infection when malaria relapses after an infection has been cleared [23]. This stage of the lifecycle is known as the pre-erythrocytic stage and is followed by the blood stage [21].

When schizont-infected hepatocytes rupture they release thousands of merozoites into the bloodstream which subsequently invade erythrocytes and undergo another asexual reproductive cycle (erythrocytic schizogony) [20, 22]. Here, merozoites feed on haemoglobin and develop into immature trophozoites, then to mature trophozoites and finally to schizonts. These then rupture along with the erythrocyte, releasing yet more merozoites, vastly increasing the parasitaemia; this is responsible for the clinical manifestations of malaria [20, 21]. Merozoites continue to infect erythrocytes and keep cycling to reproduce more; however, a small number differentiate into gametocytes, either female macrogametocytes or male microgametocytes. During a blood meal mosquitoes take up gametocytes into their midgut where the cycle enters its third and final stage [20, 21].

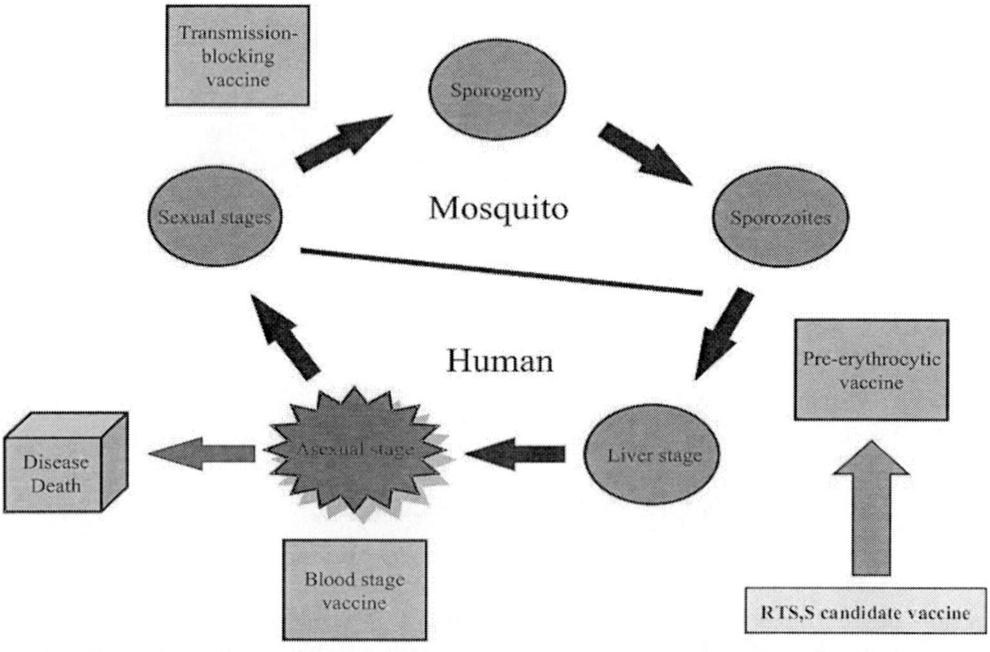

Figure 2. Schematic life cycle of *Plasmodium falciparum,* indicating where vaccination may be expected to intervene. A pre-erythrocytic vaccine, such as the RTS,S candidate, targets the parasite before asexual stages are released into the blood, causing the pathology of the disease.

In this stage macrogametocytes mature into macrogametes and microgametocytes exflagellate to form microgametes [2, 20]. Microgametes fertilise macrogametes (sexual reproduction) forming zygotes which then become motile ookinetes [20]. Ookinetes penetrate the mosquito midgut wall where they develop into oocysts, marking the beginning of the sporogenic cycle in which a large number of sporozoites are produced [2, 21]. Eventually the oocysts rupture, releasing sporozoites which make their way to the salivary glands to reinitiate the cycle.

Figure 2 illustrates this lifecycle for *P. falciparum* and shows the three stages that vaccines target – pre-erythrocytic vaccines (PEV), blood stage vaccines (BSV) and transmission blocking vaccines (TBV) (block sporogenic cycle). The various morphological events lead to the temporal expression of a great number of stage-specific antigens for which experimental vaccines are designed to target.

Pathogenesis and Pathophysiology

The classic clinical signs of acute uncomplicated malaria infection are febrile paroxysms, which are rolling fevers consisting of three stages – the cold stage (cold, rigors), hot stage (spiking temperature) and sweating stage [20]. This cyclic fever runs every two days, separated by a short period where the host feels slightly better before another cycle begins. The paroxysms are cytokine-induced and directly relate to erythrocyte rupture [2]. Paroxysms are more suggestive of a *P. vivax* or *P. ovale* infection as *P. falciparum* infections often present with continuous fever; however, individuals in endemic areas are more likely to present with atypical fever [6]. The fever is frequently accompanied by other manifestations such as headache, myalgia, malaise, confusion, anxiety and hepatosplenomegaly due to engorgement with infected erythrocytes [20, 22].

Severe *P. falciparum* infection (complicated malaria) can manifest in a number of ways including cerebral malaria, severe anaemia, renal disease and pulmonary oedema. The severe cases and their manifestations are what constitute the majority of deaths [22]. The pathogenic effects of *P. falciparum* are associated with three specific processes: cytoadherence, haemolysis of infected and uninfected erythrocytes, and production of malarial pigment (haemozoin) [20].

Pathogenesis of *P. falciparum* differs from other types of malaria mainly due to its unique ability to cytoadhere to endothelial cells of small blood vessels [13, 22]. This sequestration allows the parasite to avoid splenic clearance but subsequently reduces blood flow to other tissues which consequently experience hypoxic cell injury or even death [13, 22]. Adherence in the neurovascular system is often intense and explains delirium, irritability, convulsions and coma experienced in cerebral malaria. This is concordant with the fact cerebral malaria is only found with *P. falciparum* infections as only this species can cytoadhere [24]. Anaemia is the inevitable consequence of mass destruction of infected erythrocytes; it further compounds tissue hypoxia by reducing the oxygen carrying capacity of blood and, if severe, causes profound hypoxia to vital organs [13]. However, other processes can cause anaemia such as lysis of uninfected erythrocytes resulting from a disease-induced, complement-mediated immune response [2, 13]. Finally, haemozoin, formed from the metabolism of haemoglobin by the parasite, can also exacerbate anaemia [20]. Its accumulation locks in iron, causing an iron store depletion in the host. Iron is needed to manufacture properly functioning haem in new erythrocytes and is essential for normal oxygen carriage. All organ failure/dysfunction is related to these pathological processes; for example, cerebral anaemia is due to hypoxia of the brain, and renal disease is due to hypoxic tubular necrosis [6].

Natural Immunity

Immunity of humans to *P. falciparum* develops slowly in endemic areas and is attributed to the parasite's low immunogenic nature and high antigenic polymorphism which makes immunity strain-specific [25, 26]. Consequently, this necessitates cumulative exposure to many variants of a particular species which usually requires the first twenty years of life to develop fully [25, 27]. Infections are more severe in the young, hence the majority of malaria-related deaths are in children [6, 28]. Repeated exposure elicits non-sterile immunity whereby individuals effectively form a commensalism with the parasite; subsequent infection is therefore often asymptomatic and is known as stable malaria [29, 30]. Although the adult immune system can control infections, asymptomatic individuals are still reservoirs of infection; furthermore, immunity wanes rapidly unless an individual is continually re-infected, making immunity imperfect [29-31]. Individuals with waning immunity or irregular infection therefore have unstable malaria [6]. These reasons further highlight the need for an effective vaccine which would induce sterile immunity without requiring years of exposure and debilitating illness.

The Need for a Vaccine

Control of malaria comes in three forms, pharmacological, vector control and vaccines, and the strategy of the GMEP was based on the former two [15]. Despite its failure, the same constituent methods continue to be employed. These are still effective and prompted the RBM partnership in 1998 to declare a drive to halve morbidity and mortality by 2010, and again by 2015 [15, 32]. The former deadline has passed and the latter target, while still theoretically possible, is highly ambitious and therefore very unlikely to be achieved.

There are ample ways to prevent or lessen the risk of contracting malaria. However, malarious areas are concentrated mainly in developing countries where the economic resources to implement effective and sustained nationwide coverage are often lacking. Furthermore, poor education, living conditions and malnourishment, for example, exacerbate the situation. There are also problems with drug resistance within the parasite and insecticide resistance within the mosquito due to selection pressures imposed by their overuse and misuse [33]. Novel agents are developed but resistance eventually emerges, thus new ones will always be needed [16]. These also incur greater expenditure due to high unit prices to cover research and development (R&D) costs. Unfortunately, since economic hardship is commonplace in most nations that need new agents it adds further to the financial strain; even a relatively small added expense constitutes a large economic burden. Accordingly, current hope rests with the development of a vaccine.

Vaccinology

Developing a vaccine is based upon identifying a candidate, formulating and enhancing it and eventually putting it through clinical trials. However, a number of hurdles can hinder vaccine development, making the process very challenging. Firstly, an incomplete understanding of the human immune system makes selecting candidates difficult. They are often chosen on empirical evidence, making long term investment by pharmaceutical companies a risky proposition [34]. Secondly, health and safety restrictions mean that a lot of time and money is needed to trial each candidate, thereby restricting RandD to the small number of pharmaceutical companies who can afford it [34]. In fact, the cost of trialling a vaccine candidate can amount to around $1 billion, can take over a decade and use as many as 100,000 volunteers [35, 36]. Furthermore, many candidates fail to progress through the phases of development, meaning that arguably an enormous amount of money is wasted. Consequently, there are likely to be many potential candidates effectively sitting on the shelf waiting for when the time and money can be invested.

An ideal malaria vaccine would have a high efficacy in all ages of recipient, be safe to administer, safe inside the host and not have any serious side-effects [35]. It should also reproduce, or even better, improve upon naturally acquired immunity and be long-term without necessary boosters or interference from other vaccines. Finally, it should be inexpensive to manufacture and purchase. Unfortunately, malaria vaccines are unlikely to fulfil some of these ideological properties. Instead, it is more probable that they will be moderately effective, confer short-term immunity and be difficult and expensive to make [35].

Vaccine Targets

In 2004, the world's foremost health organisations including the WHO, MVI, BAMGF and the Wellcome Trust embarked on a new strategy to accelerate the development of a malaria vaccine [34]. Through their collaboration, in 2006 the Malaria Vaccine Technology Roadmap was created. This outlined a highly ambitious new goal to attain a vaccine by 2025 that has a protective efficacy of over 80% against clinical disease caused by *P. falciparum* and lasts for over four years [34]. An important milestone was outlined that by 2015 the vaccine should be 50% effective against severe disease and death and should last for over a year.

Pharmaceutical companies are fully committed to finding a potentially viable product and, despite the hurdles to development, in September 2009 there were 70 candidate vaccines in 23 trials for *P. falciparum* [19]. Therefore, there is formidable competition and hopefully enough collective drive to make meeting this goal a reality and potentially revolutionising the fight against malaria. The three areas vaccines target are the three stages of the lifecycle; pre-erythrocytic, asexual blood and sexual stages (Figure 2).

Candidate vaccines aimed at the pre-erythrocytic stage intend to prevent invasion of erythrocytes by targeting either the sporozoites or the intrahepatic parasite [37]. They are designed to induce sterile immunity against antigens found on inoculated sporozoites or expressed by schizont-infected hepatocytes; examples of such antigens and vaccine candidates are explained later. Their effectiveness is based on preventing hepatocyte invasion and so the development of merozoites, which would otherwise invade erythrocytes [22]. With a relatively large period within which to operate (seven days for *P. falciparum*) and a small number of infectious organisms with which to deal, it makes this a good stage to target [38]. This is a clinically silent stage and so an effective vaccine would prevent clinical symptoms developing plus halt transmission.

History of Pre-Erythrocytic Vaccine Development

The drive for PEV development started with the successes achieved in a rodent model system in the 1960s. These demonstrated that immunisation of mice with the bites of radiation-attenuated infected mosquitoes could protect against challenge with infectious sporozoites [39]. Subsequently, a series of human studies in the 1970s showed induction of complete immune protection in approximately 90% of malaria-naïve volunteers inoculated with *P. falciparum* radiation-attenuated sporozoites (RAS) [40-42]. The underlying mechanism is through induction of antibodies against the conserved circumsporozoite protein (CSP) that coats the surface of *P. falciparum* sporozoites [43]. Together with the induction of $CD4^+$ and $CD8^+$ T cells that recognise antigens displayed by schizont-infected hepatocytes, a very effective immune response was provoked [43]. Furthermore, CSP is involved in binding to hepatocytes plus sporozoite development within the mosquito, thus making it essential to the parasite and therefore a prime vaccine target [44]. Attenuated sporozoites induce a much better immunity than do killed sporozoites because they can infect hepatocytes; killed sporozoites merely induce the humoral response whereas infected hepatocytes induce the cellular response too [45]. The observation of a high level of protection in humans showed promise as a proof of principle that sterile immunity can be induced. However, subsequent development of this approach encountered a number of problems and hence the reason the search for a PEV is still ongoing. These setbacks are based on several logistical and strategic impracticalities. Firstly, obtaining irradiated sporozoites is possible but the process produces a large quantity of mosquito impurities which, if injected, can induce serious medical problems [45]. Consequently, each subject instead had to be bitten by hundreds of irradiated mosquitoes over several months [39]. Secondly, sporozoites could not be cultured nor mass-produced, meaning the methodology required to initiate a large-scale vaccination programme was lacking [43].

Although RAS seemed like a dead end, research continued with the next step being genetically attenuated sporozoites (GAS). Here, the expression of several virulence genes such as *UIS3* are "knocked out", which induces immunity but ultimately arrests intrahepatic sporozoite development, thus preventing progression of the parasite to the blood stage [46]. These experiments showed promising results but did not solve the problem of how to manufacture and administer sporozoites in large quantities. However, in 2003 the biotechnology company Sanaria Inc. finally developed a way to mass produce sporozoites [47]. The product is safe and this process has been shown to generate sufficient quantities to meet demands needed to make a paediatric vaccine for Africa [48]. The candidate vaccine for this is known as PfSPZ and early trials are in progress with the support of MVI [49]. This new technology can also be applied to GAS [43].

Combined with the known feasibility to vaccinate against malaria and an ever-expanding hunger for scientific breakthroughs, this partial success prompted the emergence of an entirely new endeavour into vaccine development - subunit candidates. This movement created a great deal of interest in a range of antigens, such as CSP, thrombospondin-related adhesive protein (TRAP) and liver stage antigen 1 (LSA-1), which saw a number of subunit candidates emerge containing these antigens in their constructs [38, 50]. To date, the most promising subunit candidate is RTS,S.

RTS,S

With research shifted towards synthetic vaccine design, RTS,S was duly created in 1987 by Glaxo Smith Kline (GSK) and began its early development in collaboration with the Walter Reed Army Institute of Research (WRAIR) [18]. RTS,S has been shown to elicit sterile immunity in malaria-naïve and semi-immune individuals; it is based on the pre-erythrocytic antigen CSP which has been studied extensively and linked strongly to effective human immune responses [50].

What is RTS,S?

RTS,S is a hybrid molecule consisting of two recombinant segments (RTS and S) co-expressed in a *Saccharomyces cerevisiae* yeast cell [51]. RTS comprises three distinct portions, the first of which is a single polypeptide chain corresponding to a large region of the highly conserved tandem repeat (R) tetra-peptide sequence from CSP; each repeat tetra-peptide is called NANP [52, 53]. There are 19 copies of NANP and it is named for its amino acid sequence (Figure 3).

The second portion is the T cell epitope-containing (T) flanking region on the C-terminus; this region is made up of highly conserved amino acid sequences separated by immunodominant effector $CD4^{+}$ and $CD8^{+}$ epitopes known as Th2R and Th3R [50, 52]. The 'R' and 'T' components correspond to amino acids 207–395 on CSP of the 3D7 standard laboratory strain of *P. falciparum* [50, 52, 53]. Figure 4 is a simplified representation of the 'RT' portion. This RT peptide chain is then fused to the N-terminal of the Hepatitis B surface (S) antigen (HbsAg), hence RTS [51]. The second segment (S) is also a polypeptide chain and is 226 amino acids in length; it is an unfused S antigen that corresponds to HBsAg [50]. These recombinant proteins self-assemble into virus-like composite particulates, allowing for increased uptake and expression by antigen-presenting cells [51, 52].

L-Asparagine (Asn)(N)— L-Alanine (Ala)(A) — L-Asparagine (Asn)(N) — L-Proline (Pro)(P)

Figure 3. Structure of the NANP tetra-peptide sequence from *P. falciparum* circumsporozoite protein.

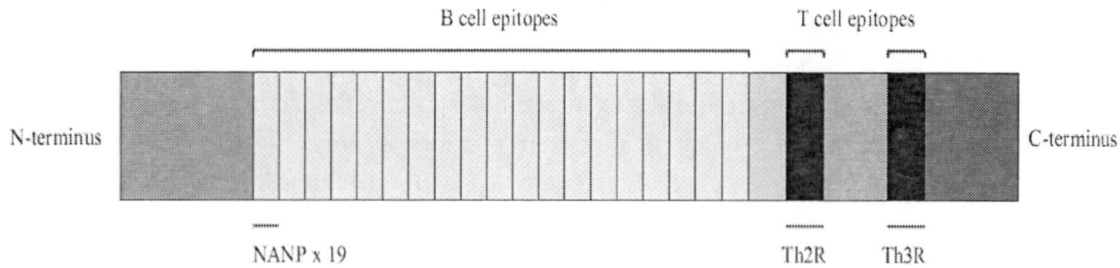

Figure 4. Schematic diagram of the 'RT' section of the RTS,S construct.

HbsAg is used for its high cell-mediated and humoral immunogenicity; this property is effectively a secondary boost to the immune response which then has a primary effect on a sporozoite challenge [54]. Furthermore, using HbsAg stimulates immunity to Hepatitis B as well, making this a potentially bivalent vaccine [12, 18].

How Does RTS,S Work?

The exact processes involved in naturally acquired pre-erythrocytic stage immunity remain poorly defined [45]. Nevertheless, it is known that the first line of defence is antibody-producing B cells that target newly inoculated sporozoites [55]. This humoral immune response is a consequence of B cell activation after recognition of the repeat tetra-peptide. The antibodies involved are predominately polyclonally produced non-specific IgM and IgG but a small number, approximately 5%, are species- or stage-specific and can interact with more of the parasite antigens [56]. The time frame for the immune system to act on the sporozoites before they infect hepatocytes is short, and they are rarely cleared in this time. Once the hepatocytes become infected the cellular immune response takes over, which involves $CD4^+$ and $CD8^+$ T cells.

$CD8^+$ T cells are implicated in the response to intrahepatocyte infection through a number of mechanisms [55, 57]. One of these uses cytolytic activity and works via the recognition of infected cells displaying parasite fragments in association with major histocompatability complex class I [58]. Recognition induces the secretion of cytotoxins and pore-forming perforins, which ultimately cause cell death, thus killing the parasite. This ability gives rise to its alternate name of cytoxic T cells; however, $CD8^+$ T cells can also produce cytokines, especially interferon gamma (IFN-γ) [58].

IFN-γ has both immunostimulatory and immunomodulatory properties and its production has been shown to play a more significant role than cytolytic activity toward infected hepatocytes [55, 57]. One of its mechanisms of action is based on the induction of the nitric oxide pathway, which is thought to be largely responsible for destroying infected hepatocytes [57, 59]. Although $CD8^+$ T cells are important, the quantities found in sporozoite-infected individuals are not high enough to account for the IFN-γ levels found [60]. Other IFN-γ-producing cells are therefore principally responsible for its production; $CD4^+$ T cells, natural killer (NK) cells, natural killer T (NKT) cells and $\gamma\delta$ T cells (a rare form of T cell) [45, 55]. In fact, $CD4^+$ cells produce the highest levels of IFN-γ and murine studies have shown $CD4^+$ cells (mainly Th1) to be essential to controlling parasitaemia [61]. Furthermore, depletion of $CD8^+$ T cells still preserves IFN-γ levels but depletion of $CD4^+$ T cells does not [62]. These observations were made during a study involving RTS,S and help to explain the reasoning behind the design of the construct.

RTS,S works in two ways to induce an immune response against a malaria infection (Figure 5). Firstly, it induces antibody-producing B cells by mimicking the repeat tetra-peptide of CSP [38, 48]. This process and the subsequent B cell proliferation and differentiation blocks sporozoite entry into hepatocytes. This induction acts effectively as an immune booster because, as discussed, the immune system alone would rarely clear all the sporozoites. The second approach is via the induction of high levels of IFN-γ by stimulating IFN-γ-producing Th1 CD4$^+$ T cells that recognise the specific T cell epitopes on the RTS construct [55, 57]. It also induces CD8$^+$ T cells but to a lesser extent [59]. As IFN-γ is involved in inhibiting parasitic development within hepatocytes its production further improves the vaccine's effectiveness. RTS,S only targets conserved antigens to avoid exerting a selection pressure which could lead to parasite resistance.

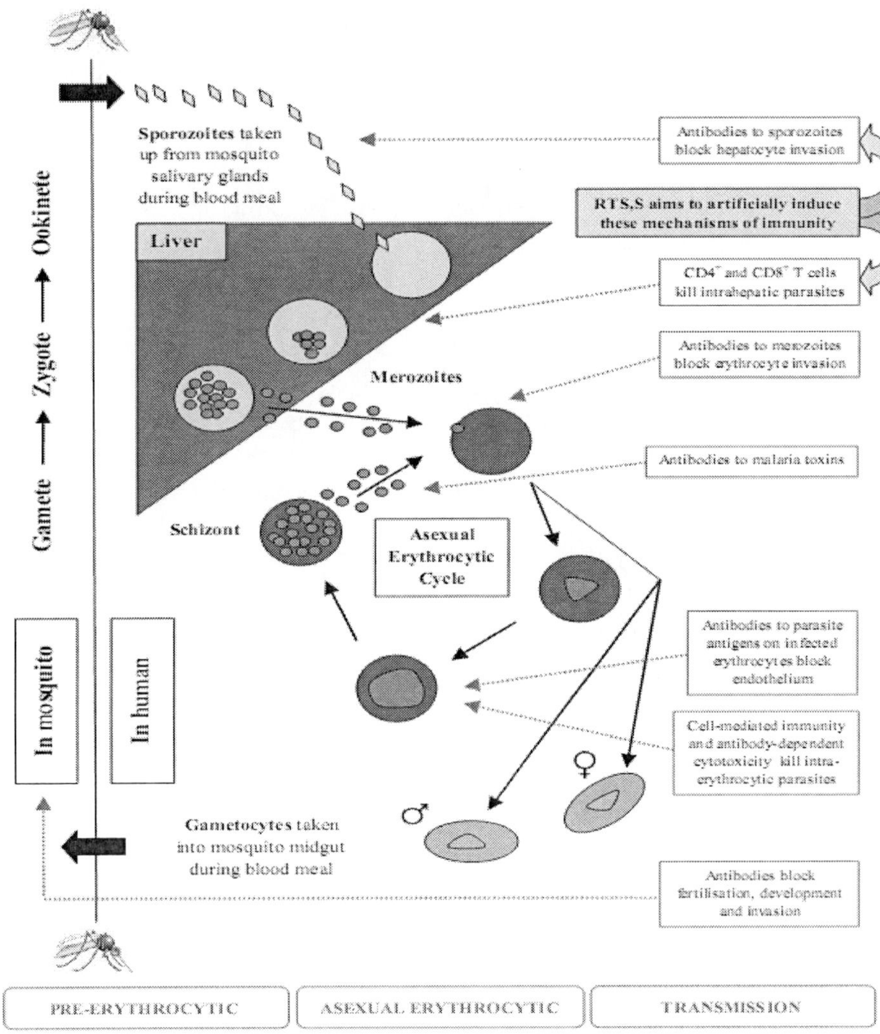

Figure 5. Schematic diagram showing the mechanisms of immunity against different life cycle stages of *P. falciparum*, highlighting those against the pre-erythrocytic parasite that RTS,S aims to induce.

Sporozoites are not particularly immunogenic and, due to its close relation to CSP, the same can be said for RTS,S. Consequently, an adjuvant system is required to boost immunogenicity, some of the best results for which have been obtained using AS01 and AS02. These are proprietary formulations of GSK's AS class of adjuvant system. AS01 uses liposomes mixed with immunostimulants 3-O-deacylated monophosphoryl lipid A (MPL) and portion 21 (QS-21) of *Quillaja saponaria,* a plant native to South America [48, 63]. AS02 uses water-in-oil in place of liposomes but retains the same immunostimulants. These adjuvants boost antibody and T cell responses, thus escalating cell-mediated immunity [64]. A specific benefit is their capacity to stimulate Th1 rather than Th2 $CD4^+$ T cells [48]. This is advantageous because the Th1 subset is the only one to produce IFN-γ.

The immune system has the ability to remove sporozoites from the blood and to prevent development within hepatocytes; however, it is not totally effective. It is not fully understood why only partial immunity to malaria is induced but it has been theorised that the shedding of CSP-antibody complexes may act to avoid detection [65]. If RTS,S is successful, it may find a way around this problem.

Timeline of RTS,S Development

To date, the majority of vaccine candidates have been aimed at CSP and TRAP. Most studies on these have given poor results which therefore makes it surprising that RTS,S, a CSP subunit candidate, has shown such promise. Furthermore, parasites rarely induce a strong immune response, meaning that parasitaemia is usually controlled rather than cleared; this makes the ability of RTS,S to induce sterile immunity (usually after only three doses) all the more impressive. This section offers an overview of the long developmental path that RTS,S has taken and its current stage of development. Figure 6 outlines the step-by-step process in vaccine development.

Combined with information gained from studies on attenuated sporozoites and new subunit technologies, a novel generation of malaria vaccines was created [66]. 1984 saw GSK and WRAIR begin preclinical trials on subunits that used portions of the central repeat region of CSP [51]. After a number of preliminary studies, four candidates were proposed, three of which contained portions of CSP fused to a tetanus toxin (R16tet32, R32tet32, R48tet32) and one fused to a tetracycline resistance gene (R32LR) [51, 67]. R32tet32 was selected and prepared with the adjuvant alum to become FSV-1. This protected one volunteer in its phase I/IIa trial, becoming the first ever subunit malaria vaccine to do so [51]. Unfortunately, despite this individual demonstration of proof of concept and the fact that it was safe and well tolerated by all subjects, overall it showed poor immunogenicity and was abandoned. Nevertheless, work continued and after several further failures a candidate called R16-HBsAg emerged that was instead combined with HBsAg [68, 69]. R16-HBsAg was also adjuvanted with alum and found to be safe and immunogenic, showing circulating antibodies in all twenty volunteers, in most cases for over 10 months [70]. Despite this, trials for this candidate were abandoned after phase I due to the realisation that by including the non-repeating flanking regions of the CSP a vaccine may be even more immunogenic [51, 69]. To this end, a new subunit construct which still contained HBsAg was formulated in 1987, marking the emergence of RTS,S [51].

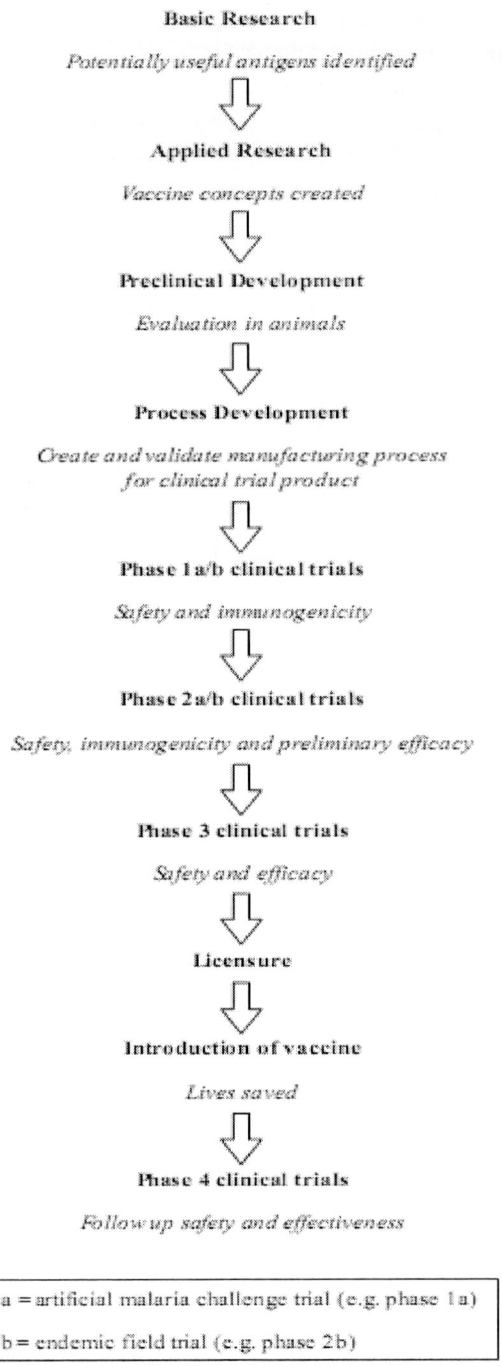

Figure 6. Flow chart of the phases of vaccine development.

Phase I/II clinical trials for vaccination of malaria-naïve volunteers with RTS,S began in 1992 at WRAIR [66, 69]. There were two formulations of the candidate – RTS,S adjuvanted with alum and RTS,S adjuvanted with MPL and alum. Results from this trial showed both to be safe and well tolerated; however, no volunteers receiving alum-adjuvanted RTS,S became immune. In contrast, two out of eight volunteers receiving the MPL and alum-adjuvanted RTS,S did become immune and were considered fully protected [69].

These initial results were encouraging but left room for improvement. Consequently, some new adjuvant systems were tried and the first human study in which they were used considered three. These were RTS,S/SBAS4 (RTS,S plus MPL and alum), RTS,S/SBAS3 (RTS,S in oil-in-water emulsion) and RTS,S/SBAS2 (RTS,S plus MPL and QS21 in oil-in-water emulsion) [71]. The phase Ib study occurred in 1996 and again involved malaria-naïve adults; one vaccine, RTS,S/SBAS2, administered in three doses over six months, conferred outstanding results showing protection in six out of seven volunteers [51, 71]. Unfortunately, subsequent testing on the volunteers showed short- lasting immunity with persistence in only one out of five of those who agreed a follow-up six months later [52]. Despite this, work continued and RTS,S/SBAS2 was soon shown to be a potent inducer of both cellular and humoral immune responses in all ten new volunteers and prompted the start of phase I/IIa trials [62]. These looked at optimisation of dosing regimens using 0, 1 and 9 month intervals followed by a sporozoite challenge 2-4 weeks after the final dose [72]. In 41 volunteers overall efficacy was 41% and two or three doses were necessary to induce protective immunity [72].

Unfortunately, it was found that RTS,S degraded in liquid formulation with its adjuvant SBAS2, thus seriously reducing its shelf-life and making long-term storage a concern. As a result, a reformulation created a lyophilised (freeze-dried) two vial system in which RTS,S and SBAS2 are reconstituted prior to administration [73]. This reformulation was renamed RTS,S/AS02A which has now been used for the bulk of research performed on RTS,S in the 21st century. The redesigned drug underwent phase I/IIa testing just as in the previous study and elicited an efficacy of 42% with no negative effects on efficacy with reformulation [73]. Phase IIa trials, conducted to improve dosing regimens, tested volunteers either with a 0, 1 and 3 month schedule or a 0, 7 and 28 day schedule; results showed efficacies of 45% and 39%, respectively [74]. The most recent finding for RTS,S/AS02A with respect to naïve adults is a study published in 2009 of a phase IIa trial testing safety, efficacy and immunogenicity of RTS,S/AS02A compared to RTS,S with a new adjuvant system AS01B which uses liposomes in place of oil-in-water [75]. Both were reported to be safe, well tolerated and immunogenic, with RTS,S/AS01B showing a significantly greater efficacy of 50% over RTS,S/AS02A, which showed 32% [75]. The need for comparative field trials was indicated. Much of the work done on RTS,S/SBAS2 (RTS,S/AS02A) has been to benefit malaria-naïve individuals entering malarious areas, such as army personnel and tourists. However, these promising results also triggered interest in the capacity of RTS,S to induce protection in residents of malarious areas. Consequently, trials began in semi-immune adults, young children and infants who reside in regions of low and high endemicity.

Trials in Semi-Immune Adults

An initial phase I safety and immunogenicity trial with RTS,S/SBAS2 was performed in The Gambia which showed it to be safe, well tolerated and immunogenic [76]. This was followed by an efficacy trial where 131 men were given three doses and followed up after 15 weeks [77]. Overall efficacy was 34%; however, it should be noted that efficacy for the first 9 weeks was determined to be 71%, but eventually decreased to 0% by the end of week 15 as immunity waned [77]. Despite this, two studies shortly after confirmed that the newly reformulated RTS,S/AS02A had the ability to induce cellular immunity in semi-immune adults and was not strain-specific [78, 79]. A further phase I study tested safety and immunogenicity in adults living in a hyperendemic region of western Kenya in order to ascertain if endemicity and ethnicity has an effect on efficacy, which was found not to be the case [80]. Soon after, the findings of a five year long safety and immunogenicity study of RTS,S/AS02A provided the first long-term indication of safety combined with persisting immunity [81]. However, the most recent data for semi-immune adults are from a phase IIb study that evaluated safety and reactogenicity of RTS,S/AS02A compared to the less studied RTS,S/AS01B [82]. Three doses over six months with a six month follow-up saw good tolerance for both formulations plus an efficacy of 29.5% for RTS,S/AS01B and 31.7% for RTS,S/AS02A [82]. Regardless of this, it was felt that RTS,S/AS01B had a more favourable immunogenicity profile.

Trials in Children

Such encouraging results meant that GSK and PATH's MVI formed a collaboration in 2001 with the aim of creating a paediatric vaccine [83]. Initial phase I studies in Mozambique showed RTS,S/AS02A to be safe, well tolerated and immunogenic in children aged 1-4 years using a 0, 1 and 2 month vaccination schedule [84]. The same overall consensus was achieved for a study involving children aged 1-11 years in The Gambia using varied dosages over a 0, 1 and 3 month vaccination schedule [85].

The first phase IIb proof of concept efficacy study used 2022 children aged 1-4 years living in Mozambique over a six month study period [86]. It was shown that RTS,S/AS02A conferred a 29.9% efficacy for protection against the first or only clinical episode. However, the efficacy against severe malaria was a much more impressive 57.7% [86]. A follow-up study extended monitoring to 21 months and when considering the studies together, only a slight waning in protection against severe malaria (48.6%) was witnessed, whereas protection against a first or only clinical episode improved (35.3%) [87]. Alongside this trial, a phase IIb safety trial using the same volunteers and lasting the full 21 months showed it to be safe and well tolerated [88].

An efficacy study of RTS,S/AS01E saw 402 Ghanaian children aged 5-17 months receive all three doses, for which an efficacy of 53% was recorded [89]. Around the same time, a phase I/IIb study looked at the possibility of developing a paediatric version of RTS,S/AS02A called RTS,S/AS02D and thus compared their safety and immunogenicity [90]. 200 children aged 3-5 years were randomly divided into two equally sized groups each receiving one of the two vaccines using a 0, 1 and 2 month schedule. This study showed that RTS,S/AS02D was as safe and immunogenic as RTS,S/AS02A and justified further evaluation in the juvenile population [90].

A recent study in Ghanaian children compared RTS,S/AS01E and RTS,S/AS02D using either a 0 and 1 month, a 0, 1 and 2 month or a 0, 1 and 7 month vaccine schedule [91]. Results from 521 children showed both to be safe and well tolerated but greater immunity with RTS,S/AS01E than RTS,S/AS02D and with three rather than two doses [91]. Another study in 180 Gabonese children aged 18 months to 4 years corroborates these findings [92].

Trials in Infants

The results obtained with the paediatric formulation RTS,S/AS02D in children prompted some of the first studies in infants with the first proof of concept study published in 2007 [93]. This trial involved 214 infants in Mozambique and produced strong results, showing 65.9% efficacy even after six months [93]. Furthermore, in 2008 a phase IIb study on RTS,S/AS02D that used a 8,12 and 16 week vaccination schedule conferred a 65.2% efficacy in the six month follow-up after the third dose was administered [94]. This trial also demonstrated that RTS,S/AS02D does not interfere with other childhood vaccinations. The latest study to be published is a phase I/IIb trial on cell-mediated responses to RTS,S/AS02D in infants [95]. This involved infants below one year of age living in Mozambique and showed responses in approximately half of the immunised infants but with very low stimulation of cytokine-producing $CD4^+$ and $CD8^+$ T cells. Despite this, responses were significantly higher than for the control. This is the first time a malaria-specific cellular immune response has been witnessed in infants below one year of age prior to immunisation [95].

Results from all the trials denote the need for further development and in May 2009, GSK commenced the first ever large-scale phase III malaria subunit vaccine trial [96]. It will eventually recruit up to 16,000 children and infant volunteers from seven African nations, which will therefore also make it the largest ever malaria vaccine trial [96, 97]. The protocol for the trial has been designed to test safety and efficacy and involves two age groups, 5-17 months and 6-12 weeks, thereby testing both children and infants [98]. The formulation RTS,S/AS01E is thought to have the greatest potential for improvement and so was selected as the candidate of choice [99]. It has been administered in three doses at 0, 1 and 2 months with a fourth 'booster' dose at 20 months to determine if it enhances the overall protective effect [98]. In collaboration with the WHO, all infants in the 6-12 week group will receive a multivalent vaccine against five childhood illnesses in conjunction with RTS,S/AS01E [97, 98]. This will determine whether RTS,S can be administered as part of a future childhood vaccine package [98]. The volunteers will be followed up for at least 30 months and if the trial is successful it could serve as a prelude to the development of the first ever licensed malaria vaccine. Publication of initial results, on efficacy in children 5-17 months of age, is expected sometime in 2012.

Problems with RTS,S

Despite the successes with RTS,S, in the opinion of some malaria researchers it has not lived up to expectations [100]. For over two decades the development of RTS,S has been littered with failures in addition to witnessing the indulgence of a vast amounts of money, time, intellect and effort. As a result, a kind of 'pseudo-hype' has been created which is likely to have originated out of desperation for a malaria vaccine and is exacerbated by the news media and relentless support from non-governmental organisations (NGOs). The work performed by NGOs is of the utmost calibre in bringing the malaria control problem to public awareness and therefore demands the highest respect. However, unfortunately their involvement has the secondary effect of placing an excessive and arguably premature expectation on RTS,S to succeed where other vaccines have failed.

Analysing objectively the end result of each study progress could be described as moderate rather than impressive. When looking at the first studies with RTS,S/SBAS2 in malaria-naive adults six out of seven people demonstrated protection which appears remarkable except for the fact that only one volunteer retained this immunity [71]. Shortly after, in 2001, an efficacy of 41% was recorded, which is an improvement. However, since then very little progress has been made with the most recent trial on malaria-naïve adults using AS01B producing only 50% protection [72]. Results are even poorer for semi-immune adults, with the greatest efficacy reaching only 34%, made worse by protection waning to 0% after only 15 weeks [77]. Paediatric trials have been more encouraging with some of the most recent data showing efficacies of 65.9% after six months [93]. However, doubt has been cast over this figure as it was subject to adjustment; some have argued that inflating figures is not best practice but also scientific propaganda [101]. Regardless, the problem with all the results obtained is the same – RTS,S has yet to produce an efficacy high enough to induce herd immunity which is ultimately necessary to eradicate malaria [16].

In addition to moderate results, there exists another major problem for RTS,S and indeed for any pre-erythrocytic vaccine. If a vaccine were not completely effective, such that only one sporozoite were allowed to develop, the resulting blood stage merozoites would be unabated as the vaccine does not act on this stage [38]. Therefore, to be successful RTS,S must be 100% effective at preventing hepatocyte invasion and/or development [50].

Those who prefer to see the cup as half full would still herald what has been attained so far in RTS,S clinical trials as an outstanding achievement when considering how much suffering could be avoided. Furthermore, like-minded economists would probably comment on a reduction in lost working hours and its positive effect on the economy. However, those not this way inclined would argue that the money could have been better invested in existing methods that already have the potential to eradicate malaria [6]. Furthermore, this area of research appears to have had more success in mice and other experimental models than in humans [100]. This was certainly realised but instead of redesigning the construct or finding better candidates at the preclinical stage of vaccine development, interest instead shifted to improving adjuvant systems for use in clinical trials. It is not an easy topic to approach but tests on humans provide more useful and realistic data than do any model system [100]. However, the ethical minefield surrounding enrolment of volunteers seriously limits and slows progress. This will have undoubtedly affected development of RTS,S and probably that of many other vaccines, too.

Although the RTS,S programme has shown consistently a good safety profile and the vaccine is well tolerated, there have been rare complications. Owusu-Agyei *et al.* (2009) administered 5315 doses of RTS,S/AS02 to 1864 children and 3149 doses of RTS,S/AS01 to 1145 children [91]. All children were under six years and in this entire cohort there were two cases of simple febrile seizures and two cases of intussusception, in which part of the intestine prolapses. While this medical condition occurs infrequently it should be noted that a vaccine against Rotavirus, called Rotashield, was withdrawn because it too caused intussusception in rare cases, despite an extremely high efficacy [102]. Results from phase III trials of RTS,S will provide more information but it should remain a consideration that withdrawal for safety reasons is a possibility.

One of the biggest problems that RTS,S has faced is the serious lack of knowledge about the human immune response to malaria. It has meant that to some extent research has had to be empirically driven; this is likely to have either hindered development or even masked potential areas of research which could have led to rational and improved vaccine design [34]. It is not surprising that despite some trials having shown good immunogenicity, some have shown poor to no induction of important arms of the immune system, such as T cells.

Genetic analysis of the *pfcs* gene (which codes for CSP in *P. falciparum*) in different isolates has shown over 20 polymorphisms in each of the regions encoding the T cell epitopes Th2R and Th3R [103]. These polymorphisms create antigenic variation that can potentially lead to immune evasion by varied isolates of *P. falciparum* [104]. The large number of differences geographically is therefore likely to impact on the efficacy of RTS,S if applied globally. Aside from this, there are other factors that impact on the ability of RTS,S to induce an immune response, including age, pregnancy, nutritional status and co-infection [105]. These all dampen the immune system and thus could skew data from clinical trials.

With an involvement in malaria vaccine design that stretches back over 25 years, GSK will have incurred vast RandD costs. As a result, if RTS,S is sufficiently successful to be marketed the unit price is likely to be high. Since most endemic countries are economically deprived, it is unlikely that their governments will be able to afford to vaccinate the population of their nation. NGOs are likely to provide financial assistance but they would never be able to afford to vaccinate the billions who are at risk. It is to be hoped that if and when the time comes, RTS,S is offered for large-scale vaccination in sub-Saharan Africa at a price at, or not much above, production costs. GSK will be acutely aware that a prohibitive pricing policy will attract widespread negative publicity. It can be argued that wealthier nations, from where most pharmaceutical companies originate, should subsidise the enormous costs of vaccine production. This could be either at the level of government or the level of the individual being charged a relatively high fee for prophylactic vaccination prior to travel to a malarious region.

The Future

Research suggests that with the current efficacy, RTS,S will more than halve the death rate and incidence around the world, meaning that approximately 500,000 deaths and around 250 million clinical cases could be prevented each year. These figures indicate that RTS,S has enormous potential to save lives and significantly reduce the socioeconomic burden of malaria.

If RTS,S is marketed within the next few years, however, it is unlikely that its efficacy will be high enough to act alone and will probably need to be combined with current control measures and implemented as part of a wider anti-malaria initiative. This makes control even more expensive plus cannot guarantee that it will help eradicate malaria. Reaching the point when RTS,S can be used independently seems to be a much more distant, if at all a realistic, prospect. Although research is likely to continue to try to achieve this goal, it appears interest has arisen in a number of novel vaccine candidates, which could be used to augment the protection given by RTS,S in other ways.

One such area is that of multi-stage vaccines that target, as the name suggests, more than one stage of the *P. falciparum* lifecycle in order to elicit an additional or synergistic response [34]. A combination of a PEV and a BSV is thought to be the most feasible route to conferring protection; recent BSV trials have shown promising results and with RTS,S having already proven to be partially effective it could be incorporated to make a new candidate [106]. Multiple epitopes are targeted in multi-stage vaccines, making the induction of both humoral and cellular immunity more likely. Furthermore, with a greater number of antigens being presented, it would provoke a greater immune response and could hopefully overcome the problems of low immunogenicity that is often found with *Plasmodium*.

On the other hand, single stage, multi-antigen vaccines have also been postulated. This would be through either vaccinating in combination or expanding the construct of RTS,S to include other conserved pre-erythrocytic antigens such as LSA-1 and TRAP which have been shown to be immunogenic [43, 51]. Unfortunately, there has been much disappointment in this area. Furthermore, combining candidates that independently have incurred huge RandD expenditures makes the new one potentially very pricey [34, 51]. Research continues and this area should still remain a possibility.

There has also been research into altering the RTS,S platform and using attenuated viral vectors such as adenovirus or poxvirus as they enter cells easily and induce a pronounced cell-mediated immunity [107]. In addition, GSK has also looked into "prime-boost" technology which "primes" a DNA vaccine, then "boosts" with a viral vector [108]. The DNA vaccine is a fragment of *P. falciparum* DNA coding for an antigen such as CSP and this primes naïve T cells to differentiate into memory T cells. The viral vector expresses a CSP antigen which, when administered, boosts the immune response by activating the memory T cells previously formed [108]. Initially, poor findings were attained when testing recombinant modified vaccinia virus with RTS,S/AS02A [51]. However, better results have been seen with adenovirus 35 expressing CSP boosted by RTS,S/AS01B [66].

The breakthroughs concerning attenuated sporozoites made possible by Sanaria Inc. could ultimately lead to the demise of RTS,S as a novel vaccine strategy. As previously mentioned, efficacies of 90% were produced and it was these results that confirmed the possibility of achieving a truly efficacious PEV. If the trials end successfully for Sanaria Inc. it is likely that their vaccine will be superior and will probably replace RTS,S as the front runner for licensing, relegating it to the history books as merely a stepping stone in the development toward a fully functional malaria vaccine.

While these are all possibilities for the future of RTS,S, they are not certain and its prospects should not be dismissed before the results of the current phase III trial are released. Any number of scientific advances, especially from an immunological perspective, could bring new ideas and radical changes to the strategy behind RTS,S. For example, a recently published study suggests a novel way to measure vaccine efficacy for RTS,S without the need for sporozoite challenge [109]. Although only a modest breakthrough, this still highlights the potential and the present need for RTS,S. Furthermore, if its future is resigned to being only a stepping stone, its implementation, if for only a few years, will still be worthwhile when considering the benefits it would convey in that time.

Conclusion

Malaria and its associated negative socioeconomic impacts have been laid bare and the need for a vaccine made clear. Whether RTS,S is reformulated, incorporated into a cocktail with other candidates or new adjuvant systems are developed, research will undoubtedly continue when considering how lucrative a vaccine it could be. Furthermore, with RTS,S specifically aimed at *P. falciparum*, most cases of which are isolated to only ten countries, it could save hundreds of thousands of lives a year and have a monumental effect on the mortality rate even if implemented in just these nations. Proof that a vaccine is feasible is based on two facts. Firstly, knowledge that repetitive exposure leads to naturally acquired non-sterile immunity, and secondly that sterile immunity can be induced using subunits, and indeed attenuated sporozoites. With this in mind and considering the mass of supportive data, a malaria vaccine seems likely within the next decade.

However, although RTS,S could be the world's first licensed malaria vaccine, it has not performed as required. Trials have yet to show that RTS,S can induce herd immunity which is ultimately necessary to meet the NGOs' goal of malaria eradication. Moreover, it may have been shown to induce sterile immunity but, as with naturally acquired immunity, it is imperfect and immunity eventually waned in many recipients. The results of the phase III trial will go a long way to determine its future. If unsuccessful, it is probable that other candidate vaccines will replace RTS,S as the centre of attention. Conversely, this would further compound the view of some protagonists in the malaria research community that vaccine development has been a waste of resources and focus on eradication by existing control measures should be the imperative.

To answer the question of whether RTS,S is the holy grail of malaria vaccines still needs more time, but to hazard a guess based on what is known at present, the answer would be a qualified no. RTS,S has undoubted provided the foremost advance in the field but it has yet to prove itself as *the* vaccine to finally unshackle humanity from the tyrannical hold of malaria.

Acknowledgements

The authors' research is supported by the Wellcome Trust and the University of Leeds.

References

[1] Wahlgren, M. and Perlmann, P. (1999). *Malaria: Molecular and Clinical Aspects.* Amsterdam: Harwood Academic.

[2] Bruce-Chwatt, L.J. (2002). *Bruce-Chwatt's Essential Malariology*, 4th edition. London: Hodder Arnold.

[3] Moya, A. and Font, E. (2004). *Evolution: From Molecules to Ecosystems*. Oxford: Oxford University Press.

[4] Singh, B., Kim Sung, L., Matusop, A., Radhakrishnan, A., Shamsul, S.S., Cox-Singh, J., Thomas, A. and Conway, D.J. (2004). A large focus of naturally acquired Plasmodium knowlesi infections in human beings. *Lancet* 363 (9414), 1017-1024.

[5] World Health Organization (2008). World Malaria Report 2008. Geneva: WHO.

[6] Breman, J.G. (2009). Eradicating malaria. *Science Progress* 92 (1), 1-38.

[7] U.S. Census Bureau. (2011). International Programs - World POPClock Projection [online]. [Last accessed 20 June 2011]. Available from: URL:http://www.census.gov/ ipc/www/ popclockworld.html.

[8] Hay, S.I., Guerra, C., Tatem, A., Noor, A. and Snow, R. (2004). The global distribution and population at risk of malaria: past, present, and future. *Lancet Infectious Diseases* 4 (6), 327-336.

[9] Guerra, C.A., Gikandi, P.W., Tatem, A.J., Noor, A.M., Smith, D.L., Hay, S.I. and Snow, R.W. (2008). The limits and intensity of Plasmodium falciparum transmission: implications for malaria control and elimination worldwide. *PLoS Medicine* 5 (2), e38.

[10] World Health Organization (2010). *Malaria* [online]. [Last accessed 20 June 2011]. Available from: URL:http://www.who.int/mediacentre/factsheets/fs094/en/.

[11] Malaria Vaccine Initiative (2010). *The PATH Malaria Vaccine Initiative* [online]. [Last accessed 20 June 2011]. Available from: URL:http://www.malariavaccines.org/ publications-factsheets.php.

[12] Malaria Vaccine Initiative (2007). *Accelerating Progress Toward Malaria Vaccines* [online]. [Last accessed 20 June 2011]. Available from: URL:http://www.malariavaccines.org/ files/ 080212_MVI_ portfolio_bro_mvilogo_ 000.pdf.

[13] Sherman, I.W. (1998). *Malaria – Parasite Biology, Pathogenesis and Protection.* Washington DC: ASM Press.

[14] Gallup, J.L. and Sachs, J.D. (2001). The economic burden of malaria. *American Journal of Tropical Medicine and Hygiene* 64 (1-2), 85-96.

[15] Greenwood, B.M. (2008). Control to elimination: implications for malaria research. *Trends in Parasitology* 24 (10), 449-454.

[16] Targett, G.A.T. and Greenwood, B.M. (2008). Malaria vaccines and their potential role in the elimination of malaria. *Malaria Journal 7* (suppl. 1), S10.

[17] Malaria Vaccine Initiative (2008). *Fighting malaria today and tomorrow* [online]. [Last accessed 20 June 2011]. Available from: URL:http://www.malariavaccines.org/ publications-factsheets.php.

[18] Malaria Vaccine Initiative (2006). *Fact Sheet: RTS,S Malaria Vaccine Clinical Trials.* [Last accessed 20 June 2011]. Available from: URL:http://www.malariavaccine.org/ files/FS_RTSS _FINAL.pdf.

[19] World Health Organization (2009). *World Malaria Report* 2009. Geneva: WHO.

[20] Markell, E.K., Voge, M. and John, D.T. (1992). *Medical Parasitology*, 7th edition. London: W.B. Saunders.

[21] Centers for Diseases Control (2011). DPDx – *Malaria* [online]. [Last accessed 20 June 2011]. Available from: URL:http://www.dpd.cdc.gov/DPDx/HTML/malaria.htm.

[22] Knell, A.J. (1991). *Malaria: a publication of the tropical programme of the Wellcome Trust.* Oxford: Oxford University Press.

[23] Mueller, I., Galinski, M.R., Baird, K., Carlton, J.M., Kochar, D.K., Alonso, P.L. and del Portillo, H.A. (2009). Key gaps in the knowledge of Plasmodium vivax, a neglected human malaria parasite. *Lancet Infectious Diseases* 9 (9), 555-566.

[24] Mühlberger, N., Jelinek, T., Gascon, J., Probst, M., Zoller, T., Schunk, M., Beran, J., Gjørup, I., Behrens, R.H., Clerinx, J., Björkman, A., McWhinney, P., Matteelli, A., Lopez-Velez, R., Bisoffi, Z., Hellgren, U., Puente, S., Schmid, M.L., Myrvang, B., Holthoff-Stich, M.L., Laferl, H., Hatz, C., Kollaritsch, H., Kapaun, A., Knobloch, J., Iversen, J., Kotlowski A., Malvy, D.J.M., Kern, P., Fry, G., Siikamaki, H., Schulze, M.H., Soula, G., Paul, M., Gómez i Prat, J., Lehmann, V., Bouchaud, O., da Cunha, S., Atouguia, J. and Boecken, G (2004). Epidemiology and clinical features of vivax malaria imported to Europe: sentinel surveillance data from TropNetEurop. *Malaria Journal* 3 (5), 1-7.

[25] Kurtis, J.D., Mtalib, R., Onyango, F.K. and Duffy, P.E. (2001). Human resistance to Plasmodium falciparum increases during puberty and is predicted by dehydroepiandrosterone sulfate levels. *Infection and Immunity* 69 (1), 123-128.

[26] Baird, J.K., Jones, T.R., Danudirgo, E.W., Annis, B.A., Bangs, M.J., Basri, H., Purnomo and Masbar, S. (1991). Age-dependent acquired protection against Plasmodium falciparum in people having two year exposure to hyperendemic malaria. *American Journal of Tropical Medicine and Hygiene* 45 (1), 65-76.

[27] Baird, J.K. (1998). Age-dependent characteristics of protection v. susceptibility to Plasmodium falciparum. *Annals of Tropical Medicine and Parasitology* 92 (4), 367-390.

[28] Smith, T.A., Leuenberger, R. and Lengeler, C. (2001). Child mortality and malaria transmission intensity in Africa. *Trends in Parasitology* 17 (3), 145-149.

[29] Abdel-Wahab, A., Abdel-Muhsin, A.M., Ali, E., Suleiman, S., Ahmed, S., Walliker, D. and Babiker, H.A. (2002). Dynamics of gametocytes among Plasmodium falciparum clones in natural infections in an area of highly seasonal transmission. *Journal of Infectious Diseases* 185 (12), 1838-1842.

[30] Schofield, L. and Mueller, I. (2006). Clinical immunity to malaria. *Current Molecular Medicine* 6 (2), 205-221.

[31] Taylor-Robinson, A.W. (2002). A model of development of acquired immunity to malaria in humans living under endemic conditions. *Medical Hypotheses* 58 (2), 148-156.

[32] Narasimhan, V. and Attaran, A. (2003). Roll Back Malaria? The scarcity of international aid for malaria control. *Malaria Journal* 2 (8), 1-8.

[33] Stevenson, M.M. and Zavala, F. (2006). Immunology of malaria infections. *Parasite Immunology* 28 (1-2), 1-4.

[34] Roadmap Working Group (2006). *Malaria Vaccine Technology Roadmap* [online]. [Last accessed 20 June 2011]. Available from: URL:http://www. malariavaccineroadmap.net/.

[35] Malaria Vaccine Initiative (2004). *Clinical Trials: Crucial Steps on the Road to a Malaria Vaccine* [online]. [Last accessed 20 June 2011]. Available from: URL:http://www malariavaccine.org/files/MVI_clinical_trials_paper.pdf.

[36] Roll Back Malaria Partnership (2008). *Global Malaria Action Plan Part II: The Global Strategy* [online]. [Last accessed 20 June 2011]. Available from: URL:http://www. rollbackmalaria.org/gmap/2-1.html.

[37] Hill, A.V.S. (2006). Pre-erythrocytic malaria vaccines: towards greater efficacy. *Nature Reviews Immunology* 6 (1), 21-32.

[38] Mikolajczak, S.A., Aly, A.S.I. and Kappe, S.H.I. (2007). Pre-erythrocytic malaria vaccine development. *Current Opinion in Infectious Diseases* 20 (5), 461-466.

[39] Hoffman, S.L., Goh, L.M., Luke, T.C., Schneider, I., Le, T.P., Doolan, D.L., Sacci, J., de la Vega, P., Dowler, M., Paul, C., Gordon, D.M., Stoute, J.A., Church, L.W., Sedegah, M., Heppner, D.G., Ballou W.R. and Richie, T.L. (2002). Protection of humans against malaria by immunization with radiation-attenuated Plasmodium falciparum sporozoites. *Journal of Infectious Diseases* 185 (8), 1155-1164.

[40] Clyde, D.F. (1990). Immunity to falciparum and vivax malaria induced by irradiated sporozoites - a review of the University of Maryland studies, 1971-75. *Bulletin of the World Health Organization* 68 (suppl.), S9-12.

[41] Egan, J.E., Hoffman, S.L., Haynes, J.D., Sadoff, J.C., Schneider, I., Grau, G.E., Hollingdale, M.R., Ballou W.R. and Gordon, D.M.. (1993). Humoral immune-responses in volunteers immunized with irradiated Plasmodium falciparum sporozoites. *American Journal of Tropical Medicine and Hygiene* 49 (2), 166-173.

[42] Rieckmann, K.H., Beaudoin, R.L., Cassells, J.S. and Sell, K.W. (1979). Use of attenuated sporozoites in the immunization of human volunteers against falciparum malaria. *Bulletin of the World Health Organization* 57 (suppl. 1), S261-265.

[43] Vanderberg, J.P. (2009). Reflections on early malaria vaccine studies, the first successful human malaria vaccination, and beyond. *Vaccine* 27 (1), 2-9.

[44] Ménard, R., Sultan, A.A., Cortes, C., Altszuler, R., van Dijk, M.R., Janse, C.J., Waters, A.P., Nussenzweig, R.S. and Nussenzweig, V. (1997). Circumsporozoite protein is required for development of malaria sporozoites in mosquitoes. *Nature* 385 (6614), 336-340.

[45] Doolan, D.L. and Martinez-Alier, N. (2006). Immune response to pre-erythrocytic stages of malaria parasites. *Current Molecular Medicine* 6 (2), 169-185.

[46] Mueller, A.K., Labaied, M., Kappe, S.H. and Matuschewski, K. (2005). Genetically modified Plasmodium parasites as a protective experimental malaria vaccine. *Nature* 433 (7022), 164-167.

[47] Sanaria Inc. (2010). *Sanaria - Malaria Eradication Through Vaccination* [online]. [Last accessed 20 June 2011]. Available from: URL: http://www.sanaria.com.

[48] Richie, T. (2006). High road, low road? Choices and challenges on the pathway to a malaria vaccine. *Parasitology* 133 (suppl.), S113-144.

[49] Malaria Vaccine Initiative (2009). *Sanaria PfSPZ malaria vaccine candidate* [online]. [Last accessed 20 June 2011]. Available from: URL:http://www.malariavaccines.org/ publications-factsheets.php.

[50] Ballou, W.R., Arevalo-Herrera, M., Carucci, D., Richie, T.L., Corradin, G., Diggs, C., Druilhe, P., Giersing, B.K., Saul, A., Heppner, D.G., Kester, K.E., Lanar, D.E., Lyon, J., Hill, A.V.S., Pan, W. and Cohen, J.D. (2004). Update on the clinical development of candidate malaria vaccines. *American Journal of Tropical Medicine and Hygiene* 71 (suppl. 2), S239-247.

[51] Ballou, W.R. and Cahill, C.P. (2007). Two decades of commitment to malaria vaccine development: GlaxoSmithKline biologicals. *American Journal of Tropical Medicine and Hygiene* 77 (6), 289-295.

[52] Stoute, J.A., Kester, K.E., Krzych, U., Wellde, B.T., Hall, T., White, K., Glenn, G., Ockenhouse, C.F., Garcon, N., Schwenk, R., Lanar, D.E., Sun, P., Momin, P., Wirtz, R.A., Golenda, C., Slaoui, M., Wortmann, G., Holland, C., Dowler, M., Cohen, J. and Ballou, W.R. (1998). Long-term efficacy and immune responses following immunization with the RTS,S malaria vaccine. *Journal of Infectious Diseases* 178 (4), 1139-1144.

[53] Waitumbi, J.N., Anyona, S.B., Hunja, C.W., Kifude, C.M., Polhemus, M.E., Walsh, D.S., Ockenhouse, C.F., Heppner, D.G., Leach, A., Lievens, M., Ballou, W.R., Cohen, J.D. and Sutherland, C.J. (2009). Impact of RTS,S/AS02(A) and RTS,S/AS01(B) on genotypes of P. falciparum in adults participating in a malaria vaccine clinical trial. *PLoS One* 4 (11), e7849.

[54] Ambroise-Thomas, P. (1997). Vaccination against malaria. Disappointments and hopes. *Bulletin of the French National Academy of Medicine* 181 (8), 1637-1648.

[55] Plebanski, M. and Hill, A.V.S. (2000). The immunology of malaria infection. *Current Opinion in Immunology* 12 (4), 437-441.

[56] Perlmann, P. and Troye-Blomberg, M. (2002). *Malaria Immunology*. 2nd edition. Basel: Karger.

[57] Reece, W.H., Pinder, M., Gothard , P.K., Milligan, P., Bojang, K., Doherty, T., Plebanski, M., Akinwunmi, P., Everaere, S., Watkins, K.R., Voss, G., Tornieporth, N., Alloueche, A., Greenwood, B.M., Kester, K.E., McAdam, K.P., Cohen, J. and Hill, A.V.S. (2004). A CD4+ T-cell immune response to a conserved epitope in the circumsporozoite protein correlates with protection from natural Plasmodium falciparum infection and disease. *Nature Medicine* 10 (4), 406-410.

[58] Cruse, J.M. and Lewis, R.E. (2004). *Atlas of Immunology*. 2nd edition. London: CRC Press.

[59] Sun, P., Schwenk, R., White, K., Stoute, J.A., Cohen, J., Ballou, W.R., Voss, G., Kester, K.E., Heppner, D.G. and Krzych, U. (2003). Protective immunity induced with malaria vaccine, RTS,S, is linked to Plasmodium falciparum circumsporozoite protein-specific CD4+ and CD8+ T cells producing IFN-gamma. *Journal of Immunology* 171 (12), 6961-6967.

[60] Nardin, E.H. and Nussenzweig, R.S. (1993). T-cell responses to pre-erythrocytic stages of malaria – role in protection and vaccine development against pre-erythrocytic stages. *Annual Review of Immunology* 11 (1), 687-727.

[61] Stevenson, M.M. and Riley, E.M. (2004). Innate immunity to malaria. *Nature Reviews Immunology* 4 (3), 169-180.

[62] Lalvani, A., Moris, P., Voss, G., Pathan, A.A., Kester, K.E., Brookes, R., Lee, E., Koutsoukos, M., Plebanski, M., Delchambre, M., Flanagan, K.L., Carton, C., Slaoui, M., van Hoecke, C., Ballou, W.R., Hill, A.V.S. and Cohen, J. (1999). Potent induction of focused Th1-type cellular and humoral immune responses by RTS,S/SBAS2, a recombinant Plasmodium falciparum malaria vaccine. *Journal of Infectious Diseases* 180 (5), 1656-1664.

[63] World Health Organization (2011). *WHO - Parasitic Diseases* [online]. [Last accessed 20 June 2011]. Available from:URL:http://www.who.int/vaccine_research/diseases/soa_parasitic /en/index4.html#pre-erythrocytic%20vaccines.

[64] Antigenics Inc. (2010). *QS-21 immune adjuvant* [online]. [Last accessed 20 June 2011]. Available from: URL:http://www.antigenics.com/products/tech/qs21/.

[65] Stewart, M.J. and Vanderberg, J.P. (1988). Malaria sporozoites leave behind trails of circumsporozoite protein during gliding motility. *Journal of Protozoology* 35 (3), 389-393.

[66] Heppner, D.G. Jr., Kester, K.E., Ockenhouse, C.F., Tornieporth, N., Ofori, O., Lyon, J.A., Stewart, V.A., Dubois, P., Lanar, D.E., Krzych, U., Moris, P., Angov, E., Cummings, J.F., Leach, A., Hall, B.T., Dutta, S., Schwenk, R., Hillier, C., Barbosa, A., Ware, L.A., Nair, L., Darko, C.A., Withers, M.R., Ogutu, B., Polhemus, M.E., Fukuda, M., Pichyangkul, S., Gettyacamin, M., Diggs, C., Soisson, L., Milman, J., Dubois, M.C., Garçon, N., Tucker, K., Wittes, J., Plowe, C.V., Thera, M.A., Duombo, O.K., Pau, M.G., Goudsmit, J., Ballou, W.R. and Cohen, J. (2005). Towards an RTS,S-based, multi-stage, multi-antigen falciparum malaria: progress at the Walter Reed Army Institute of Research. *Vaccine* 23 (17-18), 2243-2250.

[67] Anders, R.F. and Saul, A. (2000) Malaria vaccines. *Parasitology Today* 16 (10), 444-447.

[68] Rutgers, T., Gordon, D., Gathoye, A.M., Hollingdale, M., Hockmeyer, W., Rosenberg, M. and De Wilde, M. (1988). Hepatitis B surface antigen as carrier matrix for the repetitive epitope of the circumsporozoite protein of Plasmodium falciparum. *Biotechnology* 6 (9), 1065-1070.

[69] Gordon, D.M., McGovern, T.W., Krzych, U., Cohen, J.C., Schneider, I., LaChance, R., Heppner, D.G., Yuan, G., Hollingdale, M., Slaoui, M., Hauser, P., Voet, P., Sadoff, J.C. and Ballou, W.R. (1995). Safety, immunogenicity, and efficacy of a recombinantly produced Plasmodium falciparum circumsporozoite-protein hepatitis B surface-antigen subunit vaccine. *Journal of Infectious Diseases* 171 (6), 1576-1585.

[70] Vreden, S.G., Verhave, J.P., Oettinger, T., Sauerwein, R.W. and Meuwissen, J.H. (1991). Phase I clinical trial of a recombinant malaria vaccine consisting of the circumsporozoite repeat region of Plasmodium falciparum coupled to hepatitis B surface antigen. *American Journal of Tropical Medicine and Hygiene* 45 (5), 533-538.

[71] Stoute, J.A., Slaoui, M., Heppner, D.G., Momin, P., Kester, K.E., Desmons, P., Wellde, B.T., Garçon, N., Krzych, U. and Marchand, M. (1997). A preliminary evaluation of a recombinant circumsporozoite protein vaccine against Plasmodium falciparum malaria. *New England Journal of Medicine* 336 (2), 86-91.

[72] Kester. K.E., McKinney, D.A., Tornieporth, N., Ockenhouse, C.F., Heppner, D.G., Hall, T., Krzych, U., Delchambre, M., Voss, G., Dowler, M.G., Palensky, J., Wittes, J., Cohen, J., Ballou, W.R. and the RTS,S Malaria Vaccine Evaluation Group (2001). Efficacy of recombinant circumsporozoite protein vaccine regimens against experimental Plasmodium falciparum malaria. *Journal of Infectious Diseases* 183 (4), 640-647.

[73] Kester, K.E., McKinney, D.A., Tornieporth, N., Ockenhouse, C.F, Heppner, D.G. Jr., Hall, T., Wellde, B.T., White, K., Sun, P., Schwenk, R., Krzych, U., Delchambre, M., Voss, G., Dubois, M.C., Gasser, R.A. Jr., Dowler, M.G., O'Brien, M., Wittes, J., Wirtz, R., Cohen, J., Ballou, W.R. and the RTS,S Malaria Vaccine Evaluation Group (2007). A phase I/IIa safety, immunogenicity, and efficacy bridging randomized study of a two-dose regimen of liquid and lyophilized formulations of the candidate malaria vaccine RTS,S/AS02A in malaria-naive adults. *Vaccine* 25 (29) 5359-5366.

[74] Kester, K.E., Cummings, J.F., Ockenhouse, C.F., Nielsen, R., Hall, B.T., Gordon, D.M., Schwenk, R.J., Krzych, U., Holland, C.A., Richmond, G., Dowler, M.G.,

Williams, J., Wirtz, R.A., Tornieporth, N., Vigneron, L., Delchambre, M., Demoitie, M.A., Ballou, W.R., Cohen, J., Heppner, D.G. Jr. and the RTS,S Malaria Vaccine Evaluation Group (2008). Phase 2a trial of 0, 1, and 3 month and 0, 7, and 28 day immunization schedules of malaria vaccine RTS,S/AS02 in malaria-naive adults at the Walter Reed Army Institute of Research. *Vaccine* 26 (18), 2191-2202.

[75] Kester, K.E., Cummings, J.F., Ofori-Anyinam, O., Ockenhouse, C.F., Krzych, U., Moris, P., Schwenk, R., Nielsen, R.A., Debebe, Z., Pinelis, E., Juompan, L., Williams, J., Dowler, M., Stewart, V.A., Wirtz, R.A., Dubois, M.C., Lievens, M., Cohen, J., Ballou, W.R., Heppner, D.G. Jr. and the RTS,S Vaccine Evaluation Group (2009). Randomized, double-blind, phase 2a trial of falciparum malaria vaccines RTS,S/AS01B and RTS,S/AS02A in malaria-naive adults: safety, efficacy, and immunologic associates of protection. *Journal of Infectious Diseases* 200 (3), 337-346.

[76] Doherty, J.F., Pinder, M., Tornieporth, N., Carton, C., Vigneron, L., Milligan, P., Ballou, W.R., Holland, C.A., Kester, K.E., Voss, G., Momin, P., Greenwood, B.M., McAdam, K.P. and Cohen, J. (1999). A phase I safety and immunogenicity trial with the candidate malaria vaccine RTS,S/SBAS2 in semi-immune adults in the Gambia. *American Journal of Tropical Medicine and Hygiene* 61 (6), 865-868.

[77] Bojang, K.A., Milligan, P.J., Pinder, M., Vigneron, L., Alloueche, A., Kester, K.E., Ballou, W.R., Conway, D.J., Reece, W.H., Gothard, P., Yamuah, L., Delchambre, M., Voss, G., Greenwood, B.M., Hill, A., McAdam, K.P., Tornieporth, N., Cohen, J.D., Doherty, T. and the RTS,S Malaria Vaccine Trial Team (2001). Efficacy of RTS,S/AS02 malaria vaccine against Plasmodium falciparum infection in semi-immune adult men in The Gambia: a randomised trial. *Lancet* 358 (9297), 1927-1934.

[78] Pinder, M., Reece, W.H., Plebanski, M., Akinwunmi, P., Flanagan, K.L., Lee, E.A., Doherty, T., Milligan, P., Jaye, A., Tornieporth, N., Ballou, W.R., McAdam, K.P., Cohen, J. and Hill, A.V.S. (2004). Cellular immunity induced by the recombinant Plasmodium falciparum malaria vaccine, RTS,S/AS02, in semi-immune adults in The Gambia. *Clinical and Experimental Immunology* 135 (2), 286-293.

[79] Alloueche, A., Milligan, P., Conway, D.J., Pinder, M., Bojang, K., Doherty, T., Tornieporth, N., Cohen, J. and Greenwood, B.M. (2003). Protective efficacy of the RTS,S/AS02 Plasmodium falciparum malaria vaccine is not strain specific. *American Journal of Tropical Medicine and Hygiene* 68 (1), 97-101.

[80] Stoute, J.A., Heppner, D.G. Jr., Mason, C.J., Siangla, J., Opollo, M.O., Kester, K.E., Vigneron, L., Voss, G., Walter, M.J., Tornieporth, N., Cohen, J.D. and Ballou, W.R. (2006). Phase 1 safety and immunogenicity trial of malaria vaccine RTS,S/AS02A in adults in a hyperendemic region of western Kenya. *American Journal of Tropical Medicine and Hygiene* 75 (1), 166-170.

[81] Bojang, K., Milligan, P., Pinder, M., Doherty, T., Leach, A., Ofori-Anyinam, O., Lievens, M., Kester, K.E., Schaecher, K., Ballou, W.R. and Cohen, J. (2009). Five-year safety and immunogenicity of GlaxoSmithKline's candidate malaria vaccine RTS,S/AS02 following administration to semi-immune adult men living in a malaria-endemic region of The Gambia. *Human Vaccines* 5 (4), 242-247.

[82] Polhemus, M.E., Remich, S.A., Ogutu, B.R., Waitumbi, J.N., Otieno, L., Apollo, S., Cummings, J.F., Kester, K.E., Ockenhouse, C.F., Stewart, A., Ofori-Anyinam, O., Ramboer, I., Cahill, C.P., Lievens, M., Dubois, M.C., Demoitie, M.A., Leach, A.,

Cohen, J., Ballou, W.R. and Heppner, D.G. Jr. (2009). Evaluation of RTS,S/AS02A and RTS,S/AS01B in adults in a high malaria transmission area. *PLoS One* 4 (7), e6465.

[83] Malaria Vaccine Initiative (2011). *The RTS,S malaria vaccine candidate* [online]. [Last accessed 20 June 2011]. Available from: URL:http://www.malariavaccines.org/files/April 82011MVI_RTSScandidate.pdf.

[84] Macete, E., Aponte, J.J., Guinovart, C., Sacarlal, J., Ofori-Anyinam, O., Mandomando, I., Espasa, M., Bevilacqua, C., Leach, A., Dubois, M.C., Heppner, D.G., Tello, L., Milman, J., Cohen, J., Dubovsky, F., Tornieporth, N., Thompson, R. and Alonso, P.L. (2007). Safety and immunogenicity of the RTS,S/AS02A candidate malaria vaccine in children aged 1-4 in Mozambique. *Tropical Medicine and International Health* 12 (1), 37-46.

[85] Bojang, K.A., Olodude, F., Pinder, M., Ofori-Anyinam, O., Vigneron, L., Fitzpatrick, S., Njie, F., Kassanga, A., Leach, A., Milman, J., Rabinovich, R., McAdam, K.P., Kester, K.E., Heppner, D.G., Cohen, J.D., Tornieporth, N. and Milligan, P.J. (2005). Safety and immunogenicity of RTS,S/AS02A candidate malaria vaccine in Gambian children. *Vaccine* 23 (32), 4148-4157.

[86] Alonso, P.L., Sacarlal, J., Aponte, J.J., Leach, A., Macete, E., Milman, J., Mandomando, I., Spiessens, B., Guinovart, C., Espasa, M., Bassat, Q., Aide, P., Ofori-Anyinam, O., Navia, M.M., Corachan, S., Ceuppens, M., Dubois, M.C., Demoitié, M.A., Dubovsky, F., Menéndez, C., Tornieporth, N., Ballou, W.R., Thompson, R. and Cohen, J. (2004). Efficacy of the RTS,S/AS02A vaccine against Plasmodium falciparum infection and disease in young African children: randomised controlled trial. *Lancet* 364 (9443), 1411-1420.

[87] Alonso, P.L., Sacarlal, J., Aponte, J.J., Leach, A., Macete, E., Aide, P., Sigauque, B., Milman, J., Mandomando, I., Bassat, Q., Guinovart, C., Espasa, M., Corachan, S., Lievens, M., Navia, M.M., Dubois, M.C., Menendez, C., Dubovsky, F., Cohen, J., Thompson, R. and Ballou, W.R. (2005). Duration of protection with RTS,S/AS02A malaria vaccine in prevention of Plasmodium falciparum disease in Mozambican children: single-blind extended follow-up of a randomised controlled trial. *Lancet* 366 (9502), 2012-2018.

[88] Sacarlal, J., Aponte, J.J., Aide, P., Mandomando, I., Bassat, Q., Guinovart, C., Leach, A., Milman, J., Macete, E., Espasa, M., Ofori-Anyinam, O., Thonnard, J., Corachan, S., Dubois, M.C., Lievens, M., Dubovsky, F., Ballou, W.R., Cohen, J. and Alonso, P.L. (2008). Safety of the RTS,S/AS02A malaria vaccine in Mozambican children during a phase IIb trial. *Vaccine* 26 (2), 174-184.

[89] Bejon, P., Lusingu, J., Olotu, A., Leach, A., Lievens, M., Vekemans, J., Mshamu, S., Lang, T., Gould, J., Dubois, M.C., Demoitié, M.A., Stallaert, J.F., Vansadia, P., Carter, T., Njuguna, P., Awuondo, K.O., Malabeja, A., Abdul, O., Gesase, S., Mturi, N., Drakeley, C.J., Savarese, B., Villafana, T., Ballou, W.R., Cohen, J., Riley, E.M., Lemnge, M.M., Marsh, K. and von Seidlein, L. (2008). Efficacy of RTS,S/AS01E vaccine against malaria in children 5 to 17 months of age. *New England Journal of Medicine* 359 (24), 2521-2532.

[90] Macete, E.V., Sacarlal, J., Aponte, J.J., Leach, A., Navia, M.M., Milman, J., Guinovart, C., Mandomando, I., López-Púa, Y., Lievens, M., Owusu-Ofori, A., Dubois, M.C., Cahill, C.P., Koutsoukos, M., Sillman, M., Thompson, R., Dubovsky, F., Ballou, W.R., Cohen, J. and Alonso, P.L. (2007). Evaluation of two formulations of adjuvanted RTS,

S malaria vaccine in children aged 3 to 5 years living in a malaria-endemic region of Mozambique: a phase I/IIb randomized double-blind bridging trial. *Trials* 8 (11), 1-10.

[91] Owusu-Agyei, S., Ansong, D., Asante, K., Owusu, S.K., Owusu, R., Brobby, N.A.W., Dosool, D., Akoto, A.O., Osei-Kwakye, K., Adjei, E.A., Boahen, K.O., Sylverken, J., Adjei, G., Sambian, D., Apanga, S., Kayan, K., Vekemans, J., Ofori-Anyinam, O., Leach, A., Lievens, M., Demoitie, M., Dubois, M., Cohen, J., Ballou, W.R., Savarese, B., Chandramohan, D., Gyapong, J.O., Milligan, P., Antwi, S., Agbenyega, T., Greenwood, B. and Evans, J. (2009). Randomized controlled trial of RTS,S/AS02D and RTS,S/AS01E malaria candidate vaccines given according to different schedules in Ghanaian children. *PLoS One* 4 (10), e7320.

[92] Lell, B., Agnandji, S., von Glasenapp, I., Haertle, S., Oyakhiromen, S., Issifou, S., Vekemans, J., Leach, A., Lievens, M., Dubois, M., Demoitie, M., Carter, T., Villafana, T., Ballou, W.R., Cohen, J. and Kremsner, P.G. (2009). A randomized trial assessing the safety and immunogenicity of AS01 and AS02 adjuvanted RTS,S malaria vaccine candidates in children in Gabon. *PLoS One* 4 (10), e7611.

[93] Aponte, J.J., Aide, P., Renom, M., Mandomando, I., Bassat, Q., Sacarlal, J., Manaca, M.N., Lafuente, S., Barbosa, A., Leach, A., Lievens, M., Vekemans, J., Sigauque, B., Dubois, M.C., Demoitié, M.A., Sillman, M., Savarese, B., McNeil, J.G., Macete, E., Ballou, W.R., Cohen, J. and Alonso, P.L. (2007). Safety of the RTS,S/AS02D candidate malaria vaccine in infants living in a highly endemic area of Mozambique: a double blind randomised controlled phase I/IIb trial. *Lancet* 370 (9598), 1543-1551.

[94] Abdulla, S., Oberholzer, R., Juma, O., Kubhoja, S., Machera, F., Membi, C., Omari, S., Urassa, A., Mshinda, H., Jumanne, A., Salim, N., Shomari, M., Aebi, T., Schellenberg, D.M., Carter, T., Villafana, T., Demoitié, M.A., Dubois, M.C., Leach, A., Lievens, M., Vekemans, J., Cohen, J., Ballou, W.R. and Tanner, M. (2008). Safety and immunogenicity of RTS,S/AS02D malaria vaccine in infants. *New England Journal of Medicine* 359 (24), 2533-2544.

[95] Barbosa, A., Naniche, D., Aponte, J.J., Manaca, M.N., Mandomando, I., Aide, P., Sacarlal, J., Renom, M., Lafuente, S., Ballou, W.R. and Alonso, P.L. (2009). Plasmodium falciparum-specific cellular immune responses after immunization with the RTS,S/AS02D candidate malaria vaccine in infants living in an area of high endemicity in Mozambique. *Infection and Immunity* 77 (10), 4502-4509.

[96] Malaria Vaccine Initiative (2009). Phase 3 malaria vaccine trial begins—final testing of RTS,S [online]. [Last accessed 20 June 2011]. Available from: URL:http://www.malaria vaccines.org/RTSSPhase3_05-27-2009.php.

[97] Leach, A. (2008). RTS,S/AS01* phase 3 multi-centre efficacy trial. MALVAC 2008 Meeting: Measures of Malaria Vaccine Efficacy – Scientific, Regulatory and Public Health Perspectives. Geneva: WHO.

[98] Cohen, J. (2004). *Recent Advances in Malaria Vaccine Development*. Vaccines 3: Frontiers in Vaccine Development [online]. [Last accessed 20 June 2011]. Available from: URL:http:// www.pasteur.fr/applications/euroconf/vaccines3/vaccines3-abs.html.

[99] Vekemans, J., Leach, A., and Cohen, J. (2009). Development of the RTS,S/AS malaria candidate vaccine. *Vaccine* 27 (suppl. 6), G67-71.

[100] Druilhe, P. and Barnwell, J.W. (2007). Pre-erythrocytic stage malaria vaccines: time for a change in path. *Current Opinion in Microbiology* 10 (4), 371-378.

[101] Epstein, J.E. (2007). What will a partly protective malaria vaccine mean to mothers in Africa? *Lancet 370* (9598), 1523-1524.

[102] Franco, M.A. and Greenberg, H.B. (2001). Challenges for rotavirus vaccines. *Virology* 281 (2), 153-155.

[103] Kumkhaek, C., Phra-Ek, K., Rénia, L., Singhasivanon, P., Looareesuwan, S., Hirunpetcharat, C., White, N.J., Brockman, A., Grüner, A.C., Lebrun, N., Alloueche, A., Nosten, F., Khusmith, S. and Snounou, G. (2005). Are extensive T cell epitope polymorphisms in the Plasmodium falciparum circumsporozoite antigen, a leading sporozoite vaccine candidate, selected by immune pressure? *Journal of Immunology* 175 (6), 3935-3939.

[104] Aidoo, M. and Udhayakumar, V. (2000). Field studies of cytotoxic T lymphocytes in malaria infections: Implications for malaria vaccine development. *Parasitology Today* 16 (2), 50-56.

[105] Fortin, A., Stevenson, M.M. and Gros, P. (2002). Susceptibility to malaria as a complex trait: big pressure from a tiny creature. *Human Molecular Genetics* 11 (20), 2469-2478.

[106] Zhang, Q., Xue, X., Qu, L. and Pan, W. (2007). Construction and evaluation of a multistage combination vaccine against malaria. Vaccine 25 (11), 2112-2119.

[107] Li, S., Locke, E., Bruder, J., Clarke, D., Doolan, D.L., Havenga, M.J., Hill, A.V.S, Liljestrom, P., Monath, T.P., Naim, H.Y, Ockenhouse, C., Tang, D.C., Van Kampen, K.R., Viret, J.F., Zavala, F. and Dubovsky, F. (2007). Viral vectors for malaria vaccine development. *Vaccine* 25 (14), 2567-2574.

[108] Ramshaw, I.A. and Ramsay, A.J. (2000). The prime-boost strategy: exciting prospects for improved vaccination. *Immunology Today* 21 (4), 163-165.

[109] Vahey, M.T., Wang, Z., Kester, K.E., Cummings, J., Heppner, D.G. Jr., Nau, M.E., Ofori-Anyinam, O., Cohen, J., Coche, T., Ballou, W.R. and Ockenhouse, C.F. (2010) Expression of genes associated with immunoproteasome processing of major histocompatibility complex peptides is indicative of protection with adjuvanted RTS,S malaria vaccine. *Journal of Infectious Diseases* 201 (4), 580-589.

In: Malaria: Etiology, Pathogenesis and Treatments
Editors: A. M. Peterson and G. E. Calamandrei

ISBN: 978-1-62100-363-2

Chapter III

Global Malaria Eradication: Is It Still Achievable and Practicable?

Kaliyaperumal Karunamoorthi[1,2*]

[1] Unit of Medical Entomology and Vector Control, Department of Environmental Health Sciences and Technology, College of Public Health and Medical Sciences, Jimma University, Jimma, Ethiopia.

[2] Research and Development Centre, Bharathiar University, Coimbatore, Tamil Nadu, India.

''Malaria control should not be a campaign; it should be a policy, a long-term program. It cannot be accomplished or maintained by spasmodic effort. It requires the adoption of a practicable program, the reasonable continuity of which will be sustained for a long term of years''

-Boyd (1939)-

Abstract

Nearly six decades ago, the Global Malaria Eradication Programme (GMEP) (1955–1969) launched resulted with spectacular successes in terms of reduction/interruption of malaria transmission and substantially minimized the malaria burden too. Malaria eradication (malERA) and the sharp reduction of malaria incidence to zero has been achieved in a few countries by employing the world's cheapest "silver bullet", the so called DDT (Dichloro-Diphenyl-Trichloroethane) as well as by administering the low-cost antimalarial, chloroquine. However, due to several compounding factors such as emergence of insecticide resistance, drug resistance, inadequate fund, lack of political

*Corresponding author E-mail: k_karunamoorthi@yahoo.com. Mobile: +251 913 547 847 and +91 9600918524. Fax No: +251 047 11 11 450..Unit of Medical Entomology and Vector Control, Department of Environmental Health Sciences and Technology, College of Public Health and Medical Sciences, Jimma University, Jimma, Ethiopia

willingness, fragile healthcare system, inappropriate planning, lack of logistical support and poor infrastructures, the over-promised and under-delivered GMEP has been abandoned in 1969; subsequently in 1970s the strategy has been modified from eradication to control. Thereafter, even today malaria kills a poor African child for every 30 seconds and continues to be a major public health problem in the resource-constrained countries of Africa, Asia, Latin amerce, and beyond.

At the moment there is a worldwide renewed interest on malERA giving rise to the global agenda, which is purely due to countrywide global partnership and adequate support of international donors. There is a ray of hope as the malaria map shrinks and malaria incidence falls and some countries may consider attacking remaining foci with an elimination agenda by employing frontline vector control tools like insecticide-treated nets (ITNs), indoor residual spraying (IRS) and by supplementing with active case-management of potent antimalarial like artemisinin-based combination therapy (ACT).

However, in the present day scenario, malERA seems to be an over-ambitious and unrealistic target. In this perspective, this chapter describes briefly on the global public health and socio-economic impacts of malaria and also explains how to provide a comprehensive insight on the global malERA through campaigns and how efforts could to be taken to create a malaria free world. Furthermore, it also outlines some of the current potential obstacles and barriers, and how we can address the issues and challenges with the existing tools and how we can improve and exploit them effectively to attain the meaningful global malaria eradication. Indeed, shaping a better planet, suitable to every individual and in particular for children are a matter of grave concern as well as a mission and it is one of our foremost senses of duty too.

Keywords: Malaria Eradication; Vector Control; Antimalarials; Vaccines; Repellent; Genetically Modified Mosquitoes

Introduction

Despite of the several decades of control effort, arthropod-borne diseases have still been regarded as a major public health problem in the tropical and subtropical regions of the world.They are more common in the developing as well as resource-poor countries and inflict enormous burden in terms of morbidity and mortality.Regrettably, the majority of victims are from the pitiable underprivileged section of the society. Besides, the heightened health impact also contributes to the extensive poverty, under-development and school dropout etc. These diseases are also responsible for huge economic losses; both in terms of health-care costs and lost productivity, mostly in countries that can least afford them [1].

Among the insect vectors, mosquitoes play the major role on the transmission of many dreadful diseases like malaria, filariasis, dengue fever, yellow fever and Japanese encephalitis.Malaria is the most prevalent among the mosquito-borne diseases and the devastating nature of malaria in sub-Saharan Africa is indubitably unbearable [2]. Malaria is a major public health problem, observed to cause over hundreds of millions of death and morbidity every year and the recent WHO Malaria Report 2009 [3] estimated that nearly half of the world's populations are at the risk of malarial infection. It has been suggested that more of human beings have died of malaria than of any other disease [4], since its eradication is a major challenge to the international community [5].

Malaria has been known for 4000 years, but is recognized and feared only for the past 2500 years. In the 19th century, the scientific foundations of medicine were built and almost all important events in the history of malaria were observed to occur in the past 150 years. In 1880, Charles Louis Laveran discovered and described about the malaria parasites in human blood. Golgi at the University of Pavia, described *Plasmodium vivax*and *P. malariae;* Celli, Marchiafava, and Bignami in Rome studied the morphological differences between *P. falciparum* and the other species and the clinical course of *P. falciparum* infection. Sir Ronald Ross's discovery in 1897 of pigmented cysts on the stomach wall of an *Anopheles* mosquito in Secunderabad, India, revealed how the parasite infected man [6].

These researches meant that malariologists could at last explain the observed effects of traditional control measures, such as drainage of marshes and mosquito nets etc, and to develop better approaches to control malaria. Thanks to the increasing public and political support as the early days of the 20th century witnessed the deployment of an increasing number of interventions against malaria. However, large-scale implementation of most of the proposed measures had severe operational and financial limitations, and some strategies were found to be suitable only in particular social, ecological, and epidemiological conditions [7].

Malaria: A Disease of Morbidity and Mortality

Nearly half of the world's population is at the risk of malaria. There were approximately 250 million cases and 880,000 deaths per year or 3000 deaths per day and the majority in children <5 years old in sub-Saharan Africa [3].Around 90% of malaria cases are caused by *P. falciparum*, among which more than 80% occurs in children younger than 5 years of age in the sub-Saharan Africa [3]. Mixed infections caused by more than one *Plasmodium* species are frequent but are under recognized. 35 countries are responsible for the majority of the total deaths world-wide. The 5 main contributors (Nigeria, Democratic Republic of Congo, Uganda, Ethiopia and Tanzania) amount to 50% of global deaths and 47% of malaria cases [8]. Malaria is also a serious public health problem in certain regions of South East Asia and South America too [9].

Malaria remains to be a serious cause of maternal and childhood morbidity and mortality in sub-Saharan Africa [10]. Besides health impact of malaria is also one of the major obstacles to socioeconomic development as the main transmission periods coincide with the peak agricultural and harvesting season [11], and the annual Gross Domestic Product (GDP) is estimated to have reduced by as much as 1.3% in countries with high disease rates. In Africa it has been estimated that at least USD 12 billion per year is lost directly through illness, treatment and premature death [3].

In areas of high stable transmission, morbidity and mortality are high in young children whose acquired protective immunity is insufficient to protect against the severity of the disease. Areas of low or unstable transmission are subject to malaria epidemics, and people of all ages are at the risk of the disease. There is a substantial geographical overlap between malaria and HIV, and the co-infection is associated with increase in parasite density and case fatality [12]. Malaria is frequently referred to as a disease of the poverty. Evidently, poorest countries of the world, in particular those in sub-Saharan Africa are the major victims of this malicious disease [11].

The surfacing of vector resistance to insecticide, drug resistance and several other compounding factors like operational failure, inadequate fund, lack of political willingness, high operational cost, limited human resource, etc have lead to the world-wide emergence and resurgence of malaria. Due to the above said factors, subsequently in 1970s the strategy has been modified from eradication to malaria control. Thereafter, even today malaria kills a poor African child in every 30 seconds and continues to be amajor public health problem in the resource-constrained and developing countries of Africa, Asia, Latin amerce, and beyond.It needs to be addressed immediately and effectively by under-taking certain concrete steps in achieving a malaria-free world.

The past decade has seen an unprecedented surge in political commitment and international funding for malaria control. Coverage with existing control methods (i.e., vector control and artemisinin-based combination therapy) is increasing, and, in some Asian and African countries, childhood morbidity and mortality from malaria caused by *P. falciparum* have started to decline. Consequently, there is now renewed interest in the possibility of malaria elimination. But the ability of the parasite to develop resistance to antimalarial drugs and increasing insecticide resistance of the vector threaten to the progress towards elimination.*P. vivax*, with its dormant liver stage, is particularly difficult to eliminate, and access to effective and affordable treatment at community level is a key challenge. In addition, an effective and affordable vaccine against all species of malaria is still out of reach [13].

We are facing a pivotal period in the history of malaria control. Increasing intervention coverage combined with measurable evidence of effect from several countries and regions have strengthened political resolve to control the disease. There has been an unprecedented increase in international funding commitments, and has risen from \$ 0.3 billion in 2003 to \$1.7 billion in 2009 [3]. Rapid scale-up of insecticide-treated nets and ACTs has halved childhood morbidity and mortality due to malaria in some countries in Africa with stable, high transmission, reawakening interest in the prospect of malaria elimination and, in the long-term, eradication [13].

In this context, I aim to focus on the existing major challenges and issues and how the scientific community can explore the solutions to attain meaningful malaria eradication making the present chapter more significant and pertain. In the present day scenario, malaria eradication (malERA) seems to be an over-ambitious and unrealistic target. However, translating our hardly learnt lessons into reality could be an ideal approach to address the present catastrophe. The purpose of this chapter is to describe the briefly on the global public health and socio-economic impacts of malaria and explains how to provide comprehensive insight on the global malERA through campaigns and how the efforts are to be taken to create a malaria free world. Furthermore, it also outlines some of the current potential obstacles and how we can address with the existing barriers of global malaria eradication. Indeed, shaping a better planet, suitable to every individual and in particular for children are a matter of grave concern or mission and one of our foremost senses of duty as well.

Malaria Eradication (malERA)

Since the perceived failure of the Global Programme for Malaria Eradication in 1969, the idea of malaria eradication has been dropped [14]. However, after a lapse of almost 40 years, malaria eradication is back on the global health agenda, inspired by the Gates Malaria Forum in October 2007 [15,16] and this aspiration has subsequently been endorsed by WHO and Roll Back Malaria Partnership. This change in direction of malaria control has provoked a vigorous debate within the malaria research and control communities as to whether resurrection of the goal of eradication at this point in time is helpful or likely to be counterproductive [14]. Although the debate over the wisdom of this target still continues the growing impatience with the low ambitions of current efforts, fuelled by reductions in morbidity and mortality in some countries [17], and progress in the development of new drugs and the first-ever vaccine leads many decision makers to adopt eradication of malaria as the primary aim for their organizations [18].

History of Global Malaria Eradication Program (GMEP)

To understand malaria today, it is important to acknowledge the history of the disease and the previous global efforts taken in order to control and eradicate it. In the mid-19th century, malaria was endemic in most countries and territories of the world, affecting about 90% of the world's population and stretching as far north as the Arctic Circle [19]. Efforts to control and eliminate malaria on a large scale date back to the late 19th century, with the discovery of the plasmodium parasite and its transmission by anopheline mosquitoes. In 1955, WHO set out to rid the world of malaria. The campaign GMEP, focused on all the malarious countries except Madagascar and sub-Saharan Africa. The plan was to interrupt malaria transmission primarily by attacking the malaria's mosquito vector using the insecticide dicholoro-diphenyl-trichloroethane (DDT), as a vector control tool together with case management [20].

It was thought that if the parasite's cycle of transmission from human to mosquito and vice versa could be blocked for 3 years, then the parasite with the disease would also disappear. Scores of nations joined the programme and poor nations shifted substantial portions of their health budgets to malaria eradication whereas the donor nations poured billions of dollars into the effort. Eradication teams spread out around the world; wetlands were drained; forests and fields were dusted; and millions of homes were sprayed [21].

The activities of the GMEP led to the elimination of the disease from countries at the edges of global malaria distribution and where the intensity of transmission was quite low [20].There were remarkable successes. Malaria was eradicated from southern Europe as well as from parts of North Africa and the Middle East [22]. In India, for example, the number of malaria cases has reduced from an estimated 110 million in 1955 to less than 1 million in 1968, and mortality due to malaria was virtually eliminated. In Sri Lanka, the incidence of malaria was reduced to a mere 18 cases in 1966 from an estimated 2.8 million cases in 1946 [23]. But soon the effort began to falter and the insecticide resistant mosquitoes and drug-resistant parasites began to emerge and some of the countries were unsuccessful in interrupting transmission [22], which eventually slowed down the fund flow and by the end of the 1960s malaria eradication was completely abandoned giving rise to the less ambitious goal of eliminating the disease where possible and controlling where it could not be eliminated [21].

The Current Status of Global Malaria Control

The GMEP was over-promised and under-delivered [7]. Decades of pessimism followed and the malariologists were afraid to even mention the goal of this program by name [15]. Eradication of malaria remains beyond our grasp today nevertheless firmly back on the global health agenda as a long-term target [18]. Despite the exponential population growth in malaria-endemic areas during the past 60 years, an estimated 50% of the world's population live in malaria-free areas, compared with only 30% in 1950 [24,25]. Several African countries that have achieved high coverage with insecticide-treated nets (ITNs), indoor residual spraying (IRS), and effective treatment programmes have recently reported a pronounced decline in malaria burden, accompanied, in some instances, by a sharp fall in all-cause mortality in children younger than 5 years of age [26].

Progress in shrinking the malaria map (the geographical range of endemic malaria) is remarkable. Since 1945, 79 countries have eliminated malaria and the proportion of the world's population who live in malaria-endemic regions has decreased from 70% to 50% [27]. Worldwide, 109 countries are now malaria free, whereas 99 still have malaria transmission. Of these 99 countries, 32 have started to eliminate malaria, with a success prospect for the next decade provided if they are adequately supported [28].

Existing Major Issues and Challenges: Call for Concrete Actions

When we plan the elimination agenda for the next decade, the first point is to emphasize that efforts directed at shrinking the malaria map should in no way detract from control in highly endemic countries or in the development of new interventions and delivery methods. However, greater attention to shrinking the malaria map is crucial for global malERA [29]. By definition, eradication of human malaria parasites globally [18] requires the intervention options to be available that can eliminate transmission any part of the world. Leading vector control technologies such as ITNs and IRS can suppress transmission by one or even two orders of magnitude [30,31] and dramatically alleviate disease burden [32,33].

Nevertheless, these measures alone are not sufficient to eliminate transmission in large tracts of tropical Africa where the entomological inoculation rate (EIR) and the most direct measure of human exposure, can exceed a thousand of infectious bites per person per year [34,35]. If the local parasite population are entirely eliminated by mass drug administration, the transmission shall be nullified. A single infected person moving into other areas may give rise to as many as ten thousand new transmissions [35]. Under such conditions, simulations predict that even 100% coverage of an entire population with ITNs exhibiting near-ideal properties will fail to push the EIR below the threshold required for local elimination [36].

Although the 32 malaria-eliminating countries are as wealthy as the previous successful eliminators were, and have similar health-system capacity [37], they still face a formidable array of obstacles. These obstacles include the increasing movement of people across borders that prevails constant importation, the inadequate tools for fighting *P. vivax*[38], the threat of insecticide and drug resistance, and the global financial crisis creating pressure on domestic and international resources for malaria.

Future Strategies and Priorities: Essential and Inevitable

Malaria Epidemiology: Needs Better Understanding

No campaign for the control or elimination of malaria can proceed without a detailed appreciation of the epidemiology of the disease and of the host-parasite-vector interactions. As the increasing parts of the world move towards elimination, a deeper understanding of the basic science of host-parasite-vector population interactions in disease transmission and of the changes in these interactions resulting from intensified control and elimination efforts will be increasingly important [39]. A better understanding on the human response to malaria will be increasingly important as elimination proceeds. Despite many decades of studies on immune responses to malaria, there is still no consensus on immune correlate of protection [40,41].

Vector Control: A Long Serving Companion

Though, currently we are not equipped with the magic bullets to prevent malaria, the effective low-cost interventions are available for its treatment, prevention and control [11]. Over the past several decades, vector control remains to be one of the most powerful weapons in the battle against malaria. Even today, it is considered as a corner stone in the malaria control and elimination campaign under the specific set of environmental conditions. It is one of the most powerful weapons in the process of managing vector populations to reduce/interrupt transmission of disease. The existing vector control interventions have offered highly encouraging results and a unique opportunity to eliminate malaria from a few countries. Therefore, presently, there has been a world-wide renewed attention and commitment in combating with malaria [42].

The idea behind vector control is to reduce levels of mortality and morbidity by reducing/interrupting the transmission of the disease. The preventive measures like appropriate and regular deployment of nets, indoor residual spraying and application of repellents as prevention interventions can be complemented by the removal of stagnant water, the breeding site of mosquitoes [8,42-44]. The overarching goal of vector control is to reduce the vectorial capacity of the local vector populations that lie below the critical threshold level in order to prevent ongoing or epidemic transmission. After Ingestion, as it takes a relatively long time (days) for *Plasmodia* in *Anopheles* vectorsto become infective to humans, the most effective vector control strategies currently in use rely on the interventions like indoor residual insecticide spraying and ITNs that reduce vector daily survival rates [45].

Insecticide-Treated Nets (ITNs)

Insecticide-treated nets make more efficient use of insecticide than indoor spraying as nets act as baited traps to attract mosquitoes to a toxic surface of finite area [46]. Ordinary ITNs need to be retreated every year whereas it is not required with the long-lasting insecticide nets (LLINs), which are designed in such a way that the insecticide lasts as long as the net. ITNs work in two ways: first, they protect the individual user against biting, and second, they can kill mosquitoes that try to bite. Like IRS, use of ITNs can produce a community-wide reduction in transmission [47].

The effectiveness of ITN interventions in reducing the burden of malaria has been amply demonstrated in a variety of epidemiological settings. ITN use by children in several settings has been shown to be cost-effective too [48]. More of pregnant women use ITNs and the cost-effectiveness of ITN use by pregnant women is likely to be similar to that for children [9]. Randomized controlled trials in Kenya, Ghana, The Gambia, and Burkina Faso have demonstrated that wide-scale use of ITNs can reduce all-cause of child mortality by around one-fifth, saving an average of 6 lives for every 1,000 children aged between 1-59 months [49].

The pyrethroids are the only WHO approved class of insecticides for use in insecticide-treated bednets and long lasting insecticide-treated nets. Recent studies have shown a 20% drop in mortality in African settings when ITNs are used [50]. In Kenya, a study showed that one death was averted for every 140 ITNs distributed [17]. Wherever community-level ITN coverage is greater than about 60%, a community effect is seen in which non-users receive similar protection to that of ITN users [51].

Challenges and Issues

ITNs, especially long-lasting nets, are as effective as indoor residual spraying when full population coverage is achieved. The distribution of such nets is a logistical challenge, but experience has shown that they can be distributed rapidly in mass campaigns. Once if high coverage has been achieved, as in campaigns, coverage has to be maintained as a long-term intervention by routine redistribution. Communication for behavioral change is essential to ensure effective use of the nets. The average total cost of long-lasting insecticidal nets is US$ 1 per user per year. Conventional treatment of ordinary nets is difficult to achieve and is twice as expensive as using long-lasting insecticidal nets [20].

Indoor Residual Spraying (IRS)

IRS is an effective method of vector control which involves applying a long-lasting insecticide to the inside walls of houses and other structures where people sleep. It is aimed at killing mosquitoes that enter houses when they rest on sprayed surfaces (e.g. walls and ceilings). IRS is widely used in areas of seasonal transmission, including epidemic-prone areas, and increasingly in more malaria-endemic areas. The most common insecticides used are DDT and pyrethroids. IRS is appropriate in epidemiological settings where vectors mainly stay indoors and in countries where the necessary logistical capabilities can be deployed [52].

In areas with intense and perennial transmission, it is essential to maintain the population's long-term acceptance of spraying once or several times a year. In view of the difficulties encountered in maintaining indoor residual spraying, World Health Organization has invested substantially in exploring other methods, especially insecticide-treated bednets. These nets have been effective in many rigorous trials [53], especially to reduce childhood mortality in Africa. Few trials have compared insecticide-treated nets and indoor residual spraying, but the results observed reveal that the methods are more or less equal in efficacy [54]. Since only pyrethroids can be used for insecticide-treated nets, and pyrethroid resistance is emerging as a constraint on their effectiveness [55], the fact that four classes of insecticides can be used for indoor residual spraying is one of the main reasons for the justifying renewed interest in this method.

Major Challenges and Issues

Despite of its initial widespread use and contribution to the success of malaria eradication and control efforts, in recent years, the use of IRS has declined. This is due in part to the lack of commitment and financing by the government to sustain these efforts over a long term and the lack of concerns about insecticide resistance and finally due to the community acceptance in fear of its harmful effect on the environment and human health [56].

IRS requires stringent planning, management and supervision. It can be delivered only by well-staffed and well-equipped vector control services, which currently do not exist in many countries. In the long term, IRS tends to generate community fatigue, eventually resulting in increasing refusal. In areas with almost perennial malaria transmission, spraying would be difficult to conduct with existing insecticide formulations that have a short residual effect. The average total cost of indoor residual spraying is US $3.5 per person protected per year. Both ITNs and IRS methods to be effective, there must be high population coverage rates, exceeding at least 80% [20].

The most pressing challenge is the development of a coherent research agenda for discovering and developing a broader range of insecticides, with novel modes of action that can circumvent emerging resistance to existing insecticides, in particular, pyrethroid-based insecticides [57]. The second challenge is the development of interventions that affect vectors that do not rest or feed indoors and are therefore not susceptible to current tools.

Insecticide Resistance: A Debacle and Need for Innovative Approach

Insecticide resistance, by definition, is an inherited characteristic that allows an insect to survive a dose of a pesticide that would normally prove fatal. According to WHO (1957) [58] resistance has been defined as “the developed ability in a strain of insects to tolerate doses of toxicant which would prove lethal to the majority of individuals in a normal population of the same species". Insecticide resistance is the major threat to the effective prevention and control of malaria[59].

The number of available and effective pesticides for malaria vector control is also reported to be decreasing. Currently, only the pyrethroid class of insecticides is appropriate for ITNs impregnation and LLINs [59]. However, vectors have already developed resistance against pyrethroids in some areas of the world and it is a serious threat to sustained use of ITNs and IRS. Although 12 insecticides are currently recommended by the WHO for IRS, they belong only to four chemical classes namely organochlorines, pyrethroids, carbamates, and organophosphates, and the cross-resistance among insecticides is frequent [20].

Long-lasting insecticidal bednets and IRS have saved millions of lives; nevertheless we are victims of our success, as the expanding access to insecticides, combined with agricultural spraying practices, creates evolutionary pressure on mosquitoes to develop resistance. In east Africa and other areas, two species of mosquito have already been found to be resistant to the commonly used insecticides, including permethrin and DDT [60]. Worse is that there are no new classes of insecticides in late stage development. The GMEP of the 1950s and 1960s also failed in part due to insecticide resistance [29]. Therefore, we must learn from the past, and focus on research that accelerates development of new tools and the ones that support effective use of existing ones [29].

These multiple constraints mean that vector control cannot, in the long term, rely solely on the two interventions mainly IRS and ITNs. They will have to be supplemented progressively with other measures in the context of integrated vector management, which will be essential at an intermediate stage to enhance and sustain the achievements made with the existing interventions [20]. To ensure a long life of insecticides, it is essential to guard against the development of resistance.

Resistance Management

For public health use, it is essential that alternative insecticides belonging to new or different classes be developed if current scaling-up efforts are to be sustained and if local interruption of malaria transmission is to be achieved [20]. It is vital to manage pesticide programs using methods that reduce the probability of resistance, including temporal rotation of pesticide classes or developing a spatial mosaic to the juxtapose use of different pesticide classes for malaria vector control. For larval control, there is only one currently recommended organophosphate, temephos, which could be used in a rotation or as a spatial mosaic with other larvicidal agents [59]. Otherwise, the recent advances will be rapidly jeopardized, especially in the case of indoor residual spraying, which tends to lose its efficacy as soon as vectors become resistant [20].

Repellent

Generally, vector control is considered to be the most effective measure to prevent transmission of vector-borne disease. However, currently vector-borne diseases remain as a serious threat to humankind due to the emergence of the drug resistant parasites, insecticide resistant vectors and the non-availability of suitable and effective vaccines. In this context, repellents play a key role in reducing the man-vector contact and eventually reduce the vector-borne diseases [61]. Insect repellents have a unique role in regions where mosquito vectors bite in the early evening. It provides a valuable supplement to bed net use [62].Repellents are extremely useful and helpful whenever and wherever other personal protection measures are impossible or impractable [63].

N, N-Diethyl-m-methylbenzamide (DEET) has been considered to be one of the most effective synthetic repellents against mosquitoes. However, its toxic reactions have been reported in some circumstances, especially among children and the elderly. Additionally its toxic reactions have been reported in some circumstances, especially among children and the elderly [64,65]. In addition, DEET also acts as a plasticizer and has an objectionable odor to some individuals [66]. There have also been questions raised regarding its long term persistence in the body and its possible teratogenic and mutagenic effects [67].

Furthermore, mosquitoes can gradually develop resistance to synthetic repellents; therefore, using synthetic chemical shall not be the best choice [68]. Thus, research and development of alternative repellent compounds against mosquitoes with lower or no toxicity to humans are highly desired [66]. Repellents of plant origin do not pose hazards of toxicity to human and domestic animals and are easily biodegradable [69,70]. Plants have been used since ancient times to repel/kill blood-sucking insects in the human history and even now, in many parts of the world people use plant substances to repel/kill the mosquitoes and other blood-sucking insects [71].

At the moment repellent of plants origin have been receiving massive attention due to their environmental and user friendly nature and it demands more scientific survey in order to identify new repellents or insecticidal plants. Repellent plants usage custom is a result ofthousands of years of experience. This expertise has been passed down to many generations chiefly through the word of mouth. This mode of information conveyance may result in distortion or loss of indigenous knowledge and usage custom of repellent plants. Therefore, right nowdocumenting and safeguarding these practices have become a crucial core issue [72].

Skilled Personnel and Healthcare Infrastructure

An effort as large and complex as malaria elimination requires input from many researchers and practitioners- the input that is largely absent today. 40 years ago, WHO had 500 staff focusing on malaria elimination [73] - today there is only a handful around the world. This gap must be closed and more resources devoted to research and implementation should support for elimination efforts to be successful and this approach is the unique and possible path for malaria eradication [18].

We can make tremendous progress with the tools that we have today: prevention with ITNs and IRS, diagnosis with rapid diagnostic tests, and treatment with artemisinin-based combination therapy (ACTs). It is entirely feasible to eliminate malaria from countries and regions where the intensity of transmission is low to moderate, and where health systems are strong. Eliminating malaria from countries where the intensity of transmission is high and stable, such as in tropical Africa, will require more potent tools and stronger health systems than are available today [74]. The maintenance phase of elimination will be the responsibility of the once endemic countries themselves and not the international donors. There is a pressing need for capacity building in endemic nations to ensure tomorrow's leaders of elimination who shall be responsible for future decision-making, research, and management of their control and elimination programmes. Access to populations at risk is a major concern if a sustained control and elimination are to be achieved [28].

Quantitative Mathematic Models

A global malaria eradication effort will require massive changes to a complex web of interconnected biological systems. The optimal path to eradication is intrinsically unpredictable because of the potential for parasites and vectors to evolve, the waxing and waning of human immunity, and behavioural changes in human and vector populations. The range of conditions that favor malaria transmission are so varied and diverse that decisions and plans cannot be based solely on the evidence that has been acquired in randomized control trials conducted in only a few settings [39].

To succeed, eradication will require a strategic plan that is constantly updated with the latest surveillance, monitoring, and evaluation data. Moreover, planning processes involve some sort of conceptual model, and this model will necessarily consider many potential sources of uncertainty. Rational quantitative mathematical models provide the best way to synthesize information, quantify uncertainty, and extrapolate current knowledge. Such models can provide critical quantitative insights that are not otherwise possible [39].

Laboratory Diagnosis

Prompt and accurate diagnosis is the key for effective disease management, which is one of the main interventions of the Global Malaria Control Strategy to reduce morbidity and to prevent death from malaria [20]. The most commonly used diagnostic test for malaria is microscopy to detect parasites in stained blood films. Thick blood films are used in routine diagnosis and as few as one parasite per 200 μl blood can be detected. The method can be used to differentiate between different parasite species and the stages of the life cycle [75].

Rapid diagnostic 'dipstick' tests (RDTs) that detect malaria antigens in blood are easy to perform and do not require trained personnel or special equipment. However, they are relatively expensive and *P. falciparum* can only be diagnosed whereas *P. ovale*, *P. malariae* and *P. vivax* cannot be distinguished from one another while using this method. In areas where malaria transmission is high, clinical diagnosis is usually sufficient to warrant treatment. However, in areas of Southeast Asia where malaria is a less common cause of fever and where treatments are more expensive, microscopic diagnosis is preferred. Diagnostic tests can ensure more cost effective disease management and use of medications. They may also reduce drug resistance, as treatment based on clinical symptoms may alone be selected for resistance [75].

Diagnostic tests are useful for monitoring the prevalence of malaria infection, for example, in nomadic populations such as non-immune refugees entering malaria zones due to civil unrest. It is thus of concern that poor diagnosis may continue to hinder effective malaria control. This is due to a combination of factors, including non-specific clinical presentation of the disease, high prevalence of asymptomatic infection in some areas, lack of resources and insufficient access to trained health care providers and health facilities, and widespread practice of self-treatment for clinically suspected malaria. The coexistence of *P. falciparum* and *P. vivax* presents difficulties for malaria diagnosis and treatment. More over, in low malaria-endemic area, this is characterized by an annual incidence below1/1000 [20]. In such low-endemicity areas, RDTs for diagnosing *vivax*malaria are often not sensitive enough [76].

Antimalarial Drugs

Malaria control relies heavily on the use of effective anti-malarial medicines. Antimalarials are used to treat malaria illness, to prevent both infection and disease caused by *Plasmodia*, to eliminate dormant malaria parasites from the liver, and to prevent malaria transmission [77]. Although the bitter-tasting component of the bark of *Cinchona ledgeriana* from Peru, was known to be an effective anti-malarial since 15th century and an infusion of Qinghao (*Artemesia annua*) has been used for more than 2000 years in China, the active ingredients were only isolated by pharmacists in the early 19th and late 20th centuries, respectively [78].

Treatment of vivax malaria still relies on chloroquine (CQ) and primaquine and whereas CQ treatment is largely effective for vivax malaria world-wide. Despite this, the CQ–primaquine combination is still the treatment of choice for vivax malaria. In addition, CQ treatment of vivax malaria often leads to the appearance of falciparum malaria in patients due to the prevalence of mixed-species infections [79,80]. Primaquine is the only registered drug for eliminating vivax hypnozoites in the liver, but the high prevalence of glucose-6-phosphate dehydrogenase deficiency in the human populations compromises the use of this drug [81].

Artemisinin derivative-based combination therapy (ACT) has been advocated as the therapy of choice to handle widespread drug resistance in P. falciparum malaria and at the same time preventing recrudescence due to artemisinin monotherapy. However, most of the combinations are less than ideal because of side effects, pharmacokinetic mismatch, and cost [82,83].

Challenges and Issues

Artemisinin based drug combinations are highly effective, with cure rates similar to that of chloroquine 30 years ago. They seem to be a good long term choice for most African countries, being safe and well tolerated (with the caveat that their safety in early pregnancy is not yet clear). Compared with other antimalarials, ACTs can reduce gametocyte carriage thereby lowering the risk of infectiousness in those who take treatment [84]. Behind these successes, however, lies a worrying reality: the spread of drug and insecticide resistance threatens to unravel the progress. Malaria strains resistant to the cheapest and most commonly used drugs already exist in almost every endemic country. Now, irrational use and continued over-reliance on artemisinin monotherapies are undermining the gold standard for malaria treatment, ACTs. Last year, a study showed significantly longer parasite-clearance times in patients taking ACTs along the Thai–Cambodian border [85].With no new classes of drugs in late-stage development; resistance to ACTs may give rise to many of the ineffective endoperoxide drug candidates as synthetic alternatives to artemisinin [86].

ACTs are massively deployed in most falciparum-endemic countries to deal with multi drug resistance (MDR) parasites. However, circulation of counterfeit and substandard artemisinin is a major threat to the success of malaria control. Fake artemisinins, containing few or no active ingredients, are life-threatening [87], and substandard drugs encourage resistance development. The problem of drug resistance is further exacerbated by the irrational drug use (e.g., artemisinin monotherapy and its inability to adhere to treatment regimes) and the circulation of counterfeit/substandard drugs in private sectors [88], which leads to treatment failures and to promote the development of drug resistance [89]. Hence artemisinin drug quality control is urgently needed.

The drugs that are presently being used in large-scale infectious disease control and elimination programmes such as those for onchocerciasis and trachoma can be administered in a single encounter once or twice a year. Notably, however, the antimalarial drug regimens that were used with varying success to eliminate malaria from Italy [90], the former Soviet Union [91], and various islands such as the Vanuatu island of Aneityum [92], have involved complex regimens of multiple administrations of at least two drugs usually repeated at frequent intervals for prolonged periods of time. Though, multiple dosing regimens of multiple drugs have been used successfully to eliminate malaria from areas with relatively good health systems and stable populations, malaria eradication will require drugs that, ideally, can be administered in a single encounter at infrequent intervals [77].

Evidence-based mechanisms are needed to improve access to effective treatments and displace monotherapies. Today, only 3% of children under the age of 5 years receive ACTs, partly because 40–60% of patients are treated in the private sector where ACTs remain prohibitively expensive [93]. The Affordable Medicines Facility for Malaria (AMFm) is an innovative approach to reduce ACT costs. To support the AMFm and other efforts, the ACTwatch project is collecting data on market penetration for ACTs and building recommendations on how to increase access to and affordability of ACTs [94].

Antimalarial Drug Resistance

Antimalarial drug resistance has been defined as the "ability of a parasite strain to survive and/or multiply despite the administration and absorption of a drug given in doses equal to or higher than those usually recommended but within the tolerance of the subject". This definition was later modified to specify that the drug in question must "gain access to the parasite or the infected red blood cell for the duration of the time necessary for its normal action" [95]. Most researchers interpret this as referring only to persistence of parasites after treatment doses of an antimalarial rather than as a prophylaxis failure, although the latter is a useful tool for early warning of the presence of drug resistance [96].

Antimalarial drug resistance has emerged as one of the greatest challenges facing malaria control today. Drug resistance has been implicated with the spread of malaria to new areas and re-emergence of malaria in areas where the disease had been eradicated. Drug resistance has also played a significant role in the occurrence and severity of epidemics in some parts of the world. Population movement has introduced resistant parasites to areas that are previously free from drug resistance [97]. The development and spread of drug-resistant strains of malaria parasites has been identified as a key factor in this resurgence and is one of the greatest challenges to malaria control today. There is currently an increase in attention and resources aimed at malaria, including such initiatives as Roll Back Malaria [98].

The emergence of artemisinin resistant malaria along the Thai-Cambodian border has provoked global alarm that the most valuable and effective antimalarial drug is in danger of being lost; triggering a campaign to identify and eradicate resistant parasite strains [99-101]. It has been suggested that concerns about drug resistance and strategies to deter it -for example, the obligatory use of combinations of drugs with different mechanisms - may not be a priority in the context of malaria eradication, because resistance is unlikely to emerge and spread when transmission is very low in the late stages of elimination. However, evidence suggests that drug resistance can spread rapidly and become fixed in populations in settings of low malaria transmission [102]. The problem of antimalarial drug resistance is aggravated by the existence of cross resistance among drugs belonging to the same chemical family [97].

Prevention of Drug Resistance

An ideal eradication drug would have a short half life with a sustained (depot-like) release followed by rapid elimination, and would be deployed in combination with other drugs with matching pharmacokinetic and pharmacodynamic profiles both to deter resistance and to improve efficacy [103]. An intermediate goal may be to develop a safe product for delivery at a single encounter of a curative dose of a drug, shall offer 4 or more weeks of post-treatment causal prophylactic efficacy [77]. Another creative approach from the past that may hold promise for the future is the use of long-acting formulations.

Despite the emergence of artemisinin resistant malaria concerns the artemisinin resistance phenotype has been poorly characterized. Decreased parasite sensitivity to the artemisinin drugs in standardizedin vitrotests has not been reported to date from clinical trials and a molecular marker for artemisinin resistance remains elusive. The key features of the phenotype appear to have prolonged parasite clearance times and slower than expected parasite clearance rates in patients with adequate plasma drug concentrations[104]. Therefore, appropriate studies must be carried out in order to identify the molecular marker for artemisinin resistance.

Vaccine: A Future Hope for Meaningful Malaria Eradication

Vaccines are the most cost-effective tools for public health and have been instrumental in previous elimination campaigns against smallpox [105], polio [106], and measles [107,108]. The research and development agenda for the development of vaccines can serve as key components of a future arsenal of tools to eradicate malaria [109]. Malaria vaccines could be one of the most cost-effective interventions and crucial components to eradicate malaria in the poorest countries of the world. It is unlikely that malaria can be eradicated without a vaccine or another transformative tool that can be used in areas of intrinsically high malaria transmission [104].

Vaccines are potential tools for the future. Several malaria vaccines are being developed, based on the candidate antigens from the three main target stages of the life cycle of the malaria parasite: vaccines that target sporozoites, which will reduce human infection rates and, if highly effective, will prevent human infection; those that target the parasites in asexual blood stages, which will reduce the intensity of disease and mortality; and those that target the parasite in the sexual stages that develop in the mosquito, and which will reduce and interrupt the transmission of malaria [20]. The inclusion of a transmission blocking vaccine would also greatly prolong the useful life of vaccines against other stages by preventing the spread of parasites that become resistant to these vaccines [110].

Vaccines against the pathogenic asexual blood stages of plasmodium parasites are designed with the main objective of preventing clinical disease. Antibodies to region II of the *P. vivax*Duffy binding protein are associated with strain-specific immunity [111], supporting further research into this potential vaccine target. Polymorphism of the surface proteins of *P. falciparum* and variability in the parasite invasion pathways mean, however, that production of a blood-stage vaccine against this species is much more challenging. Interest in the development of a multi-antigen, multistage vaccine that targets different stages in the parasite's life cycle is now increasing [112]. This approach might confer better protection than do vaccines based on single antigens, and avoid vaccine failure caused by polymorphic variation in parasite populations [113].

Major Set-Backs and Challenges

Current efforts to develop malaria vaccines are primarily directed towards reducing the morbidity and mortality that are associated with malaria and focuses on *P. falciparum.* For example, the Malaria Vaccine Roadmap [114] has a strategic goal of developing a vaccine with 80% protective efficacy against *P. falciparum* by 2020. However, if malaria vaccines are to contribute to programs for malaria elimination, they will need to have an impact on malaria transmission. The scientific and ethical basis for the development of vaccines referred to as transmission-blocking vaccines (TBVs) that specifically target malaria sexual stage antigens with the goal of having an impact on transmission has been described previously [115,116].

TBVs are not designed to protect the vaccinated individual from contracting malaria, instead reduces the number of infectious vectors and the circulating parasite population. Research on TBVs has traditionally targeted surface proteins of mosquito stages of *P. falciparum* and *P. vivax;* phase 1 vaccine trials have shown immunogenicity of these vaccines in human beings [117]. More recent work has targeted antigens in the mosquito midgut or saliva that facilitate parasite invasion of the vector and host, respectively [118].The malERA Consultative Group on Vaccines 2011 [109] recommends that vaccine development efforts need to pay attention to *Plasmodium* species other than *P. falciparum*, especially *P. vivax*, if malaria eradication is to be achieved.

Recent advances in malaria vaccine development have heightened the possibility that, if proven effective, a new anti-malaria tool could be deployed for use alongside existing interventions [119]. A vaccine candidate targeting the most life-threatening malaria parasite, *P. falciparum*, is moving through a Phase 3 efficacy trial in Kenya and six other African countries - Burkina Faso, Gabon, Ghana, Malawi, Mozambique, and Tanzania [119]. Data from previous studies indicate that this vaccine candidate—GlaxoSmithKline Biologicals' RTS,S - may cut episodes of clinical malaria in young children by about half [120]. If the efficacy trial confirms earlier findings, the World Health Organization (WHO) has indicated that a policy recommendation for RTS,S is possible as early as 2015, paving way for implementation in countries through their expanded programs on immunization. Final results from the trial are expected in late 2014 [121].

Genetically Modified Mosquitoes (GMM)

Currently, only two types of weapons are available to fight against malaria – the drugs that kill the parasite in humans and insecticides that kill the mosquito vector. Both approaches suffer from problems of development of resistance by the target organisms and from expense and complicated logistics for the implementation of control measures. Despite intensive efforts in the last few decades, an effective vaccine has not yet been developed. Clearly, new approaches to combat malaria are urgently needed [122].

This has to be a multidisciplinary effort because no single control measure is sufficient. Mosquitoes are the obligatory vectors of malaria parasites. After a blood meal, the parasite undergoes an intricate development cycle that involves mating of the gametes, transformation into the motile ookinete, formation of the oocyst and its burst into thousands of sporozoites that colonize the mosquito salivary glands [123]. If the mosquito is able to block any of this developmental stages the *Plasmodium* cycle is interrupted and less malaria transmission would be expected. Within this thought, the genetic modification of mosquitoes to reduce their ability to transmit the disease is a strategy that needs to be further explored [124].

In the last decade, molecular biology has been a source of great hope for creating genetically-modified mosquitoes in order to resist the malaria parasite. Genetically Modified Mosquitoes that are unable to transmit pathogens offer opportunities for controlling vector-borne diseases such as malaria and dengue. Site-specific gene recombination technologies are advantageous in the development of these insects because antipathogen effector genes can be inserted at integration sites in the genome that cause the least alteration in mosquito fitness [125].

GMM applications seek to suppress or manipulate mosquito populations so as to decrease vector mosquito populations or reduce their ability to transmit disease. These applications release reared mosquitoes into the environment (as do other control strategies not using or applying GM technology to mosquitoes). These technologies are novel in mosquito control, and in the case of population manipulation representing untested concepts for vector interventions in the field. Some non-GMM control approaches are described which have common principles of rearing and releasing mosquitoes and common measures of efficacy are likely to apply [126].

Major Challenges and Issues

GMM research already has yielded the proof-of-principle demonstration that malaria-resistant and dengue-resistant mosquitoes can be produced, and that induced sterility can be generated. However, the way in which laboratory derived genetically engineered mosquito strains could be deployed effectively, efficiently and safely in the field remains to be determined. The need to control major diseases such as malaria and dengue is widely accepted, but many challenges remain unmet. These challenges encompass technical issues; funding and regulatory constraints that influence how rapidly new control tools can be developed ; anticipated economic, environmental, health and social trade-offs associated with the use of different control methods ; and social and cultural issues expected to influence acceptance of these methods. In the case of a new technology such as GMM, careful planning and preparation is required to address these challenges [126];

- There is no widely accepted regulatory or biosafety framework that provides guidance for all aspects of the implementation of GMM technologies. While national standards will necessarily take priority over any other guidance, a framework of guiding principles as recommended here could provide helpful advice to stake-holders. Such a document could foster standardization of procedures, comparability of results and credibility of conclusions, which will be useful for decision-making by funders and end users of the technologies.
- Risk analysis – Identify methods to define hazards and prioritize risks to be monitored, starting at the laboratory phase and continuing through field release. These include additional approaches to identifying environmental and ecological hazards such as fault-tree and event-tree analyses [127]. Community engagement to identify valued aspects of the environment should be used to inform this process.
- Integrated methods for risk analysis should be developed to ensure that novel and conventional control approaches are judged by common standards.
- Models to extrapolate limited testing to wider field applications – Create models that relate measurable entomological outcomes to epidemiologically-relevant impacts.

Sterile Insect Technique (SIT)

SIT is a species-specific and environmentally nonpolluting method of insect control that relies on the release of large numbers of sterile insects [128,129]. Mating of released sterile males with native females shall lead to a decrease in the females' reproductive potential and ultimately, if males are released in sufficient numbers over a sufficient period of time for the local elimination or suppression of the pest population. Highly successful, area-wide SIT programmes have eliminated or suppressed a range of major veterinary and agricultural pests around the world [130].Field trials in the 1970s and 1980s demonstrated that SIT could also be made to work against mosquitoes, even with the technology then available [131,132]. For example, *Anopheles albimanus* was successfully controlled in a trial in El Salvador using chemosterilized mosquitoes [133].

Cytoplasmic Incompatibility (CI) SIT

It was also used successfully in field experiments with *Culex pipiens fatigans* [134]. CI is caused by maternally transmitted intracellular bacteria of the genus *Wolbachia* and refers to the strongly reduced hatch rate in matings between infected males and females that are either uninfected or harbour a different infection type [135]. Therefore, infected males released into an uninfected population are sterile without the need for radiation. Interest in this incompatible insect technique (IIT) has recently revived [135,136]. However, infected females are fertile with infected males, so inadvertent release of infected females could lead to replacement of the target population with a *Wolbachia*-infected form rather than suppression [130].

Classical Radiation-Induced Sterility

The project is composed of two parts: technology development and field feasibility studies. The International Atomic Energy Agency (IAEA) is primarily involved in technology development, but it also plays a supporting role assisting national efforts in their field feasibility studies. Two field sites are being studied for the initial feasibility studies: the Nile valley in the Northern State of Sudan and Reunion Island. In both instances, *An. arabiensis* is the sole malaria vector [137]. All current SIT programmes use radiation to sterilize the insects. However, it has proven difficult to irradiate mosquitoes to near-complete sterility without significantly weakening them [138,139].

Challenges and Issues

Although the concept here is population suppression and/or local elimination, it is probably the only benchmark available at present for vector control strategies based on modern biotechnological tools [131]. The novelty of the approach thus poses challenges on several fronts [140];

- First, there are various technical hurdles affecting progress and posing challenges to the scientific community.
- Second, the transition from the laboratory to the field requires careful planning to manage the risk of project failure or premature termination.
- Third (and unknown at this stage), it remains to be seen under what ethical, legal, and societal frameworks (ELSI) adoption in Disease Endemic Countries (DECs) can be secured.

The final critical challenge is the development of novel approaches that permanently reduce the high vectorial capacities of the dominant malaria vectors in sub-Saharan Africa. Genetic control programs based on permanent reduction of the vectorial capacities of natural vector populations have received the most attention to date [141,142].

Global Malaria Eradication: Is It Achievable and Practicable?

Many malaria control strategies exist, but none of them are appropriate and affordable in all contexts. Malaria control and prevention efforts need to be designed for the specific environment in which they will be used and need to take into account the local epidemiology of malaria and the level of available resources and political will [97]. The existing methods of vector control will have to be improved if the ambitious targets for malaria control and elimination are to be reached. These will include new, longer-lasting (up to 1 year at least) and user-friendly formulations of insecticides for indoor residual spraying, especially in areas of perennial transmission, and affordable, acceptable 5-year insecticidal nets made widely available by mass production. New tools are needed for malaria control in specific situations, such as in forests in Asia and Latin America where local vectors are exophagic and exophilic, and conventional vector control with existing tools is impossible [20].

Maintaining long-term momentum in the face of success in regional elimination while waiting to achieve final eradication will be a major challenge. Shrinking the map by starting on the malaria margins with the "easy-to-eliminate" settings will boost morale initially but may bring marginal benefits to such areas at the expense of those where the burden of malaria is the highest. Any strategic plan – and here again we learn from the past – needs to be a synchronous global effort, locally adapted in all endemic areas [143]. Although we lack sufficient knowledge, systems and tools to eradicate malaria today, we do have a window of political will and financial resources to refocus on the goal of effective control through universal coverage of appropriate interventions. The prerequisites for a successful start are: (i) a process of inclusive discourse to agree on global vision, goals and strategy; and (ii) a global plan for all endemic areas describing how, where and when we move from control towards elimination; What must distinguish the new era, especially in Africa, is a real rather than rhetorical emphasis on health systems [143].

The current malaria control effort has focused on developing existing products and procedures (for example, drugs and the distribution of bednets) to reduce malaria morbidity and mortality. However, it is commonly accepted that eradication will not be achieved with current tools. Thus, we must now accelerate the development of a new generation of tools and knowledge aimed specifically at malaria eradication. As we look towards this ambitious goal, we must recognize that cutting-edge basic science, novel research strategies, and creative multidisciplinary approaches, are required to be mobilized to bridge the gap between bench, preclinical, clinical, and population-based sciences [144].

The unacceptable health burden of malaria, and its economic and social impacts on development, has made it a focal point of the international development agenda, and the world has embraced an ambitious plan for scaling up malaria control that progresses towards country-by-country and regional elimination and the ultimate goal of global eradication [145]. A key question, however, is whether elimination from all regions of the world (eradication) is feasible with the current tools and state of knowledge. For a number of reasons, we believe that the answer is ''no'' [146];

- First, malaria is not a single disease. The five Plasmodium species (falciparum, vivax, ovale, malariae, knowlesi) that cause human malaria are transmitted by more than 30 Anopheline mosquito species with diverse breeding and feeding habits, and result in different disease spectra in different population target groups and epidemiological settings.
- Second, current malaria control and elimination programs face remarkable heterogeneity of transmission dynamics of malaria in endemic areas, including differences in parasite, vector, human, social, and environmental factors.
- Third, operational limitations include underperforming health services, lack of political will, insufficient financial, social and human resources, and for some areas, inadequate tools to interrupt transmission given an exceedingly high force of transmission. Each country presents different combinations of these problems and their determinants.

Thus, a widely held view suggests that with currently available tools, much greater gains could be achieved, including elimination from a number of countries and regions, but that even with maximal effort we will fall short of elimination in many areas and of global eradication [146]. Nonetheless, global malaria eradication remains to be the ultimate goal of WHO and all malaria endemic countries. Eradicating malaria will require sustained long-term investments to fully scale-up today's tools while at the same time investing in the research requires to develop tomorrow's transformative tools. Eradicating malaria is a long-term goal that will likely take 40 years or more to achieve [74].

Acknowledgement

I am greatly indebted to Dr. K. Ilango M.Sc., Ph.D., Scientist, Zoological Survey of India, Chennai, India and Dr. S. Sabesan M.Sc., Ph.D., Scientist, Vector Control Research Center, Pondicherry, India for their constant encouragement and support. I would like to thank MrsMelitaPrakash for her sincere assistance. My last but not the least heartfelt thanks go to my colleagues of our Department of Environmental Health Science, College Public Health and Medicine, Jimma University, Jimma, Ethiopia, for their kind support and cooperation.

References

[1] M. Jacobs-lorena, and A. A. James, Genetic modification of insects of medical importance: past, present and future. *Report of the Scientific Working Group on Insect Vectors and Human Health*, TDR/SWG/VEC/03.1 P68-73.(2002).
[2] K. Karunamoorthi and K. Ilango, *Eur. Rev. Med. Pharmacol. Sci.* 14(1), 57, (2010).
[3] WHO. *World Malaria Report* 2009. The World Health Organization, Geneva, Switzerland (2009).
[4] R. M. Packard, *The making of a tropical disease: a short history of malaria*. Baltimore: Johns Hopkins University Press (2007).
[5] A. R. Butler, S. Khanand E. Ferguson, *J. R. Coll. Physicians Edinb.* 40, 72, (2010).
[6] G. Majori, *The Lancet*, 354, 31, (2000).
[7] J. A. Na′jera, M. Gonza′lez-Silva and P. L. Alonso, *PLoS Med.* 8(1), e1000412 , (2011).
[8] WHO. *World Malaria Report 2008*. The World Health Organization, Geneva, Switzerland (2008).
[9] WHO. *World Malaria Report 2005*. http://rbm.who.int/wmr. (2005) (accessed on 31st December 2010).
[10] K. Karunamoorthi, D. Bishaw and T. Yilkal, *J. Pub. Health*, 18, 559, (2010).
[11] K. Karunamoorthi and M. Bekele, *J. Infect. Pub. Health*, 2(4), 171, (2009).
[12] J. A. Berkley, P. Bejon, T. Mwangi and et al. *Clin. Infect. Dis*. 49, 336, (2009).
[13] J. Crawley, C. Chu, G. Mtove and F.Nosten, *The Lancet*, 375, 1468 (2010).
[14] B. Greenwood, *Trans. R. Soc. Trop. Med.Hyg*.103S, S2, (2009).
[15] L. Roberts and M. Enserink, *Science*, 318, 1544, (2007).
[16] Bill and Melinda Gates Foundation Malaria Forum – Day 2, 17 October 2007 [Transcript].
[17] G. W. Fegan, A. M. Noor, W. S. Akhwale and S. Cousens, *The Lancet*, 370, 1035, (2007).
[18] R. Feachem and O. Sabot, *The Lancet*, 371, 1633, (2008).
[19] Wernsdorfer. Historical review of the global malaria eradication program - Concept, achievements, shortcomings. *Presentation at WHO Informal Consultation on Global Malaria Control and Elimination,* (2008).
[20] WHO. Global malaria control and elimination: report of a technical review. Global Malaria Control and Elimination Meeting (2008). http://malaria.who.int/docs/elimination/MalariaControl EliminationMeeting.pdf.
[21] Editorial, The Lancet, 370, 1459, (2007).
[22] WHO. Malaria Control in Countries where Time-limited Eradication is Impracticable at Present: *Technical Report Series* 537. Geneva, Switzerland, (1974).

[23] WHO. *Re-examination of the global strategy of malaria eradication.* Geneva: World Health Organization. Geneva, Switzerland, (1969).
[24] S. I. Hay, C. A. Guerra, A. J. Tatem, A. M. Noor and R. W. Snow, *Lancet Infect. Dis.* 4, 327, (2004).
[25] C. A. Guerra, P. W. Gikandi, A. J. Tatem and et al., *PLoS Med.* 5, e38, (2008).
[26] I. Kleinschmidt, C. Schwabe, L. Benavente and et al., *Am. J. Trop. Med.Hyg.*80: 882 (2009).
[27] R. G. A. Feachem, A. A. Phillips, J. Hwang, et al., *The Lancet*, (2010).
[28] P. Das and R. Horton, Malaria elimination: worthy, challenging, and just possible. *The Lancet,* 376, 1515 (2010).
[29] W. Kilama and F. Ntoumi, *The Lancet*, 374, 1480, (2009).
[30] L. Molineaux and G. Gramiccia G, "*The Garki Project*". Geneva: World Health Organization. 311p, (1980).
[31] G. F. Killeen, T. A. Smith, H. M. Ferguson, S. Abdulla, H. Mshinda and et al. , *PLoS Med.* 4, e229, (2007). doi:10.1371/journal.pmed.0040229.
[32] C. Lengeler, *Cochrane Database Syst. Rev.* CD000363, (2004). doi:10.1002/14651858.CD000363.pub2.
[33] B. L. Sharp, I. Kleinschmidt, E. Streat, R. Maharaj, K. I. Barnes and et al., *Am. J. Trop. Med. Hyg.* 76, 42, (2007).
[34] D. L. Smith, J. Dushoff, R. W. Snow and S. I. Hay, *Nature*, 438, 492, (2005).
[35] D. L. Smith, F. E. McKenzie, R. W. Snow and S. I. Hay, *PLoS Biol.* 5, e42, (2007).
[36] G. F. Killeen, A. Tami, J. Kihonda, F. O. Okumu, M. E. Kotas and et al., *BMC Infect.Dis.* 7, 121, (2007).
[37] D. A. Henderson, *Smallpox: the death of a disease*. New York: Prometheus Books, (2009).
[38] A. J. Tatem, D. L. Smith, P. W. Gething, C. W. Kabaria, R. W. Snow and S. I. Hay, *Lancet,* 2010; published online Oct 29. DOI:10.1016/S0140-6736(10)61301-3.
[39] The malERA Consultative Group on Modeling, *PLoS Med.* 8, e1000403, (2011).
[40] F. H. Osier, G. Fegan, S. D. Polley, L. Murungi, F. Verra and et al., *Infect. Immun.* 76, 2240, (2008).
[41] P. D. Crompton, M. A. Kayala, B. Traore, K. Kayentao, A. Ongoiba and et al., *Proceed. Natl. Acad. Sci. USA,* 107, 6958, (2010).
[42] K. Karunamoorthi, *Clin. Microbiol. Infect.* (In Press). (2011).
[43] K. Karunamoorthi and S. Sabesan, *Parasitol. Res.* 105(3), 641, (2009).
[44] K. Kaliyaperumal and D. Yesuf, *East Afr. J. Pub. Health*, 6(2), 205, (2009).
[45] A. Enayati and J. Hemingway, *Ann. Rev. Entomol.* 55, 569, (2010).
[46] W. K. Reisen and P. F. L. Boreham, *J. Med. Entomol.* 19, 98, (1982).
[47] J. Hill, J. Lines and M. Rowland, *Adv. Parasitol.* 61, 77, (2006).
[48] WHO. Malarial and HIV/AIDS interactions and policy implications. *Report of an informal technical consultation*, 23-25 June 2004. WHO/HIV/2004.8 Geneva, Switzerland. (2004).
[49] C. Lengeler, Insecticide-treated bednets and curtains for preventing malaria (Cochrane Review). *The Cochrane Library*. Oxford: Update Software. (2002).
[50] B. Adele, The Lancet, 374, 1581, (2009).

[51] W. A. Hawley, P. A. Phillips-Howard, F. O. terKuile, D. J. Terlouw, J. M. Vulule, M. Ombok, B. L. Nahlen, J. E. Gimnig, S. K. Kariuki, M. S. Kolczak and A. W. Hightower, *Am. J. Trop. Med. Hyg*. 68(4S), 121, (2003).

[52] Roll Back Malaria. World malaria day 2010: Africa update. *Progress and impact series.* (2010).

[53] C. Lengeler, *Cochrane Database Syst. Rev*. 2, CD000363. (2004).

[54] C. Lengeler and B. Sharp, Indoor residual spraying and insecticide-treated nets. In: C. Murphy, K. Ringheim, S. Woldehanna and J. Volmink. eds. Reducing malaria's burden: evidence of effectiveness for decision makers. Washington, DC: *Global Health Council,* 17-24. (2003).

[55] J. Etang, F. Chandre, P. Guillet and L. Manga, *Malar. J*. 3, 46, (2004).

[56] WHO. Global Malaria Programme. *Indoor residual spraying Use of indoor residual spraying for scaling up global malaria control and elimination.* Geneva, Switzerland. (2006).

[57] H. Ranson, H. Abdallah, A. Badolo, W. M. Guelbeogo, C. Kerah-Hinzoumbe′ and et al., *Malar. J.* 8, 299, (2009).

[58] WHO. WHO. *Tech. Rep. Ser*. 125, (1957).

[59] USAID. Integrated Vector Management Programs for Malaria Control. *Programmatic Environmental Assessmen*t. (2007).

[60] V. Corbel, R. N'Guessan, C. Brengues and et al., *Acta Trop*. 101, 207, (2007).

[61] K. Karunamoorthi and S. Sabesan, *Eur. Rev. Med. Pharmacol. Sci*. 14(5), 443, (2010).

[62] S. J. Moore and RITAM Vector Control Group, *Guidelines for Studies on Plant-based Insect Repellents*. CRC Press LLC, p. 366, (2004).

[63] K. Karunamoorthi and S. Sabesan, *Int. Health,* 1(2), 173, (2009).

[64] R. P. Moody, F. M. Benoit, R. Riedel and L. J. Ritter, *Toxicol. Environ. Health*, 26, 137, (1989).

[65] J. R. Clem, D. F. Havemann and M. A. Raebel, *Ann. Pharmacother*, 27, 289, (1993).

[66] J. Zhu, X. Zeng, L. T. Yanma, K. Qian, Y. Han, S. Xue, B. Tucker, G. Schultz, J. Coats, W. Rowley and A. Zhang, *J. Am. Mosq. Control. Assoc*. 22(3), 515, (2006).

[67] V. I. Vashkov, S. E. Gleiberman and A. P. Volkova, *Med. Parazitol. Bolezni*. 45(6), (1976).

[68] B. Gerhardson, *Trends Biotechnol*. 20, 338, (2002).

[69] V. P. Sharma and M. A. Ansari, *Indian J. Med. Entomol*. 31(3), 505, (1994).

[70] V. P. Sharma, B. N. Nagpal and A. Srivastava, Trans. R. *Soc. Trop. Med. Hyg*. 87, 627, (1993).

[71] K. Karunamoorthi, S. Ramanujam and R. Rathinasamy, *Parasitol. Res*. 103(3), 545, (2008).

[72] K. Karunamoorthi, K. Ilango and A. Endale, *J. Ethnopharmacol*. 125(2), 224, (2009).

[73] G. Harrison, *Mosquitoes, malaria, and man: a history of the hostilities since 1880*. New York: EP Dutton, (1978).

[74] WHO, WHO Global Malaria Programme: *Q and A on malaria elimination and eradication.* (2010).

[75] C. Cross, Malaria is diagnosed using a combination of clinical observations, case history and diagnostic tests. (2004).
http://malaria.wellcome.ac.uk/doc_WTD023886.html.

[76] C. Wongsrichanalai, I. Arevalo, A. Laoboonchai K. Yingyuen, R. S. Miller, A. J. Magill, J. R. Forney and R. A. GasserJr, *Am. J. Trop. Med. Hyg*. 69, 26, (2003).
[77] The malERA Consultative Group on Drugs. *PLoS Med*. 8(1), e1000402, (2011).
[78] G. Lewison and D. Srivastava, *Acta Trop*. 106, 96, (2008).
[79] M. Mayxay, S. Pukritrayakamee, K. Chotivanich, M.Imwong, S. Looareesuwan and N. J. White, *Am. J. Trop. Med. Hyg*. 65, 588, (2001).
[80] S. Krudsood, P. Wilairatana, D. P. Mason, S. Treeprasertsuk, P. Singhasivanon, and S. Looa- reesuwan, *Southeast Asian J. Trop. Med. Pub. Health*, 30, 623, (1999).
[81] V. Wiwanitkit, *J. Vector Borne Dis*. 45, 98, (2008).
[82] S. Yeung, W. Pongtavornpinyo, I. M. Hastings, A. J. Mills, and N. J. White, *Am. J. Trop. Med. Hyg*. 71, 179, (2004).
[83] P. G. Kremsner, and S. Krishna, *The Lancet*, 364, 285, (2004).
[84] Editorial, *BMJ*, 331, 706, (2005). doi: 10.1136/bmj.331.7519.706.
[85] A. M. Dondorp, F. Nosten, Y. Poravuth, and et al., *N. Engl. J. Med*. 361, 455, (2009).
[86] T. A. Wells, A question of quality: interview with Chris Hentschel, President and CEO of MMV. October, 2008. http://www.mmv.org/IMG/pdf/FINAL_mmv08_news17_A4pgs.pdf.
[87] P. N. Newton, R. McGready, F. Fernandez, M. D. Green, M. Sunjio, C. Bruneton, S. Phanouvong, P. Millet, C. J. Whitty, A. O. Talisuna, S. Proux, E. M. Christophel, G. Malenga, P. Singhasivanon, K. Bojang, H. Kaur, K. Palmer, N. P. Day, B. M. Greenwood, F. Nosten and N. J. White, *PLoS Med*. 3, e197, (2006).
[88] P. Newton, S. Proux, M. Green, F. Smithuis, J. Rozendaal, S. Prakongpan, K. Chotivanich, M. Mayxay, S. Looareesuwan, J. Farrar, F. Nosten and N. J. White, *Lancet,* 357, 1948, (2001).
[89] L. Cui and et al., *Acta Trop*. (2011). Doi:10.1016/j.actatropica.2011.04.006.
[90] F. M. Snowden, *The conquest of malaria*. Italy 1900-1962. New Haven: Yale University Press. (2005).
[91] L. J. Bruce-Chwatt, *Bull. World Health Organ*. 21, 737, (1959).
[92] A. Kaneko, G. Taleo, M. Kalkoa, S. Yamar, T. Kobayakawa and et al., *Lancet*, 356, 1560, (2000).
[93] MMV. *Medicines for Malaria Venture*. Understanding the antimalarials market: Uganda 2007—an overview of the supply side. Nov 6, 2008. http://www.mmv.org/article.php3?id_article=536.
[94] ACT watch. http://www.actwatch.info/home/home.asp (accessed Oct 12, 2010).
[95] L. J. Bruce-Chwatt and et al., *Chemotherapy of malaria*, Geneva, World Health Organization, (1986).
[96] H. O. Lobel and C. C. Campbell, *Clin. Trop. Med. Commun. Dis*. 1, 225, (1986).
[97] P. B. Bloland, *Drug resistance in malaria*. WHO/CDS/CSR/DRS/2001.4, (2001).
[98] D. N. Nabarro and E. M. Talyer, *Science*, 280, 2067, (1998).
[99] M. Enserink, Malaria's drug miracle in danger. *Science*. pp. 844, (2010).
[100] N. J. White, *Lancet,* 376, 2051, (2010).
[101] C. Wongsrichanalai and S. R. Meshnick, *Emerg. Infect. Dis*. 14, 716, (2008).
[102] J. F. Cortese, A. Caraballo, C. E. Contreras and C. V. Plowe, *J. Infect. Dis*. 186, 999, (2002).
[103] M. M. Nyunt and C. V. Plowe, *Clin. Pharmacol. Ther*. 82, 601, (2007).

[104] WHO. *Global Report on Antimalarial Drug Efficacy and Drug Resistance*: 2000-2010. Geneva: WHO, (2010).
[105] D. A. Henderson, *Bull. World Health Organ.* 65, 535, (1987).
[106] J. John, *Expert. Rev. Vaccines*, 8, 5, (2009).
[107] W. J. Moss and D. E. Griffin, *Nat. Rev. Microbiol.* 12, 900, (2006).
[108] J. G. Breman, C. A. de Quadros, W. R. Dowdle, W. H. Foege, D. A. Henderson and et al., *PLoS Med.* 8, e1000405, (2011).
[109] The malERA Consultative Group on Vaccines. *PLoS Med.*, 8(1), e1000398, (2011).
[110] UNDP/World Bank/WHO (TDR). *Malaria transmission blocking vaccines*: an ideal public good. TDR/RBM/MAL/VAC/2000.1. (2001).
[111] J. L. Cole-Tobian, P. Michon, M. Biasor, and et al., *Infect. Immun.* 77, 4009, (2009).
[112] D. Butler, Nature, 462, 19. (2009).
[113] A. Saul and M. P. Fay, *PLoS One,* 2, e850, (2007).
[114] *Malaria Vaccine Technology Roadmap Final Report* (2006) Available: http://www.malariavaccineroadmap.net.
[115] WHO. Malaria transmission blocking vaccines: An ideal public good. Geneva: World Health Organization. (2000) Available: http://www.who.int/vaccine_research/feuille_1_4-1pdf.
[116] R. Carter, *Vaccine*, 19, 2309, (2001).
[117] Y. Wu, R. D. Ellis, D. Shaffer and et al., *PLoS One,* 3, e2636, (2008).
[118] R. R. Dinglasan and M. Jacobs-Lorena, *Trends Parasitol.* 24, 364, (2008).
[119] PATH Malaria Vaccine Initiative: *The PATH Malaria Vaccine Initiative [fact sheet].* Seattle: PATH; 2010. [http://www.malariavaccine.org//files/March182011MVIfactsheet_backgrounder.pdf].
[120] K. P. Asante, S. Abdulla, S. Agnandji, J. Lyimo, J. Vekemans, S. Soulanoudjingar, R. Owusu and et al., Safety, immunogenicity and efficacy of the RTS,S/AS01E malaria vaccine candidate integrated in EPI: extended follow-up of a randomized controlled Phase 2 infant trial in Gabon, Ghana and Tanzania. *Presented at: 59th annual meeting of the American Society of Tropical Medicine and Hygiene*, Atlanta; November 5, (2010).
[121] D. I. Ojakaa, P. Ofwar, Y. W. Machira, E. Yamo, Y. Collymore, A. Ba-Nguz, P. Vansadia and A. Bingham, *Malar. J.* 10, 147, (2011).
[122] M. Jacobs-Lorena. *J. Vect. Borne Dis.* 40, 73, (2003).
[123] A. Ghosh, M. J. Edwards and M. Jacobs-Lorena, *Parasitol. Today* 16, 196, (2000).
[124] L. A. Moreira and M. Jacobs-Lorena, *Neotrop. Entomol.* 32(4), 531, (2003).
[125] D. A. Amenya, M. Bonizzoni, A. T. Isaacs, N. Jasinskiene, H. Chen, O, Marinotti, G. Yan and AA. James, *Insect Mol. Biol.* 19(2), 263, (2010).
[126] WHO. Progress and prospects for the use of genetically modified mosquitoes to inhibit disease transmission. *World Health Organization*, Geneva, Switzerland, 4-6 May 2009.
[127] B. A. Ayyub. *Risk analysis in engineering and economics*. Boca Raton, USA, Chapman and Hall/CRC, (2002).
[128] V. Dyck, J. Hendrichs and A. Robinson, eds. Sterile insect technique: *principles and practice in area-wide integrated pest management.* Dordrecht, Springer, (2005).
[129] E. Knipling, *J. Econ. Entomol.* 48, 459, (1955).

[130] L. Alphey. Population suppression strategies for dengue virus vector control (Aedes). Progress and prospects for the use of genetically modified mosquitoes to inhibit disease transmission. *World Health Organization*, Geneva, Switzerland, 4-6 May 2009.
[131] M. Q. Benedict and A. S. Robinson, *Trends Parasitol.* 19, 349, (2003).
[132] W. Klassen and C. Curtis. History of the sterile insect technique, In: V. Dyck, J. Hendrichs, A. Robinson, eds. Sterile insect technique: *principles and practice in area-wide integrated pest management.* Dordrecht, Springer, pp 53, (2005).
[133] C. Lofgren, and et al., *Am. J. Trop. Med. Hyg.* 23, 288, (1974).
[134] H. Laven, *Nature*, 216, 383, (1967).
[135] S. Dobson, C. Fox and F. Jiggins, *Proceed. R. Biol. Soc.* 269, 437, (2002).
[136] C. Brelsfoard, Y. Sechan and S. Dobson, *PLoS Negl. Trop. Dis.* 2, e129, (2008).
[137] M. Q. Benedict. Conventional sterile insect technique against Anopheles arabiensis. Progress and prospects for the use of genetically modified mosquitoes to inhibit disease transmission. *World Health Organization*, Geneva, Switzerland. (2009).
[138] M. H. Andreasen and C. F. Curtis, *Med. Vet. Entomol.* 19, 238, (2005).
[139] M. Helinski, A. Parker and B. Knols, *Malar. J.* 5, 41, (2006). doi:10.1186/1475-2875-5-41
[140] B. G. J. Knols, H. C. Bossin, W. R. Mukabana and A. S. Robinson, *Am. J. Trop. Med.Hyg.* 77(6), 232, (2007).
[141] S. P. Sinkins and F. Gould, *Nat. Rev. Genet.* 7, 427, (2006).
[142] O. Terenius, O. Marinotti, D. Sieglaff and A. A. James, *Cell Host Microbe.* 13: 417, (2008).
[143] M. Tanner and D. de Savign. Malaria eradication back on the table. http://www.who.int/bulletin/volumes/86/2/07-050633/en/ (accessed on 2nd June 2011).
[144] The malERA Consultative Group on Basic Science and Enabling Technologies. *PLoS Med.* 8(1), e1000399. (2011).
[145] Roll Back Malaria Partnership (2008) The global malaria action plan for a malaria free world. Geneva: RBM, Available: http://www.rollbackmalaria.org/gmap/gmap.pdf.
[146] K. Mendis, A. Rietveld, M. Warsame, A. Bosman, B. Greenwood and et al., *Trop. Med. Int. Health*, 14, 802, (2009).

In: Malaria: Etiology, Pathogenesis and Treatments
Editors: A. M. Peterson and G. E. Calamandrei
ISBN: 978-1-62100-363-2

Chapter IV

Malaria: An Infection with Global Impact

Ritesh G. Menezes[1], Sadip Pant[2], Tanuj Kanchan[3], S. Senthilkumaran[4], Magdy A. Kharoshah[5], Ramadas Naik[6], Y. P. Raghavendra Babu[3], P. P. Jagadish Rao[3], and Abul Fazil[7]

[1] Department of Forensic Medicine, Srinivas Institute of Medical Sciences and Research Centre, Mangalore, India
[2] Department of Internal Medicine, University of Arkansas for Medical Sciences, Little Rock, Arkansas, US
[3] Department of Forensic Medicine, Kasturba Medical College, Mangalore, India
[4] Department of Emergency and Critical Care Medicine, Sri Gokulam Hospital and Research Institute, Salem, India
[5] Forensic Medicine Authority, Ministry of Justice, Egypt
[6] Department of Pathology, Kasturba Medical College, Mangalore, India
[7] Department of General Medicine, Kasturba Medical College, Mangalore, India

Abstract

Malaria is a major public health problem in developing countries and is the top ranked priority tropical disease of the World Health Organization. It is a leading cause of disease and death among children under five years, pregnant women and non-immune travellers/immigrants. Every year, there are about 500 million clinical attacks of malaria. Of these, 2-3 million are severe and about 1 million people die (about 3000 deaths every day). Malaria in pregnancy accounts for about 25% of cases of severe maternal anemia and 10-20% of low birth weight. About 40% of the world's population is at risk of malaria. According to the World Malaria Report, malaria is prevalent in 108 countries of the tropical and semitropical world (Africa; Amazon, central and southern America; central, south and southeast Asia; Pacific). The economic burden of malaria is huge, estimated to be $12 billion a year in Africa alone. Known since millennia, malaria continues to upsurge in incidence till date due to a variety of factors including but not limited to drug resistance, global climate change, changing agricultural practices, insecticide resistance mosquitoes, population movements and poverty, and political instability.

Malaria is caused by the protozoa Plasmodium (P) and transmitted by the bite of an infected female anopheline mosquito. There are five species known to cause infection namely, P. falciparum, P. vivax, P. ovale, P. malariae, and P. knowlesi. Infection due to P species other than P. falciparum is called non-falciparum malaria. P. falciparum causes the most severe disease and patients with this form of malaria may progress to life-threatening illness within hours. The P life cycle consists of an exoerythrocytic (asymptomatic) stage and erythrocytic (symptomatic) stage. Several human genetic polymorphisms and mutations have been observed to influence either clinical attack or severity of the disease, particularly hemoglobin and red cell antigens. Individuals living in endemic areas appear to develop partial immunity to malaria following repeated infections. Although malaria classically presents as a febrile paroxysm with headache, myalgia, nausea, vomiting, malaise, splenomegaly, anemia and thrombocytopenia, it is a great imitator and trickster with varied and dramatic manifestations especially in endemic regions. Malaria diagnostic tools include clinical criteria, light microscopy, rapid diagnostic tests (RDTs), and molecular diagnostic techniques. Light microscopy remains the gold standard for diagnosis of malaria; it permits determination of the infecting species as well as quantification of parasitemia, facilitating monitoring the response to therapy. Malarial target antigen for RDTs includes histidine-rich protein 2 of P. falciparum, a pan-malarial Plasmodium aldolase, and the parasite specific lactate dehydrogenase. Molecular technologies have been developed to improve the diagnosis of malaria, although these methods are limited by a number of factors including specialized equipment, continuing supplies, operator expertise, turnaround time and cost. Treatment of chloroquine sensitive non-falciparum malaria comprises administration of chloroquine followed by standard course of primaquine for radical cure. Therapeutic options for chloroquine resistance non-falciparum malaria include mefloquine, atovaquone-proguanil or a combination of quinine and tetracycline or doxycycline. Parenteral antimalarial is often required for falciparum malaria and includes artmisinin derivative or qunine/quinidine along with doxycycline or clindamycin. Artesunate is the preferred therapy for treatment of severe falciparum malaria in adults and children wherever intravenous artesunate is available. Strategies for malaria control include mosquito vector control, personal protection from mosquito bites and chemoprophylaxis. Malaria vaccine is still under trial.

Although mortality is rare with non-falciparum malaria, for patients with complicated falciparum malaria the mortality approaches 10-20%. Medico-legal autopsies in cases of sudden unexpected natural deaths have revealed malaria as the cause of death in a few cases. In a study conducted at Government Wenlock District Hospital in Mangalore, a malaria endemic area in South India, autopsy files revealed 5 cases of sudden death due to malaria diagnosed by histopathology between September 2004 and August 2008. Cerebral malaria, acute renal insufficiency, acute pulmonary edema and acute respiratory distress syndrome are possible mechanisms of sudden death due to malaria.

1. Introduction

The history of malaria predates humanity. No disease has afflicted the mankind history and settlement patterns as much as malaria. The causal association of malaria with marshy land can be found in the literature as old as 1740 by Horace Walpole which was responsible for its nomenclature (Italian "mala" bad and "aria" air). In 1800, a French army surgeon Charles Louis Alphonse Laveran noticed motile parasites in the blood of a patient suffering from malaria. Since then, a lot of effort has been made to understand the biology of this parasite and uncover effective prevention and control measures. Four Nobel prizes have been awarded for malaria related research so far. Yet, malaria continues to inflict havoc on millions, predominantly in the poorest regions of the world. In regards to overall mortality from infectious diseases worldwide, malaria stands fifth after respiratory infections, HIV/AIDS, diarrheal diseases, and tuberculosis. However, in Africa it is second only to HIV/AIDS in inflicting deaths [1-5]. It is the topmost cause of disease and death worldwide in children aged less than 5 years of age, pregnant women and travellers/non immune immigrants. Malaria is a major public health problem in developing countries and is the top ranked priority tropical disease of the World Health Organization (WHO). There are approximately 500 million clinical attacks of malaria worldwide annually. Among them, 2-3 million cases are severe and about a million people die a year (about 3000 deaths every day) [1 4]. Malaria in pregnancy accounts for about 25% of cases of severe maternal anaemia and 10-20% of low birth weight. About 40% of the world's population is at risk of malaria. According to the World Malaria Report, the disease is prevalent in 108 countries of the tropical and semitropical zones including Africa, Amazon, central and southern America, central, south and south-east Asia, and the Pacific [1]. The global economic burden of malaria is huge and estimated to be $18 million annually; $12 billion a year in Africa alone [6]. It continues to upsurge in incidence till date due to a variety of factors including but not limited to drug resistance, global climate change, changing agricultural practices, insecticide resistance mosquitoes, population movements, and poverty and political instability.

2. Epidemiology

2.1. Agent

Malaria is caused by Plasmodium (P), which is an obligate intracellular protozoa. Five species of Plasmodium are responsible for diseases in humans: P. falciparum (malignant tertian malaria); P. vivax (benign tertian malaria); P. ovale (ovale malaria); P. malariae (quartan malaria) and P. knowlesi (this species has not yet been proven to be transmitted from humans to mosquitoes and a monkey reservoir may be required to infect mosquitoes) [6]. P. falciparum accounts for nearly all deaths and severe disease due to malaria. A comparison table of important characteristics of different Plasmodium species is given below in table 1 [7-15].

2.2. Transmission Pattern

The epidemiology of malaria can be viewed as being stable or unstable based on transmission patterns and intensities. Stable malaria refers to high transmission intensities without marked fluctuation over years although seasonal fluctuations may occur. Different areas can experience different levels of transmission intensities. These areas (Table 2) are designated as hypoendemic, mesoendemic, hyperendemic, or holoendemic based on prevalence of infection in children aged 2 to 9 years of age (which in turn has been traditionally defined by spleen or parasite rates) [15,16].

Table 1. Salient Features of Different Plasmodium Species [7-15]

Species	P. *vivax*	P. *falciparum*	P. *malariae*	P. *ovale*	P. *knowlesi*
Geographic Distribution	70-90% of cases in most of Asia and South America, 50-60% of cases in South East Asia and western Pacific, 1-10% in Africa.	80-90% of cases in Africa, 40-50% of cases in western Pacific and South East Asia, 4-30% in South Asia, South America and rest of tropics.	2-3% in Africa, sporadic in Asia and South America	Even more uncommon and rare outside Africa.	Identified by molecular techniques in patients in Malaysia, the Philippines, Thailand, and Myanmar.
Distinguishing microscopic features	Commonly rings only; Maurer's clefts; crescentic gametocytes	Schuffner's dots, irregular trophozoites	Band forms	Large nuclei; Schuffner's dots, irregular trophozoites	Resembles P. malariae
Exo-erythrocytic cycle (Days)	8	5.5	15	9	8-9
Erythrocytic cycle (Hours)	48	36-48	72	48	24
Number of merozoites per hepatic schizonts	10000	40000	2000	15000	Unknown
Persistent exo-erythrocytic cycle	Yes	No	No	Yes	No
Fever pattern	Tertian	Tertian	Tertian	Quartan	Quotodian
Relapses	Yes	No	No	Yes	No
Recrudescence	No	Yes	Yes	No	No
Erythrocyte preference	Reticulocytes	All	Only mature RBCs	Reticulocytes	Unknown
Severe malaria	Up to 24%	Up to 22 %	Very rare	Very rare	6-10%
Drug resistance	Yes	Yes	No	No	No

Table 2. Epidemiological Classification of Malaria [15,16]

- Hypoendemic: spleen rate or parasite rate 0–10%
- Mesoendemic: spleen or parasite rate 10–50%
- Hyperendemic: spleen or parasite rate 50–75%
- Holoendemic: spleen or parasite rate over 75%

People dwelling in highly endemic areas exhibit a high immunity level and tolerate the infection well. Endemicity is relatively insensitive to changes in climate or local habitats and epidemic is unlikely. Conversely, unstable malaria refers to fluctuating transmission pattern from year to year. In such areas of low endemicity, population is non immune and thus morbidity and mortality from infection can be high. Outbreaks of disease can occur in such areas due to changes in the ecology like human migration and resettlement, natural disasters, construction works like road building, etc.

2.3. Transmission Modes

Malaria is spread to humans by bite of an infected female anophiline mosquito. Blood meal is required by female mosquitoes to lay eggs. Male mosquitoes do not suck blood but feed on plant sap. Other rare modes of malaria transmission include blood transfusion, transplacental route (congenital malaria), through contaminated needles and organ transplantation [17]. There are more than 480 species of anophiline mosquitoes of which approximately 50 are proven vectors. Important vectors include *An. gambiae* complex and *An. funestus* in Africa, *An. freeborni* in North America, *An. culicifacies, An. fluviatilis, An. minimus, An. philippinensis, An. stephensi,* and *An. sundaicus* in the Indian subcontinent [18, 19].

2.4. Host

Humans are the only significant parasite reservoir and sustained transmission is dependent on maintaining a pool of infected individuals and contact between them and the mosquitoes. Various factors influence the susceptibility to infection. These include immune status of the individual and prior exposure to malaria, certain genetic diseases and polymorphisms, pregnancy, and HIV infection. These factors are discussed elsewhere in the present chapter.

2.5. Environment

Transmission of malaria is profoundly influenced by climate. The optimal conditions are environmental temperatures between 20 and 30 degree Celsius and relative humidity of at least 60%. Malaria transmission does not occur at temperatures below 16 degree Celsius or above 33 degree Celsius and at altitudes more than 2000 meters because development of malaria parasite in mosquito (sporogony) fails to take place [15-20]. Malaria is common during rainy season because stagnant water and high humidity favor mosquito breeding and survival. Streams, water tanks, pits, cisterns, and overhead tanks are favored breeding sites of a mosquito. *An. gambiae* prefers small, open, clean water bodies, including those created by cattle hoofprints or tracked by vehicle tyres. *An. funestus* breeds in larger, open, clean water bodies such as small ponds. .*An. fluviatalis* breeds in moving water, while *An. sundicus* prefers brackish (salty) water [15]. Irrigation schemes, dams, deforestation, agricultural practice, natural disasters, etc. can influence mosquito population and alter patterns of malaria transmission.

3. Life Cycle of Malaria Parasite

The life cycle of Plasmodium shuttles between human and the female anopheles mosquito. It has three stages:

3.1. Preerythrocytic (Exo-Erythrocytic Schizogony) or Hepatic (Tissue) Phase

Infection begins with the introduction of sporozoites (the infective stage of the parasite) into the host circulation when a female anopheles takes a blood meal. 8-15 sporozoites are typically injected in one bite and within 30-45 minutes of the bite, sporozoites disappear from the blood stream. Some enter hepatocytes while others are cleared by phagocytes. Sporozoites themselves do not produce the disease but multiply profusely over a period of 6-16 days to form a very large number of merozoites (about 10,000-30,000 in each infected hepatocyte) [21,22,23]. The swollen hepatocyte ruptures releasing the merozoites into the circulation. These merozoites invade erythrocytes but cannot infect hepatocytes or start a fresh cycle of pre-erythrocytic schizogony. This phase is asymptomatic and constitutes the incubation period of malaria [24]. In P. vivax and P. ovale infections some of the intrahepatic sporozoites do not develop immediately but rather remain dormant for months to upto five years before reproduction begins. These are known as hypnozoites or "sleeping forms" and are responsible for relapses associated with these species. On the other hand, P. falciparum and P. malariae have no persistent liver forms and therefore relapses do not occur in infection with these species. But they can cause recrudescence of infection due to persistent erythrocytic forms [15].

3.2. Erythrocytic Schizogony

Merozoites enter erythrocytes via multiple receptor ligand interactions rapidly (seconds to a few minutes). Attachment of the parasite is mediated by specific erythrocyte surface receptors e.g. Duffy binding protein and reticulocyte homology protein for P. vivax and glycophorins for P. falciparum [25, 26]. Different plasmodium species target erythrocytes of different age, e.g. P. vivax and P. ovale primarily invade mature erythrocytes, P. malariae invades only mature erythrocytes, and P. falciparum invades both. Thus, parasitemia (number of infected erythrocytes) in the cases of P. vivax, P. ovale and P. malariae species is generally less than 2%. By contrast, parasitemia as high as 60% can occur with P. falciparum. Once inside the RBCs, the young trophozoites appear as "ring forms" during the early phase of development (<12 hours). The parasites rapidly consume hemoglobin within RBCs and grow into an irregular and amoeboid form. Approximately 36 hours after merozoites invasion, repeated nuclear division occurs (merogony) and erythrocytes burst to release 6-32 daughter merozoites. These invade uninfected erythrocytes and the cycle is repeated until it is contained by the host's own immunity, antimalarial drugs, or a combination of two [15, 25]. The cycle repeats every 48 hours in P. vivax, P. ovale, and P. falciparum infection (tertian) and every 72 hours (quartan) in P. malariae infection. Generally it requires 5-7 days before a sufficient number of schizonts rupture at the same time and infection becomes synchronized. Hence malaria paroxysm is often absent in the initial days of the illness. Further, cases where more than one brood of the parasite is developing in the blood at different times, periodicity is not found and fever may occur daily (quotidian). This is particularly true for P. falciparum infection where fever may never regularize to a tertian or subtertian (every 36 hours) patterns. After a period of erythrocytic schizogony, a small proportion of merozoites differentiate into sexual forms known as microgametocytes (male) and macrogametocytes (female) necessary for completing the cycle in the mosquitoes.

3.3. Sexual Development

The gametocytes are taken up by the mosquito during the blood meal. They move to the stomach (midgut) of the mosquito where further development occurs. Microgametocytes divide into 4-8 microgametes; each of which fuse with a macrogamete to form a zygote. Zygote develops into a motile ookinete within 18-24 hours. Ookinete penetrates the gastric epithelium to lie between the epithelial cells and the basal lamina and develops into oocyst. The oocyst grows in size by repeated meiotic divisions called sporogony to form sporozoites. This generally takes 8-35 days depending on external temperature and species of parasite and mosquito. Finally, the oocyst ruptures releasing thousands of motile sporozoites into the coelomic cavity of the mosquito from where they migrate to the salivary glands. Humans are infected at the next bite, thus completing the life cycle [27].

4. Pathogenesis

The pathophysiology of malaria is complex and results from red cell destruction and the host's response to this phenomenon. Only blood stage of the parasite is involved in the pathogenesis of malaria.

4.1. Cytokine Storm

At the end of each erythrocytic schizogony, the rupture of infected erythrocytes releases numerous known and unknown substances which induce the release of cytokines in much the same way as bacterial endotoxin. These products, particularly the glycosylphosphatidyl inositol act directly on macrophages and endothelial cells to secrete inflammatory mediators like TNF alpha, IL-1, IL-6, IL-10, interferon-γ, macrophage inflammatory protein chemokines MIP1α and MIP1β, lymphotoxin and nitric oxide (NO). Many studies have indicated the GPI anchor which is common to several merozoite surface proteins such as MSP-1, MSP-2, and MSP-4, as the major parasite toxin [28-30]. The GPI anchor covalently links proteins including the malaria parasite surface antigens to the cell membrane lipid bilayer. Similarly, the plasmodial DNA is also highly proinflammatory. This DNA (presented by hemozoin) is produced during the parasite development inside RBCs. It interacts with Toll-like receptor-9 intracellularly causing release of proinflammatory mediators that in turn induce COX-2-upregulating prostaglandins leading to the induction of fever [31, 32]. Hemozoin related induction of apoptosis in budding erythroid cells in the bone marrow has been linked to anemia [33, 34]. Cytokines are responsible for multisystem pathology and explain diverse features such as fever, malaise, dyserythropoiesis, hypoglycemia, placental dysfunction, vascular damage, and upregulation of intracellular adhesion molecules (particularly ICAM-1 thereby promoting cytoadherance).

4.2. Cytoadherence, Resetting and Sequestration

These are central to the pathogenesis of falciparum malaria. The trophozoite and schizont stages of P. falciparum induce the formation of thousands of sticky electron dense protuberances on the surface of erythrocytes. These bind via receptor ligand interactions to venular and capillary endothelium (called cytoadherence) and to unaffected erythrocytes called (rosette formation) [35-41]. The knobs are primarily composed of P. falciparum erythrocyte membrane protein-1 (P*f*EMP-1). *Pf*EMP-1 is the product of a highly variable (*var*) gene family with at least 60 different genes. This antigenic variation associated with the surface exposed *Pf*EMP-1 allows the parasite to evade the immune system [19]. Some of the important host receptors for such interactions include ICAM-1 (vascular endothelium), CD36 (on endothelium and platelets), and CSA (in the placenta) and Complement Receptor 1 (CR1 on erythrocytes mediates rossetting). Cytoadherence and rosetting leads to sequestration of infected red cells within the microvasculature resulting in partial blood flow obstruction, endothelial barrier breakdown, and inflammation. Sequestration often leads to the disappearance of infected erythrocytes containing mature forms of P. falciparum from circulation. This is the reason why the mature forms of P. falciparum are hardly found in the peripheral smears and the degree of parasitemia may be greatly underestimated. Sequestration occurs in the venules of various organs, being greatest in the brain followed by the heart, liver, kidneys, and intestine and least in the skin [35-41].

4.3. Immune Response to Malaria

Host response to malaria is complex and not completely understood. Both specific and non specific cell mediated and humoral mechanisms are activated in response to infection. As a result, a person from endemic region is protected from severe illness but not from infection and develops tolerance to infection (cessation of clinical phenomenon despite parasitemia). This state of partial immunity is known as permunition. It is species and strain specific and is believed to result from less production of cytokines by macrophages for a given load of parasite. Therefore asymptomatic parasitemia is common among older children and adults in areas of high transmission intensities [42-44]. Immune persons have a polyclonal increase in serum IgM, IgG2, and IgA, although much of these antibodies are not protective in nature. The factors that prevent the development of effective immune response against malaria include lack of MHC class I and class II molecules on the surface of infective erythrocytes, enormous diversity of malarial strains, periodic alteration of the antigenic protein composition on the erythrocyte surface and non specific activation of the immune system that interfere with the development of specific cellular immunity ('immunological smokescreen') [27]. In endemic regions, newborns and young infants are protected against malaria by antibodies acquired transplacentally and through breast milk, and fetal hemoglobin (HbF) which retards the development of the parasite. Finally, HIV infection is associated with increased susceptibility, higher parasitemia, and an increased risk for recurrent malaria infection, particularly in patients with CD4 counts <200 cells/μL [45].

4.4. Genetics

Human genetic polymorphism is one of the important host factors modulating malaria infection. People who are heterozygotes for sickle cell anemia, thalassemia, glucose-6-phosphate dehydrogenase (G6PD) deficiency, and hereditary ovalocytosis are resistant to malaria [25]. The relative protection conferred against malaria in heterozygotes living in endemic areas has ensured the survival of a gene that is generally fatal in homozygotes (balanced polymorphisms). The probable mechanisms include: 1] Poor penetration of erythrocytes by merozoites. 2] Diminished growth of parasite. 3] Rapid clearance by the reticuloendothelial system. 4] Oxidative injury to erythrocytes membrane in heterozygotes may be responsible for premature death of the malaria parasite [27]. Similarly, individuals lacking the Duffy antigens (largely observed in West and sub Saharan Africa are resistant to infection with the P. vivax because of lack of surface receptors required for entry into RBCs [27]. Further a convincing association has been reported between HLA polymorphism and susceptibility to an infection. The presence of HLA Class I antigen BW 53 and HLA Class II halotype (DRB1 1302-DQB1 0501) has been found to confer protection against P. falciparum malaria [15]. Finally, polymorphisms in tumor necrosis factor (TNF) genes appear to influence the severity of P. falciparum infection. In a large case controlled study in Gambian children, a sevenfold increased risk of severe neurological sequelae or death from cerebral malaria was observed among those who were homozygous for a polymorphism in the promoter region of the TNF gene (TNF2 allele) [46,47].

4.5. Itching and Immunity

There has been a speculation that the itching mechanism confers relative protection against malarial infection among residents of malaria endemic regions as their daily peak of itch sensitivity overlaps with the peak biting phase of female Anopheles mosquitoes. On the other hand, there could be an increased susceptibility to malaria in individuals visiting endemic regions from different time zones during the phase of jet-lag due to the disturbed circadian rhythm controlling the itch mechanism. Therefore, it is hypothesized that individuals suffering from jet-lag are more prone to malaria as their peak protective daily behavioral itch sensitivity does not overlap with the peak biting phase of female Anopheles mosquitoes when compared to the residents of endemic regions [48]. However, whether this hypothesis in actuality operates not to confer malaria protection to jet-lagged travelers when compared to endemic residents and more importantly, if at all it doesn't, how significant it is in comparison to the more evident lack of preformed circulating antibodies in jet-lagged travelers when compared to preformed circulating antibody mediated relative protection among pre-sensitized endemic residents, is an area of further research [49].

5. Clinical Features

The incubation period (time from sporozoite inoculation to the onset of fever) ranges from 12-35 days (shortest for P. falciparum and longest for P. malariae). This, however, can be prolonged by chemoprophylaxis and host immunity. In areas of high P. falciparum transmission, severe disease is mainly confined to children below 5 years of age and infrequent with increasing age (also known as stable malaria) [42-44]. On the other hand, with lower or seasonal transmission pattern, and when non immune person visits endemic areas, severe malaria can affect both children and adults (unstable malaria). While malaria is thought to a be a febrile illness with a classical pattern and related symptoms, in malaria endemic regions it can present with such varied and dramatic manifestations that it needs to be considered as a differential diagnosis for almost all the clinical problems.

5.1. Uncomplicated Malaria

The clinical picture of uncomplicated malaria is common to all four species. The classical malarial paroxysm consists of three successive stages, namely, the cold stage, the hot stage, and the sweating stage [15]. Cold stage is characterized by a sudden rise in temperature and may last anywhere from 15 minutes to 90 minutes. Chills and rigors are the hallmark feature of this stage. This is followed by a hot stage where the patient develops high grade fever (which may even reach beyond 106 F) with severe headache, anorexia, lethargy, myalgia, nausea, and vomiting. The hot stage lasts 2-6 hours. Profuse sweating and rapid fall in temperature over 2-3 hours constitute the final stage (the sweating stage). The entire paroxysm may last upto 8-12 hours and between the episodes, the patient appears well. In cases of infection with P. vivax and P. ovale malaria, this typical pattern of fever recurs once every 48 hours and this is called *benign tertian malaria.* In falciparum infection, this pattern may *(malignant tertian malaria)* or may not be seen and the paroxysms tend to be more frequent *(sub-tertian malaria).* In P. malariae infection, recurrence of fever occurs every 72 hours and is called *quartan malaria.* This classical malarial pattern is not seen in early infection, immune individuals (residents of endemic regions), following drug treatment, and infection with two or more species.

The hallmark physical finding is splenomegaly. Spleen becomes palpable towards the end of the first week of illness; it is soft and occasionally tender. The liver may be enlarged, soft and sometimes tender. There may be anemia and slight jaundice. Absence of lymphadenopathy and skin rash is useful negative finding in malaria [27].

5.2. Acute Severe (Complicated) Malaria

Severe malaria is defined as acute malaria with high levels of parasitemia (>5% in low transmission areas and >10% in high transmission areas) and/or major signs of organ dysfunction [27,50,51]. One or more of the following features in the presence of asexual parasitemia defines severe malaria: 1] Cerebral malaria. 2] Severe anemia (hemoglobin <5 g/dl or hematocrit <15%). 3] Acute renal failure. 4] Pulmonary edema or ARDS. 5] Hypoglycemia (blood glucose <40 mg/dl). 6] Shock. 7] Disseminated intravascular coagulation (DIC). 8] Repeated generalized convulsions (>2 episodes a day). 9] Acidemia. 10] Hemoglobinuria. Almost all severe morbidity and mortality in malaria is caused by P. falciparum. Severe malaria is a medical emergency.

5.3. Cerebral Malaria

Cerebral malaria is a complex clinicopathologic syndrome characterized by an unarousable state (Blantyre coma score ≤ 2) in the setting of P. falciparum parasitemia demonstrable in the peripheral blood and all other causes of altered neurological status (e.g. hypoglycemia, febrile seizures, bacterial meningitis and viral encephalitis) ruled out [50-52]. The Blantyre coma score is a clinical indicator of severity in children with altered consciousness due to malaria. It was developed based on modifications of Glasgow coma score because some key Glasgow indicators are not appropriate for evaluation of altered consciousness in pediatric malaria [53,54]. Although the cerebral malaria definition demands presence of unarousable coma, it should be noted that in a patient with P. falciparum malaria, any degree of neurological manifestation should be treated as a case of cerebral malaria until proven otherwise. It is the most dreaded complication of P. falciparum infection with 15-20% mortality despite treatment [52].

The onset is generally sudden with high fever for a few days followed by cerebral dysfunction including altered level of consciousness, abnormal neurological signs, delirium, seizures, and coma. There may be pallor, jaundice, and hepatosplenomegaly. Cerebral malaria is a state of diffuse, symmetric encephalopathy. Neurological signs are variable and include deep coma, variable muscle tone and tendon reflexes, absent abdominal reflexes, upgoing plantar in half the patients, opisthotonus, and decerebrate or decorticate posturing. Mild neck stiffness may be present but meningeal signs, cranial nerve abnormalities, and signs of raised intracranial tension are absent. Papilledema is rare but retinal hemorrhages are found in 15% of cases with indirect ophthalmoscopy and 30-40% of cases with papillary dilatation [55]. A variety of transient eye movement abnormalities is common, the commonest being disconjugate gaze [15].

With treatment, the recovery is fast. Most of the children regain consciousness within 24-48 hours. Neurological sequel in the form of hemiparesis, ataxia, cortical blindness, mental retardation and aphasia are seen more in children (10%) than in adults (3%) [15].

5.4. Severe Anemia

Profound anemia can develop rapidly in malaria which may lead to high output cardiac failure and death. Anemia in malaria is attributed to several mechanisms including destruction of parasitized as well as unparasitized erythrocytes (by immune mechanisms), dyserythropoiesis, hypersplenism and hemolysis associated with drug treatment. The problem is often compounded by pre-existing anemia secondary to malnutrition and helminthiasis in the developing nations. Anemia is normocytic, normochromic and reticulocyte count is often low or normal.

5.5. Blackwater Fever

This is characterized by sudden massive intravascular hemolysis, not explicable by G6PD deficiency, which occurs following P. falciparum infection. While this mystifying entity has been classically attributed to quinine related immune hemolysis, the results are inconclusive [15]. As a result, there is a passage of dark colored urine due to hemoglobinuria, hence the name 'blackwater fever'. Due to hemolysis, the hemoglobin estimation is unreliable and so is the parasite load estimation. Blackwater fever is usually transient, devoid of any renal impairment and resolves without any complication. However, in severe cases acute renal failure and peripheral circulatory failure may ensue [15].

5.6. Hypoglycemia

It is a common biochemical abnormality in severe malaria and may lead to general deterioration and death within a short very span of time. It is common in children (up to 25%) and pregnant women. Factors responsible for hypoglycemia include cytokine-induced suppression of gluconeogenesis, increased glucose consumption by the host (and to a lesser extent by the parasite) and quinine-stimulated pancreatic insulin secretion. It is not possible to detect hypoglycemia clinically as the manifestations are indistinguishable from those due to severe malaria itself [15,27]. Therefore, frequent blood glucose monitoring should be done in all cases of severe malaria. Quinine stimulated hypoglycemia can be prevented by administering quinine infusion slowly over 4 hours in 5% or 10% dextrose solutions.

5.7. Algid Malaria

The term algid malaria is obsolete now (L."algidus"=cold). Majority of patients with severe malaria remain well perfused and warm, but some develop shock with cold periphery. This is known as algid malaria and most of the time results from secondary gram negative bacteremia. Severe malaria predisposes to bacterial infections due to transient immunosuppression and altered macrophage function [56,57]. In endemic areas, Salmonella bacteremia has been associated with P. falciparum infections [57]. Catheter-induced urinary tract infections and chest infections are common. Splenic rupture can also cause shock in patients with malaria due to hypovolemia.

5.8. Other Features

Renal failure, pulmonary edema, jaundice, DIC and metabolic acidosis are other important manifestations of severe malaria. Renal failure is caused by acute tubular necrosis secondary to interference of renal microcirculation by sequestered erythrocytes [58]. Glomerulonephritis is very rare and reported following P. malariae malaria [15,58]. Pulmonary edema arises due to cytokine induced increased permeability of pulmonary capillary, a finding not observed in other vascular beds [27,59,60]. It may be precipitated by excessive potential fluid therapy. Severe jaundice due to hemolysis, hepatic dysfunction and/or cholestasis may occur with P. falciparum malaria. While thrombocytopenia and mild coagulopathy are common with falciparum malaria, frank DIC with evidence of bleeding may occur in <5% of patients with severe falciparum malaria [15,27]. It is the consequence of activation of the coagulation cascade by the parasitized erythrocyte and cytokines with or without secondary bacterial infection. Metabolic acidosis, an important cause of death, is attributed to anaerobic glycolysis in host tissue, hypovolemia, failure of renal and hepatic clearance of lactate and lactate production by the parasite.

5.9. Congenital Malaria

Congenital malaria is rare with occurrence rate of around 0.3% in immune mothers and 7.4% in non immune mothers [61-66]. It can be caused by all 4 species of the parasite. Symptomatic congenital malaria is rare despite parasitemia in endemic areas due to transplacental transfer of protective maternal IgG antibodies and a high proportion of HbF which inhibit parasite development. It usually manifests between the second and eighth weeks of life although presentation as early as day one or as late as months have been reported. Clinical features include fever, irritability, poor feeding, lethargy, anemia, jaundice, and hepatosplenomegaly (closely resembling neonatal sepsis and TORCH infection). Further, it is an important cause of abortion, stillbirths, premature births, and intrauterine growth retardation in endemic areas [61-67]. Placenta may be black in colour due to malarial pigment with or without the presence of parasites in tissue sections. Since there is no exoerythrocytic stage in congenital P. vivax and P. ovale infection, radical cure with primaquine is not required [15,27,61-67].

5.10. Chronic Complications of Malaria

Repeated infection with malaria can cause chronic complications like tropical splenomegaly syndrome, nephrotic syndrome (secondary to P. malariae and is called quartan malaria nephropathy), endemic Burkitt's lymphoma, and possibly endomyocardial fibrosis.

5.11. Tropical Splenomegaly Syndrome

It is also known as hyper-reactive malarial splenomegaly and is considered to be an abnormal immune response to repeated malarial infection. It is not specific to any species. Constant stimulation of the reticuloendothelial system by the circulating antigen antibody complexes results in its hyperplasia leading to progressive enlargement of the liver and spleen [15]. This is marked by residence in malaria endemic region, massive splenomegaly, mild to moderate hepatomegaly, elevated serum IgG and IgM malarial antibody level, normocytic normochromic anemia, leucopenia and thrombocytopenia due to hypersplenism are prominent features [68,69]. The spleen exhibits dilated sinusoids with lining reticulum cells showing marked erythrophagocytosis and the pulp shows lymphocytic infiltration. Similarly, the liver shows sinusoidal dilatation with infiltration and Kupffer cell hyperplasia with phagocytosis of cellular debris and erythrocytes. Parasites are absent in the peripheral blood. Therapy consists of administration of appropriate antimalarial prophylaxis for a prolonged period (at least 1 year) [70,71]. Chemoprophylaxis acts by removing the antigenic stimulus from repeated malarial infections, thus permitting the patient's immune system to return to normal. Response is generally seen within 3 months. There is no role of splenectomy. Complications include splenic infarct, increased susceptibility to infections, and severe anemia. Portal hypertension is not marked and variceal bleeding is rare.

5.12. Relapses and Recrudescence

Both relapse and recrudescence is characterized by return of infection after its apparent termination. The main importance of differentiating relapse from recrudescence is that, recrudescence is amenable to standard chemotherapy, whereas relapses require specific treatment with primaquine to eradicate the infection (radical cure). Relapse results from release of persistent parasites (hypnozoites in the liver) into the circulation. Only P. vivax and P. ovale can produce hypnozoites and hence, capable of producing relapse. Relapse occurs in approximately half of those infected and although occurs after weeks to months, may occur as long as five years after initial infection. P. falciparum and P. malariae infections, on the other hand, may remain dormant in the bloodstream for years (upto 50 years has been noted for P. malariae) either due to ineffective treatment or host immune response or both and give rise to repeated episodes of parasitemia called recrudescence [15,27,72,73].

6. Laboratory Diagnosis

6.1. Peripheral Blood Smear

This is the most economic, sensitive (can detect parasites at densities as low as 5 to 10/μL of blood by trained staffs) and reliable method for diagnosis of malaria. It is considered as the gold standard test [15,27,74]. There are two types of smears, the thick smear and the thin smear. Each type has its own significance; hence both should be prepared in a suspected case of malaria. Thick smear is at least 20 times more sensitive for detection of the parasite than thin film; therefore, it is used primarily for the parasite detection. On the other hand, thin smear is used for species identification since parasite morphology is better appreciated in such preparation. The timing of blood smears with fever spikes is less important. More important is to conceptualize the fact that a single negative smear does not rule out the diagnosis of malaria. Therefore, if an initial smear comes negative, repeated smears should be obtained every 6-12 hours for at least 48-72 hours in a clinically suspected case unless an alternate diagnosis is robustly established.

P. falciparum schizonts and trophozoites are usually not visible in peripheral smear as they are sequestered mainly in the microvasculature unless in cases of overwhelming parasitemia. When present, they are characterized by small ring forms sometimes with double chromatin specks, "accole" forms (parasites adhered to RBC membrane), crescent shaped gametocytes, intense parasitemia (>2%), involvement of RBCs of normal size (mature RBCs) and multiple infections in a single erythrocyte [15,27,75,76]. Other species of parasites have all stages in peripheral blood and infect less than 1% of RBCs. Even in the absence of parasitemia, the diagnosis of acute malaria can be suggested by the presence of malarial pigment (hemozoin) in monocytes or neutrophils.

6.2. Quantitative Buffy Coat (QBC) Method

This technique involves staining the centrifuged and compressed red cells with acridine orange and visualizing the parasite using fluorescence microscopy. This method is faster and more sensitive than routine microscopy but species identification is less accurate [27,75,76].

6.3. Rapid Diagnostic Tests (RDTs)

Immunochromatographic tests are based on parasite antigen capture using monoclonal or polyclonal antibodies and are popular in fields as they do not require microscope or experienced laboratory staffs for interpretation. Currently used antigen targets are histidine-rich protein 2 of P. falciparum, a pan-malarial Plasmodium aldolase, and the parasite specific lactate dehydrogenase. The threshold of detection by these rapid diagnostic tests is in the range of 100 parasites/μl of blood compared to 5 parasites/μl by thick film microscopy [77-80]. Parasight F test is a dipstick antigen capture assay which detects P. falciparum histidine rich protein 2 (*Pf*HRP2) in blood. Optimal is another antigen-based test which detects parasite lactate dehydrogenase (pLDH). It is not species specific. The only RDT approved by the US Food and Drug Administration for detection of malaria in United States so far is the BinaxNOW® Malaria test kit, which is based on the antigens HRP-2 and aldolase. The sensitivity and specificity of this test is 95% and 94% respectively for P. falciparum and 69% and 100%, respectively for P. vivax [81]. In non immune individuals, symptomatic malaria can occur at parasite densities which are much below the detection threshold of dipstick tests currently available. Further, the sensitivity and specificity of these RDTs is influenced by a multitude of factors including the type of the parasite, the level of parasitemia, the target antigen, the expression of the target antigens on the parasites, the presence of gametocytes, persistent antigenemia, cross-reactions with other malaria species and other autoantibodies, and prior treatment [82,83]. Finally, all dipstick tests are qualitative tests and cannot determine the degree of parasitemia.

6.4. Polymerase Chain Reaction

This is a highly sensitive and specific method. Although expensive, its potential to unravel the diagnosis of malaria even in the face of low parasitemia cannot be overlooked (around 10 fold more sensitive than microscopy). Similarly, it is an important tool to identify genes which confer drug resistance [84-87].

6.5. Serology

While antimalarial antibodies are of little diagnostic help in clinical practice, it is a useful aid in epidemiological surveys and for screening potential blood donors. Detection of protective antibodies following vaccination will be of importance in assessing response to malaria vaccines in the future [84-87].

7. Treatment

The need for hospitalization for management of malaria includes severe disease, infection with P. falciparum or P. knowlesi in a non immune host and patient's inability to tolerate oral medications due to persistent vomiting. Hospitalization permits clinical observation for tolerance of antimalarial therapy, monitoring for falling parasitemia (reflecting efficacy of therapy), and advanced management in the case of progression to severe disease. Follow up smears to demonstrate declining parasitemia with subsequent clearance is the accepted clinical practice. The gametocytes may persist for several weeks after successful treatment. This would clear eventually and does not represent treatment failure. Patients should be informed that malaria can recrudesce, and if they have febrile episodes in the future that repeat evaluation for malaria should be pursued. Malaria is a notifiable disease in many nations and all cases should be reported to the respective public health authority.

7.1. Treatment of Chloroquine Sensitive Malaria

The drug regimens used in an acute clinical attack of malaria with P. vivax, P. malariae, P. ovale and chloroquine susceptible P. falciparum is outlined in table 3 [15,27,88]. Chloroquine sensitive regions include Haiti, the Dominican Republic, many areas in the Middle East, and Central America west of the Panama Canal. Middle Eastern countries with eminent chloroquine-resistance include Iran, Oman, Saudi Arabia, and Yemen [4,15,27,89,90]. A rule of thumb is to administer chloroquine resistant P. falciparum treatment in any case of uncertain exposure history, known exposure to a chloroquine resistant region or unknown prevalence of chloroquine resistance.

Table 3. Treatment of Acute Malaria other than Chloroquine Resistant Variety [15,27,88]

In patients who can take orally	Chloroquine 600 mg base (=1000 mg salt) stat followed by 300 mg base (=500 mg) at 6, 24 and 48 hours. Or Hydroxychloroquine 620 mg base (=800 mg salt) stat, followed by 310 mg base (=400 mg salt) at 6, 24, and 48 hours.
In patients who cannot take orally	Chloroquine IV 10mg/kg base over 4 hours followed by 5mg/kg base (given in a 2 hour infusion) every 12 hours (total dose not to exceed 25mg/kg)

Since latent exoerythrocytic forms persist in the liver in infections with P. vivax and P. ovale, delayed true relapses occur in the majority of patients. In such cases, radical cure can be obtained by adding primaquine in the dose of 7.5-15 mg daily for 14 days [88]. Primaquine can cause severe hemolysis in G6PD deficient individuals. Therefore, G6PD screening test should be performed before starting this drug. There is no point in administering antirelapse treatment in highly endemic regions because the chance of reinfection is very high and a subsequent attack may be falsely labeled as failure of radical cure.

7.2. Treatment of Chloroquine Resistant Malaria

Chloroquine resistance is abundant in all malarious regions now except those specified above as chloroquine-sensitive areas. Chloroquine resistance should be suspected: 1] In all patients with severe malaria. 2] In any patient who has already received a standard chloroquine therapy in the last one month. 3] In cases where no clinical/microbiological evidence of improvement is seen within 48 hours of treatment. The treatment of uncomplicated chloroquine resistant malaria is outlined in table 4 [15,27,88,90]. Artemisinin combination therapies (ACTs) are recommended by the WHO as the first line treatment of uncomplicated falciparum malaria [88].

7.3. Treatment of Severe Malaria

7.3.1. Antimalarial Therapy

7.3.1.1. Artemisinins

Intravenous artesunate of 2.4 mg/kg as the first dose, followed by 2.4 mg/kg at 12 and 24 hours, followed by 2.4 mg/kg once daily is the drug of choice for severe malaria [88,90]. Data indicates a clear and significant mortality benefit of artesunate over quinine and lesser incidence of adverse effect [91-93]. Following four doses of intravenous artesunate, oral antimalarial treatment may be administered if the patient is able to tolerate oral therapy. After the patient is no longer critically ill, oral combination therapy is typically used to complete the course of treatment. Intravenous therapy for more than 3 days may be indicated in very ill patients. Artesunate dosing need not be adjusted for hepatic or renal failure, nor for concomitant or previous therapy with other medications. The most common adverse effects associated with artemisinins include nausea, vomiting, anorexia, and dizziness [93].

Table 4. Treatment of uncomplicated chloroquine resistant malaria [15,27,88,90]

1. Artemisinin Combination Therapy (ART)
a. Artemether+ Lumefantrine (Coartem) 1 tablet = 20 mg artemether and 120 mg lumefantrine) Dosage: For adults, 4 tabs stat followed by 4 tabs at 8 hour, then 4 tabs twice daily for 2 days. b. Artesunate + Amodiaquine 1 tablet = 50 mg of artesunate and 153 mg base of amodiaquine Dosage: 4 mg/kg of artesunate and 10 mg/kg of amodiaquine given once a day for 3 days. c. Artesunate + Mefloquine 1 tablet= 50 mg of artesunate and 250 mg base of mefloquine Dosage: 4 mg/kg of artesunate given once a day for 3 days and 25 mg base/kg of mefloquine (usually split over 2 or 3 days to minimize vomiting). d. Artesunate + Sulfadoxine-Pyrimethamine 1 tablet of artesunate= 50mg of artesunate; 1 tablet sulfadoxine-pyrimethamine= 500mg of sulfadoxine and 25 mg of pyrimethamine. Dosage: 4 mg/kg of artesunate given once a day for 3 days and a single administration of sulfadoxine-pyrimethamine (25/1.25mg base/kg) on day 1.
2. Atovaquone-Proguanil (Malarone) 1 tablet= 250mg of Atovaquone and 100 mg of Proguanil Adult Dosage: 4 tablets once daily for 3 days.
3. Quinine plus Doxycycline/Tetracycline/Clindamycin Quinine 600mg thrice daily for 7 days followed by a. doxycycline 100mg twice daily for 7 days or, b. tetracycline 250mg four times daily for 7 days or, c. clindamycin 600 mg thrice daily for 7days
4. Mefloquine +/- Doxycycline 1 tablet = 250mg of mefloquine Mefloquine: 750 mg as initial dose, followed by 500 mg given 6-12 hours after initial dose Plus doxycycline 100mg twice daily .... 5. In patients who cannot take orally: Quinine hydrochloride by IV infusion 20mg/kg in 500ml of 5-10 % dextrose over 4 hours followed by 10mg/kg over 2 hours in 5-10% dextrose every 8 hours for 7 days.

7.3.1.2. Quinine/Quinidine

Intravenous quinine dihydrochloride 20 mg salt/kg (in 5% dextrose) loading dose over 4 hours, followed by 10 mg salt/kg (over 2 hours in 5% dextrose) at 8 hour intervals (maximum 1800 mg salt/day) should be used for treatment of severe malaria only when artesunate is unavailable. Quinidine is as effective as quinine in the treatment of severe malaria and is an acceptable alternative wherever parenteral quinine is not available (e.g. USA). Intravenous quinidine gluconate 10 mg salt/kg loading dose (maximum 600 mg salt) in normal saline over 1 hour, followed by 0.02 mg/kg/minute continuous infusion. For patients with malaria acquired in south-east Asia, parenteral treatment with quinine (or quinidine) should be combined with one of the following: doxycycline, tetracycline or clindamycin. For children with malaria acquired in Africa, clinical management consists of administering parenteral quinine (at least 3 doses) until the child can swallow, followed by oral therapy with an artemisinin combination drug. Both quinine and quinidine can act as pancreatic secretagogues, leading to hyperinsulinemic hypoglycemia. Tinnitus, reversible hearing loss, nausea, vomiting, dizziness, and visual disturbances may occur with quinine and is called cinchonism. Quinidine can cause QT prolongation and should be administered with electrocardiographic monitoring. Infusions should be done with care and the rate should be reduced if the corrected QT interval becomes prolonged by more than 25% of the baseline value. Such monitoring is not necessary in the setting of quinine administration in patients without cardiac abnormalities [15,27,59,88,90,94,95].

7.3.2. Supportive Therapy

Fluid and electrolyte requirements should be individualized. Dehydration and shock should be corrected. It is also important to remember that the administration of excess parenteral fluids during the period of unrecognized renal impairment can precipitate acute water intoxication and fatal pulmonary edema. Packed red cells are transfused for severe anemia. Fever is controlled by paracetamol and tepid sponging. Acid base disturbances should be corrected. Blood sugar should be checked 3-4 times a day to detect hypoglycemia. Exchange transfusion should be considered for patients with parasite density of >10% with end organ complications. Renal failure is managed appropriately. Seizures are controlled with parenteral diazepam or phenobarbitone or phenytoin. Management of coma is similar to that of coma due to other causes. There is no role of steroids, heparin or low molecular weight (LMW) dextrans in the treatment of cerebral malaria. Similarly, the role of mannitol in cerebral malaria is uncertain. With appropriate therapy, patients show signs of clinical and laboratory improvement within 48-72 hours [15,27,59,94-95].

7.4. Treatment of Malaria in Pregnancy

Malaria in pregnancy should be treated with chloroquine or quinine in the usual doses. Mefloquine is probably safe in the second and third trimesters and may be used when benefit outweighs the risk. Primaquine and tetracycline should be avoided. Associated anemia needs administration of iron and folic acid [96].

8. Prevention of Malaria

Primary prevention of malaria involves personal protection against mosquito bites and appropriate chemoprophylaxis before entering a malaria endemic region. Personal protection measures include limiting outdoor activity between dusk and dawn, staying in screened rooms, wearing protective clothing (long pants, tucked in boots or socks and long-sleeved shirts), use of insect repellents, mosquito nettings sprayed with or soaked in an insecticide such as permethrin, flying-insect spray indoors around sleeping areas and last but not the least, avoiding malaria endemic areas whenever possible (particularly recommended for higher risk individuals including pregnancy and very young or very old age group).

8.1. Chemoprophylaxis

Non-immune persons travelling to endemic areas require chemoprophylaxis; the choice of which depends on whether the type of malaria prevalent in that region is chloroquine sensitive or not (Table 5) [15,27,97]. Therefore, whenever possible, it is recommended to learn about the risk of malaria in that geographic region and the most appropriate prophylaxis agent to be taken by contacting the Center for Disease control official website ww.cdc.gov/malaria/travel/index.htm or its toll-free phone number (1-800-232-4636) before making an international travel [98].

Table 5. Drug Regimens for Malaria Prophylaxis [15,27,97]

Chloroquine sensitive malaria	Chloroquine base (300mg) once a week
Chloroquine resistant malaria	Mefloquine 250mg once a week Or, Doxycycline 100mg daily Or, Malarone (Atovaquone 250mg + Proguanil 100mg) 1 tablet daily.

Prophylaxis is begun 1 week prior to entering the area (except for doxycycline and malarone which are started 1-2 days before departure) and continued for 4 weeks after leaving the transmission area. It is worth noting that chemoprophylaxis does not confer 100% protection; hence the diagnosis of malaria should still be considered in a patient returning from endemic areas with fever who was on appropriate chemoprophylaxis.

8.2. Mosquito Repellents

Some of the popular mosquito repellents are DEET (N,N-diethyl-m-toluamide), icaridin (also known as picaridin, KBR3023), permethrim and IR 3535 and essential oil of the lemon eucalyptus (P-MENTHANE-3,8-DIOL or PMD). For protection against mosquitoes, the US Center for Disease Control issued a statement in May 2008 recommending equally DEET, picaridin, oil of lemon eucalyptus and IR3535 for skin [99-101]. Permethrin is recommended for clothing, gear, or bed nets. As with all chemicals in general, these should be kept out of reach of children and the children should not be allowed to use them on their own. Pregnant women should try to avoid the use of repellents as far as possible, as the fetus may be vulnerable.

8.3. Malaria Vaccines

Despite intensive efforts, an effective malaria vaccine is not in being till date. Current research is focused on 3 developmental stages of the malaria parasites – the sporozoite, the merozoite, and the gamete. Sporozoite vaccine would prevent infection, merozoite vaccine would prevent the invasion of erythrocytes by merozoites, and gametocyte vaccine would block transmission of infection by blocking the parasite development in the mosquito. Although the vaccines have shown good results in laboratory models, human trials have been disappointing in most instances. Only two vaccines have gone beyond phase I clinical trials. The first subunit vaccine was prepared using a portion of circumsporozoite protein (CSP) which is produced in abundance by the sporozoites. This antigen is the basis for the "RTS,S" vaccine ('RTS' stands for 'repeat T epitopes' derived from the circumsporozoite protein; 'S' stands for the S antigen derived from hepatitis B). Phase II trials of this vaccine demonstrated a 30 to 60% reduction in the incidence of malaria infection with a favorable safety profile and phase III trial is underway in Africa [102-104]. Another vaccine containing Spf66 antigen is undergoing phase III clinical trials. This vaccine is called "cocktail vaccine" as it includes a combination of multiple epitopes from different malarial antigens and from different stages of parasites. In a study conducted in Columbia, the vaccine gave an overall protective efficacy of 33.6% (77% in children) [105]. Research has concentrated on vaccine against all stages of parasites life cycle. Special emphasis is on merozoite surface antigen (MSP1 and MSP 2) vaccines. Other antigens currently under study as vaccine candidates include erythrocyte binding antigen 175 and gametocyte antigens (Pfs25). While vaccine based on MSP1 should be able to prevent initial infection, Pfs25 will be helpful in reducing the disease transmission only. DNA vaccines have just made a beginning [106].

8.4. Mosquito Vector Control

Mosquito vector control methods include use of insecticide treated nets (ITNs), household insecticide residual spraying (IRS), larval control, and genetic control methods. Since effective insecticides for use against adult Anopheles have become available, ITNs and IRS have become the most important measures for mosquito vector control [107].

9. Sudden Unexpected Natural Malarial Deaths and Medico-Legal Autopsy

Sudden unexpected natural deaths especially those unwitnessed can be suspicious and lead to forensic questions necessitating the need for a medico-legal autopsy to discover the cause and manner of death [108,109]. Such deaths are primarily attributed to the cardiovascular system. Nonetheless, medico-legal autopsies have revealed parasitic infections like malaria as the occasional cause of sudden death. Though malaria is well recognized in antemortem settings, there have been only a few cases reported in forensic literature where malaria has been diagnosed posthumously in suspicious circumstances requiring a medico-legal autopsy [109-113]. This bars forensic pathologists from including malaria in the differential diagnosis for sudden death in most of the situations. Although not a common cause of sudden death, malaria can masquerade a variety of disorders and hence can easily be missed if this possibility is not kept at the back of mind while performing an autopsy especially if there is a travel history to malaria endemic areas. Moreover, in highly endemic areas where asymptomatic parasitemia is common, clinical diagnosis may be missed and confirmation of the diagnosis of malaria as the cause of death often has to rely on postmortem findings. Hence, forensic pathologists should give due importance to malaria as one of the important causes of unexplained death in the context of travel to endemic areas or sudden unexpected death in malaria-endemic regions itself [109,111]. Cerebral malaria, acute renal insufficiency, acute pulmonary edema and acute respiratory distress syndrome are possible mechanisms of sudden death due to malaria [109,110].

In a study conducted at Government Wenlock District Hospital in Mangalore, a malaria endemic coastal city in South India, autopsy files revealed 5 cases of sudden death due to malaria diagnosed by histopathology between September 2004 and August 2008 [113]. Macroscopic findings during autopsy are often unspecific. Histopathology confirms sequestration of parasitized erythrocytes with malarial pigment in the blood capillaries of most organs [109]. Microscopy of cadaveric blood smears may reveal remnants of intraerythrocytic parasites. Presence of this postmortem finding of parasitemia in sudden death due to malaria varies considerably from 25% to 80% [114,115]. Microbiological analysis may be compromised or impossible due to autolysis in some cases. Rapid diagnostic tests are of utmost significance in such cases and are considered a valuable tool in postmortem diagnosis of malaria [110,116]. Even in the setting of microbiological evidence of malaria in cadaveric blood, it is prudent to go ahead and perform the complete autopsy in order to ascertain the cause of death and distinguish fatal malaria from incidental parasitemia [110,116,117].

References

[1] World Malaria Report, Geneva: *WHO*; 2008.

[2] Hay SI, Guerra CA, Tatem AJ, Noor AM, Snow RW. The global distribution and population at risk of malaria: past, present and future. *The Lancet Infectious Diseases* 2004; 4: 327-336.

[3] Hay SI, Snow RW. The malaria Atlas Project: developing global maps of malaria risk. *PLoS Medicine* 2006; 3: e473.

[4] Guerra CA, Snow RW, Hay SI. Mapping the global extent of malaria in 2005. *Trends in Parasitology* 2006; 22: 353-358.

[5] The Global HIV/AIDS Epidemic: Fact Sheet. *Kaiser Family Foundation*. April, 2009.

[6] Sachs J, Malaney P. The economic and social burden of malaria. *Nature* 2002; 415: 680-685.

[7] Singh B, Kim LS, Matusop A, Radhakishnan A, Shamsul SS, Cox-Singh J, et al. A large focus of naturally acquired Plasmodium knowlesi infections in human beings. *Lancet* 2004; 363: 1017-1024.

[8] Dhangadamajhi G, Kar SK, Ranjit MR. High prevalence and gender bias in distribution of Plasmodium malariae infection in central east-coast India. *Tropical Biomedicine* 2009; 26: 326-333.

[9] Matteelli A, Castelli F, Caligaris S. Life cycle of malaria parasites. In: Carosi G, Castelli F (Eds). Handbook of Malaria Infection in the Tropics. Bologna: Associazione Italiana 'Amici di R Follereau' *Organizzazione per la Cooperazione Sanitaria Internazionale;* 1997.p.17-23.

[10] Rogerson SJ, Carter R. Severe vivax malaria: newly recognised or rediscovered. *PLoS Medicine* 2008; 5: e136.

[11] Genton B, D'Acremont V, Rare L, Baea K, Reeder JC, Alpers MP, et al. Plasmodium vivax and mixed infections are associated with severe malaria in children: a prospective cohort study from Papua New Guinea. *PLoS Medicine* 2008; 5: e127.

[12] Tjitra E, Anstey NM, Sugiarto P, Warikar N, Kenangalem E, Karyana M, et al. Multidrug-resistant Plasmodium vivax associated with severe and fatal malaria: a prospective study in Papua, Indonesia. *PLoS Medicine* 2008; 5: e128.

[13] Chin W, Contacos PG, Collins WE, Jeter MH, Alpert E. Experimental mosquito-transmission of Plasmodium knowlesi to man and monkey. *The American Journal of Tropical Medicine and Hygiene* 1968; 17: 355-358.

[14] Garnham PCC. *Malaria parasites and other haemosporidia*. Oxford: Blackwell; 1966.

[15] Warrell DA. Malaria. In: *Weatherall DJ, Ledingham JGG*, Warrell DA. (eds). Oxford Textbook of Medicine. 3rd ed. Oxford: Oxford University Press; 1996.p.3306.

[16] MacDonald G. *The epidemiology and control of malaria*. London: Oxford University Press; 1957.

[17] Filler S, Causer LM, Newman RD, Barber AM, Roberts JM, MacArthur J, et al. Malaria surveillance- United States, 2001. Morbidity and Mortality Weekly Report: *Surveillance Summaries* 2003; 52: 1-14.

[18] http://www.cdc.gov/malaria/about/biology/mosquitoes/index.html.

[19] http://www.anobase.org/species/MalariaSpecies.html.

[20] Barillas-Mury C, Kumar S. Plasmodium-mosquito interactions: a tale of dangerous liaisons. *Cellular Microbiology* 2005; 7: 1539-1545.

[21] Kebaier C, Voza T, Vanderberg J. Kinetics of mosquito-injected Plasmodium sporozoites in mice: fewer sporozoites are injected into sporozoite-immunized mice. *PLoS Pathogens* 2009; 5: e1000399.

[22] Amino R, Thiberge S, Martin B, Celli S, Shorte S, Frischknecht F, et al. Quantitative imaging of Plasmodium transmission from mosquito to mammal. *Nature Medicine* 2006; 12: 220-224.

[23] Jones MK, Good MF. Malaria parasites up close. *Nature Medicine* 2006; 12: 170-171.

[24] Vaughan AM, Aly AS, Kappe SH. Malaria parasite pre-erythrocytic stage infection: gliding and hiding. *Cell Host and Microbe* 2008; 4: 209-218.

[25] Weatherall DJ, Miller LH, Baruch DI, Marsh K, Doumbo OK, Casals-Pascual C, et al. Malaria and the red cell. *Hematology* 2002; 1: 35-57.

[26] Mayer DC, Cofie J, Jiang L, Hartl DL, Tracy E, Kabat J, et al. Glycophorin B is the erythrocyte receptor of Plasmodium falciparum erythrocyte-binding ligand, EBL-1.

Proceedings of the National Academy of Sciences of the United States of America 2009; 106: 5348-5352.

[27] White NJ, Breman JG. Malaria. In: Kasper D, Braunwald E, Fauci AS, Hauser SL, Longo DL, Jameson JL (Eds). *Harrison's Principles of Internal Medicine*. 17th ed. New York: McGraw Hill Co; 2008: 1280-1294.

[28] Mackintosh CL, Beeson JG, Marsh K. Clinical features and pathogenesis of severe malaria. *Trends in Parasitology* 2004; 20: 597-603.

[29] Chakravorty SJ, Hughes KR, Craig AG. Host response to cytoadherence in Plasmodium falciparum. *Biochemical Society Transactions* 2008; 36: 221-228.

[30] Clark IA, Budd AC, Alleva LM, Cowden WB. Human malarial disease: a consequence of inflammatory cytokine release. *Malaria Journal* 2006; 5: 85.

[31] Parroche P, Lauw FN, Goutagny N, Latz E, Monks BG, Visintin A, et al. Malaria hemozoin is immunologically inert but radically enhances innate responses by presenting malaria DNA to Toll-like receptor 9. *Proceedings of the National Academy of Sciences of the United States of America* 2007; 104: 1919-1924.

[32] Schumann RR. Malarial fever: Hemozoin is involved but Toll-free. *Proceedings of the National Academy of Sciences of the United States of America* 2007; 104: 1743-1744.

[33] Lamikanra AA, Theron M, Kooij TW, Roberts DJ. Hemozoin (malarial pigment) directly promotes apoptosis of erythroid precursors. *PLoS One* 2009; 4: e8446.

[34] Awandare GA, Ouma Y, Ouma C, Were T, Otieno R, Keller CC, et al. Role of monocyte-acquired hemozoin in suppression of macrophage migration inhibitory factor in children with severe malarial anemia. *Infection and Immunity* 2007; 75: 201-210.

[35] Miller LH, Baruch DI, Marsh K, Doumbo OK. The pathogenic basis of malaria. *Nature* 2002; 415: 673-679.

[36] Chen Q, Schlichtherle M, Wahlgren M. Molecular aspects of severe malaria. *Clinical Microbiology Reviews* 2000; 13: 439-450.

[37] Bonnefoy S, Ménard R. Deconstructing export of malaria proteins. *Cell* 2008; 134: 20-22.

[38] Vogt AM, Barragan A, Chen Q, Kironde F, Spillmann D, Wahlgren M. Heparan sulfate on endothelial cells mediates the binding of Plasmodium falciparum-infected erythrocytes via the DBL1alpha domain of PfEMP1. *Blood* 2003; 101: 2405-2411.

[39] Maier AG, Rug M, O'Neill MT, Brown M, Chakravorty S, Szestak T, et al. Exported proteins required for virulence and rigidity of Plasmodium falciparum-infected human erythrocytes. *Cell* 2008; 134: 48-61.

[40] Horata N, Kalambaheti T, Craig A, Khusmith S. Sequence variation of PfEMP1-DBLalpha in association with rosette formation in Plasmodium falciparum isolates causing severe and uncomplicated malaria. *Malaria Journal* 2009; 8: 184.

[41] Chookajorn T, Ponsuwanna P, Cui L. Mutually exclusive var gene expression in the malaria parasite: multiple layers of regulation. *Trends in Parasitology* 2008; 24: 455-461.

[42] Dondorp AM, Lee SJ, Faiz MA, Mishra S, Price R, Tjitra E, et al. The relationship between age and the manifestations of and mortality associated with severe malaria. *Clinical Infectious Diseases* 2008; 47: 151-157.

[43] Osier FH, Fegan G, Polley SD, Murungi L, Verra F, Tetteh KK, et al. Breadth and magnitude of antibody responses to multiple Plasmodium falciparum merozoite

antigens are associated with protection from clinical malaria. *Infection and Immunity* 2008; 76: 2240-2248.

[44] Doolan DL, Dobano C, Baird JK. Acquired immunity to malaria. *Clinical Microbiology Reviews* 2009; 22:13-36.

[45] Hewitt K, Steketee R, Mwapasa V, Whitworth J, French N. Interactions between HIV and malaria in non-pregnant adults: evidence and implications. *AIDS* 2006; 20: 1993-2004.

[46] McGuire W, Knight JC, Hill AV, Allsopp CE, Greenwood BM, Kwiatkowski D. Severe malarial anemia and cerebral malaria are associated with different tumor necrosis factor promoter alleles. *The Journal of Infectious Diseases* 1999; 179: 287-290.

[47] McGuire W, Hill AV, Allsopp CE, Greenwood BM, Kwiatkowski D. Variation in the TNF-alpha promoter region associated with susceptibility to cerebral malaria. *Nature* 1994; 371: 508-510.

[48] Kumar CJ, Sharma VK, Kumar A. Jet lag and enhanced susceptibility to malaria. *Medical Hypotheses* 2006; 66: 671.

[49] Lobo SW, Menezes RG, Bodhe AV, Kanchan T, Pillay VV, Pant S. Jet-lagged individual vis-à-vis local resident and susceptibility to malaria. *Medical Hypotheses* 2008; 70: 458-460.

[50] WHO *Guidelines for the Treatment of Malaria*. Geneva; WHO: 2010.

[51] Field JW. Blood examination and prognosis in acute falciparum malaria. *Transactions of the Royal Society of Tropical Medicine and Hygiene* 1949; 43: 33-48.

[52] Mung'Ala-Odera V, Snow RW, Newton CR. The burden of the neurocognitive impairment associated with Plasmodium falciparum malaria in sub-saharan Africa. *The American Journal of Tropical Medicine and Hygiene* 2004; 71: 64-70.

[53] Newton CR, Chokwe T, Schellenberg JA, Winstanley PA, Forster D, Peshu N, et al. Coma scales for children with severe falciparum malaria. *Transactions of the Royal Society of Tropical Medicine and Hygiene* 1997; 91: 161-165.

[54] Molyneux ME, Taylor TE, Wirima JJ, Borgstein A. Clinical features and prognostic indicators in paediatric cerebral malaria: a study of 131 comatose Malawian children. *The Quaterly Journal of Medicine* 1989; 71: 441-459.

[55] Lewallen S, Bronzan RN, Beare NA, Harding SP, Molyneux ME, Taylor TE. Using malarial retinopathy to improve the classification of children with cerebral malaria. *Transactions of the Royal Society of Tropical Medicine and Hygiene* 2008; 102: 1089-1094.

[56] Berkley JA, Bejon P, Mwangi T, Gwer S, Maitland K, Williams TN, et al. HIV infection, malnutrition, and invasive bacterial infection among children with severe malaria. *Clinical Infectious Diseases* 2009; 49: 336-343.

[57] Morpeth SC, Ramadhani HO, Crump JA. Invasive non-Typhi Salmonella disease in Africa. *Clinical Infectious Diseases* 2009; 49: 606-611.

[58] Barsoum RS. Malarial acute renal failure. *Journal of the American Society of Nephrololgy* 2000; 11: 2147-2154.

[59] Severe and complicated malaria. World Health Organization, Communicable Diseases Cluster. *Transactions of the Royal Society of Tropical Medicine and Hygiene* 2000; 94: S1-S90.

[60] Stanley J. Malaria. E*mergency Medicine Clinics of North America* 1997; 15: 113-155.

[61] Valecha N, Bhatia S, Mehta S, Biswas S, Dash AP. Congenital malaria with atypical presentation: a case report from low transmission area in India. *Malaria Journal* 2007; 6: 43.

[62] Hashemzadeh A, Heydarian F. Congenital malaria in a neonate. *Archives of Iranian Medicine* 2005; 8: 226-228.

[63] Emad S, Saira L, Seema H, Shahina H. Congenital malaria. *Pakistan Journal of Medical Sciences* 2008; 24: 765-767.

[64] Menendez C, Mayor A. Congenital malaria: the least known consequence of malaria in pregnancy. *Seminars in Fetal and Neonatal Medicine* 2007; 12: 207-213.

[65] Lesko CR, Arguin PM, Newman RD. Congenital malaria in the United States: a review of cases from 1966 to 2005. *Archives of Pediatrics and Adolescent Medicine* 2007; 161: 1062-1067.

[66] Sotimehin SA, Runsewe-Abiodun TI, Oladapo OT, Njokanma OF, Olanrewaju DM. Possible risk factors for congenital malaria at a tertiary care hospital in Sagamu, Ogun State, South-West Nigeria. *Journal of Tropical Pediatrics* 2008; 54: 313-320.

[67] Orogade AA, Falade CO, Okafor HU, Mokuolu OA, Mamman AI, Ogbonu TA, et al. Clinical and laboratory features of congenital malaria in Nigeria. *Journal of Pediatric Infectious Diseases* 2008; 3: 181-187.

[68] Moraes MF, Soares M, Arroz MJ, Do Rosario VE, Da Graca JP, Abecasis P. New concepts in hyperactive malarial splenomegaly. *Acta Medica Portuguesa* 2003; 16: 41-46.

[69] Mothe B, Lopez-Contreras J, Torres OH, Munoz C, Domingo P, Gurgui M. A case of hyper-reactive malarial splenomegaly: the role of rapid antigen-detecting and PCR-based tests. *Infection* 2008; 36: 167-169.

[70] Gupta OP, Bajaj S, Gupta SC. A study on tropical splenomegaly syndrome and chloroquine prophylaxis. *The Journal of the Association of Physicians of India* 1989; 37: 570-575.

[71] Vriend WH, Hoffman SL, Silaban T, Zaini M. Splenectomy in massive tropical splenomegaly: two-to six-year follow-up in 14 patients. *Tropical and Geographical Medicine* 1988; 40: 298-303.

[72] Schwartz E, Parise M, Kozarsky P, Cetron M. Delayed onset of malaria- implications for chemoprophylaxis in travelers. *The New England Journal of Medicine* 2003; 349: 1510-1516.

[73] Joshi H, Prajapati SK, Verma A, Kanga S, Carlton JM. Plasmodium vivax in India. *Trends in Parasitology* 2008; 24: 228-235.

[74] Moody A. Rapid diagnostic tests for malaria parasites. *Clinical Microbiology Reviews* 2002; 15: 66-78.

[75] Castelli F, Carosi G. Diagnosis of malaria infection. In: Castelli F, Carosi G (Eds). *Handbook of Malaria Infection in the Tropics*. Bologna: Organissazione per la Cooperazione Sanitaria Internazionale; 1997.p.114.

[76] Warhurst DC, Williams JE. ACP Broadsheet No 148. July 1996. Laboratory diagnosis of malaria. *Journal of Clinical Pathology* 1996; 49: 533-538.

[77] Makler MT, Hinrichs DJ. Measurement of the lactate dehydrogenase activity of Plasmodium falciparum as an assessment of parasitemia. *The American Journal of Tropical Medicine and Hygiene* 1993; 48: 205-210.

[78] Makler MT, Piper RC, Milhous WK. Lactate dehydrogenase and the diagnosis of malaria. *Parasitology Today* 1998; 14: 376-377.

[79] Brown WM, Yowell CA, Hoard A, Vander-Jagt TA, Hunsaker LA, Deck LM, et al. Comparative structural analysis and kinetic properties of lactate dehydrogenases from the four species of human malarial parasites. *Biochemistry* 2004; 43: 6219-6229.

[80] Forney JR, Wongsrichanalai C, Magill AJ, Craig LG, Sirichaisinthop J, Bautista CT, et al. Devices for rapid diagnosis of malaria: evaluation of prototype assays that detect Plasmodium falciparum histidine-rich protein 2 and a Plasmodium vivax-specific antigen. *Journal of Clinical Microbiology* 2003; 41: 2358-2366.

[81] Stauffer WM, Cartwright CP, Olson DA, Juni BA, Taylor CM, Bowers SH, et al. Diagnostic performance of rapid diagnostic tests versus blood smears for malaria in US clinical practice. *Clinical Infectious Diseases* 2009; 49: 908-913.

[82] The Role of Laboratory Diagnosis to Support Malaria Disease Management: Focus *on the Use of Rapid Diagnostic Tests in Areas of High Transmission*. Geneva; WHO: 2006.

[83] Bisoffi Z, Gobbi F, Angheben A, Van den Ende J. The role of rapid diagnostic tests in managing malaria. *PLoS Medicine* 2009; 6: e1000063.

[84] Hawkes M, Kain KC. Advances in malaria diagnosis. *Expert Review of Anti-Infective Therapy* 2007; 5: 485-595.

[85] Bronzan RN, McMorrow ML, Kachur SP. Diagnosis of malaria: challenges for clinicians in endemic and non-endemic regions. *Molecular Diagnosis and Therapy* 2008; 12: 299-306.

[86] Boonma P, Christensen PR, Suwanarusk R, Price RN, Russell B, Lek-Uthai U. Comparison of three molecular methods for the detection and speciation of Plasmodium vivax and Plasmodium falciparum. *Malaria Journal* 2007; 6: 124.

[87] Shokoples SE, Ndao M, Kowalewska-Grochowska K, Yanow SK. Multiplexed real-time PCR assay for discrimination of Plasmodium species with improved sensitivity for mixed infections. *Journal of Clinical Microbiology* 2009; 47: 975-980.

[88] *Guidelines for the Treatment of Malaria*. Geneva; WHO: 2006.

[89] http://wwwn.cdc.gov/travel/yellowBookCh4-Malaria.aspx.

[90] http://www.cdc.gov/malaria/pdf/treatmenttable.pdf.

[91] Dondorp AM, Fanello CI, Hendriksen IC, Gomes E, Seni A, Chhaganlal KD, et al. Artesunate versus quinine in the treatment of severe falciparum malaria in African children (AQUAMAT): an open-label, randomised trial. *Lancet* 2010; 376: 1647-1657.

[92] Dondorp A, Nosten F, Stepniewska K, Day N, White N. Artesunate versus quinine for treatment of severe falciparum malaria: a randomised trial. *Lancet* 2005; 366: 717-725.

[93] Rosenthal PJ. Artesunate for the treatment of severe falciparum malaria. *The New England Journal of Medicine* 2008; 358: 1829-1836.

[94] Trampuz A, Jereb M, Muzlovic I, Prabhu RM. Clinical review: severe malaria. *Critical Care* 2003; 7: 315-323.

[95] Severe and complicated malaria. World Health Organization, Division of Control of Tropical Diseases. *Transactions of the Royal Society of Tropical Medicine and Hygiene* 1990; 84: S1-S65.

[96] Gitau GM, Eldred JM. Malaria in pregnancy: clinical, therapeutic and prophylactic considerations. *The Obstetrician and Gynaecologist* 2005; 7: 5–11.

[97] http://www.cdc.gov/travel/yellowBookCh4-Malaria.aspx.

[98] http://ww.cdc.gov/malaria/travel/index.htm.

[99] Debboun, M, Frances, SP, Strickman, D. Insect Repellents. Boca Raton; CRC Press: 2007.

[100] Hill N, Lenglet A, Arnez AM, Carneiro I. Plant based insect repellent and insecticide treated bed nets to protect against malaria in areas of early evening biting vectors: double blind randomised placebo controlled clinical trial in the Bolivian Amazon. *British Medical Journal* 2007; 335: 1023.

[101] Rowland M, Downey G, Rab A, Freeman T, Mohammad N, Rehman H, et al. DEET mosquito repellent provides personal protection against malaria: a household randomized trial in an Afghan refugee camp in Pakistan. *Tropical Medicine and International Health* 2004; 9:335-342.

[102] Bejon P, Lusingu J, Olotu A, Leach A, Lievens M, Vekemans J, et al. Efficacy of RTS,S/AS01E vaccine against malaria in children 5 to 17 months of age. *The New England Journal of Medicine* 2008; 359: 2521-2532.

[103] Agnandji ST, Asante KP, Lyimo J, Vekemans J, Soulanoudjingar SS, Owusu R, et al. Evaluation of the safety and immunogenicity of the RTS,S/AS01E malaria candidate vaccine when integrated in the expanded program of immunization. *The Journal of Infectious Diseases* 2010; 202: 1076-1087.

[104] Abdulla S, Oberholzer R, Juma O, Kubhoja S, Machera F, Membi C, et al. Safety and immunogenicity of RTS,S/AS02D malaria vaccine in infants. *The New England Journal of Medicine* 2008; 359: 2533-2544.

[105] Valero ML, Amador LR, Galindo C, Figueroa J, Bello MS, Murillo LA, et al. Vaccination with SPf66, a chemically synthesised vaccine, against Plasmodium falciparum malaria in Colombia. *Lancet* 1993; 341: 705-710.

[106] Le TP, Coonan KM, Hedstrom RC, Charoenvit Y, Sedegah M, Epstein JE, et al. Safety, tolerability and humoral immune responses after intramuscular administration of a malaria DNA vaccine to healthy adult volunteers. *Vaccine* 2000; 18: 1893-1901.

[107] Barat LM. Four malaria success stories: how malaria burden was successfully reduced in Brazil, Eritrea, India, and Vietnam. *The American Journal of Tropical Medicine and Hygiene* 2006; 74: 12-16.

[108] Bhagavath P, Rastogi R, Menezes RG, Valiathan M, Kumar TSM, Babu YPR, et al. Sudden death due to pulmonary aspergillosis. *Journal of Forensic and Legal Medicine* 2009; 16: 27-30.

[109] Menezes RG, Kanchan T, Rai S, Rao PPJ, Naik R, Shetty BSK, et al. An autopsy case of sudden unexplained death caused by malaria. *Journal of Forensic Sciences* 2010; 55: 835-838.

[110] Alunni-Perret V, Vandenbos F, Kechkekian A, Marty P, Legros F, Michiels JF, et al. Fatal cerebral malaria diagnosed after death in a French patient. *The American Journal of Forensic Medicine and Pathology* 2010; 31: 269-272.

[111] Ette HY, Koffi K, Botti K, Jouvet A, Effi AB, Honde M. Sudden death caused by parasites: postmortem cerebral malaria discoveries in the African endemic zone. *The American Journal of Forensic Medicine and Pathology* 2002; 23: 202-207.

[112] Peoch MY, Gyure KA, Morrison AL. Postmortem diagnosis of cerebral malaria. *The American Journal of Forensic Medicine and Pathology* 2000; 21: 366-369.

[113] Rastogi P, Nagesh KR, Kanchan T, Menezes RG, Rao PPJ. Study of sudden death due to malaria in Mangalore- a malaria endemic zone in South India. *Journal of Forensic Medicine and Toxicology* 2010; 27: 29-31.

[114] Muehlethaler K, Scheurer E, Zollinger U, Markwalder R, Nguyen XM. Fulminant cerebral malaria in a Swiss patient. *Infection* 2005; 33: 33-35.

[115] Wichmann O, Loscher T, Jelinek T. Fatal malaria in a German couple returning from Burkina Faso. *Infection* 2003; 31: 260-262.

[116] Chappuis F, Loutan L, Samii K, Rougemont AL. The use of a rapid diagnostic test to determine malaria as a cause of death. *Journal of Travel Medicine* 2003; 10: 356-357.

[117] Lyke KE, Diallo DA, Dicko A, Kone A, Coulibaly D, Guindo A, et al. Association of intraleukocytic Plasmodium falciparam malaria pigment with disease severity, clinical manifestations, and prognosis in severe malaria. *The American Journal of Tropical Medicine and Hygiene* 2003; 69: 253-259.

In: Malaria: Etiology, Pathogenesis and Treatments
Editors: A. M. Peterson and G. E. Calamandrei
ISBN: 978-1-62100-363-2

Chapter V

Malaria in the Archaic Greek World: Links among Myth, Archeological Finds and Paleopathological Researches

Sergio Sabbatani and Sirio Fiorino
S. Orsola Hospital, Bologna, Italy

Myths are often the remote mirror
of really occurred historical events

Abstract

Malaria influenced human natural selection and, in particular, Plasmodium Falciparum exerted a major impact on human genome in comparison with every other pathogen. Different and discussed opinions exist, concerning the period in which Plasmodium Falciparum infection appeared in Hellenic peninsula, although it was stated that this protozoan came from central Africa and reached Mediterranean and Egyptian coasts through Nile Valley. Paleopathology is providing some convincing responses, by means of the biomolecular analysis on bone remains, a methodology introduced with increasing frequency in the last ten years. Unfortunately some limits, such as the very ancient age of the remains, cannot be overcome and in addition the state of preservation of samples may influence the sensibility of laboratory methodologies. It is also to remember that previously only the macroscopic study of skeleton was performed.

On the ground of a largely shared valuation that the myths may be the remote mirror of really occurred historical events and that the mythical tails, arising from the archaic history as well as from the pre-historic age, are frequently represented in the ancient artistic manifactures [Corinthian and Athenian ceramics], the Authors endeavoured to establish a link between some archeological remains of Hellenic origin and mythical events concerning Hercules. In particular it was considered the tale recording the second labour of the Hero, when the Hydra of Lerna was defeated and killed.

In accordance with some theories, the fight of Hercules against monster endowed with multiple-heads, which both were reproducing and doubling after their excision, would be the clear memory of the attempt to reclaim the marshes in malarial district of

Lerna. This area in Argolis, during the Neolithic age, would be an healthy place and some communities of fishers probably settled here, since fresh water from a coast lake were available. Subterrean rivers, coming from mountains in Argolis, supplied this lake. Nevertheless, an environmental change caused the lake to be covered with sand and the apperance of a marsh with subsequent likely disappearance of human settlements, approximately in 1250 b.C. This decline would have been caused by the appearance of Plasmodium Falciparum malaria. The study of epidemics, from an historical point of view, might benefit by archeological contribution and, in addition, by works of the crafstmen and artists, who depicted, in their manufactures, remarkable mythical events for ancient people.

However, paleopathological study possibly along with the integration of biomolecular analysis remain not replaceable approaches.

Introduction

Mirko Gremek and Danielle Gourevitch open their volume entitled "The Diseases in the Ancient Art" in such a way: "The History is a reconstruction of the ancient events, starting from the current signs of the past times, however, It is conditioned by what we are and we know. With regard to both the History and the History of Medicine these marks are represented not only by the written documents, but also by all the other products of human activity, such as oral tradition, whenever it is available, buildings, changes of the natural environment and, at last, works of art and remains of human body. These data were neglected by historians for a long time" [1].

The Paleopathology, which studies human body remains, beginning from the early studies carried out by Sir Arthur Ruffer in Alexandria in the first decades of twentieth century [2], had, in particular in the second half of the century, an interesting development and contributed to explain the appearance of infectious diseases, as a consequence of the introduction, in the Mesolithic and Neolithic ages, of livestock in human activities. The use of moleculary biology in the study of human and animal remains [3] and, more recently, of immune-detection tecniques on specimens [dental pulp and bone marrow], which were obtained and treated with standardized methods [4,5], enabled a better understanding of the epidemics appearance and evolution (plague, tuberculosis, typhus etc), bringing the historical and medical knowledge "as evidence" to enter, with full dignity, the contemporary scientific debate. In historical and prehistorical times many infectious diseases, due to the rapid development, caused the death or otherwise gave rise to a complete recovery. With the exception of tuberculosis, brucellosis and osteomyelitis, infectious diseases rarely left their signs in the bones, therefore, since skeletal remains represented the main source for the examination, the Paleopathologists had little chances to study infectious diseases. Owing to these problems, Scholars obtained useful informations by means of literary texts analysis [6,7,8] and by means of observation of artworks and handiworks [1].

As Mirko Grmek and Danielle Gourevitch suggested, useful clues may be obtained from ancient works of art, including sculptures, fresco and vase paintings, glyptics [semiprecious stone engraving], numismatics, mirror engraving, the art of the coroplast [terracotta working tecnique] and mosaic art. These signs also may promote a scientific, historical and medical interpretation of myth. In addition it should be thought that in Greek-Roman classical world the myth inspired not only immortal literary works by Homer, Virgil, Lucretius and Ovid

[6,7,8] but also it contributed to establish, inside each human society, custom and behaviour. These habits were the basis of rules and laws, which then persisted for several centuries, albeit these norms were modulated, reviewed and, not infrequently, simply embedded in Western Christian culture. Nevertheless, even if the elapsed time damaged the artworks in several circumstances, a lot of remains, not only minor art manufactures, reached our Age and they may show how the ancient people viewed, regarded and filtered the disease through their unconscious. A lot of examples may be observed in Grmek and Gourevitch's quoted text: wounds, pathological thinness, madness, obesity, abnormal height, pathologies affecting chest, spine, head, neck, eyes, limbs, as well as sex-related diseases, are the most glaring examples, which show the weight that the Art could have in depicting the illness. According to the assumption that the origin of infectious diseases was unknown in the ancient time -it should be observed that this knowledge become a common heritage in the scientific world only with the microbiological revolution in nineteenth century- both the poisoning, in all its causes and manifestations, and the pathological condition that we now know to be induced by an infectious agent were considered to have a common genesis [1].

In other words both a plant and a root ingestion[1] could induce a clinical course similar to the tetanic infection, caused by Clostridium Tetani, which was characterized by spastic contraction of the face muscles with the presence of a sardonic laugh (figure 1), an event which was quite possible in a world where the agriculture and the sheep-breeding were the predominant human activities. Because of the knowledge of the microbial as well as submicrobial world was lacking in the ancient times, only the magic or rather the spell, practised by a god, could justify the appearance of an epidemic or the death of a hero. Therefore this kind of spell appeared to have the characteristics and the traits of a poisoning to those who had a naturalistic approach to reality. Hurting the feelings of Apollo, of Jupiter, of Minerva, or of any other gods on polytheistical Olympus could stir up the wrath of the gods and the ultimate vent, that their anger could have, was represented by the "poisoning" of a victim or of a group of persons and/or animals. For example, the poison, in comparison with wound caused by a stab, -an event with an evident relation of cause and effect - possessed a part of mystery which resulted essential to go quickly into the supernatural dimension. This opinion was quite congenial to ancients because they did not possess advanced knowledge of physics, biology and chemistry. We have to recall, incidentally, that the Egyptian civilization, which preceded Greek and Roman civilizations, was practically soaked in magic [9]; everything was magic, the nature and the human activities, in particular, were influenced by this dimension of mystery which, according to this view, made hieroglyphics, engraved on stones or painted on a wall or written on a papyrus, magical, if, on these manufactures, ritual formulas were reported. Therefore, in the ancient world, the use of the word "poisoning" appeared to be referred to infection almost automatically as well as, in return, to the onset of epidemics which, now and then, afflicted the cities.

[1] Anemone coronaria [in greek Batrachion], as reported by Pausanias, is "shrill taste " to the palate and once it is eaten "this herb causes the withdrawing of the nerves so that the mouth is sprained and those who eat it, while they are dying, seem to laugh". The plant, that is particularly abundant in Sardinia, took the popular name of sardonic or sardonic grass, when this herb is put into the mouth it induces teeth grind, causing sardonic laugh [Figure 1], as it may be observed in tetanus because of muscle spasm induced by the tetanic toxin.

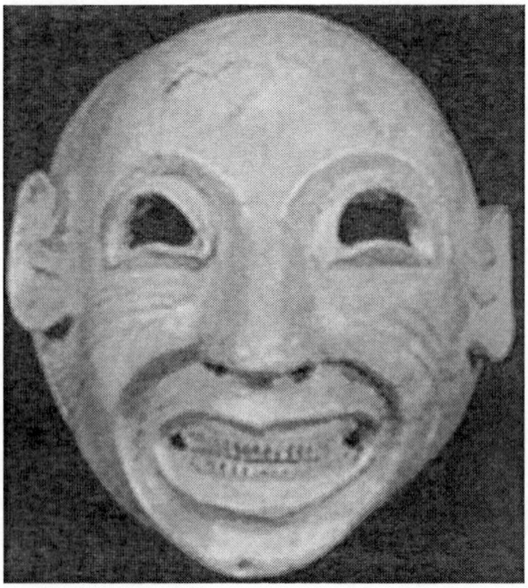

Figure 1.

These "poisonings" could be easily attributed to human responsibility, individual or collective, which had hit the gods' susceptibility. It has to be considered the classic episode concerning Apollo, who, with his arrows, caused the plague in the ranks of the Greek army during the siege of Troy [10], or the case of Philoctetes, who was bitten by a snake and abandoned by his fellows on the island of Lemnos [11]. This case will give rise to different interpretations, both with respect to the causality of the event [12] and in relation to developments of the Homeric tale. Our paper links three elements: classical myth, archaeological remains accurately representing it and medical-scientific interpretation[2]: The aim of this work is to describe infectious features in paleopathology, because, as we reported, with regard to classical world, either a relationship or an identification exists among "poisoning/magic" and infectious diseases, according to our modern conception.

Hercules'myth[3]

Angelo Brélich wrote: "Hercules is the Greek hero for excellence, because he is the symbol of Greek human condition and of the themes of Greek life": the continuous presence of sorrow and pain, the ineluctability of the death, the relationships among women and men, the travels and the spreading of knowledge to new lands. For these reasons and for a cosmic dimension of winner, Hercules, "lion-hearted"-as he was defined by Homer -was certainly among the gods and heroes of the ancient times, the most beloved and the most represented in art [13]. *Hercules' peculiar position takes its origin from ancient times, since the beginnings*

[2] A complementarity between archeology and medicine may exist. During the excavations in Mycenae, which began on August 7, 1879, Heinrich Schliemann was already supported by the great pathologist Rudolf Virchoff to better understand the structure of the excavations and to obtain valuable information on human remains inside the tombs.

[3] For an extensive exposition of of Hercules' myth, see the book: Ercole, l'Eroe, il Mito, edited by Stefano De Caro [13]. In our brief summary, we referred to this text..

of Hellenic civilization, when the Dori reported to be descended from Heraclids, hero's sons, and in the archaic period, when the aristocratic society of the whole Greece made them the model of heroic and warrior virtues, on which the aristocratic society was based. This mythical feature was not only inherited in the Ancient Classical Greece, but it was transmitted to the Etruscan and Roman world-it has to be thought that Tarquinii considered him as their mythical ancestor-, and he eventually became a symbol of victory for the Macedonians of Alexander the Great. It's interesting to note that the victories of Alexander in remote lands allowed an easy transfer of the Hercules' myth and he was adopted as a deity by the peoples and nations that were gradually subjugated in his great empire[4]*. The Hercules' popularity in Rome was great (both cities and emperors used the title of Herculean), while some cities in the Gulf of Naples (Pompeii and Herculaneum) boasted of having been founded by the legendary hero. His great charm, even with the advent of Christianity and despite the destruction of pagan temples, in some ways remained in the experience of the early Christian world –it is interesting the similarity with the biblical Samson- and, after the Middle Ages, it gave rise to an intense flowering of artistic works in the Renaissance [13]. We come now to the presentation of some features of the Hercules' myth, that presents a relationship with the subject matter*[5]*.*

A giant dragon with nine snake-shaped heads lived in the marshy plain of Lerna, but according to different versions, it had 50 golden heads. Any head was cut off, two grow back, in addition also the breath and blood of the Hydra (the Dragon was called in a such way) were deadly poisons. The myth says that the Hydra was slain by Hercules during the second of his labours. Hercules crushed the beast while it digested its meal in the cave where it went to rest. Hydra rushed at the hero and knocked him down, but he counter-attacked and cut all the Hydra's heads (Figure 2). He discovered, however, that from the stump of every severed head two others grow back. With the aim to escape the terrible stench, emitted from the mouth of the monster, Hercules caught his breath, while in order to prevent the regrowth of heads, he asked his nephew Iolaus to cauterize the wounds by means of fire. But the last head was immortal and it could be neutralized only by burying it, together with the body, under a huge boulder. Finally Heracles dipped the tip of his arrows in the very poisonous blood of Hydra, to make the infected-wounds incurable, once darts were thrown. There is one more tragic implication that is linked to this event as the poison of the Hydra was later the cause of the hero' death. Hercules was traveling with his wife Deianira and he came to a river, near which there was a centaur, his name was Nessus and he acted as a ferryman. Hercules was the first to be ferried, whereas Deianira was the second. During the carriage, the centaur tried to rape the woman. As soon as Nessus reached the bank of the river, he was mortally wounded in the heart by the hero (figure 3). Centaur's revenge, before his death, was terrible: he predicted to Deianira that one day her husband would have stopped loving her and, while he was talking like this, he suggested that she collected the blood, that was oozing from his wound. He said

[4] A king of Commagene, in the remote region of Antitauro, included among the gods, who protected his mausoleum on the top of Nimrud Dagh, a strange Iranian-Greek god called Heracles-Ares-Verethragna, the legend reports that the union of Heracles with fifty virgins, the Daughters of Thespis, produced a race that, under the guidance of his nephew Iolaus, crossed the Mediterranean and colonized Sardinia. According to an epigram, this would have been his thirteenth fatigue [!] [13].

[5] The myth of Hercules is one of the most complex, coming from the Greek world, therefore it will not reported here in its entirety. Different versions of this myth were elaborated and included in this tale over a very long period of time, from the Mycenaean and perhaps pre-Mycenaean ages to the Hellenistic-Roman age; this complex story occurred in relatively distant geographical environments.

that later it would have turned to an useful filter of love, but Nessus' blood, became a potent poison, by means of the Hercules' arrow. Afterwards Deianira, deceived by the centaur Nessus, used the blood that she had collected as a love potion. She permeated a clothing and she took care that it was worn by her husband. The poisoned blood caused hero to suffer an unenduable burning sensation, also the garment, clung to his skin, prevented him to remove it.

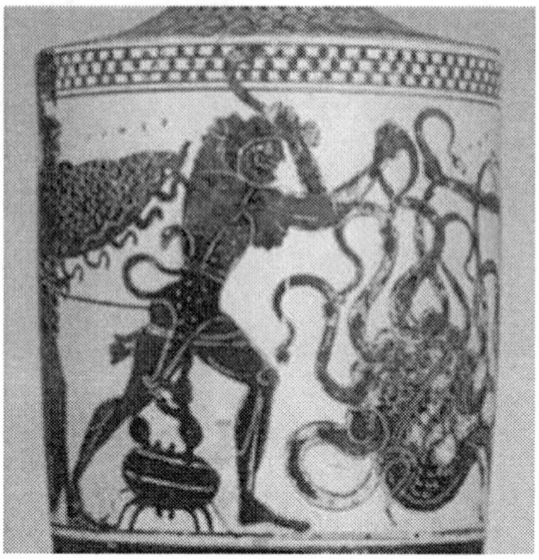

Figure 2.

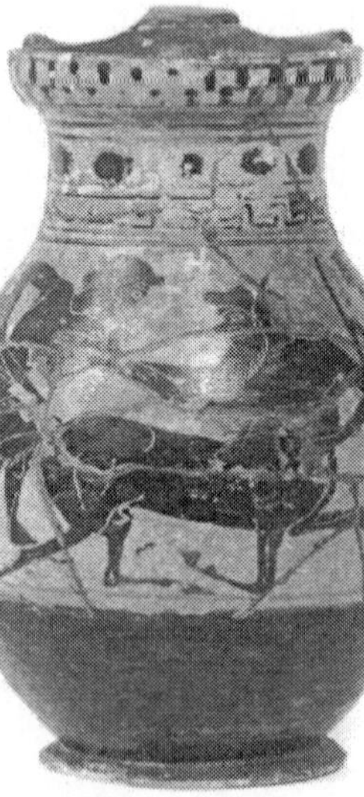

Figure 3.

As we saw, Hercules' myth has its roots in early times, however, in the course of time, the story's end concerning the hero was not accepted by the Greeks and as early as seventh century the following idea emerged: at the time of human death the hero was taken up into Olympus, hailed as a god among other gods[6].

[6] Although Greek Heroes had a special consideration, however they were mortal. Hercules himself, earlier on, although he had a divine parent, was not allowed to be immortal. In the Homer's poems no reference to the

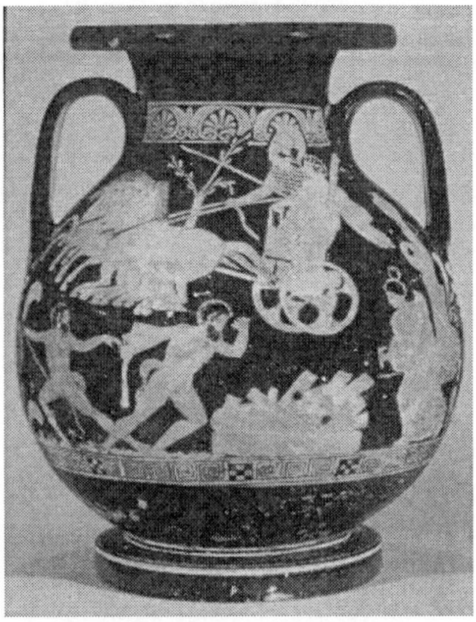

Figure 4.

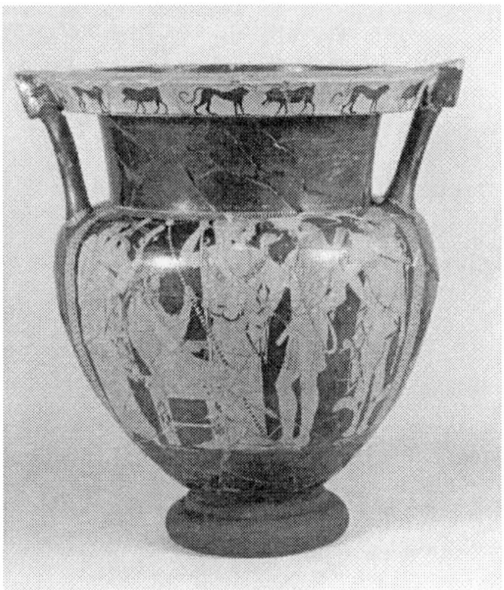

Figure 5.

The myth was reworked out like this: Hercules, while he felt was dying from the poison, got himself to carry to the top of Mount Oeta in Thessaly, not far from Thermopylae, and ordered to erect a huge wooden pyre. Then the hero climbed over it, after he convinced Peante, father of Philoctetes, to set the pyre to fire with the promise to give Peante his bow and arrows. Therefore the Hercules' mortal part was burned (Figure 4), whereas, according to the wishes of his father Zeus, who wrapped him in a cloud of thunder, the immortal part

hero's immortality was made. In the Iliad Achilles says: "Not even the powerful Hercules, dear to lord Zeus, Kronos' son, escaped death, but he was knocked down by the Fate and by the cruel wrath of Hera." The same conception, suggesting Hercules' death, was originally expressed in the eleventh book of the Odyssey, when Odysseus remembers that he saw the hero in his descent to Hades. [13].

ascended into Olympus (figure 5)], where the now-deified hero had a house and a wife, Hebe, Hera's daughter. [13].

Bibliographic Excursus in the Context of Paleopathological, Historical and Medical Researches

Only after both the malarial parasite and the vector that transmits the infection to humans were identified, reliable theories about the presence of malaria in the South of Europe and particularly in Greece and southern Italy in the classical period could be developed [14]. Mirko Grmek states that the first well-based notions which consider this interesting topic date back to the beginning of the twentieth century and have to be ascribed to Angelo Celli with regard to the Roman world [15] and to Ronald Ross with regard to the Greek world [16]. The philologist W. H. Samuel Jones in 1907, after development of a critical re-reading concerning the ancient literary sources and after taking into account the new scientific knowledge, expressed his viewpoint concerning the presence and the spreading of malaria in Greece and in Aegean islands [17]. His thesis can be summarized in these terms. Malaria was introduced into Greece during the classical period and in particular, in Attica only at about 430 BC. The African origin was probably[7] because at that time the contacts with Egypt[8] were constant and frequent, the author explained the severity of the infectious disease with the following consideration: the new pathocenosis hit a population that had not previously known this disease. The second proposed thesis concerns the evidence that the epidemic struck the most fertile regions of Greece, corrupting men's health, changing the characteristics of the country, with devastating effect in terms of demography, finally, significantly descreasing the economic development of the country. According to Jones's opinion, malaria would have been the decisive factor, causing the decline of classical civilization. Moreover, this scourge since the Hellenistic period and until the beginning of the twentieth century would have been the decisive factor which restrained the economic and demographic development of the countries in eastern Mediterranean basin for a long time [23, 24, 25].

---

[7] According to studies conducted by Livingston in 1958 [18] the first people in Africa who had to deal with the strong increase in incidence of malaria were the Bantu when, during the Iron Age, they introduced agriculture. Previously, about 10 000 years ago, at the onset of the Neolithic age, with the final withdrawal of ice from Europe a profound and rapid climate variation occurred; and at this stage in North Africa and in the Middle East the man switched from an hunting economy to an agricultural economy. This step caused nucleation phenomena [concentration of the population] that allowed the development of a social organization, initially based on individual households, and then progressively extended to include an aggregation of groups, giving rise to clans and tribes [alliances among families]. The new lifestyle and the resulting increase in population, with a concentration of people in stable areas] would have allowed a moderate spread of malaria. In the ancient Egypt, where traces of an rural society dating back to 5000 BC were found, malaria was certainly very common in the south of the Nile Valley, an area that allowed access to most of Tropical Africa; perhaps the disease was less common in the northern part of Egypt, in this area macroscopic paleopathological traces have been found in the recent past in some mummies in which the presence of splenomegaly was observed. There is also a papyrus dating back to 1570 BC in which fever and splenomegaly are mentioned [19].

[8] For a comprehensive account on the origin of malaria according to the Paleopathology and especially to the evolution of primates during the Quaternary period, see the works of Luigi Capasso [21,22, 23].

In relation to the first point Jones based his opinion on the lack of data concerning fevers in Greek texts before the fifth century BC and on the finding that the major Greek cities were located in areas particularly exposed to malaria [24]. The Author believed that if the epidemic had shown its own signs at the time of the foundation of the original settlements, those sites would have not been good candidates, since they were close to areas exposed to unhealthy countries and they would have, inevitably, exposed people to recurrent fevers. At that time this thesis was largely accepted by the scientific world [14], but several Greek physicians, who knew the problem by direct experience, questioned such a viewpoint by saying that in Greece malaria was endemic even before the human race arrived in this country; nevertheless they admitted that there were historical variations of endemic disease with the appearance of critical episodes of epidemic in the classical period and recognized that the deleterious effects would have also occurred in the historical periods marked by the decline [26, 27]. Among the causes of recrudescence of this endemic disease, the great Italian malariologist Angelo Celli hypothesized a cyclical variation in the virulence of the pathogenic micro-organism, as well as ecological environmental factors. Deforestation, dryness and reversion of the country to marshland as well as the shortage of watercourses maintenance, especially in central Italy and in southern Italy were the major outer factors affecting climate changes in the considered places [28, 29, 30, 31, 32]. With respect to this issue the positions were articulated: Felix Regnault believed that the changes were related mainly to human activities [29], while Elisworth attributed more importance to large geophysical cycles that would have affected the local microclimate [14]. As it may be observed at the time the debate already predicted the modernity of our times.

Plinio Fraccaro believed that the bad influence of malaria also extended to the social dimension, the decline of rural agriculture would have wasted the agriculture, causing both a demographic impoverishment of the country and, in a perverse circuit, making the malaria worse [33]. Sigerist suggested a strengthening synergy between biological and social factors [34], while more recent researches, with regard to the eastern Mediterranean, considered the biological aspects more important than the social dimension [14]. Since the thirties of the twentieth century the attention was concentrated on the role of Plasmodium falciparum in comparison to the role of other Plasmodia, since this species has certainly a more important role on morbidity and mortality than other forms [35, 36]. Since 1964, the development of paleopathology, thanks to researches by Lawrence Angel [37, 38, 39], allowed to establish important connections among porotic hyperostosis(IO) and certain hereditary anemias, and in particular between thalassemia and malignant malaria.[9] Through the study of sets of historical skeletal remains it was possible to suggest a link among the frequency of these blood disorders and the onset or reoccurrence of the epidemic, although it should be noted that the

[9] John Lawrence Angel [1915-1986] has a great merit, thanks to his studies in Greece, between 1937 and 1967, he correlated the morphological anthropological evolution with paleopathological anthropological evolution, linking the mankind with his environment. In 1971, Angel realized a monograph devoted to the population of the city of Lerna, where the most of the skeletons are dated to the Bronze Age. In this basic text he was the first to propose a paleo-demographic study of the necropolis. This idea allows to carry out studies on the whole of numerous human remains and not only on some isolated cases. He also, overcoming the previous practice, introduces in the paleopathological research the comprehensive study of the skeleton, whereas previously only the study of the Skull was performed. With this new approach very different diseases were described, such as congenital dislocation of the hips, of the feet, fractures, infections, rachitism and bone tumors. Between 1937 and 1986, Angel studied more than 2,300 skeletons dating from the Paleolithic to the present day. As he wrote in his seminal text The People of Lerna, a major purpose of his visit to Greece was to carry out anthropological studies directed against the Nazi racial theories [40].

porotic hyperostosis can be caaused by iron acquired deficiency or alimentary deficit in the course of famines. If it may be supposed that the frequency of the I.O. in the skeletons found in Greece and on the Aegean coasts of Anatolia, in broad terms, reflects the evolution of malarial epidemic in these areas, it has been hypothesized that there would have been three periods of hyperendemic, respectively in the Neolithic era, in the Roman age and in modern times, while the epidemic would have minimal impact during the Paleolithic era, on the eve of the fifth century and in the Byzantine age. Grmek, rightly, points out that the epidemic outbreaks would have occurred in the times when the balance of the pathocenosis in the ancient Greek world broke [14]. Grmek, on the basis of these considerations, replaced the viewpoint of Jones, that suggested that the first introduction of malaria in Greece was in the fifth century BC, with the hypothesis of an early reintroduction of malaria, in particular of malaria caused by Plasmodium Falciparum, in this age [41, 42]. According to his opinion, only the great cultural maturation, which occurred in that period, allowed the writings, reporting the presence of recurrent fevers, to attain our epoch. These events are described in the texts of Hippocrates [Books I and III of the Epidemics] and in the chronicles of Thucydides. We recall that the great Athenian general reports events concerning the Athenian expeditionary force, engaged in the siege of Syracuse in Sicily, in 413 BC.

In this context it is necessary to recall the role played by the vector in the spreading of Plasmodium Falciparum[10]. The presence of the species Anopheles (A.) Labranchiae and A. Sakharov has been proved to be crucial for the onset of the epidemic; it would appear that these species settled into the Aegean basin, into Italy and Spain only after the massive deforestation occurred in these countries during Hellenistic and Roman eras. Based on these considerations, Leonard J. Bruce-Chwatt [43, 44] and Julian de Zulueta [45] believed that the absence of these forms in the geographical areas considered would have made impossible the spreading of Plasmodium falciparum during the mentioned periods, since the documented presence of the only A. Atroparvus in southern Europe, would have not allowed, in that period of the history, the spreading of species Plasmodium Falciparum of tropical origin. On the basis of these entomological considerations, the comparison among the proposed theories could come to nothing, only the discovery of mosquito fossils of the Anopheles genus [with their genetic characterization] in the southern Europe would have enabled to overcome this crucial controversy. In this complex plot of issues fortunately the studies of Robert Sallares came out [46] and, thanks to his researches, it was possible to point out the ecology of the ancient Greek world beyond the impasse, which we have referred to. The researches on paleoclimate have indeed confirmed the difficulty of survival of species of mosquitoes able to resist and to transmit malignant malaria in eras characterized by a strong drop in temperature in Europe [11]. In addition, the significant prevalence of the I.O. in the detected skeletons, since

[10] With an effective witticism the mosquito has been defined the most important enemy of the human species, as it, being the carrier of many infections, has conditioned, in the course of time, human evolution. A more purposeful and evolutionistic interpretation may be considered: the mosquito would have effectively helped the human species in its evolutionary adaptation to the environment.

[11] In Europe, certainly the cold climate of the Pleistocene did not favour the spreading of malaria, it has to be considered that fauna and flora that then could be found in the Southern Europe were similar to those that nowadays are found in the Northern Europe. Only Plasmodium vivax and Plasmodium malariae survival was allowed by such a climate, whereas Pl falciparum lifecycle was impossible. In the same way the presence of genus Anopheles mosquitos was prevented in Europe and it was restricted to Northern Africa and Asia [20]. Only at the end of the fourth millennium BC. people coming from the countries of Asia Minor and of the Eastern Mediterranean Sea promoted agriculture diffusion in Europa; the possible spreading of the most

it can be also associated with dietary deficiency conditions, to date it is no longer recognized as a reliable sign of the presence of malaria, as it was shown that the acquired anemias also, such as those derived from food shortages, may give rise to these stigmata. These findings have led to remodulate the knowledge, which previously was considered as acquired, about the presence of malaria in the Eastern Mediterranean basin during the Neolithic and Mesolithic ages. Grmek point out, however, that if it is true that in modern times only malaria caused by Plasmodium Falciparum may exert a so important selective pressure as to determine the frequency, in a given population, of thalassemia, and then of the I.O., whereas with regard to both historical and even to prehistorical periods, the approach should be substantially different [14]. He, in 1994, re-formulated his thesis and admitted that other diseases, in addition to food shortages and to benign forms of malaria, could have acted synergistically, when co-present, increasing the prevalence of hereditary anemias. He also suggested a hypothesis that cannot be excluded: the Plasmodium vivax and Plasmodium malariae [benign species] could have presented major changes in virulence, causing a possible increase in I.O. development.

While the opinion of de Zulueta, who denied the presence of Plasmodium Falciparum in prehistoric Europe, was now being shared, on the other hand Gremek reported to be convinced that the malignant malaria invaded Greece in the fifth century BC. His opinion was based on two points: the Hippocratic description of clinical cases, in which "black urine" was observed in association with remittent fevers, and Thucydides' historical citation concerning the attacks of fever during the previously mentioned siege of Syracuse in 413 BC The historiographer and physician concluded his argument, hypothesizing that the malignant malarial hyperendemic would have emerged late in antiquity, and would have modified pathocenosis and only in the Roman period, it would have caused a really tangible damage. In particular, the pressure exerted by malarial endemic would have conditioned the social and economic development, especially in central and southern Italy, in the late empire [14]. After this review, his opinion was substantially coincident with that of Robert Sallares [46]. This scholar in 2004 [after 10 years from Grmek's publication] concluded its most recent and ponderous work, noting that if the Greeks, who founded colonies in southern Italy from the beginning of eighth century, had brought with them the most common mutation of beta-thalassemia [12] in the eastern Mediterranean Sea, this might mean that the falciparum malaria had already produced its adverse effects in some of the most densely populated districts of Greece. It is right to wonder whether these regions of Greece were the same areas from where the settlers, who searched new lands, had their origin[13]. [46]. Now, we come back to the onset

benign forms of malaria in the Southern European Countries was favoured by the appearance of some propitious conditions such as lifestyle change and demographic increase.

[12] One of the most frequent mutations of the beta-thalassemia in modern populations in the Mediterranean basin, is the B + IVSnt 110 [GA]. It may be detected in the Italian areas of Greek colonization, and it has its highest frequency in the lands of the Eastern Mediterranean; it is very common in Greece and it is also associated with a high level of haplotype diversity in Turkey. Consequently it has been suggested that this mutation originated in Greece or Anatolia, and it was spread to the West and particularly in Italy, due to the Greek colonization from the eighth century b.C. onwards [47].

[13] Sallares reports in his work that a number of quotations concerning intermittent fevers characteristic of malaria are recorded in ancient literature: the Hippocratic Corpus, dating back to the fourth and fifth centuries B.C., the ancient Indian texts difficult to date and the Chinese literature dating to the end of the first millennium B.C. These evidences leave no doubt that the benign tertian fever [caused by Plasmodium vivax] and quartan fever [caused by Plasmodium malariae] were endemic in the old world and particularly in Greece, as well as in India and China from 500 BC

of malignant malaria caused by Plasmodium Falciparum. It is well known that relations with the Nile Valley were frequent and the prospects of an epidemic spreading from that country were very likely. Recently, a letter was published by Andreas G. Nerlich et al. in "Emerging Infectious Diseases", which reports the unambiguous identification of ancient DNA of Plasmodium Falciparum, extracted from tissues of Egyptian mummies [48]. The two positive samples were obtained from individuals who were buried in the tomb complexes in Thebes-West and who lived in an epoch comprised between the New Kingdom and late period (1500 - 500 BC). Each sample was obtained from adults who had pathological evidence in bone of chronic anemia[14]. In February 2010 an interesting original contribution was published in JAMA. The authors, studying the paleopathology of Egyptian mummies of pharaohs and of some family members, respectively belonging to dynasties of 18th, 19th and 20th and dating back to the New Kingdom (1550 BC-1295 BC), detected the presence of Plasmodium Falciparum infection in 4 human remains [49]. They found plasmodial DNA, by use of genetic tests including PCR primers that specifically amplify small subtelomeric variable open reading frame (STEVOR), merozoite surface protein 1 (MSP1) and apical membrane antigen 1 (AMA1) gene fragments. It is interesting to note that among the four mummies found to be suffering from malaria, there is also that of Pharaoh Tuthankhamen. These important findings confirm that malaria epidemic was widespread in the Nile Valley at least since the sixteenth century BC.

Currently this scientific achievement is the earliest genetic evidence of malaria in mummies with confirmed date. Previously, immunological assays were used to detect antigens related to the Plasmodium Falciparum including the PARA Sight-F test and ICT Malaria PF test. The first test is a dual antibody immunoassay, designed to retrieve the antigen of histidine-rich protein-2, descending from the *Plasmodium falciparum* trophozoites. This method yielded very promising results because the antigen was proved in 7 out of 18 mummies dating back from 3200 BC to about AD 550., but there is the likelihood that this was a false positive result because later the antibody reactivities were not confirmed by PCR. In the considered circumstance the antibody reactivities are directed towards ancient proteins, it is known that they deteriorate over time as all the biomolecules, thus they lose their shape. Sallares points out that very little is known about how reliable are immunological tests when they are used to detect ancient deteriorated proteins [50]. There are also specific medical conditions that may generate false positive results with the test PARA Sight, used for diagnosis of malaria: it was recently reported that patients with rheumatoid factor, and several other immunological disorders showed false positive results using this technique [50]. The contribution of ELISA tecniques that use monoclonal antibodies is questionable, interesting results have been reported for the diagnosis of infection caused by schistosoma in Egyptian mummies, but their application for diagnosis of malaria in ancient human remains, provided (in this case) disappointing results. [50]. With regard to the geographical Hellenic context, unfortunately the mummification was never performed and, in consideration of the limitations due to immunological techniques, only bio-molecular studies on skeletal remains, obtained

[14] The author analyzed a total of 91 samples of bone tissues belonged to subjects who lived between 3500 and 2800 BC, and who were buried at Abydos [7 cases], and remains found in a Middle Kingdom tomb in Thebes West dating back to 2050 - 1650 BC [42 cases], and in various burial complexes in Thebes West used between the Middle Kingdom and the late period [42 cases]. The bio-molecular analysis on the subjects who lived in earlier periods [predynastic] and during the Middle Kingdom were negative [48].

from the burials, will help to determine when and where the infection caused by Plasmodium Falciparum took root in the Hellenic peninsula.

The Site of Lerna

Lerna was an ancient urban settlement in Greece, in the South East of Argolis (Figure 6), on the western shore of a bay, about 10 km from Argos; Arcadia and Argolis together constitute the Peloponnese peninsula. The site, inhabited since the sixth millennium BC (Neolithic), reveals, in ruins, precious artifacts and important aspects of the ancient civilization of Hellas[15]. The archaeological site is important for the documentation of private dwellings from the Neolithic period until the Mycenaean age [51]. During the early stages of occupation in the Neolithic, it is likely that the site was distant from the sea, but as the levels of costs continued to rise, significant parts of the Argive plain were covered with water, giving rise to the lake. This basin had a diameter of about 4.7 km. and it was surrounded by a swampy environment [52, 53]. The lake, separated from the open sea by a barrier of sand, had originated when the sea level had dropped at the end of the last glaciation, reaching its maximum extent early in the Bronze Age [52].

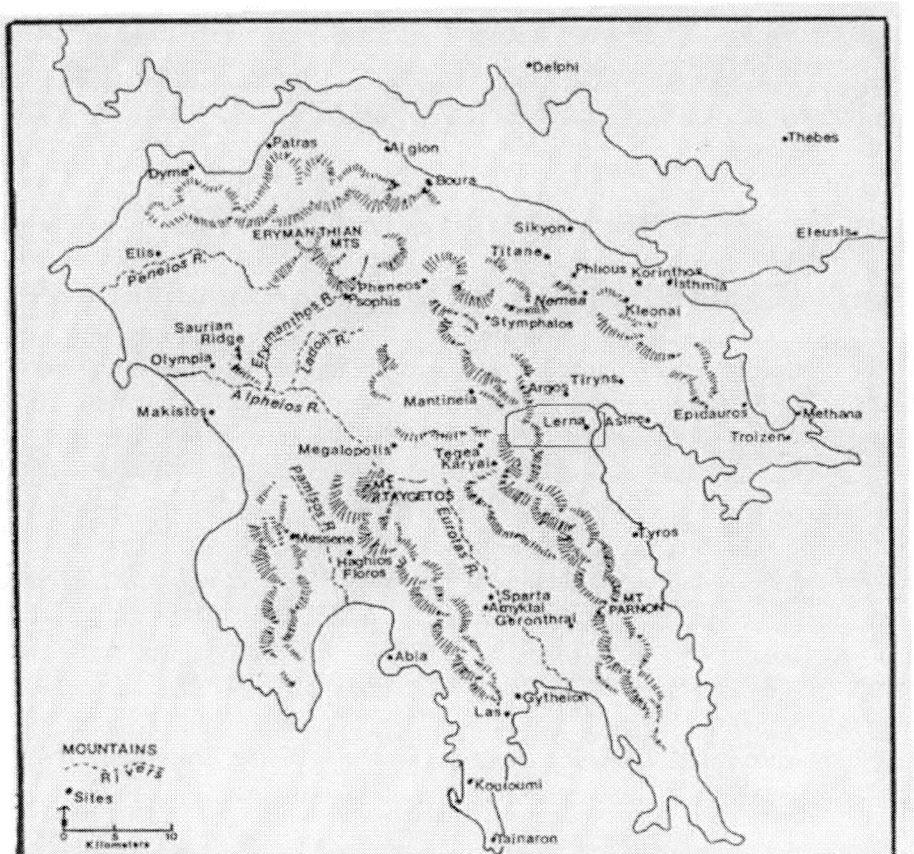

Figure 6.

[15] The excavations were conducted between 1952 and 1958.

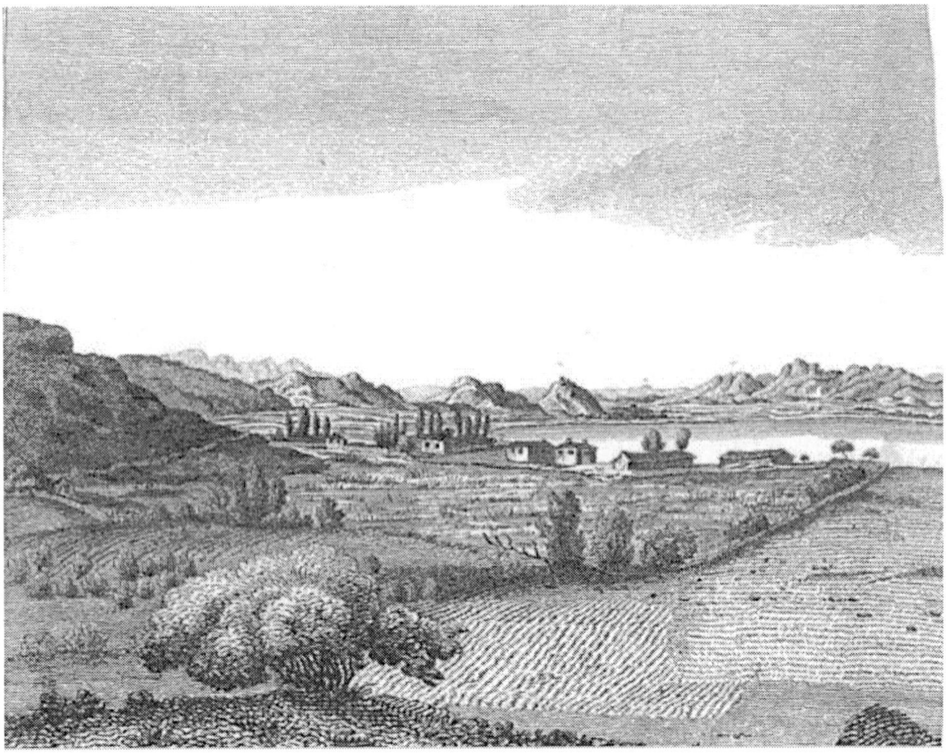

Figure 7.

The lake of Lerna[16] was fed through karst conduits, first and foremost from the river Erasinos, coming from the Argolis mountains with fresh water that gushed out, famous for its quality, especially in the early Bronze Age [54]. According to Pausanias, the waters continued to flow in summer, even if the other surface waters dried up [54]. Baird ruled that even in the middle of the nineteenth century the subterranean reappearance of underground river Erasinos occurred with "burst from the rocks with great violence," while Boblaye pointed out that abundant bubbles emerged from the waters, a phenomenon probably related to the associated release of carbon dioxide [54]. Around 1250 BC the site, near the lake, was definitively abandoned because of the changing conditions of the country, having the appearance of the marsh made it uninhabitable. Despite both the covering with sand and the erosion of the soil, the remains of Lake Lerna were visible until the late nineteenth century [52] and were visited by many travelers who reported accurate descriptions of this place [54]. Figure 7 shows what remained of the lake of Lerna when, in 1810, Sir William Gell, an English traveler, writer and artist, arrived in the Peloponnese [55]. Now we come back to consider the archaeological excavations concerning the site of Lerna and in particular its necropolis, 9 burials were of the Neolithic period, most of these tombs dated back to the Middle Bronze Age (2050/2000-1700/1650 BC), whereas no Late Bronze Age burials were discovered, the later graves were

[16] In the fourth century BC, the karst features of the Arcadian rivers were described by the greek philosopher Aristotle. In his treatise entitled Meteorology [350 BC] he argued that since Arcadia is surrounded by mountains, its waters could reach the sea only through underground channels. Modern science has ascertained Arcadian karst nature [54].

rare. The tombs of the Middle Bronze Age were generally found near the houses but, some of the infant burials were detected under the floors of the dwellings [53].

There are many findings in the Attic ceramics concerning the Hercules myth'[17] and whereas it may be shared the thesis suggesting that the painted figures on Greek vases constitute one of the most classic examples of ancient visual communication, it is also interesting the interpretation of the myths most frequently depicted. Grmek and Gourevitch explained the vase-paintings, on the Corinthian pottery dating back to 630-570 BC, which represent Hercules, whereas he is killing the Hydra, the snake with many heads, as an attempt to reclaim the malarial swamps of Lerna by the mythical hero [1]. Lerna, probably, before the deterioration of the lake area was a place with a mild climate and a favourable environment to human settlements. Later, in Corinth, just a few kilometers far from Lerna, an Asclepeion was erected and it is known that these sanctuaries were in countries favoured by nature. A prerequisite for the building of a sanctuary was the presence of a source of pure water, which frequently was thermal.[18] In these sacred places the medical knowledge was provided by Asclepiades[19], physicians-priests who boasted of having Asclepius as their ancestor; it is interesting to note that this knowledge was handed down only within their progeny.

Biomolecular Study of the Bone Remains Found in Lerna

Biomolecular studies on ancient DNA of malarial parasite in human remains and the determination of globin gene mutations could potentially confirm whether the skeletal signs of anemia [porotic hyperostosis] observed in some Aegean prehistoric skeletons, are secondary to genetic thalassemia rather the result of acquired anemia due to alimentary iron deficiency. Unfortunately, even the most sophisticated search techniques have to face the possibility of survival of DNA in ancient human skeletons; it was established that the most important factor, influencing DNA survival, is not the chronological age of the specimens, but their thermal history, namely either the refrigeration state [in ideal conditions] or exposure to hot environment [in unfavourable contexts]. Since the degradation of DNA occurs more rapidly at higher temperatures, the index used is the so-called "thermal age". This parameter is calculated from the historical evolution of the temperature in a site and in relation to its geographical location [53]. Scholars who dealt with these issues have made clear that the limit of the DNA breakdown, which included data on the extraction of ancient authenticated DNA, would be approximately 19000 years, if the temperature remained relatively constant in the course of time and around 10 ° C. Based on this assumption, it is unlikely that samples,

[17] Hercules is the most represented character in the Attic black-figures vase-paintings, which represent the earlier Athenian ceramic production [seventh century BC.], while Theseus is represented in the later Athenian red-figures vase-paintings production; the first specimen of red-figures vase-paintings dated back to about 575 BC. [Approximately].

[18] In the Hellenistic sanctuary of Asclepius in Corinth, the term Lerna was attributed to the water-containing tank, used by sick subjects who take baths not only for religious purposes. It is interesting to note that in the Hellenistic period the term Lerna, was not only referred to a geographical entity, as in the Archaic period, but it was also attributed to a place [the tank] of the sanctuary haunted by patients. [56].

[19] These physicians-priests, although they took care of the patients and performed some medical and surgical practices, were only the god's intermediaries but they did not possess an independent thought. Therefore this concept of Medicine remarkably differs from the precepts of Hippocratic doctrine.

obtained from any site with a thermal age normalised to approximately 10 ° C for a period of more than 19000 years, contain ancient DNA. When the proposed calculations are applied to the study of Eastern Mediterranean Sea, it may be obtained that a thermal age of 19 000 years at 10° C corresponds to approximately 3600 chronological years, therefore on the basis of this assumption it is unlikely that ancient DNA is detectable in human remains found at Neolithic sites of this area, which pre-date 2000 BC[20]. Nevertheless other problems should be examined; it is crucial to consider also the poor preservation of human remains caused by their exposure to water for the time that elapsed from their excavation, as well as the possibility that the methodologies, used for DNA detection, induced false positive results. This pitfall might be occurred in special manner before the adoption of rigorous criteria for study of specimens. The use of standard methodologies, in this context, prevent the event that the bone remains may be contaminated by modern biological material. Furthermore it is possible that some samples which gave negative results in previous researches would have detected the presence of ancient DNA if the highly-sensitive polymerase chain reaction (PCRs), now available, had been used [53]. Chilvers recently published data of a biomolecular-paleopathological research, performed in 8 sites dating back to the Neolithic and Bronze Age in Greece and Crete. Among the published data he also included those related to bones (Figure 8) found in Lerna, dating back to 2050-1675 BC, thus these specimens dated to the expected 3600-year age limit, beyond which these remains are unlikely to contain ancient DNA. Nevertheless the bio-molecular investigation of these authors did not allow to detect DNA in the eight samples studied although the most of them are closely linked to 3600-year age period [53].

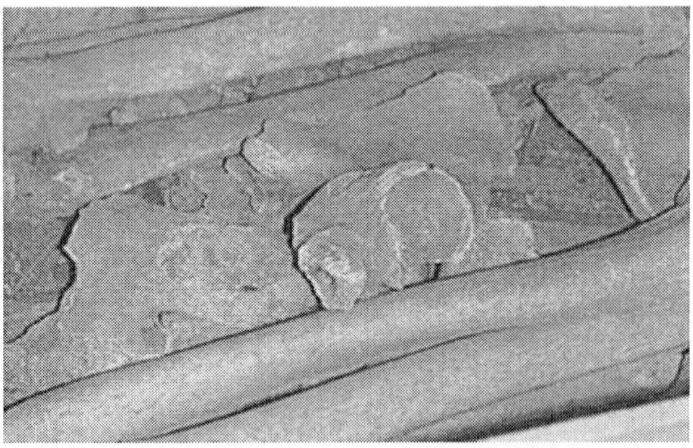

Figure 8.

The authors noted that the marshy conditions, which likely prevailed near to Lerna, for at least part of the considered period and in the ground, where these skeletons were buried, would suggest the presence of a high moisture content. Unfortunately, this abundance of water would have facilitated the degradation of ancient bone DNA [53].

[20] On the basis of this consideration it results that the sites of the Bronze Age of Minoan Palatial Period [about 2000-1450 BC] and of Mycenaean Greece, dating from about 1650 to 1150 BC, represent the maximum limit for the preservation of ancient DNA [53].

Discussion

Malaria was one of the most common diseases in the "ancient world" and it still afflicts heavily, causing a high morbidity and mortality, a large part of mankind. Certainly the pressure of natural selection by different species of plasmodia, and in particular by Plasmodium Falciparum induced a greater impact on the human genome than any other pathogen [50]. In Greece, from the beginning of fifth century BC, the reports of the authors, who wrote about malaria, became more and more frequent. All the Greek medical literature, in a remarkable way, has been concerned with malarial fevers, in addition many poets and prose-writers (Sophocles and Aristophanes) mentioned the presence of fevers associated with chills [27]. From a literary point of view with regard to malaria in the writings of the authors who lived before 500 BC (Homer Il. XXII, 31 and Theognis, v. 173-4) only two references may be found, although, according to Plinio Fraccaro's opinion, these reports are enough questionable [27]. According to several modern authors who are interested in this topic, the spreading of malaria from the sixth century onwards played a significant role in the decline of the Hellenic world, in fact, on closer inspection, the Greeks mentioned by Polybius did not have any more the courage, the love for hard work, intelligence, the patriotism of their ancestors. At the beginning of the twentieth century, Plinio Fraccaro asked an interesting question: *".... then, has malaria led to the decline of Greece or rather has the decline of Greece allowed the spread of malaria? " [*27].

With the aim to obtain a definite answer to such a question to date, it may be theoretically used the scientific evidence provided by molecular biology, which establishes an accurate dating of the detected paleopathological remains. The aim of our work was to include in a bibliographic, comprehensive review, which is focused on the paleopathology of malaria, an analysis of the meaning of the Hercules'myth in ancient Greece in relation to some of the numerous archaeological findings, where it was represented. In general, a scientific interest concerning the nature of the myth rose between the seventeenth and eighteenth centuries, when philosophers, philologists and historians began to look at its origin and function. In the nineteenth and twentieth century the debate flared up and the topic became a theme of discussion for various schools of thought (naturalistic, anthropological with its various components, psychological, philosophical-symbolist, functionalist). They provided interesting but inconclusive observations for the development of a comprehensive theory. However, it is commonly accepted the concept that in myth and legend, frequently fragments of truth may be present, and it is also through and thanks to the myth that ancient people transcribed and coded natural phenomena for which they often were unable to find an explanation. In other words if the ancients did not understand what was happening when the lightning flashed in the sky, it was easier and more useful to think that Jupiter was angry and he was hurling his thunderbolts to punish men.

In this context, the degradation of the plain of Lerna as well as of the lake which was progressively becoming a marsh, caused by climatic and geo-morphological modifications, was "justified" and explained by those who lived in those places, by means of the emergence, in the newly formed marsh, of a monster with seven heads. It is interesting to note that the Hydra, according to myth, gave out a mephitic exhalation, a miasma, but there is no evidence to suggest that in ancient times the Hellenes had developed a relationship between the unhealthiness of the place and the miasma[21].

Hercules, the hero for excellence, killing the monster, fights successfully against those environmental conditions, causing a serious danger to people. The identification of the Hydra with the malaria, in this view, becomes plausible. The only possible cure/clean to the minds of an archaic people is that performed by Heracles, a hero endowed with superhuman strength and courage. He provides his prerogatives and turns them to obtain beneficial ends, moreover in his second labour he utilizes his tremendous strength and in this endeavor he is helped by his nephew Iolaus to prevent the re-growing of the heads. In this shared action an example, albeit primitive, of medical culture may be observed. Iolaus, cauterizing the stumps of severed heads, prevents their regeneration. Hercules does not use brute force alone, otherwise he assumes the characteristics of the civil hero, he uses his knowledge and, most interestingly, he takes care that his nephew Iolaus, the most cherished person to him, exerts this knowledge. In his generosity, however, Hercules paid for his commitment with his life, the monster's infected blood by fraud is used by a wild natural entity, the centaur Nessus, to poison the hero. It is interesting to note that both the centaur Nessus' and the Hydra's blood is identified as the carrier of poison. The archaic Greeks did not have, as we have pointed out, the concept of infection and identified it with the poisoning. Hercules, when he wore the tunic, which was soaked with the Nessus' blood, felt a sensation of burning skin, that caused him considerable sufferings. The pain was so unbearable that he had to be sacrificed on the pyre because the poisoned garment, which was wasting him, could not be removed. Does not that burning, that consumes the hero, look like a malignant fever, the typical fever caused by malaria due to Plasmodium Falciparum? And yet does not the fire of the pyre evoke a death induced by a severe hyperthermia? In the archaic Greece the rational approach of Hippocratic medicine is still far-off, the cause of the disease is attributed to a monstrous being that, by means of a poison, takes possession of the hero's body, forcing him to the final sacrifice.

The archaeological remains and the artistic representations in particular, as detectable in the paintings of black and red-figure vases, are able to suggest, through the representative images of the myth, that at Lerna, a marshy area developed in the Archaic period. This event occurred as a result of major environmental changes, which made the country unhealthy and induced the crisis of human survival in that region. The main elements which are characteristic of the myth include the representations of the monster of Lerna, the Hercules' fight with this natural wicked entity and his victory, the Hero's sacrifice and death, caused by Nessus' infected blood and finally his divinization, after the body was burnt on the pyre. It is a metaphorical representation of the new environmental reality, it is therefore clear that the pictures, which show the heroes' deeds, report the language of that time with immediacy. In the archaic Attic pottery and then in ceramics, belonging to classical Athenian period, the most sensible representations of the collective imaginary may be observed. These frames allow us to understand the meaning of that age. Edward Dodwell[22], a traveler of the early decades of the nineteenth century, was the first to pay attention to the several stories about the lake in early stage. In a chapter of his book [58] entitled the "Lake of Lerna" he indicated in

[21] Only in the fifth century BC, in his work entitled : "About the Air, Water and Places", Hippocrates [Kos Larissa 351 BC-458 BC] suggested the influence of the environment on human health, through the action of sun, soil, water, air, hot, cold.

[22] Dodwell described the malarial fevers that occured in that place and he was a victim of an infection contracted during these trips [54].

an appropriate way the relevant historical sources [Herodotus, Strabo and Pausanias], who had described the lake[23] and reported vivid descriptions of the Hydra. Comparing all the above quotations with what he observed at the beginning of the nineteenth century, he came to the conclusion that the lake in the mythological view coincided with Hydra, "entered the flat and devastated the country and the flocks" [58]. In this metaphor the regrowing heads of the Hydra corresponded to water courses and, over time, having the channels of these tributaries silted up with sand, the waters of karstic origin, coming from the mountains of Argolis, through hidden culverts, would have run elsewhere. Dodwell also suggested that the number of Hydra's heads changes, due to the fact that the number of watercourses, feeding the lake, would have varied with the seasons. This opinion was shared by other travelers who visited the plain of Argos in the early decades of the nineteenth century and soon became the accepted viewpoint [54]. Now, coming back to modern studies, paleopathological researches and bio-molecular investigations, which unequivocally confirm the view of Angel, published in the sixties of last century in the famous volume Lerna [56] and in other articles [37, 38, 39], unfortunately, to date, did not achieve the expected results.

Although the molecular techniques are now very sensitive, the objective limits that we have presented briefly, by reviewing the recent literature, do not allow us to obtain the evidence that, as they say, the circle can be closed permanently. With the aim to reconstruct the Hellenic pathocenosis and in particular the evolution of the malaria epidemic in the ancient Greece, to date, we can only put together the pieces provided by the literary narrative[24], by the myth, by the art expressed in the archaeological findings, by the investigation on Paleoclimate, by the study, through geo-morphological scientific methods, of the region and, in the last analysis, by a key proof (with the known limits), represented by macroscopic investigation on skeletal remains, identifying the classic signs of porotic hyperostosis. Paleo-entomological investigations could confirm what it is suspected, however, there is a limit dictated by the evidence that only the discovery of fossils belonging to genus Anopheles could give us the opportunity to know with certainty the evolution of the different species involved in transmission of Plasmodium malaria. This is very suggestive the idea of providing a link among informations obtained from literature and from myth, from manufactures and from archaeological remains that represent them and exquisitely scientific disciplines such as paleopathology, bio-molecular research on ancient human remains and, when available, on paleo-entomological findings. Beyond the results achieved by our attempt to correlate and integrate these data, our viewpoint seems very interesting and promising to us.

---

[23] In the Archaic period in central Boeotia there was another central karst lake, in the west of Thebes, near Orchomenos, it was Lake Copaide and it was fed by the river Cephisus. When the Lake turned into a marsh attemps of land reclamation were initiated by Alexander the Great. According to the famous malariologist Ronald Ross, in a speech he gave on November 29, 1909 at the Oxford Medical Society, the turning into a marsh of this sheet favoured the strong spread of malaria in a region of Greece, which had been densely populated till then, where there were flourishing cities. Malaria progressively "... sapped the energies of the race, attacking the rural population, killing babies, catching the rising generation ..." [33].

[24] The Homeric poems are of considerable importance in documenting the process of development of the ancient Hellenic culture, and they also allow to obtain valuable information and details on the early formation of the Medicine. It has to be observed that description of traumatic injuries [about 180] has a prominent place in the Homeric poems.

Pictures

1) Sneering mask, “sardonic laugh” from Tharros (Oristano). V century b.C. National Archeological Museum -Cittadella dei Musei. Cagliari (Italy)
2) Black-figures vase-painting: Hercules is attacking Hydra, while Iolaus is cauterizing the stumps of cut heads. It was found in Euboea (Greece). Vase number 461, from Louvre Museum.
3) Black-figures olpe-painting: Hercules is attacking Nessus with a sword. Athenian manufacture (510-500 BC). It was found in Certosa’s necropolis, Bologna (Etruria Padana, Italy), tomb number 318, from Municipal Archeological Museum, Bologna, Italy.
4) Red-figures vase-painting: Hercules’ apotheosis following his suffering at the stake. Pelike found at Vulci [Tuscia], Staatliche Antikensammlungen und Glyptothek. 2366 (J 384), Munich.
5) Red-figures crater-painting: Hercules, taken by goddess Athena, his patroness, is admitted by his father Zeus to the presence of gods in Olympus. Athenian manufacture (470-460 BC). It was found in Arnoaldi’s necropolis, Bologna (Etruria Padana, Italy), tomb number 78, from Municipal Archeological Museum, Bologna, Italy.
6) Map of the Peloponnese peninsula
7) Picture, by Sir W. Gell, showing the Lake Lerna, at the beginning of XIX century
8) Skeletal remains found at Lerna, dating back between 2050 and 1675 BC.

Acknowledgments

The Authors thank Dr. Laura Minarini, Dr. Daniela Ferrari and Dr. Marco Mengoli [Municipal Archeological Museum in Bologna, Italy] for their fruitful suggestions and interesting comments.

Photographic reproductions of pictures, number 3 and 5, were courteously provided from Photographic Archives of Municipal Archeological Museum in Bologna, Italy.

Bibliografia

[1] Grmek M., Gourevitch D. *Le malattie nell’arte antica*.Giunti Editore, 2000 Firenze.

[2] A Ruffer. *Histological studies on Egyptian mummies*. 1911, Le Caire.

[3] Drancourt M., Raoult D., Molecular insights into the history of plague. *Microbes and Infection* 4, 105-109, 2002.

[4] Bianucci R., Rahalison L., Rabino Massa E., Peluso A., Ferroglio E., Signoli M. Technical Note: A rapid Diagnostic Test Detects Plague in Ancient Human Remains: An Example of the Interaction Between Archeological and Biological Approaches [Southeastern Frence, 16th-18th Centuries]. *Am. J. Phis. Anthrop.*,136 (3), 361-367, 2008.

[5] Bianucci R., Rahalison L., Peluso A., Rabino Massa E., Ferroglio E., Signoli M., Langlois J.-Y., Gallien V. Plague Immunodetection in remains of religious exhumed from burial sites in central France. *J. Archael. Sci.* 36, 616-621, 2009.

[6] Dirckx J.H., Pestilence Narrative in Classical Literature: a study in creative imitation I. Homer, Sophocles, Thucydides and Lucretius. *Am. J. Dermatopathol.* 22, 197-202, 2000.

[7] Dirckx J.H., Pestilence Narrative in Classical Litterature: A Study in Creative Imitation II. Virgil, Ovid, Seneca, and Silius Italicus. Am. J. Dermatopathol. 22, 459-464, 2000.

[8] Carmelo U., The Different Originality of Homer and Thucydides *Am. J. Dermapath.* 23, 274-275, 2001.

[9] Ferrari D. Gli amuleti dell'antico Egitto. *Editrice La Mangragora.* 1996 Imola.

[10] Urso C. Ipotesi sul morbo acheo. *Pathologica* 86, 441-443, 1993.

[11] Stefanato C.M., Rotoli M. Il <Filottete di Sofocle> Chron. Derm. Anno XVII, 6, 915-927, 1986.

[12] Urso C., Farella V. An Inquiry on Philoctetes's Disease. *Am. J. Dermatopathol.* 18, 326-329, 1996.

[13] Ercole. L'eroe, il mito. (A cura di Stefano De Caro) *Biblioteca di via Senato Edizioni.* 2001.Milano.

[14] Grmek M.D. La malaria dans la mediterranee orientale prehistorique et antique. *Parassitologia* 36, 1-6, 1994.

[15] Celli A. Malaria. *Longmans Green*, 1900 London.

[16] Ross R. Malaria in Greece. *J. Trop. Med.* 9, 341-347, 1906.

[17] Jones WHS, Malaria. *A neglected factor in the history of Greece and Rome.* Macmillan Bowes and Bowes, 1907 Cambridge.

[18] Livingston. F.B. Anthropological implication of Sickle Cell Gene. Distribution in West africa. Americ. *Anthrologist.* 60, 533-562, 1958.

[19] http://www.demarchi.org/tesi.htm [visitato il g. 07/10/2010].

[20] Capasso L. Fossil mosquitoes and the spread of infectious diseases in man's ancestors. *J. Paleopathol.* 3: 171-201,1991.

[21] Capasso L. The origin of human malaria. *Int. J. Anthropol.* 13 (n.3-4), 165-175, 1998.

[22] Capasso L. Dalla Pozza G., Di Tota G. Culex Tanzaniae, sp.n.: a new fossil mosquito of the Pliocenic coppal from Moa Moa, near Dar-el-Salaam (Tanzania, East Africa). *Bollettino della Società Paleontologica Italiana* (1998) (citazione ripresa da Capasso-21).

[23] Jones WHS. Malaria and History. *Ann. Trop. Med. Parasit.* 1, 529-546, 1908.

[24] Jones WHS. Malaria and Grek history. With Withington ET. *The history of Grek therapeutics and the malaria theory.* Manchester University Press, 1909 Manchester.

[25] Jones WHS. Dea Febris; a study of malaria in a ancient Italy. *Ann. Archaeol. Anthrop.* 2, 97-124, 1909.

[26] Kouzis A. Quelques notes sur les fièvres paludéennes d'après les anciens médicins grecs. *Atti Soc. Studi Malaria* 9: 81 sq., 1909.

[27] Cawadias A. Le paludisme dans l'histoire de l'ancienne Grèce. *Bull. Soc. Franc. Hist. Med.*8,158-165, 1909.

[28] Huntington E. The burial of Olympia: a study in climate and history. *Geogr. J.*, 36: 657-675 1910.

[29] Regnault F. Le role du dépleuplement, du déboisement et de la malaria dans la décadence de certaines nations. *Rev. Scient.* 52: 46 sq., 1914.

[30] Cardamatis JP. Du paludisme dans la Grèce continentale depuis les temps les plus reculés jusqu'à la période macédonienne. *Arch. Schiff. Trop. Hyg.* 19: 273-301, 1915.

[31] Pais E. *Storia della Sardegna e della Corsica durante il periodo romano*. Vol 2, 549 sq., Attilio Nardecchia editore. 1923 Roma.

[32] Celli A. Storia della malaria nell'Agro Romano. *Accademia dei Lincei.* 1923 Città di Castello.

[33] Fraccaro P. La malaria e la storia degli antichi popoli classici. *Atene e Roma*. 22, 57-88, 1919.

[34] Sigerist H.E. *Civilization and Disease*. University of Chicago Press. 1962 Chicago.

[35] Belios G.D. L'Histoire du paludisme en Grèce depuis l'antiquité jusq'à la decouverte de Laveran. *Jouve,* 1933 Paris.

[36] Sorre M. Complexes pathogènes et géographie médicale. *Ann. Gèogr*. 42, 1-18, 1933.

[37] Angel J.L. Osteoporosis, thalassemia. *Amer. J. Phis. Anthrop*. 22, 369-372, 1964.

[38] Angel J.L. Porotic hyperostosis, anemias, malarias, and marshes in the prehistoric Eastern Mediterranean. *Science* 153, 760-763, 1966.

[39] Angel J.L. Ecology and population in the Eastern Mediterranean. *World Ecology* 4, 88-105, 1972.

[40] Charlier P. L'anthropologie grecque comme cheval de bataille: l'affrontement des écoles francaise et américaine dans l'étude des restes humains en Grèce (1943-1985). Eur. Rev. Hist.: *Revue europeenne d'histoire*. 13 (4), 643-680, 2006.

[41] Grmek M.D. Les maladies à l'aube de la civilization occidentale. *Payot,* 1983 Paris.

[42] Grmek M.D. *Diseases in the ancient Greek world*. (Translaction M. and L. Muellner) Johns Hopkins University Press, 1988 Baltimore.

[43] Bruce-Chwatt L.J. Essential malariology. *Heinimann.* 1985 London.

[44] Bruce-Chwatt L.J. History of malaria from prehistory to eradication. In Wensdorfer W.L., McGregor I Sir (Eds) Malaria. *Principles and practice of malariology*. Vol. 1 Churchill Livingstone, 1988 pp. 1-59 Edinburgh.

[45] De Zulueta J. Changes in the geographical distribution of malaria throughout history. *Parassitologia* 29, 193-205, 1987.

[46] Sallares R. *The ecology of the ancient Greek world.* Duckworth 1991 London.

[47] Sallares R., Bouwman A., Anderung C. The spread of malaria to Southern Europe in antiquity: new approaches to old problems. *Med. Hist*. 48, 311-328, 2004.

[48] Nerlich A. G., Schraut B., Dittrich S., Jelinek T., Zink A. R. Plasmodium falciparum Ancient Egypt. *Emerg. Infect. Dis*. 8, 1317-1319, 2008.

[49] Hawass Z., Gad Y.Z., Ismail S., et al. Ancestry and pathology in King Tutankhamun's family. *JAMA* 303 (7), 638-647, 2010.

[50] Sallares R., Gomzi S. Biomolecular archaelogy of malaria. *Anc. Biomol.* 3, 195-213, 2001.

[51] www.marcianum.it (visitato il g. 07/10/2010).

[52] Zangger E. Prehistoric coastal environments in Greece: the vanished landscapes of Dimini bay and Lake Lerna. *J. Field Arch.* 18 (1), 1-15, 1991.

[53] Chilvers E. R., Bouwman A. S., Brown K.A., Arnott R. G., Prag A.N.W., Brown T. A. Ancient DNA in human bones from Neolithic and Bronze age sites in Greece and Crete. *J. Arch. Sci*., 35, 2707-2714, 2008.

[54] Clendenon C. Karst hidrology in ancient myths from Arcadia and Argolis, Greece. *Acta Carsologica* 38/1, 145-154, 2009.

[55] Gell W. The itinerary of Greece with a commentary on Pausanias and Strabo and an account of the monuments of antiquity at present existing in that country compiled in the years M DCCC I:II:V:VI by W Gell esq: MA: FRS : FSA printed for T Payne, 1810 London.

[56] Melfi M. I *Santuari di Asclepio in Grecia*, Vol. 1, pg. 211. L'Erna di Bretschneider Editore, Roma, 2007.

[57] Angel J. L. *The People of Lerna, Analysis of a Prehistoric Aegean Population*. Vol. II. Princeton, NJ: American School of Classical Studies at Athens, Princeton, and Washington, DC: Smithsonian Institution Press, 1971.

[58] Dodwell E. *A classical and topographical tour through greece, during the years* 1801, 1806, and 1806 (2 vols). Rodwell and Martin, vol.2, 223-228, 1819.

In: Malaria: Etiology, Pathogenesis and Treatments
Editors: A. M. Peterson et al, pp. 151-174
ISBN: 978-1-62100-363-2

Chapter VI

Role of Human Matrix Metalloproteinases in Malaria Pathogenesis

Mauro Prato[1,2*]

[1] Dipartimento di Genetica, Biologia e Biochimica, Università di Torino, Torino, Italy.

[2] Italian Malaria Network - Centro Interuniversitario di Ricerche sulla Malaria (CIRM).

Abstract

Human matrix metalloproteinases (MMPs) are a family of proteolytic enzymes able to destroy endothelial tight junctions, disrupt the subendothelial basement membrane, and modulate the activity of pro-inflammatory molecules and other MMPs. The regulation of balances between MMPs and their endogenous inhibitors (tissue inhibitors of metalloproteinases, TIMPs) plays a key role in either physiological processes, such as wound repair; or pathological, including tumor angiogenesis and neuroinflammation. Interestingly, in the last decade, growing evidence, in vivo and in vitro, on the involvement of MMPs and TIMPs in severe and complicated malaria has been emerging. In the present chapter, the data on altered levels MMPs and TIMPs available from human and murine models of malaria will be reviewed; and the well-established relationship between the host MMP-9 and parasite haemozoin (HZ), the lipid-enriched ferriprotoporphyrin IX crystal produced by Plasmodium parasite after haemoglobin catabolism, will be analyzed. Therefore, the functional role of deregulated balances between MMPs and TIMPs in the clinical progress towards complicated malaria (cerebral, lung and placental malaria), as well as the potential use of MMP inhibitors as an adjuvant treatment, will be discussed.

* Correspondance to: Prof. Mauro Prato, Dipartimento di Genetica, Biologia e Biochimica, Università di Torino, Via Santena 5 bis, 10126 Torino, Italy; Phone: +39-011-790-5850; Fax: +39-011-790-5845; e-mail: mauro.prato@unito.it.

Keywords: haemozoin (HZ), matrix metalloproteinases (MMPs), tissue inhibitors of metalloproteinases (TIMPs), *Plasmodium falciparum*, malaria, cerebral malaria (CM)

1. Introduction

Despite the huge amount of data available from basic and clinical research, the mechanisms underlying malaria pathogenesis are not fully understood yet. This is sadly true, especially for the etiology of clinical progress towards complicated malaria, as well as for the following prognosis; both of which are not easily predictable. Indeed, it is not clear how patients might develop and/or recover from cerebral malaria (CM), anaemia, respiratory distress, renal failure or placental malaria (Murphy SC et al. 2001). It is commonly accepted that these complications are associated with the cytoadherence of parasitized red blood cells (pRBCs) to microvascular endothelium (Chulay JD and Ockenhouse CF 1990; Sherman IW et al. 2003). The parasite rarely crosses the endothelial barriers, however, even though they appear to be leaky and more permeable. It is likely that the host factors produced as a response to the parasite infection, such as inflammatory molecules, might induce symptoms like fever and following organ failure (Nyangoto EO 2005; Clark IA et al. 2006; Clark IA et al. 2008).

In the last decade, growing evidence on the possible involvement of a specific family of human proteolytic enzymes, matrix metalloproteinases (MMPs) in malaria pathogenesis, became available (Szklarczyk A et al. 2007; Prato M et al. 2011a). These molecules are strictly related to inflammatory responses and endothelial barrier permeability (Nagase H and Woessner JF 1999; Rosenberg GA 2002; Rosenberg GA et al. 2007).

In the following sections of this chapter, an updated overview of the data, currently available, on the involvement of MMPs in malaria, along with their endogenous inhibitors (Tissue Inhibitors of Metalloproteinases, TIMPs) will be given; the role of these molecules when determining disease severity will also be addressed. Furthermore, future possible therapeutic perspectives will briefly be considered.

2. Biochemistry and Biology of MMPs and TIMPs

Human MMPs are a family of 23 proteolytic enzymes produced by a broad spectrum of different cells, including fibroblasts, endothelial cells, lymphocytes, monocytes, macrophages, and smooth muscle cells (Nagase H and Woessner JF Jr. 1999; Woessner JF Jr 2002). These enzymes have been studied and characterized for almost 50 years: the first MMP was discovered in 1962 (Gross J and Lapiere CM 1962), whereas the later one dates at 2001 (Lohi J et al. 2001). Concerning the nomenclature rules, MMPs are generally indicated by nearly sequencial numbers (from MMP-1 to MMP-28, with few numbering gaps); alternatively, they can be classified according to the sub-family to which they belong (gelatinases, collagenases, stromelysins, matrilysins, membrane-type MMPs and macrophage metalloelastase, so-called depending on specific matrix substrates) (Nagase H and Woessner JF 1999). MMP names according to both nomenclature criteria are notated in Table 1.

MMPs can be selectively inhibited by TIMPs, a well known group of endogenous small molecules (with weight around 20-kDa). The TIMP-family includes four members (from TIMP-1 to -4), which are produced by several cells, similarly as MMPs (Brew K and Nagase H 2010).

Table 1. Nomenclature of human MMPs

MMP	common name
MMP-1	collagenase-1 (interstitial collagenase)
MMP-2	gelatinase A
MMP-3	stromelysin-1
MMP-7	matrilysin-1
MMP-8	collagenase-2 (neutrophil collagenase)
MMP-9	gelatinase B
MMP-10	stromelysin-2
MMP-11	stromelysin-3
MMP-12	macrophage metalloelastase
MMP-13	collagenase-3
MMP-14	MT1-MMP
MMP-15	MT2-MMP
MMP-16	MT3-MMP
MMP-17	MT4-MMP
MMP-18/19	MMP-19
MMP-20	enamelysin
MMP-21/22	MMP-23B
MMP-23	MMP-23A
MMP-24	MT5-MMP
MMP-25	MT6-MMP
MMP-26	matrilysin-2
MMP-27	MMP-27
MMP-28	MMP-28

2.1. Biochemical Structure of MMPs

Structurally, all MMPs share four conserved domains: a signal sequence, a pro-domain, an active domain, and a Zn-binding domain. The active domain and the Zn-binding domain are essential for the catalytic activity, occurring through the coordination of the Zn^{2+}-ion by three histidines in the active domain and a fourth cysteine present in a conserved sequence of the pro-domain (Tallant C et al. 2010). Until the cysteine participates in the Zn^{2+}-ion coordination, the enzyme remains inactive. After its removal by proteolysis or distording by substrate binding ("cysteine-switch" mechanism), the Zn^{2+}-ion becomes available to bind to a hydrolytic water molecule and to the substrate,. Consequently, the enzyme is functionally active (Van Wart HE and Birkedal-Hansen H 1990). Additionally, all MMPs, except matrilysins (MMP-7 and MMP-26), share a carboxyterminal haemopexin-like domain, whose functions range from binding TIMPs for gelatinases to substrate specificity for collagenases (Overall CM 2001). Moreover, gelatinases contain a gelatin-binding fibronectin-like domain between the active domain and the haemopexin-like domain; after the haemopexin-like domain, gelatinase B (MMP-9) also contains a serine-, threonine- and proline-rich collagen type V-like domain, related to binding multiple O-linked glycans (Van den Steen PE et al. 2002). Finally, all membrane-type MMPs show an additional membrane anchor domain at the end of the sequence, and four of them (MT1-, MT2-, MT3- and MT5-MMP) also have a cytoplasmic domain. In contrast, MT4-MMP and MT6-MMP are membrane anchored through a glycosyl-phosphatidil-inositol anchor (Itoh et al. 1999; Kojima et al. 2000). Figure 1 summarizes the main structures of different MMP-family members.

	Signal sequence	Prodomain	Active domain	Fibronectin-like domain	Zn-binding domain	Collagen V-like domain	Haemopexin-like domain	Membrane anchor domain	Cytoplasmic domain
Collagenases	+	+	+	-	+	-	+	-	-
Gelatinases	+	+	+	+	+	±	+	-	-
Stromelysins	+	+	+	-	+	-	+	-	-
Matrilysins	+	+	+	-	+	-	-	-	-
Metalloelastase	+	+	+	-	+	-	+	-	-
MT-MMPs	+	+	+	-	+	-	+	+	±

Figure 1. Structure of MMP-subfamilies members.

2.2. Regulation and Biological Functions of MMPs

MMP gene expression can be either constitutive or inducible. The factors able to promote MMP transcription include: pro-inflammatory molecules, growth factors, nitric oxide (NO), cell-cell interactions, cell-matrix interactions, UV radiations (Nagase H and Woessner JF Jr. 1999). Following protein expression, MMP pro-forms can then be activated through different mechanisms: for example, pro-MMP-9 is activated through a proteolytic cascade sequentially involving plasminogen, MMP-3 and MMP-1 (Van den Steen et al. 2002); while activating MMP-2 requires a previous formation of a multimeric pro-MMP-2/TIMP-2/MT1-MMP complex (Nagase H 1998). Thus, after removing or distorting the pro-peptide, MMPs are functionally active.

In earlier studies, MMPs were mainly related to the degradation of structural proteins in the extracellular matrix (ECM) and sub-endothelial basement membranes. However, aside from their initial role as ECM modifiers, MMPs are presently known also to be responsible for the cleavage of a large spectrum of other substrates, such as: cytokines; chemokines; growth factors; adhesion molecules; intercellular junctions; as well as other proteases, including some haemostasis-related molecules; and MMPs themselves (Somerville RP et al. 2003; Cauwe B et al. 2007).

Therefore, in either physiological or pathological processes, MMPs might play an essential role in the promotion or inhibition of cell survival, proliferation, migration, invasion, haemostasis and inflammation. In physiology, MMPs are involved in mechanisms of wound repair and pregnancy. In pathology, the first research on MMPs focused on their role in cancer (growth, metastasis and angiogenesis); however, during the last decades, the MMPs involvement has been suggested for a large number of other pathologies, including: cardio-vascular diseases, atherosclerosis, emphysema, acute renal failure, ophthalmic pathologies, neuro-inflammation, neuro-degenerative disorders, auto-immune diseases, osteo- and rheumatoid arthritis, and reproductive complications (Nagase H et al. 2006; Cauwe B et al. 2007).

Notable, a role for MMPs in malaria pathogenesis has also been suggested quite recently (Szklarczyk A et al. 2007; Khadjavi A. et al 2010; Prato M et al. 2011a), opening a new unexplored research field, discussed in dedicated sections. Even though the available data is still incomplete, evidence of altered levels of several MMPs in different malaria models is growing constantly. Furthermore, in severe malaria, speculating on the possible consequences of deregulated balances between MMPs and their endogenous inhibitors appears undoubtedly intriguing.

2.3. Structure, Functions and Regulation of TIMPs

In TIMP structures, some conserved cysteines in the N-terminal domain allow these molecules to act as chelators of the zinc in the active site of MMPs, contrasting the effects of removing the MMP pro-peptide and blocking enzyme activity. The crystal structure of MMP-3/TIMP-1 complex shown by Gomis-Ruth et al. represents an adequate model, explaining MMP-TIMP interactions (Gomis-Rüth FX et al. Nature 1997). However, TIMP levels (which usually exceed those of MMPs in organs and fluids in order to contain MMP-triggered proteolysis) are mandatory for MMP inhibition.

Indeed, at low doses these molecules have also been shown to play a role in the activation of gelatinase pro-forms (pro-MMP-2 and pro-MMP-9), through the formation of a trimeric complex involving a specific TIMP, one MT-MMP, and the pro-gelatinase itself. A representative example is given by the TIMP-2/pro-MMP-2/MT-1MMP complex, required for pro-MMP-2 activation. In this case, the C-terminal domain of TIMP-2 is involved in binding the pro-MMP-2 haemopexin domain (Nagase H 1998).

Similarly to MMPs, the transcription of TIMPs is dependent on several soluble factors, including cytokines and growth factors (Brew K and Nagase H 2010). Interestingly, some TIMPs possess additional growth-stimulatory or pro-apoptotic properties, independent of the MMP-blocking effects (Stetler-Stevenson WG 2008).

3. MMP Levels in Malaria Models

In the last decade, growing evidence of enhanced levels of MMPs in several malaria models, either human or murine, became available. In this section, an updated overview of the literature associated with this data will be given, as according to different models.

3.1. Human Models

The majority of works investigating the modulation of MMPs in human malaria models in vitro has been performed by investigating the detrimental effects on the phagocytic and endothelial cells of malarial pigment haemozoin (HZ), a lipid-enriched ferriprotoporphyrin IX produced by Plasmodium falciparum after haemoglobin catabolism (Egan TJ 2008). Little evidence on the involvement of MMPs in human malaria, in vivo, is available from organ autopsy studies and from the fluid analysis of patients with uncomplicated or severe malaria. Unfortunately, in the latter case, data is still conflicting, and often incomplete.

3.1.1. Models in vitro

In a series of studies performed with human adherent or immunopurified monocytes from peripheral blood, phagocytosis of free HZ or HZ-containing trophozoites was shown to enhance MMP-9 mRNA and protein expression, as well as activate MMP-9 protein release (Prato M et al. 2005; Prato M et al. 2008; Prato M et al 2010a; Giribaldi G et al. 2010; Giribaldi G et al. 2011a). This observation was also extended to the THP-1 monocytic cell line (Dell'Agli M et al. 2010). Consequently, total gelatinolytic activity (Prato M et al. 2011b) and invasion abilities (Prato M et al. 2005) of HZ-fed monocytes were increased.

The enhancement of MMP-9 in human monocytes appeared to be mediated by the HZ-dependent overproduction of several pro-inflammatory molecules, including TNFalpha (Prato M et al. 2005), IL-1beta (Prato M et al. 2008) and MIP-1alpha (Giribaldi G et al. 2011a). This was demonstrated by experiments with blocking antibodies, abrogating the effects of HZ on MMP-9; and by those with recombinant cyto/chemokines, mimicking HZ-dependent MMP-9 up-regulation. Further experiments aimed to determine which component of HZ was responsible for these effects showed that the dependence on the lipid moiety of HZ enhanced TNFalpha (Prato M et al. 2010), IL-1beta, and MMP-9 (Prato M et al. 2008), but not MIP-1alpha (Giribaldi G et al. 2010). In these studies, a major role for 15-hydroxyeicosatetraenoic acid (15-HETE), a potent lipoperoxidation derivative generated by HZ autocatalysis (Schwarzer et al. 1999), was suggested. TNF levels were also causally related to an increased release by human adherent monocytes of the active lysozyme, an enzyme stored in gelatinase granules with MMP-9 (Prato M et al. 2009). Furthermore, in this case, dependence on the lipid moiety of HZ was demonstrated, and a major role for 15-HETE was suggested (Prato M et al. 2011b). On the other side, the haem core of HZ has been shown to bind the haemopexin domain of MMP-9 and to prime the activation of the zymogen by other MMPs, such as MMP-3 (Geurts et al. 2008).

Mechanisms underlying the HZ-dependent enhancement of MMP-9 and related molecules may involve NF-kappaB activation, as suggested by parallel works performed with adherent monocytes from peripheral blood (Prato M et al 2010a; Prato M et al. 2011b) and the THP-1 cell line (Dell'Agli M et al. 2010). In these works, the HZ-induced the ehancement of producing MMP-9, lysozyme, TNFalpha and IL-1beta, as well as following the total gelatinolytic and lysozyme activities that were abrogated by using different NF-kappaB inhibitors showing anti-malarial properties (quercetin, artemisinin, parthenolide, and extracts from *Punica Granatum*). However, additional mechanisms cannot be excluded, and a role for MAP-kinases, which are putatively required for HETE-dependent activation of NF-kappaB pathway (Di Mari JF et al 2007) and which have been recently directly related to HZ-dependent MIP-1alpha production (Lucchi NW et al. 2011), is likely. The putative mechanisms, through which HZ up-regulates MMP-9, and the related molecules in human monocytes are represented in Figure 2.

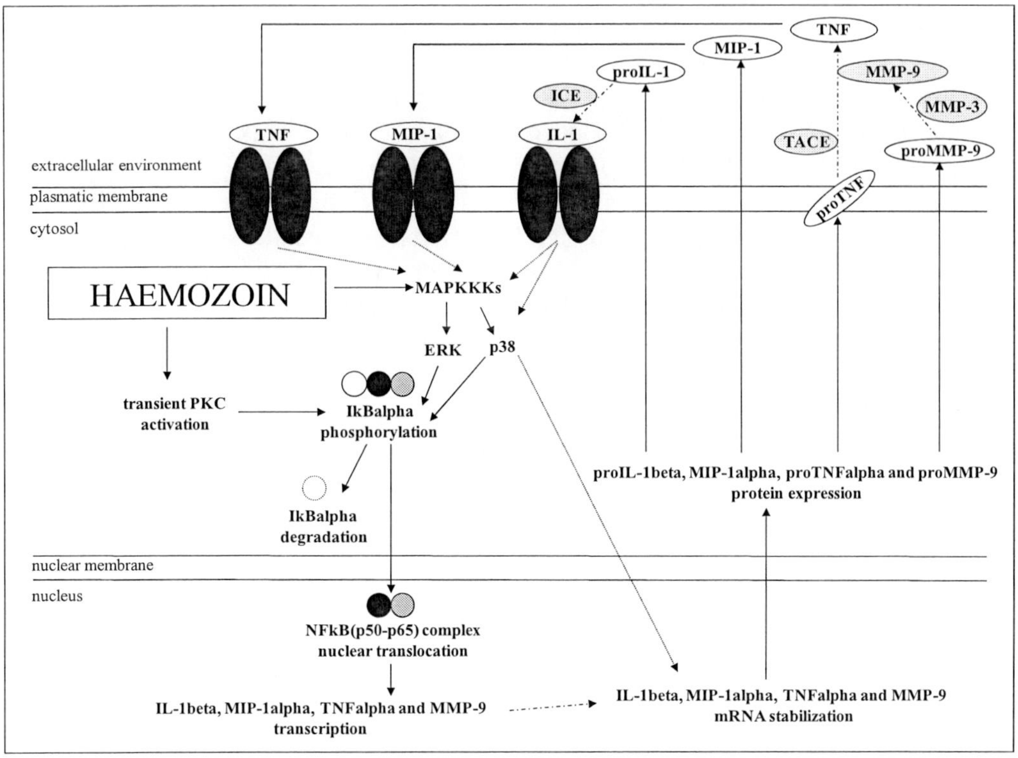

Figure 2. Putative mechanisms underlying the HZ-dependent up-regulation of MMP-9 and related pro-inflammatory molecules.

Little data on MMP regulation is available from studies with HZ-treated endothelial cells. In a human microvascular endothelial cell line (HMEC-1), HZ induced de novo pro-MMP-9 and active MMP-9 protein release without altering basal levels of MMP-2. Interestingly, HZ also enhanced protein levels of basal MMP-1 and MMP-3, two MMPs sequencially involved in pro-MMP-9 activation. Consequently, total gelatinolytic activity and cell invasion abilities were increased (Prato M et al. 2011c). Another evidence of active MMP-9 protein release enhancement, triggered by HZ, comes from studies with human endothelial cells from large calibre vessels (Prato M et al. 2011a). As suggested for human monocytes, it is also suggested that in endothelial cells likelya role for the lipid moiety of HZ is played(Prato M et al. 2011c).

3.1.2. Models in vivo

Accumulations of a pro-angiogenic urokinase-type plasminogen activator receptor (uPAR) (Fauser S et al. 2000), MMP-1 and VEGF (Deininger MH et al. 2003) in Durck granulomas, along with a lack of anti-angiogenic endostatin/collagenXVIII in ring haemorrhage areas (Deininger MH et al. 2002), were observed in the brains of patients with fatal CM, suggesting that the pro-MMP-9 proteolytic machinery is activated in areas of intense parasite sequestration and vascular damage.

Sera of patients with uncomplicated or severe malaria displayed higher levels of MMP-8 but not of MMP-9 (Armah HB et al. 2007; Dietmann A et al. 2008); however, a microarray analysis performed on blood, as a whole, from children with severe malaria showed an activation of the human MMP-9 gene by *P. Falciparum* (Griffiths MJ et al. 2005). It has been suggested that serum levels might not be an ideal source for reliable data concerning MMP levels, since their release from blood cells during sampling process might give a highly non-specific background result, interfering with the determination of true concentrations of circulating MMPs (Yung K 2008). This observation could thus explain the apparently conflicting data from these different works.

Perhaps, research of MMP levels in cerebrospinal fluid (CSF) should also not be recommended. A series of works performed by different independent authors reported that any MMP-9 increases in CSF levels of patients with different severity grades of malaria were not apparent, possibly because of the enzyme's tight association with the extracellular matrix (Armah HB et al. 2007; Dietmann A et al. 2008; Green JA et al. 2011). In the most recent of these studies, MMP-1, MMP-2, and MMP-3 levels in CM patients were also measured, and they were not different from healthy controls. However, since the evidence previously cited on an MMP-1 increase from a *post mortem* analysis of brains with CM (Deininger MH et al. 2003) is quite convincing, it is likely that MMP levels in CSF of patients with CM do not necessarily reflect organ or serum levels.

3.2. Murine Models

The effects of the differential components of HZ on MMP-9 regulation in murine macrophages are available from a series of studies performed in vitro, using a RAW 264.7 cell line. Concerning the works in vivo, a huge amount of data on MMP regulation in mice infected by P. berghei is available from few excellent works performed by using different CM and non-CM models.

3.2.1. Models in vitro

Similarly to previous observations obtained from the human model, phagocytosis of HZ had impaired the expression of several inflammatory molecules (Carney CK et al. 2006), andafter a minor down-regulatory peak, also increased the long-term mRNA expression of MMP-9 in murine macrophages. Likewise, since the lipid-free synthetic HZ (beta-haematin) did not modulate an MMP-9 expression, this effect was related to the lipid moiety of HZ (Schrimpe A et al. 2009a). The HZ-dependent enhancement of MMP-9 transcription and protein release was mimicked by 4-hydroxy-2-nonenal (4-HNE) (Schrimpe A et al. 2009a), another molecule generated by HZ from polyunsaturated fatty acids, in addition to 15-HETE

(Miller CM et al. 2005). However, contrasting from evidence observed in HZ-fed human monocytes (Prato M et al. 2008), 15-HETE did not mimic the HZ effects on MMP-9 in murine macrophages (Schrimpe A et al. 2009b). This evidence suggests the necessity of caution when extrapolating data obtained from murine models to human malaria.

3.2.2. Models in vivo

In the excellent work performed by Van den Steen and his group, by using CM-sensible C57B1/6 mice infected with *P. Berghei* ANKA (CM model) or *P. Berghei* NK65 (non-CM model) and CM-resistant Balb/C mice infected with P. berghei ANKA (CM-resistant model) (Van den Steen PE et al. 2006), the mRNA expression of a large pattern of MMPs, along with a protein release or pro-enzyme activation in selected cases, wasinvestigated in five different organs (brain, lung, spleen, liver, and kidney). Table 2 resumes the results obtained from the CM model; for major completeness, additional data from the work by Szklarczyk et al. (Szklarczyk A et al. 2007) on MMP-7 protein expression in a brain of a similar murine model of CM have been included in the Table.

Table 2. MMP organ levels in murine CM models (adapted from data shown in: Van den Steen PE et al. 2006; Szklarczyk A et al. 2007). ER: enhanced mRNA expression; DR: down-regulated mRNA expression; UR: unaltered mRNA expression; EP: enhanced protein expression; DP: down-regulated protein expression; UP: unaltered protein expression; A: pro-enzyme activation; ND: not detected

MMPs	Brain	Liver	Spleen	Lung	Kidney
MMP-2	enhanced protein	unaltered protein	down-regulated protein	unaltered protein	down-regulated protein
MMP-3	enhanced mRNA	not detected	enhanced mRNA	unaltered mRNA	not detected
MMP-7	enhanced protein	enhanced mRNA	not detected	not detected	not detected
MMP-8	enhanced mRNA	enhanced mRNA	enhanced mRNA	enhanced mRNA	not detected
MMP-9	proenzyme activation	enhanced mRNA	unaltered mRNA	enhanced mRNA	enhanced mRNA
MMP-11	unaltered mRNA	not detected	not detected	down	regulated mRNA
MMP-12	down-regulated mRNA	enhanced mRNA	not detected	not detected	not detected
MMP-13	enhanced mRNA	enhanced mRNA	enhanced mRNA	not detected	not detected
MMP-14	unaltered mRNA	enhanced mRNA	unaltered mRNA	enhanced mRNA	enhanced mRNA
MMP-15	unaltered mRNA	down-regulated mRNA	not detected	unaltered mRNA	down-regulated mRNA
MMP-16	unaltered mRNA	not detected	not detected	not detected	not detected
MMP-17	unaltered mRNA	not detected	not detected	not detected	not detected
MMP-24	unaltered mRNA	not detected	not detected	not detected	not detected

Briefly, in the work by Van den Steen's group, the enhanced expression and activation of monocytic (CD11b+) MMP-9 were observed in the brains of CM mice; such an increase appeared to be specific for CM, as suggested by comparison with non-CM models. Additionally, significant alterations in mRNA expression were found for several MMPs: MMP-3, -4, -8, and -13 were increased in the spleen; MMP-8, -12, -13, and -14 in the liver; MMP-8 and -13 in the brain. These increases were more pronounced in the CM model. In the CM-resistant model, MMP-3 expression was significantly enhanced, suggesting a protective role for this MMP in CM. Moreover, in the experiments shown by Szklarczyk's group, MMP-7 protein expression was increased in the brains of CM mice. Although, reasserting, at any rate, that caution should be taken in translating murine models to humans, this data clearly shows a huge global deregulation of MMP balances. This should certainly be taken in account, at least until more convincing data from human patients become available.

4. TIMP Levels in Malaria Models

Little evidence on TIMP regulation in malaria models is available. In this section, the effects of HZ on human and murine cells in vitro, as well as TIMP levels in human and murine malaria models in vivo, will be listed.

4.1. Human Models

HZ's effects on TIMPs have been investigated in human monocytes and microvascular endothelial cells in vitro. Additionally, among the documents investigating MMP levels in human fluids of malaria patients, TIMP levels were measured in some cases.

4.1.1. Models in vitro

In human adherent monocytes, phagocytosis of HZ promoted mRNA expression and protein release of TIMP-1, and similarly to MMP-9, the effect was mediated by inflammatory molecules TNFalpha, IL-1beta and MIP-1alpha through NF-kappaB activation (Giribaldi G et al. 2011b). The lipid moiety of HZ was necessary for TIMP-1 up-regulation, and a major role for 15-HETE was suggested. However, TIMP-1 enhancement was not sufficient to block the increase of total gelatinolytic activity (Prato M et al. 2011b) and cell invasiveness (Prato M et al. 2005), suggesting that the deregulated balance between MMP-9 and TIMP-1 favors MMP-9 effects.

In HMEC-1 HZ did not alter basal levels of the released TIMP-1 protein, whereas it increased those of TIMP-2, an endogenous inhibitor of MMP-2. Also, in this case, the total gelatinolytic activity and cell invasiveness were increased, as a result of a major induction of MMP-9 (Prato M et al. 2011c). This evidence is consistent with data from another study, analyzing through a microarray approach the mRNA expression of several molecules induced by parasitized red blood cells (pRBCs) in human brain microvascular endothelial cells (HBMECs) and showing that TIMP-1 levels were not altered by pRBCs (Tripathi AK et al. 2009).

4.1.2. Models in vivo

Little evidence on TIMP modulation in human malaria is available from analysis of fluid samples from malaria patients. Sera of patients with severe and uncomplicated malaria displayed increased levels of TIMP-1, which was significantly higher in patients with CM than in those with uncomplicated malaria. For this reason, the authors suggested to potentially use theserum TIMP-1 as a marker of malaria severity (Dietmann A et al. 2008). In the same study, serum TIMP-2 levels were analyzed, but no differences between controls and malaria patients were observed. In another study (Green JA et al. 2011), TIMP-1 and TIMP-2 levels were analyzed in CSF of patients with CM, but any increases were not detected. This latter observation suggests that TIMP levels in CSF might not reflect blood levels.

4.2. Murine Models

The effects of differential component of HZ on TIMP-1 regulation in murine macrophages were investigated in vitro by using a RAW 264.7 cell line. In vivo, the regulation of TIMP mRNA expression was investigated in CM and non-CM models.

4.2.1. Models in vitro

The effects of the lipid components of HZ on TIMP-1 modulation were analyzed in a RAW 264.7 macrophage cell line. However, the results obtained contrast with recent evidence from human monocytes, since HZ strongly inhibited TIMP-1 mRNA expression; the effect appeared to be due to 4-HNE, but not to 15-HETE (Schrimpe A et al. 2009a; Schrimpe A et al. 2009b).

4.2.2. Models in vivo

In the previously cited work by Van den Steen's group, mRNa levels of all four TIMPs were analyzed by Ribonuclease Protection Assay and if deemed necessary by additional Real Time RT-PCR. In murine CM model (C57Bl/6 mice infected with *P. berghei* ANKA), a marked increase of TIMP-3 and TIMP-1 was observed in the liver and spleen at days 6 and 8 after infection, while no changes in the expression of TIMPs were detected in the lungs and kidneys. Since TIMP-1 remained below the detection limit of the Ribonuclease Protection Assay in the brain, RT-PCR was performed, and a four-fold increase in TIMP-1 mRNA expression was documented. TIMP-2 and TIMP-4 mRNA levels were not significantly altered in any organs. In Balb/C mice infected with *P. berghei* ANKA (murine CM-resistant model), a larger increase in TIMP-1, in comparison with C57Bl/6 mice (murine CM-sensitive model), was found, suggesting a potential protective role for TIMP-1 (Van den Steen PE et al. 2006).

5. Role of MMPs in Malaria Complications

Complications of malaria affect several organs and tissues, including the brain (CM) (Idro R et al. 2010), lungs (respiratory distress) (Mohan A et al. 2008), kidneys (renal failure) (Ehrich JH et al. 2007), spleen (anaemia) (Buffet PA et al. 2010), and placenta during pregnancy (placental malaria) (Okoko BJ et al. 2003). Mechanisms underlying these complications are not fully understood, but generally they appear to be directly related to: local parasite sequestration to endothelial cells, enhanced permeability of endothelial barriers, recruitment of immune cells, and major inflammatory response. As previously noticed, the kaleidoscope of substrates processed by MMPs is quite extensive, including adhesion molecules, intercellular junctions, receptors, cytokines, chemokines, structure proteins, and other proteases (Somerville RP et al. 2003; Cauwe B et al. 2007). Interestingly, several molecules playing a crucial role in the clinical progress from uncomplicated towards severe malaria have also been indicated as MMP substrates. In Table 3, a representative list, not yet exhaustive, of MMP substrates putatively involved in malaria pathogenesis is shown. In the following paragraphs, some examples of MMP substrates possibly relevant in malaria will be analyzed in the context of three important malaria complications (CM, lung pathology and placental malaria).

Table 3. MMP substrates which might be relevant in malaria pathogenesis

SUBSTRATE	FUNCTION	MMP	REFERENCE
occludin	intercellular junction	MMP-2; MMP-9 MMP-3 MMP-7	Giebel SJ et al. 2005 Gurney KJ et al. 2006 Gorodeski GI 2007
ZO-1	intercellular junction	MMP-9	Asahi M et al. 2001
connexin 43	intercellular junction	MMP-7	Lindsey ML et al. 2006
claudin-1	intercellular junction	MMP-9	Ichiyasu H et al. 2004
claudin-5	intercellular junction	MMP-3	Gurney KJ et al. 2006
E-cadherin	intercellular junction	MMP-3; MMP-7 MMP-14 MMP-24	Steinhusen U et al. 2001 Covington MD et al. 2006 Monea S et al. 2006
VE-cadherin	intercellular junction	MMP-7	Ichicawa Y et al. 2006
ICAM-1	adhesion molecule	MMP-9	Fiore E et al. 2002
L-selectin	adhesion molecule	MMP-1; MMP-3	Preece G et al. 1996
integrin alphaVbeta4	adhesion molecule	MMP-7 MMP-14	von Bredow DC et al. 1997 Ratnikov BI et al. 2002
IL-2Ralpha	receptor	MMP-9	Sheu BC et al. 2001
uPAR	receptor	MMP-2; MMP-3; MMP-8; MMP-9; MMP-12; MMP-13; MMP-14; MMP-19; MMP-25	Andolfo A et al. 2002
pro-TNF	cytokine pro-form	MMP-1; MMP-2; MMP-3; MMP-9; MMP-14; MMP-15; MMP-17	Gearing AJ et al. 1995
pro-TGFbeta	cytokine pro-form	MMP-2; MMP-3; MMP-9; MMP-14	Yu Q et al. 2000
pro-IL-1beta	cytokine pro-form	MMP-2; MMP-3; MMP-9	Schonbeck U et al. 1998
IL-1beta	cytokine	MMP-1; MMP-2; MMP-3; MMP-9	Ito A et al. 1996
Fractalkine/CX3CL1	chemokine	MMP-2	Overall CM et al. 2006
IL-8/ CXCL8	chemokine	MMP-9	Van den Steen PE et al. 2003a
MIG/ CXCL9	chemokine	MMP-9	Van den Steen PE et al. 2003b
IP-10/ CXCL10	chemokine	MMP-9	Van den Steen PE et al. 2003b
GROalpha/CXCL1	chemokine	MMP-9	Van den Steen PE et al. 2000
ENA-78/ CXCL5	chemokine	MMP-9	Van den Steen PE et al. 2003a

5.1. Cerebral Malaria

CM is an encephalopathy, characterized by pRBCs sequestration in the microvascular blood vessels, thrombocytopenia and thrombosis, recruitment of phagocytic cells in the area of erythrocyte and platelet sequester, production of inflammatory molecules, leakage of the blood-brain barrier (BBB), and leukocyte extravasation (this latter event being dominant in murine models, but definitively less extensive in human patients). These events lead to: fever; hypoxia; high pressure; oedema; coma; and, in some cases, death. In recovering patients, neurological sequelae may occur (Pongponratn E et al. 1991; Van der Heide HC et al. 2006; Medana IM et al. 2006; Idro R et al 2010; de Souza JB et al. 2010).

During the development of CM, MMPs could play an active role in several steps occurring. As shown in Table 3, MMPs proteolytically cleave the pro-forms of many pro-inflammatory molecules known to be enhanced in CM, such as TNFalpha, IL-1beta, IL-8. As a result of cleavage, these molecules are shed, activated or functionally potentiated. Thus, MMPs could contribute to triggering the uncontrolled inflammatory response that is typical of CM. According to this theory, a HZ-dependent pathological auto-enhancing loop, between MMP-9 and TNFalpha, has been proposed in a human malaria model *in vitro* by using adherent monocytes (Prato M et al. 2005).

Moreover, in the recent years, a growing number of inter-endothelial tight junctions, including occludin, ZO-1, and claudins, have been shown to be substrates of MMPs, enhancing the permeability of endothelial barriers by destroying these junctions. Therefore, enhanced levels of MMPs in malaria might facilitate the BBB leakage. This hypothesis is consistent with data showing that HZ-containg pRBCs reduced BBB permeability in a human model *in vitro* (Tripathi AK et al. 2007), and that HZ enhanced the MMP-1, MMP-3 and MMP-9 production by human microvascular endothelial cells (Prato et al. 2011c).

Finally, MMPs can also influence haemostasis. It has been reported,either tPA/uPA molecules responsible for conversion of plasminogen to plasmin, as well as the tPA/uPA inhibitor, PAI-1, can be processed by MMPs (Lijnen HR 2001; Lijnen HR et al. 2002; Santos-Martinez MJ et al. 2008). Consequently, fibrin degradation by plasmin might be influenced by altered levels of MMPs, perhaps explaining the thrombotic events frequently occurring during CM.

5.2. Lung Pathology

Acute respiratory distress syndrome (ARDS) is an important complication in *P. falciparum* malaria, and has been described in *P. vivax* and *P. ovale* malaria, as well. It is more common in adults than in children; pregnant women and non-immune individuals, such as travellers from non-endemic areas are more susceptible to develop this condition. The key pathophysiological mechanisms appear related to increased alveolar capillary permeability, resulting in microvascular fluid loss into the lungs; patients show acute onset dyspnoea which can rapidly progress to respiratory failure. ARDS is a disease with a high mortality rate and is common cause of admission into intensive care units all over the world (Mohan A et al. 2008).

Autopsy studies in patients found dead after severe *falciparum* malaria and coma had displayed: heavy oedematous lungs, congested capillaries, thickened alveolar septa, intra-alveolar haemorrhages, hyaline membrane formation, and serous pleural and pericardial effusions (Pinheiro BV et al. 2007; Morales MM et al. 2011).

Likewise, in CM, malarial parasites promote the release and activation of cytokines, such as TNFalpha and IL-1beta from macrophages and monocytes in ARDS. These cytokines are, in turn, postulated to induce thr release of other pro-inflammatory cytokines like IL-6 and IL-8, up-regulating the endothelial expression of vascular ligands that promote cytoadherence of infected erythrocytes in the venules of infected lungs (Mohan A et al. 2008). Moreover, the association of pulmonary oedema with CM in *P. falciparum* malaria points to an involvement of pro-inflammatory molecules.

As shown in Table 3, several among these molecules are MMP substrates. Notably, the proteolytic activity of many MMPs promotes the shedding of membrane-bound pro-TNFalpha, therefore enhancing TNFalpha circulation levels. Such an event might be particularly detrimental in ARDS. Indeed, TNFalpha has been found to reduce epithelial sodium channel (ENaC) expression in alveolar epithelial cells, altering alveolar fluid clearance by acting on its classical receptor; additionally, TNFalpha triggers the release of NO, which can reduce alveolar epithelial sodium transport by reducing the function of ENaC and the sodium potassium ATPase (Eisenhut M 2006). Therefore, in this context, the role of MMPs could be crucial.

5.3. Placental Malaria

Millions of women who become pregnant in malaria-endemic areas are at an increased risk of contracting the malaria infection, jeopardizing the outcome of pregnancy. The complications of this infection for mother and fetus are considerable. It has been shown that the placenta provides an ideal environment for the development of a subpopulation of malaria parasites that adhere to receptors in the placental syncytiotrophoblast. In most cases, the parasites remain on the maternal side of the placenta; but this maternal-fetal syndrome, known as pregnancy-associated malaria (PAM), has adverse effects on both mother and fetus, causing low birth weight and high rate of death (Costa FT et al. 2006).

In PAM, parasite adhesion on placental receptors, such as chondroitin sulphate A, may trigger an inflammatory process involving cytokine-secreting mononuclear cells. Inflammation is associated with: cytotrophoblast proliferation, cytotrophoblast membrane thickening, massive cell deposition, local blood flow alteration, impairment of metabolic pathways, and compromission of nutrients between mother and fetus (Beeson JG and Duffy PE 2005).

The precise mechanism by which PAM parasites evade the immune system remains unknown. It has been shown that massive sequestration of the parasite in the placenta leads to a switch in the cell-mediated immune response, from Th2 to Th1, resulting in the clinical manifestations of PAM, characterized by an increase in the levels of released cytokines. High levels of TNFalpha, mainly secreted by placental macrophages, are associated with poor clinical outcomes in patients and with concentrations of HZ in the placenta (Fried M et al. 1998). Also, in this case, it is tempting to speculate a role for MMP-9, which has been shown to be enhanced in HZ-fed human monocytes, triggering an auto-enhancing positive loop involving TNFalpha and MMP-9, itself (Prato M et al. 2005).

Additionally, placental infection increases the levels of alpha- and beta-chemokines, including MIP-1alpha, MIP-1beta, IP-10, MCP-1, IL-8, which, in turn, increases the immune cell recruitment to the placenta. Furthermore, levels of chemokines correlate with monocyte density in the placental intervillous space, and chemokine production by HZ-laden maternal macrophages has been observed (Suguitan AL et al. 2003; Abrams ET et al. 2003). Interestingly, MIP-1alpha was shown to enhance the MMP-9 gene in HZ-fed monocytes (Giribaldi G et al. 2011a), whereas IP-10 and IL-8 are known substrates of MMP-9 (see Table 3). Thus, the chemokine/MMP axis in placental malaria should be further investigated in future studies.

6. Therapeutic Perspectives

MMP inhibition might be a future challenge to prevent malaria complications. Because of the involvement of MMPs in a large number of pathologies other than malaria, several specific synthetic MMP inhibitors are in trial or are already available (Coussens LM et al. 2002; Nuti E et al. 2007; Devel L et al. 2010). Additionally, molecules with anti-MMP properties have also been picked out from anti-malarial drugs.

6.1. Anti-Malarial Drugs Showing MMP-Inhibiting Properties

Current anti-malarial drugs are grouped in seven classes: 4-aminoquinolines, arylaminoalcohols, antifolates, 8-aminoquinolines, artemisinins, inhibitors of the respiratory chain, and antibiotics (Khadjavi A. et al. 2010). Interestingly, in the context of studies aimed to find new anti-cancer drugs among already available drugs currently used for other pathologies, several molecules belonging to these families showed MMP-inhibiting properties.

Artemisinin down-regulated MMP-2 in human melanoma cells (Buommino E et al. 2009), and MMP-1, MMP-2 and MMP-9 in murine embryonic stem-cell derived embryoid bodies (Wartenberg M et al. 2003). Also, artemisinin-derived drugs were shown to be able to block MMPs: dihydroartemisinin inhibited expression and activity of MMP-2, MMP-9 and MMP-14 in human fibrosarcoma cells (Hwang YP et al. 2010) and MMP-9 expression in human umbilical vein endothelial cells (Wang SJ et al. 2011), whereas artesunate downregulated MMP-2 and MMP-7 expression in human non-small cell lung cancer (Rasheed SA et a. 2010). Among 4-aminoquinolines, chloroquine reduced the serum levels of MMP-9 in patients with systemic lupus erythematosus (Lesiak A et al. 2010). Furthermore, doxycycline antibiotic has been reported as an MMP inhibitor, since it reduced MMP-2, MMP-7 and MMP-9 in rat prostate epithelial cells (Bruni-Cardoso A et al. 2010).

Back to the malaria context, artemisinin, quercetin, and extracts from Punica granatum were shown to inhibit the HZ-dependent enhancement of MMP-9 in human monocytes through blocking the NF-kappaB pathway in two human models in vitro (Prato M et al. 2010; Dell'Agli M et al. 2010).

Taken altogether, these data reinforce the theory that the MMP expression pattern may be altered during malaria, and several anti-malarial drugs might restore basal MMP levels, at least partially. Thus, the use of synthetic MMP inhibitors could be useful in strengthening the anti-MMP properties of available anti-malarial drugs, as will be discussed in the following paragraph.

6.2. Synthetic MMP Inhibitors

The possible use of synthetic MMP inhibitors, which are presently in advanced trials or already commercially available (Coussens LM et al. 2002; Nuti E et al. 2007; Devel L et al. 2010) as adjuvant therapy to cure or prevent complicated malaria, is certainly intriguing. At present, few data on the effects of MMP inhibitors in malaria models have been reported.

In vitro, the use of a specific synthetic inhibitor of MMP-9 abrogated the HZ-dependent increase of TNFalpha in human monocytes, suggesting that MMP inhibition might be useful to contrast the pathological inflammation,characteristic of malaria complications such as CM.

However, blocking only one specific MMP might be not sufficient *in vivo*. Indeed, MMP-9 knock-out mice infected with *P. berghei* ANKA did not show protection from CM development, suggesting that the redundant functions of MMPs might compensate for the effects of the missing MMP-9 (Van den Steen PE et al. 2006). Interestingly, in the same work, the authors showed an improvement in the survival of mice with CM after treated with the broad spectrum MMP inhibitor, BB-94. This data appears to be more promising, and future research on the effects of broad-spectrum MMP inhibitors, as well as on the protective/detrimental roles of differential MMPs in malaria models, is certainly required.

7. Conclusion

Along with their ability in ECM degradation, MMPs play a crucial role in inflammatory response, increasing the permeability of endothelial barriers and deregulating haemostasis, all events which might occur during complicated malaria. Thus, the involvement of these enzymes in malaria pathogenesis is likely. However, such a research topic has only recently been started to be investigated: up until now, the available evidence on measuring MMP levels in malaria models is still incomplete, their correlation with disease severity is not clear yet, and mechanisms underlying their deregulation are not fully understood. At present, the more convincing data comes from murine models of CM, showing a large pattern of deregulated MMPs in several organs, and from *in vitro* studies aimed to clarify the effects of HZ on the production of MMP-9, and related molecules, in human monocytes and endothelial cells. Among the required studies that are still missing, an *in vivo* analysis of a complete panel of MMPs and related molecules in human organs of patients with uncomplicated or severe malaria appears to be quite urgent, in order to better understand the feasibility and the potential effectiveness of an adjuvant therapy with synthetic MMP inhibitors, possibly helping to prevent or cure CM, lung pathology, and placental malaria. Additionally, it would be interesting to enlarge the amount of measurements of MMP and TIMP levels in fluid samples from malaria patients, clarifying if they could be useful as potential markers of disease severity. Nevertheless, the results presently available, even though partially contrasting in some cases, are certainly promising, and are opening intriguing new research perspectives in the malaria field.

Acknowledgements

Thanks are due to Dr. Giuliana Giribaldi, Prof. Paolo Arese, Dr. Philippe E. Van den Steen, Prof. Ghislain Opdenakker, Dr. Nicoletta Basilico, and Prof. Donatella Taramelli for their stimulating discussions on malaria pathogenesis, HZ biology and MMP biochemistry in the recent years. The financial support by Mrs. Franca Squazza is also strongly acknowledged.

References

Abrams ET, Brown H, Chensue SW, Turner GD, Tadesse E, Lema VM, Molyneux ME, Rochford R, Meshnick SR, Rogerson SJ. Host response to malaria during pregnancy: placental monocyte recruitment is associated with elevated beta chemokine expression. *J Immunol.* 2003; 170:2759-64.

Andolfo A, English WR, Resnati M, Murphy G, Blasi F, Sidenius N. Metalloproteases cleave the urokinase-type plasminogen activator receptor in the D1-D2 linker region and expose epitopes not present in the intact soluble receptor. *Thromb Haemost.* 2002; 88:298-306.

Armah HB, Wilson NO, Sarfo BY, Powell MD, Bond VC, Anderson W, Adjei AA, Gyasi RK, Tettey Y, Wiredu EK, Tongren JE, Udhayakumar V, Stiles JK. Cerebrospinal fluid and serum biomarkers of cerebral malaria mortality in Ghanaian children. *Malar. J.* 2007;6:147.

Asahi M, Wang X, Mori T, Sumii T, Jung JC, Moskowitz MA, Fini ME, Lo EH. Effects of matrix metalloproteinase-9 gene knock-out on the proteolysis of blood-brain barrier and white matter components after cerebral ischemia. *J. Neurosci.* 2001;21:7724-32.

Beeson JG, Duffy PE. The immunology and pathogenesis of malaria during pregnancy. *Curr. Top Microbiol. Immunol.* 2005;297:187-227.

Brew K, Nagase H. The tissue inhibitors of metalloproteinases (TIMPs): an ancient family with structural and functional diversity. *Biochim. Biophys. Acta.* 2010;1803:55-71.

Bruni-Cardoso A, Augusto TM, Pravatta H, Damas-Souza DM, Carvalho HF. Stromal remodelling is required for progressive involution of the rat ventral prostate after castration: identification of a matrix metalloproteinase-dependent apoptotic wave. *Int. J. Androl.* 2010;33:686-95.

Buffet PA, Safeukui I, Milon G, Mercereau-Puijalon O, David PH. Retention of erythrocytes in the spleen: a double-edged process in human malaria. *Curr. Opin. Hematol.* 2009;16:157-64,

Buommino E, Baroni A, Canozo N, Petrazzuolo M, Nicoletti R, Vozza A, Tufano MA. Artemisinin reduces human melanoma cell migration by down-regulating alpha V beta 3 integrin and reducing metalloproteinase 2 production. *Invest New Drugs.* 2009;27:412-8.

Carney CK, Schrimpe AC, Halfpenny K, Harry RS, Miller CM, Broncel M, Sewell SL, Schaff JE, Deol R, Carter MD, Wright DW. The basis of the immunomodulatory activity of malaria pigment (hemozoin). *J. Biol. Inorg. Chem.* 2006;11:917-29.

Cauwe B, Van den Steen PE, Opdenakker G. The biochemical, biological, and pathological kaleidoscope of cell surface substrates processed by matrix metalloproteinases. *Crit. Rev. Biochem. Mol. Biol.* 2007 May-Jun;42(3):113-85.

Chulay JD, Ockenhouse CF. Host receptors for malaria-infected erythrocytes. *Am. J. Trop. Med. Hyg.* 1990;43:6-14.

Clark IA, Alleva LM, Budd AC, Cowden WB. Understanding the role of inflammatory cytokines in malaria and related diseases. *Travel Med. Infect. Dis.* 2008;6:67-81.

Clark IA, Budd AC, Alleva LM, Cowden WB. Human malarial disease: a consequence of inflammatory cytokine release. *Malar. J.* 2006;5:85.

Costa FT, Avril M, Nogueira PA, Gysin J. Cytoadhesion of Plasmodium falciparum-infected erythrocytes and the infected placenta: a two-way pathway. *Braz. J. Med. Biol. Res.* 2006;39:1525-36.

Coussens LM, Fingleton B, Matrisian LM. Matrix metalloproteinase inhibitors and cancer: trials and tribulations. *Science.* 2002;295:2387-92.

Covington MD, Burghardt RC, Parrish AR. Ischemia-induced cleavage of cadherins in NRK cells requires MT1-MMP (MMP-14). *Am. J. Physiol. Renal Physiol.* 2006;290:F43-51.

de Souza JB, Hafalla JC, Riley EM, Couper KN. Cerebral malaria: why experimental murine models are required to understand the pathogenesis of disease. *Parasitology.* 2010;137:755-72.

Deininger MH, Fimmen B, Kremsner PG, Meyermann R, Schluesener HJ. Accumulation of endostatin/collagenXVIII in brains of patients who died with cerebral malaria. *J. Neuroimmunol.* 2002;131:216-21.

Deininger MH, Winkler S, Kremsner PG, Meyermann R, Schluesener HJ. Angiogenic proteins in brains of patients who died with cerebral malaria. *J. Neuroimmunol.* 2003;142:101-11.

Dell'agli M, Galli GV, Bulgari M, Basilico N, Romeo S, Bhattacharya D, Taramelli D, Bosisio E. Ellagitannins of the fruit rind of pomegranate (Punica granatum) antagonize in vitro the host inflammatory response mechanisms involved in the onset of malaria. *Malar. J.* 2010;9:208.

Devel L, Czarny B, Beau F, Georgiadis D, Stura E, Dive V. Third generation of matrix metalloprotease inhibitors: Gain in selectivity by targeting the depth of the S1' cavity. *Biochimie.* 2010;92:1501-8.

Di Mari JF, Saada JI, Mifflin RC, Valentich JD, Powell DW. HETEs enhance IL-1-mediated COX-2 expression via augmentation of message stability in human colonic myofibroblasts. *Am. J. Physiol. Gastrointest Liver Physiol.* 2007;293:G719-28.

Dietmann A, Helbok R, Lackner P, Issifou S, Lell B, Matsiegui PB, Reindl M, Schmutzhard E, Kremsner PG. Matrix metalloproteinases and their tissue inhibitors (TIMPs) in Plasmodium falciparum malaria: serum levels of TIMP-1 are associated with disease severity. *J. Infect. Dis.* 2008;197:1614-20.

Egan TJ. Recent advances in understanding the mechanism of hemozoin (malaria pigment) formation. *J. Inorg. Biochem.* 2008;102:1288-99.

Ehrich JH, Eke FU. Malaria-induced renal damage: facts and myths. *Pediatr. Nephrol.* 2007;22:626-37.

Eisenhut M. Changes in ion transport in inflammatory disease. *J. Inflamm. (Lond).* 2006;3:5.

Fauser S, Deininger MH, Kremsner PG, Magdolen V, Luther T, Meyermann R, Schluesener HJ. Lesion associated expression of urokinase-type plasminogen activator receptor (uPAR, CD87) in human cerebral malaria. *J. Neuroimmunol.* 2000;111:234-40.

Fiore E, Fusco C, Romero P, Stamenkovic I. Matrix metalloproteinase 9 (MMP-9/gelatinase B) proteolytically cleaves ICAM-1 and participates in tumor cell resistance to natural killer cell-mediated cytotoxicity. *Oncogene.* 2002;21:5213-23.

Fried M, Muga RO, Misore AO, Duffy PE. Malaria elicits type 1 cytokines in the human placenta: IFN-gamma and TNF-alpha associated with pregnancy outcomes. *J. Immunol.* 1998;160:2523-30.

Gearing AJ, Beckett P, Christodoulou M, Churchill M, Clements JM, Crimmin M, Davidson AH, Drummond AH, Galloway WA, Gilbert R, et al. Matrix metalloproteinases and processing of pro-TNF-alpha. *J. Leukoc. Biol.* 1995;57:774-7.

Geurts N, Martens E, Van Aelst I, Proost P, Opdenakker G, Van den Steen PE. Beta-hematin interaction with the hemopexin domain of gelatinase B/MMP-9 provokes autocatalytic processing of the propeptide, thereby priming activation by MMP-3. *Biochemistry.* 2008;47:2689-99.

Giebel SJ, Menicucci G, McGuire PG, Das A. Matrix metalloproteinases in early diabetic retinopathy and their role in alteration of the blood-retinal barrier. *Lab. Invest.* 2005;85:597-607.

Giribaldi G, Prato M, Ulliers D, Gallo V, Schwarzer E, Akide-Ndunge OB, Valente E, Saviozzi S, Calogero RA, Arese P. Involvement of inflammatory chemokines in survival of human monocytes fed with malarial pigment. *Infect. Immun.* 2010;78:4912-21.

Giribaldi, Valente E, Khadjavi A, Polimeni M, Prato M. Macrophage Inflammatory Protein-1alpha mediates Matrix Metalloproteinase-9 enhancement in human adherent monocytes fed with malarial pigment. *Asian Pac. J. Trop. Med.* 2011a; in press.

Giribaldi G, Ulliers D, Valente E, Khadjavi A, Mandili G, Polimeni M, Prato M. Malarial pigment promotes expression and release of TIMP-1 in human monocytes: role of MIP-1alpha chemokine and NF-kappaB pathway. *Proceedings of the 1st French-Italian Joint Meeting on Subcellular Trafficking,* Padua, Italy, 25-28 May 2011. 2011b; P28:96.

Gomis-Rüth FX, Maskos K, Betz M, Bergner A, Huber R, Suzuki K, Yoshida N, Nagase H, Brew K, Bourenkov GP, Bartunik H, Bode W. Mechanism of inhibition of the human matrix metalloproteinase stromelysin-1 by TIMP-1. *Nature.* 1997;389:77-81.

Gorodeski GI. Estrogen decrease in tight junctional resistance involves matrix-metalloproteinase-7-mediated remodeling of occludin. *Endocrinology.* 2007;148:218-31.

Griffiths MJ, Shafi MJ, Popper SJ, Hemingway CA, Kortok MM, Wathen A, Rockett KA, Mott R, Levin M, Newton CR, Marsh K, Relman DA, Kwiatkowski DP. Genomewide analysis of the host response to malaria in Kenyan children. *J. Infect. Dis.* 2005;191:1599-611.

Green JA, Thi Hong Chau T, Farrar JJ, Friedland JS, Thwaites GE. CNS infection, CSF matrix metalloproteinase concentrations, and clinical/laboratory features. *Neurology.* 2011;76:577-579.

Gross J, Lapière CM. Collagenolytic activity in amphibian tissues: a tissue culture assay. *Proc. Natl. Acad. Sci. U S A.* 1962;48:1014-22.

Gurney KJ, Estrada EY, Rosenberg GA. Blood-brain barrier disruption by stromelysin-1 facilitates neutrophil infiltration in neuroinflammation. *Neurobiol. Dis.* 2006;23:87-96.

Hwang YP, Yun HJ, Kim HG, Han EH, Lee GW, Jeong HG. Suppression of PMA-induced tumor cell invasion by dihydroartemisinin via inhibition of PKCalpha/Raf/MAPKs and NF-kappaB/AP-1-dependent mechanisms. *Biochem. Pharmacol.* 2010;79:1714-26.

Ichikawa Y, Ishikawa T, Momiyama N, Kamiyama M, Sakurada H, Matsuyama R, Hasegawa S, Chishima T, Hamaguchi Y, Fujii S, Saito S, Kubota K, Hasegawa S, Ike H, Oki S, Shimada H. Matrilysin (MMP-7) degrades VE-cadherin and accelerates accumulation of beta-catenin in the nucleus of human umbilical vein endothelial cells. *Oncol. Rep.* 2006;15:311-5.

Ichiyasu H, McCormack JM, McCarthy KM, Dombkowski D, Preffer FI, Schneeberger EE. Matrix metalloproteinase-9-deficient dendritic cells have impaired migration through tracheal epithelial tight junctions. *Am. J. Respir. Cell Mol. Biol.* 2004;30:761-70.

Idro R, Marsh K, John CC, Newton CR. Cerebral malaria: mechanisms of brain injury and strategies for improved neurocognitive outcome. *Pediatr. Res.* 2010;68:267-74.

Itoh Y, Kajita M, Kinoh H, Mori H, Okada A, Seiki M. Membrane type 4 matrix metalloproteinase (MT4-MMP, MMP-17) is a glycosylphosphatidylinositol-anchored proteinase. *J. Biol. Chem.* 1999;274:34260-6.

Jung K, Measurement of matrix metalloproteinases and their tissue inhibitors in serum produces doubtful results. *J. Infect. Dis.* 2008;198:1722-3.

Khadjavi A, Giribaldi G, Prato M. From control to eradication of malaria: the end of being stuck in second gear? *Asian Pac. J. Trop. Med.* 2010;3:412-420.

Kojima S, Itoh Y, Matsumoto S, Masuho Y, Seiki M. Membrane-type 6 matrix metalloproteinase (MT6-MMP, MMP-25) is the second glycosyl-phosphatidyl inositol (GPI)-anchored MMP. *FEBS Lett.* 2000;480:142-6.

Lesiak A, Narbutt J, Sysa-Jedrzejowska A, Lukamowicz J, McCauliffe DP, Wózniacka A. Effect of chloroquine phosphate treatment on serum MMP-9 and TIMP-1 levels in patients with systemic lupus erythematosus. *Lupus.* 2010;19:683-8.

Lijnen HR. Elements of the fibrinolytic system. *Ann. N Y Acad. Sci.* 2001;936:226-36.

Lijnen HR. Matrix metalloproteinases and cellular fibrinolytic activity. *Biochemistry (Mosc).* 2002;67:92-8.

Lindsey ML, Escobar GP, Mukherjee R, Goshorn DK, Sheats NJ, Bruce JA, Mains IM, Hendrick JK, Hewett KW, Gourdie RG, Matrisian LM, Spinale FG. Matrix metalloproteinase-7 affects connexin-43 levels, electrical conduction, and survival after myocardial infarction. *Circulation.* 2006;113:2919-28.

Lohi J, Wilson CL, Roby JD, Parks WC. Epilysin, a novel human matrix metalloproteinase (MMP-28) expressed in testis and keratinocytes and in response to injury. *J. Biol. Chem.* 2001;276:10134-44.

Lucchi NW, Sarr D, Owino SO, Mwalimu SM, Peterson DS, Moore JM. Natural hemozoin stimulates syncytiotrophoblast to secrete chemokines and recruit peripheral blood mononuclear cells. *Placenta.* 2011;32:579-85.

Medana IM, Turner GD. Human cerebral malaria and the blood-brain barrier. *Int. J. Parasitol.* 2006;36:5.

Miller CM, Carney CK, Schrimpe AC, Wright DW. beta-Hematin (hemozoin) mediated decompostion of polyunsaturated fatty acids to 4-hydroxy-2-nonenal. *Inorg. Chem.* 2005;44:2134-6.

Mohan A, Sharma SK, Bollineni S. Acute lung injury and acute respiratory distress syndrome in malaria. *J. Vector Borne Dis.* 2008;45:179-9.

Monea S, Jordan BA, Srivastava S, DeSouza S, Ziff EB. Membrane localization of membrane type 5 matrix metalloproteinase by AMPA receptor binding protein and cleavage of cadherins. *J. Neurosci.* 2006;26:2300-12.

Morales MM, Pires-Neto RC, Inforsato N, Lanças T, da Silva LF, Saldiva PH, Mauad T, Carvalho CR, Amato MB, Dolhnikoff M. Small airway remodeling in acute respiratory distress syndrome: a study in autopsy lung tissue. *Crit. Care.* 2011;15:R4.

Murphy SC; Breman JG. Gaps in the childhood malaria burden in Africa: cerebral malaria, neurological sequelae, anemia, respiratory distress, hypoglycemia, and complications of pregnancy. *Am. J. Trop. Med. Hyg.* 2001;64:57-67.

Nagase H. Cell surface activation of progelatinase A (proMMP-2) and cell migration. *Cell* Res. 1998;8:179-86.

Nagase H, Woessner JF Jr. Matrix metalloproteinases. *J. Biol. Chem.* 1999;274:21491-4.

Nagase H, Visse R, Murphy G. Structure and function of matrix metalloproteinases and TIMPs. *Cardiovasc Res.* 2006;69:562-73.

Nuti E, Tuccinardi T, Rossello A. Matrix metalloproteinase inhibitors: new challenges in the era of post broad-spectrum inhibitors. *Curr. Pharm. Des.* 2007;13:2087-100.

Nyangoto, EO. Cell-mediated effector molecules and complicated malaria. *Int. Arch. Allergy Immunol.* 2005;137:326-42.

Okoko BJ, Enwere G, Ota MO. The epidemiology and consequences of maternal malaria: a review of immunological basis. *Acta Trop.* 2003;87:193-205.

Overall CM. Molecular determinants of metalloproteinase substrate specificity: matrix metalloproteinase substrate binding domains, modules, and exosites. *Mol. Biotechnol.* 2002;22:51-86.

Overall CM, Dean RA. Degradomics: systems biology of the protease web. Pleiotropic roles of MMPs in cancer. *Cancer Metastasis Rev.* 2006;25:69-75.

Pinheiro BV, Muraoka FS, Assis RV, Lamin R, Pinto SP, Ribeiro PJ Jr, Oliveira JC. Accuracy of clinical diagnosis of acute respiratory distress syndrome in comparison with autopsy findings. *J. Bras Pneumol.* 2007;33:423-8.

Pongponratn E, Riganti M, Punpoowong B, Aikawa M. Microvascular sequestration of parasitized erythrocytes in human falciparum malaria: a pathological study. *Am. J. Trop. Med. Hyg.* 1991;44:168-75.

Prato M, Giribaldi G, Polimeni M, Gallo V, Arese P. Phagocytosis of hemozoin enhances matrix metalloproteinase-9 activity and TNF-alpha production in human monocytes: role of matrix metalloproteinases in the pathogenesis of falciparum malaria. *J. Immunol.* 2005;175:6436-42.

Prato M, Gallo V, Giribaldi G, Arese P. Phagocytosis of haemozoin (malarial pigment) enhances metalloproteinase-9 activity in human adherent monocytes: role of IL-1beta and 15-HETE. *Malar. J.* 2008;7:157.

Prato M, Giribaldi G, Arese P. Hemozoin triggers tumor necrosis factor alpha-mediated release of lysozyme by human adherent monocytes: new evidences on leukocyte degranulation in P. *falciparum* malaria. *Asian Pac. J. Trop. Med.* 2009;2(3):35-40.

Prato M, Gallo V, Giribaldi G, Aldieri E, Arese P. Role of the NF-κB transcription pathway in the haemozoin- and 15-HETE-mediated activation of matrix metalloproteinase-9 in human adherent monocytes. *Cell Microbiol.* 2010a;12:1780-91.

Prato M, Gallo V, Arese P. Higher production of tumor necrosis factor alpha in hemozoin-fed human adherent monocytes is dependent on lipidic component of malarial pigment: new evidences on cytokine regulation in P. *falciparum* malaria. *Asian Pac. J. Trop. Med.* 2010b;3:85-89.

Prato M, Giribaldi G. Matrix metalloproteinase-9 and haemozoin: wedding rings for human host and *Plasmodium falciparum* parasite in complicated malaria. *J. Trop. Med.* 2011a; 2011:ID ID628435.

Prato M, Valente E, Ulliers D, Khadjavi A, Giribaldi G. Quercetin, artemisinin and parthenolide abrogate the haemozoin- and 15-HETE-enhanced activity of enzymes released from gelatinase granules by human monocytes. Proceedings of the Antimal Conference – Antimalarial Drugs: *Chemistry, Development and Future Challenges,* London, UK, 15-16 March 2011. 2011b; P27:49.

Prato M, D'Alessandro S, Van den Steen PE, Opdenakker G, Arese P, Taramelli D, Basilico N. Natural haemozoin modulates matrix metalloproteinases and induces morphological changes in human microvascular endothelium. *Cell Microbiol.* 2011c; 13:1275-85.

Preece G, Murphy G, Ager A. Metalloproteinase-mediated regulation of L-selectin levels on leucocytes. *J. Biol. Chem.* 1996;271:11634.

Rasheed SA, Efferth T, Asangani IA, Allgayer H. First evidence that the antimalarial drug artesunate inhibits invasion and in vivo metastasis in lung cancer by targeting essential extracellular proteases. *Int. J. Cancer.* 2010;127:1475-85.

Ratnikov BI, Rozanov DV, Postnova TI, Baciu PG, Zhang H, DiScipio RG, Chestukhina GG, Smith JW, Deryugina EI, Strongin AY. An alternative processing of integrin alpha(v) subunit in tumor cells by membrane type-1 matrix metalloproteinase. *J. Biol. Chem.* 2002;277:7377-85.

Rosenberg GA. Matrix metalloproteinases in neuroinflammation. *Glia.* 2002;39:279-91.

Rosenberg GA, Yang Y. Vasogenic edema due to tight junction disruption by matrix metalloproteinases in cerebral ischemia. *Neurosurg. Focus.* 2007;22:E4.

Santos-Martínez MJ, Medina C, Jurasz P, Radomski MW. Role of metalloproteinases in platelet function. *Thromb Res.* 2008;121:535-42.

Schönbeck U, Mach F, Libby P. Generation of biologically active IL-1 beta by matrix metalloproteinases: a novel caspase-1-independent pathway of IL-1 beta processing. *J. Immunol.* 1998;161:3340-6.

Schrimpe AC, Wright DW. Comparative analysis of gene expression changes mediated by individual constituents of hemozoin. *Chem. Res. Toxicol.* 2009a;22:433-45.

Schrimpe AC, Wright DW. Differential gene expression mediated by 15-hydroxyeicosatetraenoic acid in LPS-stimulated RAW 264.7 cells. *Malar. J.* 2009b;8:195.

Schwarzer E, Ludwig P, Valente E, Arese P. 15(S)-hydroxyeicosatetraenoic acid (15-HETE), a product of arachidonic acid peroxidation, is an active component of hemozoin toxicity to monocytes. *Parassitologia.* 1999;41:199-202.

Sherman IW, Eda S, Winograd E. Cytoadherence and sequestration in Plasmodium falciparum: defining the ties that bind. *Microbes Infect.* 2003;5:897-909.

Sheu BC, Hsu SM, Ho HN, Lien HC, Huang SC, Lin RH. A novel role of metalloproteinase in cancer-mediated immunosuppression. *Cancer Res.* 2001;61:237-42.

Somerville RP, Oblander SA, Apte SS. Matrix metalloproteinases: old dogs with new tricks. *Genome Biol.* 2003;4:216.

Steinhusen U, Weiske J, Badock V, Tauber R, Bommert K, Huber O. Cleavage and shedding of E-cadherin after induction of apoptosis. *J. Biol. Chem.* 2001;276:4972-80.

Stetler-Stevenson WG. Tissue inhibitors of metalloproteinases in cell signaling: metalloproteinase-independent biological activities. *Sci. Signal.* 2008;1:re6.

Suguitan AL Jr, Leke RG, Fouda G, Zhou A, Thuita L, Metenou S, Fogako J, Megnekou R, Taylor DW. Changes in the levels of chemokines and cytokines in the placentas of women with Plasmodium falciparum malaria. *J. Infect. Dis.* 2003;188:1074-82.

Szklarczyk A, Stins M, Milward EA, Ryu H, Fitzsimmons C, Sullivan D, Conant K. Glial activation and matrix metalloproteinase release in cerebral malaria. *J. Neurovirol.* 2007;13:2-10.

Tallant C, Marrero A, Gomis-Rüth FX. Matrix metalloproteinases: fold and function of their catalytic domains. *Biochim. Biophys. Acta.* 2010;1803:20-8.

Tripathi AK, Sullivan DJ, Stins MF. Plasmodium falciparum-infected erythrocytes decrease the integrity of human blood-brain barrier endothelial cell monolayers. *J. Infect. Dis.* 2007;195:942-50.

Tripathi AK, Sha W, Shulaev V, Stins MF, Sullivan DJ Jr. Plasmodium falciparum-infected erythrocytes induce NF-kappaB regulated inflammatory pathways in human cerebral endothelium. *Blood.* 2009;114:4243-52.

Van den Steen PE, Proost P, Wuyts A, Van Damme J, Opdenakker G. Neutrophil gelatinase B potentiates interleukin-8 tenfold by aminoterminal processing, whereas it degrades CTAP-III, PF-4, and GRO-alpha and leaves RANTES and MCP-2 intact. *Blood.* 2000;96:2673-81.

Van den Steen PE, Opdenakker G, Wormald MR, Dwek RA, Rudd PM. Matrix remodelling enzymes, the protease cascade and glycosylation. *Biochim. Biophys. Acta.* 2001;1528:61-73.

Van den Steen PE, Dubois B, Nelissen I, Rudd PM, Dwek RA, Opdenakker G. Biochemistry and molecular biology of gelatinase B or matrix metalloproteinase-9 (MMP-9). *Crit. Rev. Biochem. Mol. Biol.* 2002;37:375-536.

Van Den Steen PE, Wuyts A, Husson SJ, Proost P, Van Damme J, Opdenakker G; Gelatinase B/MMP-9 and neutrophil collagenase/MMP-8 process the chemokines human GCP-2/CXCL6, ENA-78/CXCL5 and mouse GCP-2/LIX and modulate their physiological activities. *Eur. J. Biochem.* 2003a;270:3739-49.

Van den Steen PE, Husson SJ, Proost P, Van Damme J, Opdenakker G. Carboxyterminal cleavage of the chemokines MIG and IP-10 by gelatinase B and neutrophil collagenase. *Biochem. Biophys. Res. Commun.* 2003b;310:889-96.

Van den Steen PE, Van Aelst I, Starckx S, Maskos K, Opdenakker G, Pagenstecher A. Matrix metalloproteinases, tissue inhibitors of MMPs and TACE in experimental cerebral malaria. *Lab. Invest.* 2006;86:873-88.

van der Heyde HC, Nolan J, Combes V, Gramaglia I, Grau GE. A unified hypothesis for the genesis of cerebral malaria: sequestration, inflammation and hemostasis leading to microcirculatory dysfunction. *Trends Parasitol.* 2006;22:503-8.

Van Wart HE, Birkedal-Hansen H. The cysteine switch: a principle of regulation of metalloproteinase activity with potential applicability to the entire matrix metalloproteinase gene family. *Proc. Natl. Acad. Sci. U S A.* 1990;87:5578-82.

von Bredow DC, Nagle RB, Bowden GT, Cress AE. Cleavage of beta 4 integrin by matrilysin. *Exp. Cell Res.* 1997;236:341-5.

Wang SJ, Sun B, Cheng ZX, Zhou HX, Gao Y, Kong R, Chen H, Jiang HC, Pan SH, Xue DB, Bai XW. Dihydroartemisinin inhibits angiogenesis in pancreatic cancer by targeting the NF-κB pathway. *Cancer Chemother Pharmacol.* 2011 Apr 9. (Epub ahead of print).

Wartenberg M, Wolf S, Budde P, Grünheck F, Acker H, Hescheler J, Wartenberg G, Sauer H. The antimalaria agent artemisinin exerts antiangiogenic effects in mouse embryonic stem cell-derived embryoid bodies. *Lab. Invest.* 2003;83:1647-55.

Woessner JF Jr. MMPs and TIMPs--an historical perspective. *Mol. Biotechnol.* 2002;22:33-49.

Yu Q, Stamenkovic I. Cell surface-localized matrix metalloproteinase-9 proteolytically activates TGF-beta and promotes tumor invasion and angiogenesis. *Genes Dev.* 2000;14:163-76.

In: Malaria: Etiology, Pathogenesis and Treatments
Editors: A. M. Peterson et al, pp. 175-191
ISBN: 978-1-62100-363-2

Chapter VII

Artemisinin Combination Therapy for the Treatment of Childhood Malaria in Sub-Saharan Africa: Efficacy, Safety and Policy Considerations.

C. J. Uneke

Department of Medical Microbiology/Parasitology, Faculty of Clinical Medicine, Ebonyi State University, Abakaliki Nigeria.

Abstract

Malaria remains the most severe public health challenge facing most of the countries of the tropical and sub-tropical regions of the world. The disease is known to be associated with underdevelopment, poverty and ignorance. The World Health Organization has described malaria as a major contributor to high rate of the global infectious disease–related mortality and morbidity particularly in sub-Saharan Africa. Almost all of the malaria deaths in sub-Saharan Africa occur in children below five years of age and this translates to the child mortality of nearly 1 million each year. Early and effective treatment of childhood malaria is imperative because the majority of children who die from malaria do so within 48 hours of onset of illness. In addition, to the high malaria transmission intensity in sub-Saharan Africa, limited access to adequate treatment, increasing parasite resistance to affordable and safe medicines (chloroquine, sulphadoxine-pyrimethamine and amodiaquine); and inappropriate treatment at home or at community level, aggravate the malaria burden. The relentless increase in malaria parasites resistance to many conventional antimalarial drugs necessitated the introduction of artemisinin-based combination therapy (ACT). There is a growing international consensus that wide-scale, systematic implementation of ACT is one of the few effective measures that will enable malaria-endemic countries to achieve the ambitious goals set in Abuja in 2000 to 'roll back malaria'. The derivatives of artemisinin plant, Artemisia annua (Qinghao, Asteraceae) are currently considered the cornerstone of Plasmodium falciparum malaria treatment due to their potency and rapid action. Numerous evidence abound indicating that ACTs were very efficacious in the treatment of uncomplicated malaria among children in sub-Saharan Africa. These ACTs include; artemether-lumefantrine, artesunate-mefloquine, artesunate-amodiaquine, artesunate-sulphadoxine-pyrimethamine, artesunate-chlorproguanil-dapsone, and dihydroartemisinin-piperaquine. Most of the studies however acknowledged that more investigations are required for continuous safety monitoring and on the pharmacokinetics of these ACT varieties to provide more scientific information on the profiles of the drugs. There is need for continuous research to evaluate the tolerability, efficacy, effectiveness and cost of various combination therapy strategies, particularly relating to their potential use in Africa south of the Sahara, is imperative.

Introduction

Malaria remains the most severe public health challenge facing most of the countries of the tropical and sub-tropical regions of the world. The disease is known to be associated with underdevelopment, poverty and ignorance (Worral *et al.,* 2005). The World Health Organization (WHO) has described malaria as a major contributor to high rate of the global infectious disease–related mortality and morbidity particularly in Africa (WHO, 2008). Recent estimates of the World Malaria Report (WMR) of 2009 indicated that 243 million cases of malaria occurred worldwide in 2008, and majority of the cases (85%) occurred in the African Region (WHO, 2009). According to the WMR malaria accounted for an estimated 863000 deaths in 2008, of which 89% were in the African Region particularly sub-Saharan Africa (WHO, 2009). In areas of high malaria endemicity in sub-Saharan Africa, most of the malaria-associated morbidity and mortality are recorded in young children (Uneke, 2009a; Snow *et al.,* 2004). Almost all of the malaria deaths in sub-Saharan Africa occur in children below five years of age and this translates to the child mortality of nearly 1 million each year (DFID, 2004; Hopkins *et al.,* 2007; WHO, 2008). Indeed, a child dies of malaria every 30 seconds, a death toll of about 3000 children every day in the sub region alone (WHO, 2003, 2008).

There is sufficient evidence indicating that about 80% of deaths due to childhood malaria take place within the first 24 hours of admission (Schellenberg *et al.,* 1999; Breman, 2001; WHO 2002; DFID, 2004; Idro *et al.,* 2006). Numerous reports have shown that in highly endemic areas of sub-Saharan Africa severe *P. falciparum* infection is very rare after the age of 5 years and this is because the acquisition of malaria immunity is closely linked to the level of transmission (Newton and Krishna, 1998; Murphy and Breman, 2001; Dzeing-Ella *et al.,* 2005; Rowe *et al.,* 2006). Early and effective treatment of childhood malaria is imperative because the majority of children who die from malaria do so within 48 hours of onset of illness (Uneke, 2009). This acknowledged time element is critical to saving the lives of African children, and reducing severe malaria morbidity and mortality (Newton and Krishna, 1998; Baume, 2002; Were, 2004).

According to WHO, some of the countries in sub-Saharan Africa including Burkina Faso, Chad, Niger, Mali and Nigeria recorded more than 8 childhood deaths per 1000 in the year 2006 (WHO, 2008). In 2006, there were an estimated 881 000 (610 000–1212 000) deaths worldwide due to malaria of which 90% were in the African Region and an estimated 85% of deaths occurred in children under 5 years, but the proportion is much higher in the African (88%) than in other regions (WHO, 2008). The WHO noted in their report that up to 18 countries accounted for 90% of deaths due to malaria in sub-Saharan Africa. These countries included Malawi, Zambia, Guinea, Chad, Mozambique, Côte d'Ivoire, Angola, Cameroon, Mali, Ghana, Burkina Faso, Kenya, Niger, United Republic of Tanzania, Ethiopia, Uganda, Democratic Republic of the Congo, and Nigeria (WHO, 2008). Findings from studies conducted in some of these 18 countries have shown that children recorded the highest admission parasite densities and proportion of patients with life threatening features (Idro *et al.,* 2006; Abdalla *et al.,* 2007; Bassat *et al.,* 2008; Eliades *et al.,* 2006; Mabunda *et al.,* 2008).

Roca-Feltrer and colleagues estimated that 545 000 (uncertainty interval: 105 000–1 750 000) children under the age of five in SSA experienced an episode of severe malaria for which they were admitted to hospital, while a total of 24 000 (interquartile range: 12 000–37 000) suffered from persistent neurological deficits as a result of cerebral malaria and the number of malaria fevers associated with high parasite density in under-5s in SSA in 2000 was estimated as 115 750 000 (uncertainty interval: 91 243 000–257 957 000) (Roca-Feltrer *et al.,* 2008). The childhood malaria case-fatality rate greater than 0.6% has been recorded in most endemic areas of sub-Saharan Africa (WHO, 2008). Since nearly all childhood deaths due to malaria takes place in the first 24 hours of admission, there is therefore the dire need for early recognition and prompt treatment of the most severely ill children (WHO, 2002). This is a key RBM strategy and is based on the widespread recognition that untreated *P. falciparum* malaria contributes both directly and indirectly to death, particularly in the non-immune (Were, 2004). In addition, to the high malaria transmission intensity in sub-Saharan Africa, limited access to adequate treatment, increasing parasite resistance to affordable and safe medicines (chloroquine, sulphadoxine-pyrimethamine and amodiaquine); and inappropriate treatment at home or at community level, aggravate the malaria burden (Ajayi *et al.,* 2008a, 2008b; Tiono *et al.,* 2008; WHO, 2008; Hopkins *et al.,* 2007).

The relentless increase in malaria parasites resistance to many conventional antimalarial drugs necessitated the introduction of artemisinin-based combination therapy (ACT) (WHO, 2001). There is a growing international consensus that wide-scale, systematic implementation of ACT is one of the few effective measures that will enable malaria-endemic countries to achieve the ambitious goals set in Abuja in 2000 to 'roll back malaria', particularly that of halving malaria morbidity and mortality by 2010 (Ogbonna and Uneke, 2008). By June 2006, 37 countries in Africa had adopted ACT as the first- or second-line treatment policy (WHO, 2007). Currently there are a number of registered co-formulated ACTs that are produced to internationally recognized good manufacturing practice standards that are used in sub-Saharan Africa. These include; artemether-lumefantrine (AL), artesunate-MQ (AS + MQ), artesunate-amodiaquine (AS + AQ) and artesunate-SP (AS + SP) (Adjuik et al., 2004).

Overview of Artemisinin-Based Combination Therapies

The Derivatives of artemisinin plant, Artemisia annua (Qinghao, Asteraceae) are currently considered the cornerstone of falciparum malaria treatment due to their potency and rapid action (WHO, 2006). The discovery artemisinin for the treatment of malaria in the 1970s by Chinese scientists was one of the most outstanding scientific accomplishments in the battle against malaria (Klayman 1985). A detailed account of the process in the discovery of artemisinin is provided in the book entitled A Detailed Chronological Record of Project 523 and the Discovery and Development of Qinghaosu (Artemisinin) (Zhang, 2005). According to Cui and Su (2009), artemisinin represents a new class of antimalarial agent, and is a sesquiterpene lactone characterized by an endoperoxide bridge essential for its antimalarial activity. They further noted that because the parent drug of artemisinin is poorly soluble in water or oil, the carbonyl group of artemisinin was reduced to obtain dihydroartemisinin (DHA) and its derivatives such as the water-soluble artesunate and oil-soluble artemether and arteether, which also show greater antimalarial activity. Thus artemisinin a sesquiterpene lactone endoperoxide is extremely potent against chloroquine CQ- and sulphadoxine SP-resistant Plasmodium falciparum in vitro and in vivo and can produce faster parasite clearance and fever resolution times than any other licensed antimalarial, including quinine (White, 2008). Although efforts to produce the drug using bioengineered microbes have been reported (Li and Wu 2003; Zeng et al., 2008), the commercial source of artemisinin still remains the Artemisia plant (Kuhn and Wang, 2008). A number of earlier reports indicated that artemisinins are among the most potent antimalarial agents, effective against nearly all asexual and sexual parasite stages (Skinner et al., 1996; Kumar and Zheng, 1990; Chen et al., 1994). They have been shown to be able to kill the malaria parasites within minutes with a parasite reduction ratio of approximately 10,000 per erythrocytic cycle, resulting in rapid clinical responses (White 2008; Woodrow et al., 2005).

Artemisinin and its derivatives (artesunate, artemether, artemotil, and dihydro-artemisinin) produce rapid clearance of parasitaemia and rapid resolution of symptoms and they reduce parasite numbers by a factor of 10-100 times when compared to other antimalarials (WHO, 2006; Njuguna and Qader, 2008). Artemisinin compounds are active against all the four species of Plasmodium that infect humans and a public health advantage of ACT is that they reduce gametocyte carriage and thus transmissibility of malaria (Price et al., 1996; WHO, 2006; Snow et al., 2003). This plays a prominent role in malaria control in areas of low transmission, though this may not be so in areas of high transmission intensity where a large reservoir exists in asymptomatic people (Snow et al., 2003; Njuguna and Qader, 2008). The success recorded in the treatment of CQ- and SP-resistant malaria using artemisinin-based combination therapies (ACTs) has prompted the WHO to recommend ACTs as the preferred first-line antimalarials against *P.falciparum* malaria and has elicited substantial funding and logistical support from, among others, The Global Fund to Fight AIDS, Tuberculosis, and Malaria, The World Bank, Roll Back Malaria, the President's Malaria Initiative, the Medicines for Malaria Venture, and the Bill and Melinda Gates Foundation (Eastman and Fidock, 2009). Their outstanding efficacy, together with complementary interventions that reduce transmission, such as long-lasting insecticide-treated bed nets and indoor residual insecticide spraying, has led to a renewed call for eradicating malaria (Feachem and Sabot, 2008). Indeed, the introduction of artemisinin-based combination therapy (ACT) interventions decreased morbidity and mortality associated with malaria in several parts of the world (Ogbonna and Uneke, 2008). This explains why ACTs have now been widely adopted across sub-Saharan Africa (Eastman and Fidock, 2009).

The current ACTs use the artemisinin derivatives including artemether (ATM), artesunate (AS) or dihydroartemisinin (DHA) and these have been shown to improve oral bioavailability compared with that of artemisinin (Eastman and Fidock, 2009). These derivatives of artemisinin rapidly achieve peak plasma levels in humans and possess elimination half-lives of approximately 1–3 hrs (German and Aweeka, 2008; White, 2008). It is pertinent however to state that artemisinin and its derivatives possess short half-lives and poor pharmacokinetic properties and these translate into substantial treatment failure rates when used as monotherapy (Woodrow and Krishna, 2006). According to Eastman and Fidock (2009), combining a member of this class with a longer-lasting partner drug assures sustained anti-malarial pressure after the plasma concentrations of the ART derivatives have fallen below therapeutic levels and this increases the antimalarial treatment efficacy and reduces the selective pressure for resistance. Eastman and Fidock (2009) further noted that ideally, antimalarial combination drug partners would have similar pharmacokinetic properties so that no drug is left 'unprotected' by the other. Thus ACTs benefit substantially from the ability of the ART derivative to rapidly reduce the parasite biomass, resulting in few parasites to be cleared by the partner drug and reducing the pool of parasites from which resistance can emerge (Eastman and Fidock, 2009).

The practice of Combination drug treatment in malaria is not a new phenomenon. It has been deployed in the treatment of diseases like tuberculosis, leprosy, cancers and HIV/AIDS because it delays emergence of resistance and increases efficacy (WHO, 2004). Thus the rationale behind ACT is that the chance of parasites simultaneously developing resistance as a result of genetic mutations to two drugs with different modes of action is much lower than the chance of parasites developing resistance to single drugs (White, 1999; Nosten and White, 2007; Cui and Su, 2009). According to White (1999), the probability of a parasite arising that is resistant simultaneously to two drugs with unrelated modes of action is the product of the per parasite mutation frequencies multiplied by the total number of parasites exposed to drugs. Therefore, if the probability of a parasite being resistant to drug A is one in 10^9 and to drug B is one in 10^9 then the probability that a parasite will be simultaneously resistant to both is one in 10^{18}, representing a billion-fold reduction in probability (White, 1999; Yeung et al., 2004). Yeung et al. (2004) noted that artemisinins taken on their own as monotherapy must be taken for seven days for radical cure, but adherence to seven-day regimens is extremely low and a three-day regimen is generally regarded as the maximum because most people discontinue treatment when they feel better usually after a couple of days, and this can result in late recrudescences with monotherapy. Nosten et al. (1994) earlier observed that used in combination with another effective drug, a three-day course is sufficient and better adhered to and has the important advantage of protecting these valuable drugs.

Efficacy of Artemisinin Combination Therapy for Childhood Malaria Treatment

The efficacy of ACT in the treatment of childhood malaria has been evaluated in many parts of sub-Saharan Africa. In Tanzania, Ngasala et al. (2011) performed an open-label randomized trial of artemether-lumefantrine with supervised (n=180) and unsupervised intake (n=179) in children <5 years of age with uncomplicated falciparum malaria. They observed that the PCR-corrected cure rate after initial treatment was 98.1% (95% confidence interval [CI], 94.2%-99.4%) after supervised and 95.1% (95% CI, 90.7%-98.1%) after unsupervised intake (P=.29). After retreatment of recurrent infections, the cure rates were 92.9% (95% CI, 81.8%-97.3%) and 97.6% (95% CI, 89.3%-98.8%), respectively (P=.58). Authors concluded that artemether-lumefantrine was highly efficacious even after unsupervised administration, despite significantly lower lumefantrine concentrations, compared with concentration achieved with supervised intake, and was well-tolerated and safe after initial and repeated treatment. In another study conducted in Guinea-Bissau, Ursing et al. (2011) investigated the efficacy of artemether-lumefantrine for treatment of uncomplicated malaria among children in a randomized open-label clinical trial. Authors noted that the polymerase chain reaction-adjusted day 28 and 42 treatment efficacies were 162 (97%) of 168 and 155 (97%) of 161, respectively, for artemether-lumefantrine and concluded that the treatment achieved the World Health Organization-recommended efficacy for antimalarials that will be adopted as policy.

In a study from Nigeria, Michael et al. (2010) assessed the early variations in plasmodium falciparum dynamics in Nigerian children after treatment with artemether-lumefantrine (AL) and artesunate-amodiaquine (AA) using an open label, randomized controlled clinical trial. They reported that in children that received both medications, early response of peripheral parasitaemia showed that 42% of children who received AL and 36.7% of those who received AA had an immediate rise in peripheral parasitaemia (0-4 h after treatment) followed by a rapid fall. The study showed the high efficacy of AL and AA in Nigerian children. In another study from Nigeria, the efficacy of two artemisinin-based combinations (artemether-lumefantrine and artesunate plus amodiaquine) for acute uncomplicated malaria was evaluated among children by Falade et al. (2008). The study was an open label, randomized controlled clinical trial and the aim of the study was to test the hypothesis that artesunate plus amodiaquine (ASAQ) is as effective as artemether-lumefantrine (AL) in the treatment of acute uncomplicated malaria in Nigerian children. The PCR corrected day 28 cure rate for per protocol populations were 98.4% for ASAQ and 100% for AL. Author concluded therefore that both drugs were efficacious and well-tolerated.

In a related study conducted in Gabon, Bouyou-Akotet et al. (2010) performed a clinical trial to evaluate the efficacy, safety and tolerability of a novel pediatric fixed-dose granule formulation of artesunate-mefloquine and a new co-blister tablet formulation. In the study a total of 71 children aged 1-13 years suffering from uncomplicated falciparum malaria were stratified into two groups according to weight and all the children were treated once daily for three days. The PCR-corrected cure rate on day 28 was evaluated and there was no reappearance of parasitemia during the follow-up period and the day-28 cure rate was therefore 100% in per-protocol analysis. Authors concluded that their findings confirmed the excellent efficacy and tolerability profile of the novel pediatric artesunate-mefloquine formulation for treatment in African children. The efficacy of non-artemisinin- and artemisinin-based combination therapies for uncomplicated falciparum malaria among children was evaluated in Cameroon by Whegang et al. (2009) according to the standard World Health Organization protocol. Using a meta-analysis the findings from this study suggested that artesunate-amodiaquine (AS-AQ) is as effective as other drugs (artesunate-sulphadoxine-pyrimethamine [AS-SP], artesunate-chlorproguanil-dapsone [AS-CD], artesunate-mefloquine [AS-MQ], dihydroartemisinin-piperaquine [DH-PP], artemether-lumefantrine [AM-LM], amodiaquine, and amodiaquine-sulphadoxine-pyrimethamine [AQ-SP]). Authors noted that although AM-LM appeared to be the most effective with no treatment failure due to recrudescence, it requires six doses, rather than three doses for other artemisinin-based combinations, but has potential advantages over other forms of ACT for childhood malaria treatment.

The above studies clearly indicate that ACT is very efficacious against uncomplicated childhood malaria in sub-Saharan Africa. However, which therapies are optimal is a matter of debate. There are numerous studies that have investigated the efficacy of other ACT varieties apart form artemether-lumefantrine. In a multi-country study involving Burkina Faso, Kenya, Mozambique, Uganda and Zambia Bassat et al. (2009) evaluated the non-inferiority of dihydroartemisinin-piperaquine (DHA-PQP) versus artemether-lumefantrine (AL) in children 6-59 months old with uncomplicated P. falciparum malaria. Efficacy analysis was performed and DHA-PQP was shown to be as efficacious as AL in treating uncomplicated malaria in African children from different endemicity settings, and shows a comparable safety profile. Authors further noted that the occurrence of new infections within the 42-day follow up was significantly lower in the DHA-PQP group, indicating a longer post-treatment prophylactic effect. In a similar study conducted in Uganda, Arinaitwe et al. (2009) in a a longitudinal, randomized trial evaluated the efficacy of Artemether-lumefantrine versus dihydroartemisinin-piperaquine for falciparum malaria in young children. A total of 113 children were randomized to artemether-lumefantrine and 119 to dihydroartemisinin-piperaquine, resulting in 320 and 351 treatments for uncomplicated falciparum malaria, respectively. Authors observed that when the duration of follow-up was extended, differences in the risk of recurrent malaria decreased such that the overall incidence of malaria treatments was similar for children randomized to artemether-lumefantrine, compared with those randomized to dihydroartemisinin-piperaquine (4.82 vs 4.61 treatments per person-year; P = .63). They thefrore concluded that artemether-lumefantrine and dihydroartemisinin-piperaquine were both efficacious and had similar long-term effects on the risk of recurrent malaria.

In Côte d'Ivoire, Toure et al. (2009) conducted a comparative, randomized clinical trial of artemisinin/naphtoquine twice daily one day versus artemether/lumefantrine six doses regimen in children uncomplicated falciparum malaria. In the study, participants were randomized to receive either artemisinin/naphtoquine or artemether/lumefantrine with variable dose according to their weight. Clinical evaluation of the 123 participants showed that cumulative PCR-uncorrected cure rate on day 28 was 100% for artemisinin/naphtoquine and 98.4% for artemether/lumefantrine. Authors therefore concluded that artemisinin/naphtoquine could prove to be suitable for use as combination antimalarial therapy. A randomized multi-centre trial on the the Efficacy and safety of a fixed dose artesunate-sulphamethoxypyrazine-pyrimethamine compared to artemether-lumefantrine for the treatment of uncomplicated falciparum malaria was conducted across some African countries by Sagara et al. (2009). In this study patients with uncomplicated falciparum malaria and over six months of age were recruited in Cameroon, Mali, Rwanda and Sudan. A total of 1,384 patients were randomly assigned to receive artesunate-sulphamethoxypyrazine-pyrimethamine (AS-SMP) three-day (once daily for 3 days) regimen (N = 476) or AS-SMP 24-hour (0 h, 12 h, 24 h) regimen (N = 458) or artemether-lumefantrine (AL), the regular 6 doses regimen (N = 450). The primary objective was to demonstrate non-inferiority (using a margin of -6%) of AS-SMP 24 hours or AS-SMP three days versus AL on the PCR-corrected 28-day cure rate. Findings indicated that AS-SMP three days or AS-SMP 24 hours are safe, are as efficacious as AL, and are well tolerated.

The efficacy of another variety of ACT, the Fixed-dose pyronaridine-artesunate combination was evaluated for treatment of uncomplicated falciparum malaria in pediatric patients in Gabon by Ramharter et al. (2008). The study was designed as an open-label dose-escalation study recruiting 60 pediatric patients sequentially in 4 treatment cohorts: study drugs were administered once daily for 3 days, as tablet coformulations (pyronaridine:artesunate ratios of 6:2, 9:3, and 12:4 mg/kg) and as a granule coformulation (pyronaridine:artesunate ratio of 9:3 mg/kg). Authors noted that the drugs had a good tolerability and safety profile, at all dose levels and the polymerase chain reaction-corrected cure rates at day 28 were 100% in per-protocol analysis, at all dose levels. Authors therefore concluded that pyronaridine-artesunate is a promising novel artemisinin-combination therapy for pediatric patients with uncomplicated Plasmodium falciparum malaria. In an open randomized clinical trial in comparing two artesunate-based combination treatments on Plasmodium falciparum malaria in Nigerian children Nigeria, Ayede et al. (2010) noted that a total of 250 children each were randomly assigned to receive three doses of artesunate/sulphamethoxypyrazine/pyrimethamine (AS + SMP) (12 hourly doses over 24 hours) or three doses of artesunate/amodiaquine (AS + AQ) (daily doses over 48 hours). Authors observed that the PCR corrected cure rates for day 28 was 97.9% in the AS + AQ arm and 95.6% in the AS + SMP arm (p = 0.15). In conclusion they noted that AS + SMP FDC given as three doses over 24 hours (12-hour intervals) has similar efficacy as AS + AQ FDC given as three doses over 48 hours (24-hour interval) for the treatment of uncomplicated *Plasmodium falciparum* malaria in children in Nigeria.

Another interesting study on the efficacy of other varieties of ACT was conducted by Rulisa et al. (2007) in Rwanda to compare different artemisinin-based combinations for the treatment of Plasmodium falciparum malaria in children. The efficacy, tolerance, and degree of re-infection of two ACTs were investigated: artesunate plus sulfadoxine/pyrimethamine (As + SP) and AS plus sulfamethoxypyrazine/pyrimethamine (As + SMP). In the study, 103 children were assigned to receive As + SP and 109 to receive As + SMP. Authors noted that in spite of the high incidence of resistance to SP, As + SP showed satisfactory results consistent with recent recommendations for ACTs (adequate clinical and parasitologic response on day 28 [ACPR] > or = 90%), but results with As + SMP fulfilled the most stringent criteria (ACPR > or = 95%). Authors therefore concluded that the absence of side effects and the low price of these drugs make them it worth to reconsider national therapies in favor of either of these two drug combinations.

These studies clearly show that all the varieties of ACTs evaluated were very efficacious in the treatment of uncomplicated malaria among children in sub-Saharan Africa. Most of the studies however acknowledged that more investigations are required on the pharmacokinetics of these ACT varieties to provide more scientific information on the profiles of the drugs.

Safety of Artemisinin Combination Therapy for Childhood Malaria Treatment

The efficacy of ACT is not in doubt as numerous studies in sub-Saharan Africa have confirmed this. According to Lefèvre et al. (2011), a wealth of evidence supports consistently high efficacy of artemether-lumefantrine, and a favorable safety and tolerability profile has been demonstrated. Furthermore Lefèvre et al. (2011) noted that the child-friendly dispersible formulation of artemether-lumefantrine has proven to be as effective and well tolerated as the standard tablets, and will encourage ease of administration and improved adherence to the drug regimen. In a randomised, single-blind, multicentre trial conducted by Abdulla et al. (2008), the safety of artemether-lumefantrine dispersible tablets compared with crushed commercial tablets was assessed in infants and children with uncomplicated malaria in Benin, Kenya, Mali, Mozambique, and Tanzania. The most common drug-related adverse event observed was vomiting (n=33 [7%] and n=42 [9%], respectively) and no signs of ototoxicity or relevant cardiotoxicity were seen. Authors therefore concluded that a six-dose regimen of artemether-lumefantrine with the new dispersible formulation is as efficacious as the currently used crushed tablet in infants and children, and has a similar safety profile. In a multicentre, randomized, controlled, investigator-blinded, parallel-group study conducted in five African centres in Cameroon, Madagascar, Mali and Senegal, Ndiaye et al. (2009) assessed the safety of ASAQ--a fixed-dose artesunate-amodiaquine combination therapy in the treatment of uncomplicated Plasmodium falciparum malaria. Authors reported that during follow-up mild and moderate adverse events including gastrointestinal and/or nervous disorders were reported in 29.3% of patients, with no difference between groups in the nature, frequency or intensity of adverse events. Authors therefore noted that the fixed-dose combination artesunate + amodiaquine (ASAQ) is safe even in young children under 5 years of age.

Sirima et al. (2009) assessed the safety of a new fixed-dose combination of amodiaquine and artesunate in young African children with acute uncomplicated *Plasmodium falciparum.* The study was a randomized, open-label trial was conducted comparing the safety of fixed (F) dose AS (25 mg)/AQ (67.5 mg) to loose (L) AS (50 mg) + AQ (153 mg) in 750, P. falciparum-infected children from Burkina Faso aged 6 months to 5 years. In the study, documented, common toxicity criteria (CTC) graded adverse events (AEs) defined safety. Authors noted that both treatments were well tolerated but there was drug-induced vomiting numbered 8/375 (2.1%) and 6/375 (1.6%) in the fixed and loose arms, respectively ($p = 0.59$) and one patient developed asymptomatic, CTC grade 4 hepatitis (AST 1052, ALT 936). Authors however concluded that fixed dose AS/AQ was efficacious and well tolerated but recommended continued safety monitoring. In Ghana, Adjei et al. (2008) evaluated the safety of Amodiaquine-artesunate (AS+AQ) vs artemether-lumefantrine (AM-L) for uncomplicated malaria in children with one year follow-up. Authors noted that the incidence of adverse events, such as pruritus, fatigue and neutropaenia were similar in the two treatment groups. No patient showed signs of hearing impairment, and no abnormal neurological signs were observed during one year of follow-up. Other adverse events were mild in intensity and overlapped with known malaria symptomatology but no adverse event exacerbation was observed in any of the subjects who received multiple treatment courses with these ACT regimens during one year follow-up. Authors concluded that AS+AQ and AM-L were efficacious for treatment of children with uncomplicated malaria in Ghana and drug-related adverse events were rare in treated subjects during one year of follow-up.

The safety and tolerability of artemether-lumefantrine versus dihydroartemisinin-piperaquine for malaria in young HIV-infected and uninfected children was evaluated by Katrak et al. (2009) in Uganda. The study was a longitudinal, randomized controlled trial conducted in a cohort of HIV-infected and uninfected children aged 4-22 months. Authors reported that Participants were randomized to treatment with artemether-lumefantrine (AL) or dihydroartemisinin-piperaquine (DP) and were actively monitored for adverse events for 28 days and then passively for up to 63 days after treatment. According to authors, most adverse events were rare, with only cough, diarrhoea, vomiting, and anaemia occurring in more than

1% of treatments. There were no differences in the risk of these events between treatment groups. The study concluded that both AL and DP were safe and well tolerated for the treatment of uncomplicated malaria in young HIV-infected and uninfected children.

In another multicentre trial conducted in Cameroon, Mali, Rwanda and Sudan, Sagara et al. (2009) evaluated the safety of a fixed dose artesunate-sulphamethoxypyrazine-pyrimethamine compared to artemether-lumefantrine for the treatment of uncomplicated falciparum malaria. In the study up to 1,384 patients were randomly assigned to receive artesunate-sulphamethoxypyrazine- pyrimethamine (AS-SMP) three-day (once daily for 3 days) regimen (N = 476) or AS-SMP 24-hour (0 h, 12 h, 24 h) regimen (N = 458) or artemether-lumefantrine (AL), the regular 6 doses regimen (N = 450). Authors observed that the most common drug-related adverse events were gastrointestinal symptoms (such as vomiting and diarrhea) which were slightly higher in the AS-SMP 24-hour group. They however noted that AS-SMP three days or AS-SMP 24 hours are safe, are as efficacious as AL, and are well tolerated. Karema et al. (2006) evaluated the safety of dihydroartemisinin/piperaquine (DHA-PQP) (Artekin) for the treatment of uncomplicated *Plasmodium falciparum* malaria in Rwandan children. Seven hundred and sixty-two children aged 12-59 months with uncomplicated P. falciparum malaria were randomly allocated to one of the following treatments: amodiaquine+artesunate; AQ+SP; or DHA-PQP. Patients were followed-up until Day 28 after treatment and adverse events and clinical and parasitological outcomes were recorded. Authors observed that the frequency of adverse events was significantly lower in patients treated with DHA-PQP than in those treated with combinations containing amodiaquine and noted that A 3-day treatment with DHA-PQP proved to be efficacious with a good safety and tolerability profile.

Although all the studies on ACTs reviewed in this section reported that the drugs were safe in childhood malaria treatment in sub-Saharan Africa, most of them acknowledged the need for continuous safety monitoring. This is largely because malaria transmission intensity is high which necessitates the frequent usage of antimalarial drugs and in such situations presumptive treatment of fever with antimalarials becomes a very regular occurrence sometimes in the absence of a confirmed diagnosis. According to Talisuna et al. (2006) the informal use of antimalarial drugs may increase the risk of incorrect dosing, inappropriate treatment, and drug interactions, which may impact negatively on drug safety. This is why pharmacovigilance, defined as "the science and activities relating to the detection, assessment, understanding and prevention of adverse effects or any other possible drug related problem", is increasingly being recognized in Africa (Talisuna et al., 2006). Staedke et al. (2008) added that although the World Health Organization has supported the development of pharmacovigilance systems in African countries deploying ACTs, additional guidance on adverse events monitoring in antimalarial clinical trials is needed, similar to the standardized recommendations available for assessment of drug efficacy.

Policy Consideration on Artemisinin Combination Therapy for Childhood Malaria Treatment

The studies reviewed in this report clearly demonstrate that in the deployment of ACT the efficacy was never in doubt, the issues that have generated prolonged debate have to do with policy implementation associated with the cost and sustainability of ACT (Ogbonna and Uneke 2008). Translating policy into practice and ensuring that ACT reaches the majority of children and vulnerable adults with malaria have proved very challenging (Whitty et al., 2008). According to Bloland and Ettling (1999), policy is usually determined through complex interactions among key stakeholders, including public agencies, private market sector, consumers, regulatory agencies and the scientific community. Furthermore, important influencing factors include perceptions of policy legitimacy, support/opposition from competing interest groups, degree of congruence with existing values, perceived logistical feasibility, and anticipated future benefits/costs if adopted. Some of the most common constraints in the deployment of ACT in sub-Saharan Africa and other malaria endemic low income settings include the complex ordering and financing procedures, unfamiliarity with the drugs among prescribers and their introduction into weak health systems with suboptimal drug management and clinical practices (Zurovac et al., 2008; Rowe et al.2003; Font et al. 2001; Nshakira et al. 2002; Armstrong Eriksen et al. 2007). Whitty et al. (2008) therefore argued that for the impact of ACT to be closer to their potential, policymakers will have to think seriously about how best to improve delivery and targeting of antimalarials.

Ogbonna and Uneke (2008) observed that challenges associated with policy change on antimalarial drug in Africa have affected the wide and effective deployment of ACT. Factors identified to affect policy change and implementation of ACT in sub-Saharan Africa include the cost ofACT which is often beyond the affordability of the poor, the rising trend of dubious drug quality which is a major challenge in the developing world, and the high level of malaria management by the informal health sector, which in most cases offers poor-quality healthcare services and contributes to poor adherence or compliance to therapy (Ogbonna and Uneke, 2008). To address some of these challenges, Whitty et al. (2008) recommended three solutions as follows: The first is to promote the use of home- or community based care. According to them the principle of this is for early recognition and treatment of malaria by volunteers or individuals with limited training and support, equipped with stocks of antimalarial drugs, which they can prescribe. Secondly, recognizing that many antimalarial treatments are distributed through the private sector, which is often used in preference to formal services even when these are easy to access, this practice can be built upon and also to improve the services of the private sector. The third solution is to improve the existing formal healthcare systems, so that people are more likely to use them, and to reduce or remove all out-of-pocket payments to reduce the direct cost of care.

Conclusion

ACT still remains the most potent antimalarial medicine till date, and its efficacy against falciparum malaria, including multidrug resistant infections, has been demonstrated in numerpus studies in sub-Saharan Africa. Although resistance to ACT by the malaria parasite has not been generally reported, it is important that effort should be geared towards prolonging the efficacy of the drug and minimize chances of resistance emerging. The issue of the cost must be urgently addressed to make ACTs affordable to the poor in sub-Saharan Africa. The need for continuous research cannot be overstated. Ogbonna and Uneke (2008) recommended that continuous research to evaluate the tolerability, efficacy, effectiveness and cost of various combination therapy strategies, particularly relating to their potential use in Africa south of the Sahara, is imperative.

Reference

Abdalla SI, Malik EM, Ali KM. The burden of malaria in Sudan: incidence, mortality and disability – adjusted life – years. *Mal. J.* 6:97.

Abdulla S, Sagara I, Borrmann S, D'Alessandro U, González R, Hamel M, Ogutu B, Mårtensson A, Lyimo J, Maiga H, Sasi P, Nahum A, Bassat Q, Juma E, Otieno L, Björkman A, Beck HP, Andriano K, Cousin M, Lefèvre G, Ubben D, Premji Z. Efficacy and safety of artemether-lumefantrine dispersible tablets compared with crushed commercial tablets in African infants and children with uncomplicated malaria: a randomised, single-blind, multicentre trial. *Lancet.* 2008; 372(9652):1819-27.

Adjei GO, Kurtzhals JA, Rodrigues OP, Alifrangis M, Hoegberg LC, Kitcher ED, Badoe EV, Lamptey R, Goka BQ. Amodiaquine-artesunate vs artemether-lumefantrine for uncomplicated malaria in Ghanaian children: a randomized efficacy and safety trial with one year follow-up. *Malar. J.* 2008;7:127.

Adjuik M, Babiker A, Garner P, Olliaro P, Taylor W, White N; International Artemisinin Study Group. Artesunate combinations for treatment of malaria: meta-analysis. *Lancet.* 2004 Jan 3;363(9402):9-17.

Ajayi IO, Falade CO, Bamgboye EA, Oduola AM, Kale OO. Assessment of a treatment guideline to improve home management of malaria in children in rural south-west Nigeria. *Malar. J.* 2008b;7:24.

Ajayi IO, Falade CO, Olley BO, Yusuf B, Gbotosho S, Iyiola T, Olaniyan O, Happi C, Munguti K, Pagnoni F. A qualitative study of the feasibility and community perception on the effectiveness of artemether-lumefantrine use in the context of home management of malaria in south-west Nigeria. *BMC Health Serv. Res.* 2008a;8:119.

Arinaitwe E, Sandison TG, Wanzira H, Kakuru A, Homsy J, Kalamya J, Kamya MR, Vora N, Greenhouse B, Rosenthal PJ, Tappero J, Dorsey G. Artemether-lumefantrine versus dihydroartemisinin-piperaquine for falciparum malaria: a longitudinal, randomized trial in young Ugandan children. *Clin. Infect. Dis.* 2009;49(11):1629-37.

Armstrong Schellenberg J, Bryce J, de Savigny D, Lambrechts T, Mbuya C, Mgalula L, Wilczynska K; Tanzania IMCI Multi-Country Evaluation Health Facility Survey Study Group. The effect of Integrated Management of Childhood Illness on observed quality of care of under-fives in rural Tanzania. *Health Policy Plan.* 2004;19(1):1-10.

Ayede IA, Falade AG, Sowunmi A, Jansen FH. An open randomized clinical trial in comparing two artesunate-based combination treatments on Plasmodium falciparum malaria in Nigerian children: artesunate/sulphamethoxypyrazine/pyrimethamine (fixed dose over 24 hours) versus artesunate/amodiaquine (fixed dose over 48 hours). *Malar. J.* 2010;9:378.

Bassat Q, Guinovart C, Sigaúque B, Aide P, Sacarlal J, Nhampossa T, Bardají A, Nhacolo A, Macete E, Mandomando I, Aponte JJ, Menéndez C, Alonso PL. Malaria in rural Mozambique. Part II: children admitted to hospital. *Malar. J.* 2008;7:37.

Bassat Q, Mulenga M, Tinto H, Piola P, Borrmann S, Menéndez C, Nambozi M, Valéa I, Nabasumba C, Sasi P, Bacchieri A, Corsi M, Ubben D, Talisuna A, D'Alessandro U. Dihydroartemisinin-piperaquine and artemether-lumefantrine for treating uncomplicated malaria in African children: a randomised, non-inferiority trial. *PLoS One*. 2009; 4(11):e7871.

Baume C. *Comparing care-seeking for childhood malaria*: lessons from Zambia and Kenya. Arlington, Basic Support for Institutionalizing Child Survival (BASICS II) for the United States Agency for International Development, Arlington, Va. 2002.

Bloland PB, Ettling M. Making malaria-treatment policy in the face of drug resistance. *Ann. Trop. Med. Parasitol.* 1999; 93: 5–23.

Bouyou-Akotet MK, Ramharter M, Ngoungou EB, Mamfoumbi MM, Mihindou MP, Missinou MA, Kurth F, Bélard S, Agnandji ST, Issifou S, Heidecker JL, Trapp S, Kremsner PG, Kombila M. Efficacy and safety of a new pediatric artesunate-mefloquine drug formulation for the treatment of uncomplicated falciparum malaria in Gabon. *Wien Klin Wochenschr.* 2010;122(5-6):173-8.

Breman JG. The ears of the hippopotamus: manifestations, determinants, and estimates of the malaria burden. *Am. J. Trop. Med. Hyg.* 2001; 64: 1-11.

Chen PQ, Li GQ, Guo XB. The infectivity of gametocytes of Plasmodium falciparum from patients treated with artemisinine. *Chin. Med. J.* 1994;74, 107:709–711.

Cui L, Su XZ. Discovery, mechanisms of action and combination therapy of artemisinin. *Expert Rev. Anti Infect. Ther.* 2009; 7(8): 999-1013.

Cui L, Su XZ.Discovery, mechanisms of action and combination therapy of artemisinin. *Expert Rev. Anti Infect. Ther.* 2009 Oct;7(8):999-1013.

Department for International Development DFID. (2004). Fact Sheet-Malaria. http://www.dfid.gov.uk/pubs/files/malaria-factsheet.pdf.

Discusses the need to coordinate a global strategy to progressively eliminate malaria.

eastern Uganda. *Trop. Med. Int. Health*. 2002; 7: 309–316.

Eastman RT, Fidock DA. Artemisinin-based combination therapies: a vital tool in efforts to eliminate malaria. *Nat. Rev. Microbiol.* 2009 Dec;7(12):864-74.

Eliades MJ, Wolkon A, Morgah K, Crawford SB, Dorkenoo A, Sodahlon Y, Hawley WA, Hightower AW, Kuile FO, Terlouw DJ. Burden of malaria at community level in children less than 5 years of age in Togo. *Am. J. Trop. Med. Hyg.* 2006;75(4):622-9.

Eriksen J, Tomson G, Mujinja P, Warsame MY, Jahn A, Gustafsson LL. Assessing health worker performance in malaria case management of underfives at health facilities in a rural Tanzanian district. *Trop. Med. Int. Health*. 2007;12(1):52-61.

Falade CO, Ogundele AO, Yusuf BO, Ademowo OG, Ladipo SM. High efficacy of two artemisinin-based combinations (artemether-lumefantrine and artesunate plus amodiaquine) for acute uncomplicated malaria in Ibadan, Nigeria. *Trop. Med. Int. Health.* 2008;13(5):635-43.

Feachem R, Sabot O. A new global malaria eradication strategy. *Lancet* 2008;371:1633–1635.

Font F, Alonso González M, Nathan R, Kimario J, Lwilla F, Ascaso C, Tanner M, Menéndez C, Alonso PL. Diagnostic accuracy and case management of clinical malaria in the primary health services of a rural area in south-eastern Tanzania. *Trop. Med. Int. Health.* 2001;6(6):423-8.

German PI, Aweeka FT. *Clinical pharmacology of artemisinin-based combination therapies.* Clin.

Hopkins H, Talisuna A, Whitty CJM, Staedke SG. Impact of homebased management of malaria on health outcomes in Africa: a systematic review of the evidence. *Mal. J.* 2007; 6, 134.

Idro R, Aloyo J, Mayende L, Bitarakwate E, John CC, Kivumbi GW. Severe malaria in children in areas with low, moderate and high transmission intensity in Uganda. *Trop. Med. Int. Health* 2006; 11: 115–124.

Idro R, Ndiritu M, Ogutu B, Mithwani S, Maitland K, Berkley J, Crawley J, Fegan G, Bauni E, Peshu N, Marsh K, Neville B, Newton C. Burden, features, and outcome of neurological involvement in acute falciparum malaria in Kenyan children. *JAMA*. 2007; 297(20):2232-40.

Karema C, Fanello CI, van Overmeir C, van Geertruyden JP, van Doren W, Ngamije D, D'Alessandro U. Safety and efficacy of dihydroartemisinin/piperaquine (Artekin) for the treatment of uncomplicated Plasmodium falciparum malaria in Rwandan children. *Trans. R. Soc. Trop. Med. Hyg*. 2006;100(12):1105-11.

Katrak S, Gasasira A, Arinaitwe E, Kakuru A, Wanzira H, Bigira V, Sandison TG, Homsy J, Tappero JW, Kamya MR, Dorsey G. Safety and tolerability of artemether-lumefantrine versus dihydroartemisinin-piperaquine for malaria in young HIV-infected and uninfected children. *Malar. J.* 2009; 8:272.

Klayman DL. Qinghaosu (artemisinin): an antimalarial drug from China. *Science* 1985; 228:1049–1055.

Kuhn T, Wang Y. Artemisinin – an innovative cornerstone for anti-malaria therapy. *Prog. Drug Res*. 2008;66(383):385–422.

Kumar N, Zheng H. Stage-specific gametocytocidal effect in vitro of the antimalaria drug qinghaosu on Plasmodium falciparum. *Parasitol. Res*. 1990;76:214–218.

Lefèvre G, Marrast AC, Grueninger H. Novartis Malaria Initiative: best practice example of pharmaceutical industry's engagement in the fight against malaria. *Ann. N Y Acad. Sci.* 2011 Mar;1222:19-29.

Li Y, Wu YL. An over four millennium story behind qinghaosu (artemisinin) – a fantastic antimalarial drug from a traditional Chinese herb. *Curr. Med. Chem.* 2003;10:2197–2230.

Mabunda S, Casimiro S, Quinto L, Alonso P. A country-wide malaria survey in Mozambique. I. Plasmodium falciparum infection in children in different epidemiological settings. *Malar. J.* 2008; 7:216.

Michael OS, Gbotosho GO, Folarin OA, Okuboyejo T, Sowunmi A, Oduola AM, Happi CT. Early variations in plasmodium falciparum dynamics in Nigerian children after treatment with two artemisinin-based combinations: implications on delayed parasite clearance. *Malar. J.* 2010; 9:335.

Murphy SC, Breman .G. Gaps in the childhood malaria burden in Africa: cerebral malaria, neurological sequelae, anemia, respiratory distress, hypoglycemia, and complications of pregnancy. *Am. J. Trop. Med. Hyg*. 2001; 64(1-2 Suppl): 57-67.

Ndiaye JL, Randrianarivelojosia M, Sagara I, Brasseur P, Ndiaye I, Faye B, Randrianasolo L, Ratsimbasoa A, Forlemu D, Moor VA, Traore A, Dicko Y, Dara N, Lameyre V, Diallo M, Djimde A, Same-Ekobo A, Gaye O. Randomized, multicentre assessment of the efficacy and safety of ASAQ--a fixed-dose artesunate-amodiaquine combination therapy in the treatment of uncomplicated Plasmodium falciparum malaria. *Malar. J.* 2009; 8:125.

Newton CR, Krishna S. Severe falciparum malaria in children: current understanding of pathophysiology and supportive treatment. *Pharm. Therap.* 1998; 79(1):1–53.

Ngasala BE, Malmberg M, Carlsson AM, Ferreira PE, Petzold MG, Blessborn D, Bergqvist Y, Gil JP, Premji Z, Björkman A, Mårtensson A. Efficacy and effectiveness of artemether-lumefantrine after initial and repeated treatment in children <5 years of age with acute uncomplicated Plasmodium falciparum malaria in rural Tanzania: a randomized trial. *Clin. Infect. Dis.* 2011;52(7):873-82.

Njuguna J, Qader S. Challenges Associated with Scaling up Artemisinin Combination Therapy in Sub-Saharan Africa A Review Article. *Libyan J. Med.*. 2008 Mar 1;3(1):42-8.

Nosten F, Luxemburger C, ter Kuile FO, Woodrow C, Eh JP, Chongsuphajaisiddhi T, White NJ, 1994. Treatment of multidrug-resistant Plasmodium falciparum malaria with 3-day artesunate-mefloquine combination. *J. Infect. Dis.* 170: 971–977.

Nosten F, White NJ. Artemisinin-based combination treatment of falciparum malaria. *Am. J. Trop. Med. Hyg.* 2007;77(Suppl 6):181–192

Nshakira N, Kristensen M, Ssali F, Whyte SR. Appropriate treatment of malaria? *Use of antimalarial drugs for children's fevers in district medical units, drug shops and homes in Pharmacokinet* 2008;47:91–102.

Ogbonna, A., Uneke, C., 2008. Artemisinin-based combination therapy for uncomplicated malaria in sub-Saharan Africa: the efficacy, safety, resistance and policy implementation since Abuja 2000. *Trans. R. Soc. Trop. Med. Hyg.* 102 (7), 621–627.

Price RN, Nosten F, Luxemburger C, ter Kuile FO, Paiphun L, Chongsuphajaisiddhi T, White NJ, 1996. Effects of artemisinin derivatives on malaria transmissibility. *Lancet* 347: 1654–1658.

Ramharter M, Kurth F, Schreier AC, Nemeth J, Glasenapp I, Bélard S, Schlie M, Kammer J, Koumba PK, Cisse B, Mordmüller B, Lell B, Issifou S, Oeuvray C, Fleckenstein L, Kremsner PG. Fixed-dose pyronaridine-artesunate combination for treatment of uncomplicated falciparum malaria in pediatric patients in Gabon. *J. Infect. Dis.* 2008;198(6):911-9.

Roca-Feltrer A, Carneiro I, Armstrong-Schellenberg JR. Estimates of the burden of malaria morbidity in Africa in children under the age of 5 years. *Trop. Med. Int. Health* 2008; 13(6):771-783.

Rowe AK, Onikpo F, Lama M, Deming MS. Risk and protective factors for two types of error in the treatment of children with fever at outpatient health facilities in Benin. *Int. J. Epidemiol.* 2003; 32, 296–303.

Rulisa S, Gatarayiha JP, Kabarisa T, Ndayisaba G. Comparison of different artemisinin-based combinations for the treatment of Plasmodium falciparum malaria in children in Kigali, Rwanda, an area of resistance to sulfadoxine-pyrimethamine: artesunate plus sulfadoxine/pyrimethamine versus artesunate plus sulfamethoxypyrazine/pyrimethamine. *Am. J. Trop. Med. Hyg.* 2007; 77(4): 612-6.

Sagara I, Rulisa S, Mbacham W, Adam I, Sissoko K, Maiga H, Traore OB, Dara N, Dicko YT, Dicko A, Djimdé A, Jansen FH, Doumbo OK. Efficacy and safety of a fixed dose artesunate-sulphamethoxypyrazine-pyrimethamine compared to artemether-lumefantrine for the treatment of uncomplicated falciparum malaria across Africa: a randomized multi-centre trial. *Malar. J.* 2009;8:63.

Sagara I, Rulisa S, Mbacham W, Adam I, Sissoko K, Maiga H, Traore OB, Dara N, Dicko YT, Dicko A, Djimdé A, Jansen FH, Doumbo OK. Efficacy and safety of a fixed dose artesunate-sulphamethoxypyrazine-pyrimethamine compared to artemether-lumefantrine for the treatment of uncomplicated falciparum malaria across Africa: a randomized multi-centre trial. *Malar. J.* 2009; 8:63.

Schellenberg D, Menendez C, Kahigwa E, Font F, Galindo C, Acosta C, Schellenberg JA, Aponte JJ, Kimario J, Urassa H, Mshinda H, Tanner M, Alonso P. African children with malaria in an area of intense Plasmodium falciparum transmission: features on admission to the hospital and risk factors for death. *Am. J. Trop. Med. Hyg.* 1999; 61(3): 431-438.

Sirima SB, Tiono AB, Gansané A, Diarra A, Ouédraogo A, Konaté AT, Kiechel JR, Morgan CC, Olliaro PL, Taylor WR. The efficacy and safety of a new fixed-dose combination of amodiaquine and artesunate in young African children with acute uncomplicated Plasmodium falciparum. *Malar. J.* 2009; 8:48.

Skinner TS, Manning LS, Johnston WA, Davis TM. In vitro stage-specific sensitivity of Plasmodium falciparum to quinine and artemisinin drugs. *Int. J. Parasitol.* 1996;26:519–525.

Snow R, Craig MH, Newton CRJC, Steketee RW. The public health burden of Plasmodium falciparum malaria in Africa: Deriving the number. *Working Paper No. 11, Disease Control Priorities Project.* Bethesda, Maryland: Fogarty International Center, National Institutes of Health; 2003.

Snow RW, Korenromp EL, Gouws, E. Pediatric mortality in Africa: Plasmodium falciparum malaria as a cause or risk? *Am. J. Trop. Med. Hyg.* 2004; 71: 16–24.

Staedke SG, Jagannathan P, Yeka A, Bukirwa H, Banek K, Maiteki-Sebuguzi C, Clark TD, Nzarubara B, Njama-Meya D, Mpimbaza A, Rosenthal PJ, Kamya MR, Wabwire-Mangen F, Dorsey G, Talisuna AO. Monitoring antimalarial safety and tolerability in clinical trials: a case study from Uganda. *Malar. J.* 2008; 7:107.

Talisuna AO, Staedke SG, D'Alessandro U. Pharmacovigilance of antimalarial treatment in Africa: is it possible? *Malar. J.* 2006; 5:50.

Tiono AB, Kaboré Y, Traoré A, Convelbo N, Pagnoni F, Sirima SB. Implementation of Home based management of malaria in children reduces the work load for peripheral health facilities in a rural district of Burkina Faso. *Malar. J.* 2008;7:201.

Toure OA, Penali LK, Yapi JD, Ako BA, Toure W, Djerea K, Gomez GO, Makaila O. A comparative, randomized clinical trial of artemisinin/naphtoquine twice daily one day versus artemether/lumefantrine six doses regimen in children and adults with uncomplicated falciparum malaria in Côte d'Ivoire. *Malar. J.* 2009;8:148.

Uneke CJ. Impact of home management of Plasmodium falciparum malaria on childhood malaria control in sub-Saharan Africa. *Tropical Biomedicine* 2009a; 26, 182–199.

Ursing J, Kofoed PE, Rodrigues A, Blessborn D, Thoft-Nielsen R, Björkman A, Rombo L. Similar efficacy and tolerability of double-dose chloroquine and artemether-lumefantrine for treatment of Plasmodium falciparum infection in Guinea-Bissau: a randomized trial. *J. Infect. Dis.* 2011; 203(1):109-16.

Were W. *Bringing malaria management closer to the home*. Supporting Agency – Roll Back Malaria, Mera 3-4. World Health Organization, Geneva, 2004.

Whegang SY, Tahar R, Foumane VN, Soula G, Gwét H, Thalabard JC, Basco LK. Efficacy of non-artemisinin- and artemisinin-based combination therapies for uncomplicated falciparum malaria in Cameroon. *Malar. J.* 2010; 9:56.

White N. Antimalarial drug resistance and combination chemotherapy. Phil. Trans. R. Soc. Lond. 1999;354:739–749.

White NJ. Qinghaosu (artemisinin): the price of success. *Science* 2008; 320:330–334.

Whitty CJ, Chandler C, Ansah E, Leslie T, Staedke SG. Deployment of ACT antimalarials for treatment of malaria: challenges and opportunities. *Malar. J.* 2008;7 Suppl 1:S7.

WHO, 2001. Antimalarial Drug Combination Therapy. *Report of a WHO Technical Consultation* WHO/CDS/RBM/2001.35. World Health Organization, Geneva.

WHO, 2007. Global AMDP Database. http://www.who.int/malaria/amdp/amdp afro.htm.

WHO, Guidelines for the treatment of malaria. Geneva: WHO; 2006.

WHO. 2004. UNICEF/UNDP/World Bank/WHO Special Programme for Research and Training in Tropical Diseases. *Social science research on tropical diseases* (CD ROM). Version 1.0 Geneva: WHO/TDR; 2004.

WHO. *Reducing malaria's impact on child health, development and survival.* Roll Back Malaria briefing document. WHO/CDS/RBM/2002.38. World Health Organization, Geneva. 2002.

WHO. *The African malaria report* 2003. WHO, 17-23. Geneva, World Health Organization. 2003.

WHO. *World Malaria Report 2008*. Geneva, Switzerland. World Health Organization. 2008.

WHO. *World Malaria Report 2009*. Geneva, Switzerland. World Health Organization. 2009.

Woodrow CJ, Haynes RK, Krishna S. Artemisinins. *Postgrad. Med. J.* 2005; 81:71–78.

WHO. Guidelines for the treatment of malaria (1st ed.). *Report no WHO/HTM/MAL*/2006.1108. World Health Organization, Geneva. 2006.

Woodrow CJ, Krishna S. Antimalarial drugs: recent advances in molecular determinants of resistance and their clinical significance. *Cell Mol. Life Sci.* 2006;63:1586–1596.

Worral E, Basu S, Hanson K. Is malaria a disease of poverty? A review of literature. *Trop. Med. Int. Health* 2005; 10: 1047-1059.

Yeung S, Pongtavornpinyo W, Hastings IM, Mills AJ, White NJ. Antimalarial drug resistance, artemisinin-based combination therapy, and the contribution of modeling to elucidating policy choices. *Am. J. Trop. Med. Hyg.* 2004 Aug;71(2 Suppl):179-86.

Zeng Q, Qiu F, Yuan L. Production of artemisinin by genetically-modified microbes. *Biotechnol. Lett.* 2008; 30:581–592.

Zhang JF. *A detailed chronological record of Project 523 and the discovery and development of qinghaosu (artemisinin).* Vol. 193. Yangcheng Evening News Publishing Company; China: 2005.

Zurovac D, Njogu J, Akhwale W, Hamer DH, Snow RW. Translation of artemether-lumefantrine treatment policy into paediatric clinical practice: an early experience from Kenya. *Trop. Med. Int. Health.* 2008;13(1):99-107.

In: Malaria: Etiology, Pathogenesis and Treatments
Editors: A. M. Peterson et al, pp. 193-213
ISBN: 978-1-62100-363-2

Chapter VIII

Climate Variations and Malaria in China: Past, Present and Future

Ying Zhang[1], *Peng Bi*[1], *Janet Hiller*[1,2], *Yuwei Sun*[3] *and Baofa Jiang*[4]

[1] Discipline of Public Health, School of Population Health and Clinical Practice, Faculty of Health Sciences, University of Adelaide, Australia.
[2] Faculty of Health Sciences, Australian Catholic University, Australia.
[3] Shenzhen Baoan Health Bureau, Guangdong, China.
[4] Centre of Climate Change and Population Health, School of Public Health, Shandong University, China.

Abstract

The incidence of malaria has decreased dramatically in 20th century China. However, there has been an evident re-emergence of malaria since 2000. The transmission of malaria is complicated, and climate variability may be one of the risk factors associated with the re-emergence of malaria. The relationship between malaria and climatic variables has been assessed in many regions, such as Africa and South America. However, limited studies have been conducted in China, and little is known about the impact of climate variations on malaria in that country. This chapter has systematically reviewed previous studies that examine the association between climatic variables and malaria in China; including research methods, findings, and limitations. Evidence has also been provided by a scenario-based study, projecting the future health burdens of malaria due to rising temperatures. Recommendations are presented at the end of the chapter for policy makers, public health practitioners, as well as clinicians to prevent and control malaria in a warming climate, not only in China but also in other developing countries.

Keywords: malaria, climate variations, burden of disease, China.

1. Introduction

Malaria is the most significant mosquito-borne disease in the world, and it is still a serious public health issue in many developing countries. Due to the great efforts made by the World Health Organization and local authorities, the worldwide prevention and control of malaria has been very successful. The incidence of malaria decreased dramatically during 20th century China. However, there has been an evident re-emergence of malaria since 2000, particularly in central and southern provinces where malaria used to be highly endemic. The transmission of malaria is complicated and can be influenced by many factors. Climate variations might be one of the drivers, suggested by previous studies, because mosquitoes play very important roles in malaria transmission and are very sensitive to climate variations [1, 2].

China faces many environmental challenges, including climate variations, which is significantly affecting population health. While there is clear evidence for the impact of global climate variations on malaria, only a few studies have actually been conducted in China. The relationship between climate variability and malaria is far from clear in the Chinese setting. This chapter has systematically reviewed previous studies, in China, associated with the impact of climatic variables on malaria. In addition, a scenario-based modelling study has been presented, projecting the future disease burden of malaria in two Chinese cities, located in temperate and subtropical climatic zones. The aim of this chapter is to provide further evidence relevant to decision-making associated with the prevention and control of malaria in China and to the reduction of potential health risks from future climate change.

1.1. Epidemiology of Malaria in China

Plasmodium vivax, primarily *P. falciparum*, is predominant in China, accounting for more than 80% of the total malaria cases [3]. *Anopheles* is the transmitting vector in most of the Chinese epidemic areas. Currently, there are 4 species of mosquitoes including *An. anthropophagus* (lesteri), *An. sinensis*, *An. minimus* and *An. dirus* [4]. The first two species are the major transmitting vectors in the central Provinces, while the other two are key malaria vectors in the Yunnan and Hainan Provinces in southern China [4]. Varying distribution malaria vectors in similar areas made vector control measurments very challenging and less effective.

The malarias have been legally notifiable diseases in China since the 1950s. The incidence of malaria decreased dramatically during 20th century China (Figure 1) because of the achievements of malaria control and prevention measures [5]. However, the degree of malaria under-reporting could be a serious problem in some regions, especially in rural and remote areas [6]. There was also a notable increase in malaria incidence after 2000. The incidence of malaria in 2004 was 3.4/100,000.

The spatial distribution of malaria incidence is presented in Figure 2 (sources: WHO). There are six affected Provinces in the 2003 re-emergence of malaria. Potential reasons for the re-emerging malaria in China may include poor capability in the township clinics; a lack of an early warning system and rapid response capability; a long incubation period of

Plasmodium vivax; and an unstability of the major transmitting vector, *An. Anthropophagus* [7]. Currently, in China, the endemic area of *falciparum* malaria was confined in the Yunnan and Hainan Provinces, with all other provinces having only imported cases.

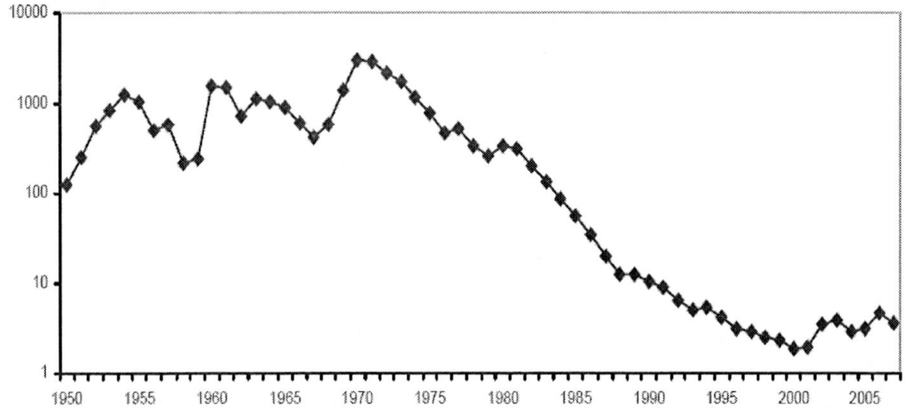

Figure 1. Annual incidence (per 100,000) of malaria 1950-2008 in China [4].

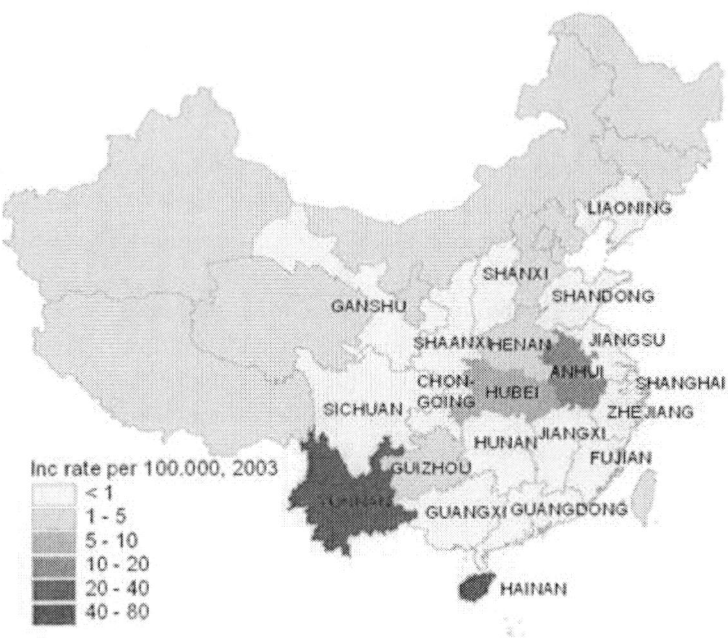

Figure 2. Incidence rate of confirmed malaria cases by Province in China, 2003 [3].

The transmission of malaria is complex, affected by socio-economic and environmental factors. Some social economic factors may include: an increasing migrant population between highly endemic Provinces and its adjacent provinces, working/travelling cross borders from infected countries, economic status (e.g. delayed treatment), occupation (e.g. raising livestock), living conditions (e.g. no screen door/window), and individual behaviors (e.g. sleeping outdoors and usage of repellent incense) [8-11]. Ecological and environmental factors play important roles in the transmission of malaria, affecting the development of mosquitoes and pathogens. Changes of the ecological environment and global warming have made a northward spread of *An. Anthropophagus* [4]. Malaria endemic also showed positive correlation with vegetation index in Huaihe River Valley [12]. The relationship between climatic variations and malaria has been reported in many tropical regions around the world [13].

1.2. Control of Malaria in China

Mosquito control has been proved to be the most effective intervention method to reduce malaria infection in China. A study reported that a mosquito net, treated with pentmethrin, could effectively prevent malaria in southern China [14]. Furthermore, new irrigation methods can sustain malaria control in southern China [15]. Health education and promotional programs can also effectively increase awareness, knowledge and appropriate behaviors in local communities [16]; thus, leading to a reduction of the disease burden of malaria. Moreover, the importance of educational programs, targeting village doctors, cannot be undermined [17].

International collaborations play a crucial role in the malaria control in China and other developing countries. Three rounds (R1, R5 and R6) of malaria programs of the Global Fund (GF) to fight AIDS, Tuberculosis and Malaria were successfully applied, with more than $62 million dollars worth of funding. R1 (2003-08) focused on the high epidemic regions in China with a target population of 9 million. R5 (2006-11) had priorities based in prevention, diagnosis and treatment, surveillance, and emergency response to roll back re-emerging malaria in central provinces. R6 (2007-12) is for malaria control across China-Myanmar border areas. These important, internationally supported, programs significantly reduce the incidence of malaria in targeted areas.

Although, in China, malaria control and prevention programs have seen a dramatic decrease in incidence over the last decades, no effective early warning system for malaria has been established nationally and locally. Given the poor health response capability at rural areas in villages and townships, it is worth having a better understanding of the spectrum of the risk factors, including climate variations, in order to provide recommendations for evidence-based policy making.

2. The Association between Climate Variations and Malaria in China (A Literature Review)

This section systematically reviews the studies which investigated the relationship between climate variations and malaria in China. Details of these studies and their limitations have been discussed.

2.1. Methods

All health outcomes related to malaria, including deaths, hospitalisation, incidence, prevalence, and number of cases were included. The target population includes all the Chinese, set at national, provincial and city levels; including studies conducted from both rural and metropolitan areas. Indicators of climate variations included: temperature, extreme heat, rainfall, relative humidity, air pressure and the Southern Oscillation Index (SOI, an index of El Nino/La Nina events). Studies published during the last 20 years, between January 1, 1990 and December 31, 2010, were included. Original studies published in academic journals, either in English or in Chinese, were also included. Review papers were excluded. The key words, in both English and Chinese, included "malaria", "climate or weather or temperature or heat or rainfall or humidity or air pressure or El Nino", and "China or Chinese". In addition to PubMed, Web of Science, Scopus, and Google Scholar, major Chinese literature search engines in China were used, including the China National Science and Technology Library (NSTL), China Knowledge Resource Integrated Database (CNKI), VP info (VIP) and Wanfang Data.

2.2. Results

There were an overall of 13 studies included in this review. Details of these studies have been summarised in Table 1. There are 62% (8 studies) of these papers published in international journals in English. Although there was only one study before 2000, the number of studies per year increased to five in 2010. The study areas cover regions with various climatic characteristics, including tropical, subtropical and temperate zones. Moreover, most of the studies have been conducted in areas where there had/has been a high incidence of malaria, i.e. Hannan Province, Yunan Province and Anhui Province.

2.3. Discussion

It is clear that there have been increased publications examining the impact of climate variations on malaria in China. However, evidence is still not robust enough to support decision making regarding malaria control in a changing environment. Moreover, there is a lack of translation of research findings, into public health practice or policy making, to fulfill the aim of malaria elimination by 2020 in China.

The results from these studies consistently support a positive association between temperature and cases of malaria across the study areas, with a lagged effect ranging from zero to two months [18, 30, 31]. However, the relationship between other meteorological variables, e.g. rainfall and humidity, varied in difference areas. For example, an increase in rainfall could lead to more malaria cases in southern China, but may not be an influencing factor in northern regions with more temperate climates [24, 28]. Moreover, malaria transmission can be related to other climatic variables, such as fog, with a one-year lag time, and the impact of El Nino [21, 22].

Table 1. Summary of reviewed studies

Authors	Year of Publication	Language	Site of study	Key analysis	Main relevant findings
1.Hu et al. [11]	1998	English	Yunnan Province (southwest)	Generalised multiple regression, 1990-1996, annual incidence	Every 1 °C increase in temperature was related to 1.2/10,000 higher incidence; 100 mm increase in rainfall was related to 100/10,000 increase in incidence
2.Bi et al. [18]	2003	English	Shuchen county of Anhui Province (southeast)	Time series analysis, 1880-1991, monthly incidence	Significant climatic variables: minimum temperature and rainfall; one month lag effect
3.Gao et al. [19]	2003	Chinese	A state in Yunan Province (southwest)	Neural network forecasting model, 1994-1999, monthly data	Climatic variables, including air pressure, temperature, relative humidity, maximum temperature, minimum temperature, rainfall, rain-day, evaporation and sunshine hours, were used to establish the model
4.Wen et al. [20]	2003	Chinese	Hainan Province (south)	Stepwise regression, 1995-2000, monthly incidence	Positive association with temperature and rainfall, with a one to two months lagged effect
5.Bi et al. [21]	2005	English	Anhui Province (east)	Correlation analysis, 1971-1992, monthly incidence	A positive correlation between the El Nino index (SOI) and the incidence
6.Tian et al. [22]	2008	English	Mengla County of Yunnan Province (southwest)	Time series analysis, 1971-1999, monthly incidence	Min and max temperatures, and days of fog frequency were positively related to malaria incidence; one year lagged effect of fog days
7.Huang et al. [23]	2009	Chinese	Hubei Province (central)	Logistic regression, 1990-2007, monthly incidence	Peak of malaria cases was correlated with temperature and precipitation, with one month lag
8.Wang et al. [24]	2009	Chinese	Anhui (east)	Spatial analysis combined with logistic regression analysis, 2004-2006	One unit increase in lowest temperature in a year may lead to a 33% increase in the probability of incidence; One unit increase in total annual rainfall may lead to 27% increase in probability of malaria incidence
9.Li et al. [25]	2010	Chinese	Three Gorges Reservoir Area	Poisson regression, 1997-2008, annual data	Positive correlation between temperature and malaria incidence
10.Xiao et al. [26]	2010	English	Hainan (south)	Time series analysis, 1995-2008, monthly incidence	Mean temperature of the previous two months could be used to predict the incidence
11.Yang et al. [27]	2010	English	676 locations across China	multinomial regression models, 1981-1995, monthly	Temperature, relative humidity and rainfall are major drivers of malaria

Authors	Year of Publication	Language	Site of study	Key analysis	Main relevant findings
				data	transmission
12.Zhang et al. [28]	2010	English	Jinan City (central north)	Time series analysis, 1959-1979, monthly number of cases	Key climatic variables: max and min temperatures; 1 °C rise in temperatures might be related to more than 15% increase in number of cases
13.Zhou et al. [29]	2010	English	Counties in Anhui Province and Henan Province (east)	Stepwise regression, 1990-2006, monthly incidence	75% changes in incidence could be contributed to changes in temperatures and rainfall

Only a few studies have attempted to quantify the association between meteorological variables and malaria, indicating that 1 °C rise in temperatures might cause a 15% increase in the number of cases in a northern area and a 33% increase in incidence in an eastern area [24, 28].

All studies used an ecological study design, i.e. analyzing data at a population level rather than at an individual level. These studies have drawn on historical disease surveillance data from local authorities, meaning that data availability and quality are curial to the study's findings. In term of data analysis, time-series analysis is the most commonly used method to examine the relationship between climatic variables and malaria. This approach is convenient to control the potential confounding factors, such as seasonal variations and long term trends, demonstrating sensitivity to changes by using just a few years of data [32]. Furthermore, generalized linear regression or Poisson regression models have been used to analyse the size of effects. However, the limitations of these models, such as controlling for auto-correlation and lagged effects, should be made known when dealing with this time series data.

Based on this review, some of the limitations of previous studies and research gaps in examining the impact of climate variations and malaria in China include: 1) not enough systematic studies to quantify the association between meteorological variables and malaria in China; 2) no attempt in detecting the threshold of temperatures for improving/developing infectious disease early warning systems; 3) a lack of focus on vulnerable subpopulations, such as the young and the elderly; 4) a lack of robust study designs in many of the previous studies; 5) that the assumptions made by previous studies had really simplified the transmission of malaria and its potential contributing factors, given the complex of this mosquito-borne disease; 6) that no local projective study forecasting the populations at risk in the future, when considering climate variations, although some currently non-endemic areas may suffer in the future.

3. Future Disease Burden of Malaria Due to Rising Temperatures (A Case Study)

This section, as a case study, projected the future disease burden of malaria due to increasing temperatures in two areas in northern and southern China, aiming to support evidence-based decision making under scenarios of global warming.

3.1. Methods

3.1.1. Selecting Study Regions

The principles for selecting the target study regions for this study included: 1) the selected regions should be from different climatic zones in China; and 2) the selected regions should have necessary data available for the analysis.

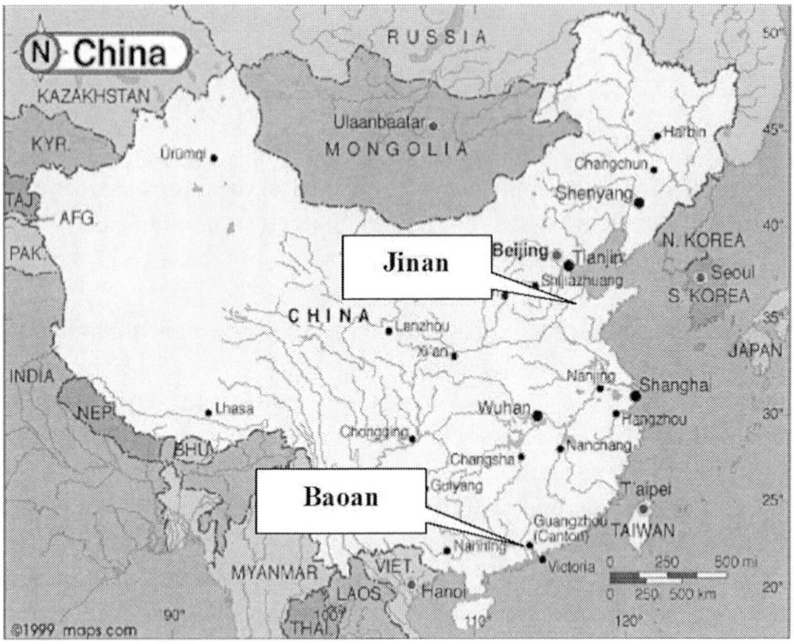

Figure 3. Geography of selected study regions.

Consequently, Jinan, the capital of Shandong Province in northern China with a population of 5.9 million and a temperate climate, and Baoan, a Special Economy District in Guangdong Province in southern China with a 3.3 million population, but a subtropical climate, were selected for the projective modelling. Geographic locations of these two study regions were indicated in Figure 3.

3.1.2. Framework for the Environmental Burden of Disease Study

The global Environmental Burden of Disease (EBD) study estimated the burden of disease from 26 major environmental risk factors, including climate change [33]. Any global environmental changes that arise in the future will tend to appear, first, in local settings where decision making usually takes place. Therefore, studies at a local level are necessary. Within the EBD framework, the assessment of the health burden attributable to climate change is proposed to estimate Disability Adjusted Life Years (DALYs) lost in the future, rather than today [34]. The method of calculating the DALYs has been published; although, weaknesses and problems still exist. DALY is a health gap measure - the gap between current health status and an ideal situation where everyone lives into old age, free of disease and disability [35]. One DALY can be thought of as one year of "healthy" life lost. DALYs are calculated by the sum of years of life lost due to premature mortality (YLL), and the equivalent "healthy" years of life lost due to disability (YLD) [36]. The estimation of the mortality burden, using a measure such as the Years of Life Lost (YLLs), has quite reliable calculation methods, based on available death registrations. Estimated YLDs, however, can be volatile, due to: (i) the parameters used in the calculation; (ii) difficulties in defining "disability"; and (iii) the observed variations in the incidence rate of infectious diseases.

3.1.3. Calculating Years Lost due to Disability

Based on the quantitative association between climatic variables and malaria, as well as future climate and population scenarios, scenario-based modeling was applied to project the future burden of malaria in the study regions of China. The YLDs, rather than the DALYs, were used to measure the burden of disease: only the incidence of malaria, and not the deaths from malaria, has been analyzed along with meteorological variables. Additionally, the mortality from malaria is very low in the study regions, and they account for only a very small proportion of the DALYs. The YLDs for malaria in 2000 were estimated and projected to 2020 and 2050 respectively.

The methods used to calculate the YLDs in this study are similar to those used in the Global EBD study, using similar age groups, disability weights, discounting, and age weighting [37]. The age groups used in this study, for both sexes, are: 0~, 5~, 10~, 15~, 20~, 30~, 40~, 50~, 60+. Age- and sex- specific incidence rates of malaria were collected from local authorities for both study regions. Case definition, disability weights (0.21), and duration (0.47 years) of a malaria episode were derived from the data of the WHO defined Western Pacific regions (including China) in the GBD study 2002 [38]. A 3% discount rate was applied in this study, calculating the YLDs to ensure consistency with the measurement of health outcomes in other analyses [36, 37]. For this study to have international comparability, uniform age weighting has been adopted. Although different discounting and age weighting could be used in burden of disease studies, such as no discounting and non-uniform age weighting - YLD(0,0) - or 3% discounting and non-uniform age weighting - YLD(3,1) -, these discounting measures and weights would not affect the potential trends between observed and projected burdens of disease based on linear regression. Therefore, only 3% discounting, without age weighting, were used for the calculation of the YLD (3,0) in this study, as used in most burden of disease studies [37, 39].

3.1.4. Climate and Demographic Scenarios

Due to the consistent positive relationship being detected between temperatures and malaria, the temperature-based scenarios were used as a proxy for future exposure to global warming. The ranges of the projections of temperatures in the temperate and subtropical regions are summarized in Table 2.

Table 2. Future temperature scenarios - range of increases in temperature (°C)

	2020	2050
Jinan (temperate region)	0.3-2.4	0.8-4.6
Baoan (subtropical region)	0.3-3.6	1.8-5.0

In addition to the change in temperature, changes in future population structures were taken into account to project the future YLDs for malaria. The scenarios for future population structures were collected from the National Bureau of Statistics of China and summarized in Table 3.

Table 3. Future demographic changes in the study regions

	Jinan (temperate)			Baoan (subtropical)		
	2000	2020	2050	2000	2020	2050
Population (thousands)	5602	6270	5720	2736	4680	4305
Population sex ratio (males per 100 females)	103.6	101.3	99.5	104.3	103.1	101.5
Percentage aged 0-4 (%)	3.33	3.15	2.79	1.66	1.35	1.14
Percentage aged 5-14 (%)	10.62	9.98	8.41	5.18	3.81	3.26
Percentage aged 15-24 (%)	29.96	27.89	26.35	20.45	17.01	14.55
Percentage aged 60 or over (%)	12.29	18.71	25.53	7.44	12.53	20.84

3.1.5. Assumptions and Uncertainties

Firstly, the quantitative association between climate variation and malaria was assumed to be maintained in the future, despite potential changes in the impact of other factors, such as socio-economic status, on disease transmission. The quantitative relationship between temperature and malaria was based on the regression models developed in our previous studies in the study regions [28]. This association was then applied to future climate and population growth scenarios. This assumption might introduce significant uncertainty to the projections.

Secondly, temperature is the key weather factor influencing the transmission of malaria. The future increases in temperature were used as a proxy for all future climate scenarios because temperature is the only climatic variable included in all the regression models developed for study diseases, and there are large variations in the predictions for other meteorological variables, such as rainfall and relative humidity. Other climatic factors, such as rainfall, may also influence disease transmission. In this study, the effects of other meteorological variables on infectious diseases have been assumed to be constant.

Thirdly, any future change in the vulnerability of population to climate change was not taken into account. Moreover, adaptation to and mitigation of climate change were assumed unchanged. For example, non-climatic factors, such as exposure to vectors or contaminated food, which affect the transmission of infectious diseases, have not been included in this projection on the assumption that they would remain constant over the study period.

This study has two major uncertainties, as has all other research on health effects of climate change. One is the uncertainty in the assessment of the quantitative relationship between meteorological variables and malaria. The other is the uncertainty in the projections of future scenarios. For the first uncertainty, as it is not yet feasible to quantify the relationship based on observed long-term effects of climate change [40], the appropriate time-series regression was applied to quantify a shorter-term exposure-effect relationship. In terms of uncertainty in the scenarios, particularly climate scenarios, projections are limited by largely unpredictable factors, both within the climate system itself and in the interaction between climate and human behavious, including population growth and economic development [41]. Therefore, a range of the morbidity burdens under various scenarios, rather than point estimation, are presented to incorporate the quantifiable uncertainties.

3.2. Results

3.2.1. Projected YLDs for Malaria in Jinan, Northern China

Table 4 shows the estimated YLDs for malaria in 2000 and projected YLDs for malaria under different scenarios in 2020 and 2050 in Jinan. It can be observed that the estimated total YLDs for malaria in 2000 were 59, with 32 from males and 27 from females. It also suggests that there may be an increase in the morbidity burden from malaria in Jinan due to a future rise in temperature and demographic changes. The projected YLDs for malaria are slightly higher in males than in females.

Table 4. The YLDs for malaria in Jinan: 2000, 2020 and 2050

		Total	Male	Female
2000		59	32	27
2020	Projection A *	72~95	39~53	33~42
	Projection B ^	81~122	49~67	42~55
2050	Projection A *	90~127	54~70	46~57
	Projection B ^	116~160	79~86	57~74

* Projection A considers future change in temperature.
^ Projection B considers future change in both temperature and population growth.

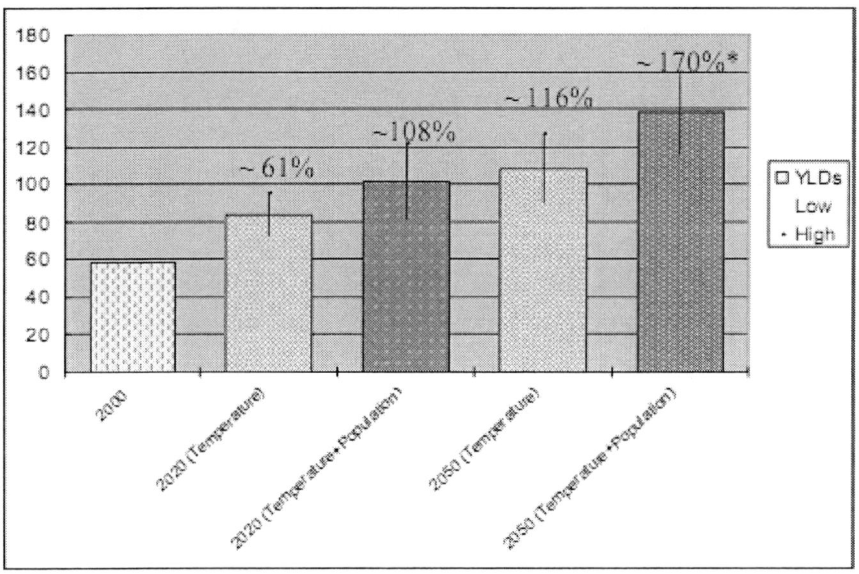

*The figures show the estimated highest percentage increase in YLDs

Figure 4. Projected YLDs for malaria in Jinan.

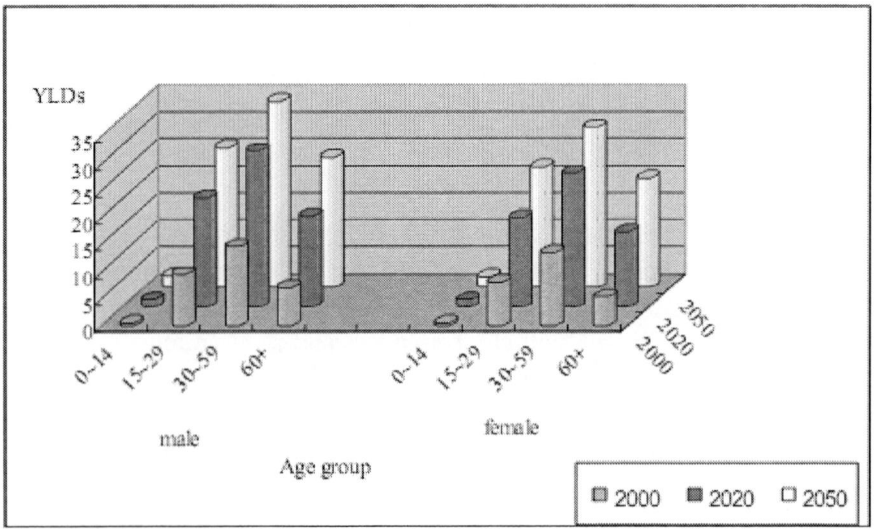

Figure 5. Projected YLDs for malaria by age and sex in Jinan.

Figure 4 demonstrates, in Jinan, the potential increasing trend in the burden of malaria under scenarios of both climate change and population growth. It indicates that if only temperature scenarios are considered, the YLDs for malaria might increase by up to 61% by 2020 and 108% by 2050, compared to 2000, if other factors remain constant. When considering future changes in both climate and population structure, however, the YLDs for malaria in Jinan would increase by up to 116% by 2020 and 170% by 2050, if other factors remain constant.

Figure 5 demonstrates, in Jinan, the age- and sex- specific YLDs for malaria in 2000 and the projected YLDs for malaria, under the scenarios with greatest temperature increase and population change, indicating that middle-aged adults account for the largest proportion of the burden. Moreover, the burden of malaria among people over 60 may have the greatest increase, compared with other age groups, due to future ageing of the population.

3.2.2. Projected YLDs For Malaria in Baoan, Southern China

The range of estimated YLDs for malaria in Baoan in 2000 and the projected YLDs in 2020 and 2050 are presented in Table 5. In 2000, the total YLDs for malaria in Baoan were 87, of which 44 were from males and 43 were from females. A clear increase in the morbidity burden from malaria has been projected under different scenarios.

Figure 6 shows the projected increasing trend in the total YLDs for malaria. The figures demonstrate that, if other factors remain constant, rising temperature alone may lead to an increase in the YLDs for malaria by up to 70% by 2020 and 130% by 2050, compared to 2000. If demographic change is considered in addition to climate change, the total YLDs for malaria in Baoan would increase by up to 144% by 2020 and 188% by 2050.

Figure 7 demonstrates the YLDs by age and sex, and projected YLDs, considering both climatic and demographic changes and indicating that the middle-aged population is going to bear the largest proportion of the increased burden of malaria. The YLDs indicate that adults and the elderly may experience a greater increase in the future morbidity burden of malaria, compared with other age groups.

Table 5. The YLDs for malaria in Baoan: 2000, 2020 and 2050

		Total	Male	Female
2000		87	44	43
2020	Projection A *	113~148	57~78	56~70
	Projection B ^	154~213	78~108	76~105
2050	Projection A *	136~200	69~101	67~99
	Projection B ^	166~250	84~126	82~124

* Projection A considers future change in temperature

^ Projection B considers future change in both temperature and population growth

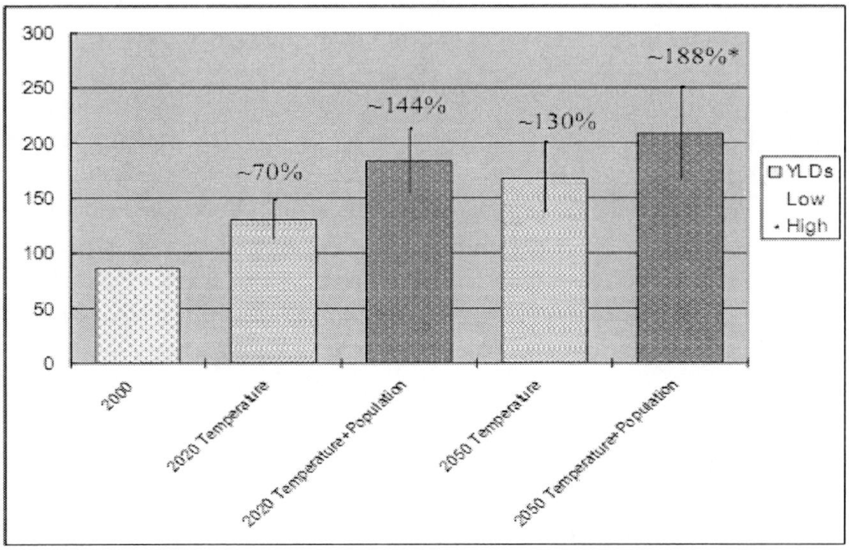

*The figures show the estimated highest percentage increase in YLDs

Figure 6. Projected YLDs for malaria in Baoan.

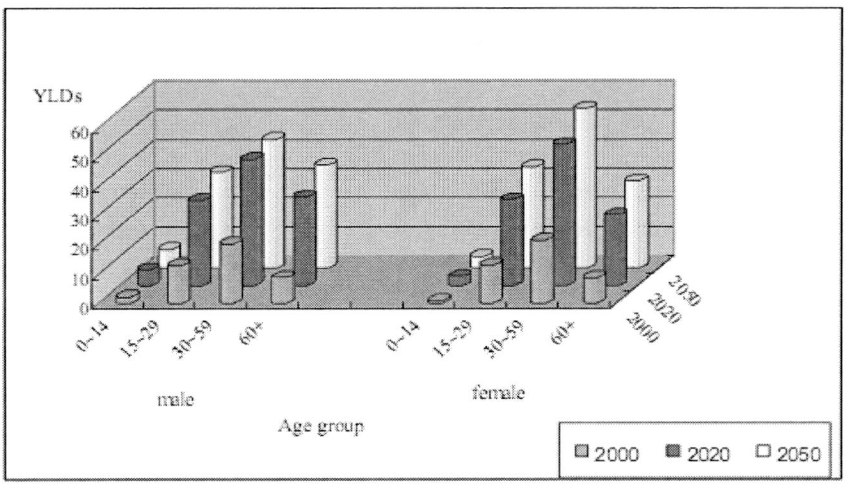

Figure 7. Projected YLDs for malaria by age and sex in Baoan.

3.3. Discussion

This is the first attempt in China at projecting the future morbidity burden of malaria, considering both climate and demographic changes. Despite the assumptions and uncertainties in the scenario-based projections, the results of this study suggest that an increasing trend in the future morbidity burden of malaria may be caused by climatic and demographic changes in China. This study also contributes to the knowledge associated with the role of climate change in the exacerbation of vector-borne diseases. The results from this study suggest that if other factors, including socio-economic status, remain constant, the morbidity burden of malaria may double by 2020, and may increase by more than 170% by 2050 in both temperate and subtropical regions in China. This study furnishes evidence that global warming may explain the resurgence of malaria in China.

In China, the potential future burden of malaria, due to climate and demographic changes, in temperate regions would be similar to that in subtropical regions. Although a higher proportion of the burden of malaria is suffered by those living in endemic regions, mainly tropical and subtropical regions, epidemics of malaria also pose a serious threat to many millions of people in non-endemic regions. Consequently, prevention in temperate regions remains a priority. Therefore, this possible geographic extension of vector-borne diseases should be noted by local public health practitioners and communities. A possible increase in the burden of malaria in the temperate regions of China should be considered in disease prevention and control. Furthermore, a possible resurgence of malaria in developed countries, which currently have only imported cases of malaria, should also receive attention. For example, it has been reported that, due to climate change, malaria may return to Great Britain by the year 2050 [42, 43].

The impact of both rising temperatures and population changes on the disease burden of malaria would be much higher than the impact of rising temperature alone. The results suggest that although middle-aged males are the subpopulation mostly suffering from malaria, both old and young people suffering from malaria would increase significantly with future changes in population structure in China. Over the next few decades, the disease burden of malaria, amongst middle-aged adults and elderly people, may show a greater rate of increase, compared with other age groups. Effective measures to mitigate the future risks of malaria should focus specifically on these vulnerable subgroups, as well as the general population.

The morbidity burden caused by future climate change could be much higher than estimated in this study if all climate-related vector-borne diseases in China are included. Other vector-borne diseases having similar transmission mechanisms to malaria may also be affected by climate change. For example, Japanese encephalitis (JE), a mosquito-borne disease with a clear seasonal distribution, occurs mainly in the tropical and temperate Asian and Pacific regions [44]. Therefore, this estimate is the first step in attempting to project the future burden of vector-borne diseases associated with climate change in China. The message from this study is based in that, in the future, the climate-related morbidity burden of vector-borne diseases in China may increase greatly if there is no effective public health adaptation to future climate change.

Due to the unavailability of data, socio-economic factors that play a role in the transmission of malaria [45] have not been included in the projection. This is a major limitation of the projection. The absence reflects the unavailability of projections of the future economic status at a local level. Improved socio-economic status can significantly reduce the burden of vector-borne diseases by providing high quality health services, environmental hygiene, health education and promotional activities. However, acceleration in economic development may lead to more energy consumption and result in a higher level of greenhouse gas emissions, the main reason for global warming. Mitigation of climate change requires sustainable development to reduce future greenhouse gas emissions; thus, generating the lowest magnitude of adverse climate scenarios. Further climate-related burden of disease studies should include other influencing factors, such as the speed of economic growth, living conditions and the state of public health services.

Other limitations on the estimates associates with the future morbidity burden of the disease include the assumptions and uncertainties in the methodology for the estimation of YLDs, and uncertainties in climatic and demographic scenarios [46]. Despite the limitations in the projection, this study provides scientific evidence for the Chinese governments and local communities regarding the potential increase in the burden of diseases related to global warming and demographic change.

4. Implications and Recommendations

The extra disease burden of malaria, including re-emergence, spatial changes and additional number of cases, may be brought to the current public health system due to future climate change. By addressing the challenges in examining the impact of climate variations on malaria, the implications and recommendations for a better adaptation to future climate change are summarized as follows.

4.1. Further Research Directions

It is still a big challenge for researchers to fully understand the impact on population health due to climate variation and future climate change, with many uncertainties in existing knowledge. The main task should be to identify key variables and thresholds of predictable impacts on the disease, in order to provide rapid and effective public health response. Integrated assessment should be performed in various climatic regions, incorporating various factors to study the impact of climatic variables (and other factors) on malaria.

In order to establish effective disease early warning systems, more studies are necessary to systematically examine the health impacts of climate variations on malaria in more target sub-populations and regions within various climatic zones across China. Projections of the mortality and morbidity burden of disease, attributable to climate change, would be of great value in current policy making. More projective studies should be conducted, based on scenarios of future climate, including changes in temperature, rainfall, humidity, and level of river flow; as well as changes in demographic and socio-economic status. Advanced statistical models which include additional influencing factors, such as vector populations and socio-economic status, would certainly enhance the power of the statistical analysis; rendering the results more reliable. Reports show that existing social inequalities in health status will be exacerbated by long-term climate change [47]. However, only a very limited number of studies have examined the relationship between social factors, climate change, and health.

4.2. Implications for Public Health and Clinical Practice

Potential extra health burdens, due to future climate change, may have a great impact on currently overloaded public health systems in both developed and developing countries. Current public health strategies lack the consideration of the changing environment, with a potential adverse effect on public health. Public health mechanisms have not, traditionally, been closely linked with other climate-related agencies, such as meteorological institutions, to allow early warning of potential changes in climate-related disease incidence. This should be remedied as early as possible. The concept of a "holistic approach" in public health should be widely adopted. Protecting populations against climate change will involve responses of different kinds, acting at various levels. They may range from biological interventions to behavior change, modifying physical environments, and altering social and economic settings.

Public health practitioners should monitor and provide rapid health responses accordingly to prevent and reduce predicted risks associated with climate change. Systematic surveillance and forecasting are of importance to reduce climate-related health burdens. Improvement of health surveillance systems will also enhance the quality of such studies. Enhanced surveillance data have multiple benefits, as the data is crucial for statistical analysis and evaluation. Disease surveillance data can be improved through active surveillance which adds information on the source of infections, onset dates and detailed individual information.
Besides disease surveillance, comprehensive surveillance systems should also improve their analysis and distribution functions, guaranteeing early accurate information sharing with relevant authorities, including government, community and clinicians. Additionally, setting up a universal disease surveillance system at a national level would be a great benefit for research and public health practice, based on which, results from different study areas could be compared. It is recommended that the surveillance or investigation of the density of local vector populations, socio-economic status, and human activities is conducted regularly, systematically and consistently by local health authorities and government. Relevant research could be undertaken involving these additional factors that influence the transmission of malaria. Integrating local meteorological variables and river flow/high tides into disease surveillance systems could improve the accuracy of early warning systems for malaria. The findings of this study, including threshold temperatures, lag times and different quantitative relationships between climate variation and malaria, imply that public health measures should consider local climatic conditions, leading to effective warning systems and faster response time to disease epidemics.

Advocacy for adapting to and mitigating climate change should be a longstanding public health activity. Advocate activities by those public health practitioners in developing policies or strategies for reduce the impact of climate change may include, but should not be limited to: lobbying decision makers for initial preventive measures in reducing climate change impact, addressing adverse impacts of climate change on population health to a wide audience, and encouraging cooperative actions from all relevant sectors. Rather than just providing information, persuasion should be another key task for public health practitioners.

Once committed to the objective of tackling climate change, public health practitioners should build-up maximum support by strategicly planning the ways that they will argue the case, including special attention to counteracting any strength of their opponents' arguments in the on-going debate on climate change. Such counteraction should be supported by high quality evidence-based research.

Public health practitioners should also take an active role in health education and promotional programs. Public health practitioners must be trained about the link between climate variations and malaria. Health education programs, aimed at public health practitioners, should be undertaken to produce information about the adverse impacts of climate variation, the potential extra health burden that climate variation may cause in the future, and preventive measures that can be implemented to reduce any future health risks of climate change. The public should be aware of how to prevent and reduce health risks associated with climate change and malaria. Information on self protection measures, such as timely preventive medicines before international travelling and the wearing of long-sleeve clothes, should be widely distributed.

The capacity of professional health workers in the root levels needs to be strengthened. Clinicians and other health professionals should also be equipped with up-to-date knowledge about the impacts of climate variations on malaria. Furthermore, clinicians play a role in educating their patients and the community because of the close relationship between them.

4.3. Implications for Policy and Economy

The results of this study indicate local consequences of climate variation and future climate change on malaria. Its implication for policy makers and governments, at all levels, is significant. Governments should take effective public health measures at an early stage to reduce any possible increase in the disease burden of malaria related to climate change. It is time to call for action, introducing public health policies based on scientific evidence and knowledge of local conditions. Scientific uncertainties are no excuse for inaction, especially recognizing that the impacts of climate change may be increasing in the future.

Communities can also facilitate the implementation of relevant policies and the adaptation to climate change in the following ways: (i) increasing the awareness of community residents and local schools of the risks of climate change and the preventive measures needed to reduce the impact of climate variation/climate change on malaria; (ii) ensuring circulation of appropriate information to respond to the potential risks of climate variation/climate change on malaria; (iii) building greenhouse-friendly communities by good community design, local traffic control, and appropriate surveillance related to climate variation/climate change; (iv) supporting people living in rural and remote regions to better adapt to future climate change.

The responsibility for a better adaptation to problems arising from future climate change should be taken by all sections of society. A shared health, environment, and development agenda could address the element of the burden of disease that is environment-related. Inter-sectoral collaboration, including governments, local communities, food industries, and professional institutions such as universities, is the most practical and effective way to a fast, effective response to future climate change. Recognizing the compelling need for national and international cooperation to reduce the severity of climate change and its health effects is required. Strategies of an international dimension should also be translated into regional and local actions. To face this global exposure to climate change, evidence-based strategic plans should be considered by policy makers and implemented at an international level.

In conclusion, the knowledge gained through this chapter will enable researchers and health policy makers, at all levels of government, to have a better understanding of the potential impact of climate variations on malaria. The Chinese Government is currently aiming for the elimination of indigenous malaria in the entire country by the end of 2020, as stated in the revised national malaria strategy. Taking the findings of this research into consideration, it is clear that climate variations play a role in transmission of malaria in China, while there is a long way to go to achieve a full understanding of the impact of climate variations on malaria and other health outcomes. It would be sustainable to incorporate climatic variables in malaria prevention and control programs and relevant policy making to eliminate malaria in China.

Refrences

[1] Kovats RS, Campbell-Lendrum DH, McMichael AJ, Woodward A, Cox JSH. Early effects of climate change: do they include changes in vector-borne disease? *Phil.Trans. R. Soc. Lond. B.* 2001;356:1057-68.

[2] Reiter P. climate change and mosquito-borne disease. *Environ. Health Perspect.* 2001;109:141-61.

[3] World Health Orgnaziation. *Malaria epidemiology in China*. http://www.wpro.who.int/sites/mvp/epidemiology/malaria/chn_profile.htm. 2011.

[4] Guan Y, China CDC National Institute of Parasitic Diseases Malaria situation and plan for elimination in China. Beijing: www.actmalaria.net/downloads/pdf/info/2009/China.pdf.

[5] Tang L. Progress in malaria control in China. *Chinese Medical Journal.* 2000;113(1):89-92.

[6] Dong Y, Li C-l, Wang X-r, Guo X-f, Li C-f, Li L, et al. Evaluation on Malaria Underreporting Degree by Capture-Recapture Method in Jiangcheng County. *Journal of Pathogen Biology.* 2007;2(3):207-9.

[7] Zhou X. *Current status of malaria in China*. wwwactmalarianet/downloads/pdf/info/2004/Chinapdf 2004.

[8] Lu L, Wu H, Liu Q-y. The impact of migrant populations on the endemic of falciparum malaria in China. *International Journal of Medicine and Parasitic Diseases.* 2006;33(5):228-31.

[9] Zhu J-m, Tang L-h, Li B-k, Jiang W-k, Wang M. Analysis of the relationship between some social factors and malaria prevalence. *International Journal Med. Parasit. Dis.* 2007;34(22):76-8.

[10] Xu J, Wang L, Liu X, al e. Analysis of factors associated with the residents' outdoor sleeping habit in malaria endemic areas in Yuanjiang County of Yunnan Province (Article in Chinese). *China Tropical Medicine*. 2003;2.

[11] Hu H, Singhasivanon P, Salazar NP, Thimasarn K, Li X, Wu Y, et al. Factors influencing malaria epidemicity in Yunnan Provinece, PR China (Analysis of spatial

pattern by GIS). *Southeast Asian Journal of Tropical Medicine and Public Health.* 1998;29(2):191-200.

[12] Zhu J-m, Tang L-h, Lib a-k, Zhang G-q, Wu S, Chang F-x. The Relationship Between Malaria Endemic and Normalized Differential Vegetation Index in Huaihe River Valley. *International Journal Med. Parasit. Dis*. 2007;34(3):122-4.

[13] Kovats S, Bouma M, Hajat S, Worrall E, Haines A. El Nino and health. *Lancet* 2003;362:1481-89.

[14] Lin R-x, Zhang X-c, Wu J, Wu X-g, Zhu D-h. Study on control strategy and surveillance of malaria in the past ten years in Guangdong. *Journal of Tropical Medicine.* 2006;6(10):1095-7.

[15] Liu Q, Kang X, Chao C, Feng S, Li Y, He R, et al. New irrigation methods sustain malaria control in Sichuan Province, *China Acta Tropica*. 2004;89(2):241-7.

[16] Dong Y, Yang Y-m, Wang X-r, Zhou Y-b, Li C-l, Wu X-h, et al. Impact of Malaria Health Education on Awareness and Behavior among Minority Nationalities in Yunnan Province. *Parasitoses and Infectious Diseases*. 2007;4(3):103-6.

[17] Xia Z, Zhang H, Cheng K, al e. Local Knowledge, Attitude and Practices (KAPs) on Malaria : A Baseline Study of Caochong Village in Hubei Province, China (Article in Chinese). *China Tropical Medicine*. 2007;7(4):492-6.

[18] Bi P, Tong S, Donald K, Parton KA, Ni J. Climatic variables and transmission of malaria: a 12-year data analysis in Shuchen County, China. *Public Health Rep.* 2003;118(1):65-71.

[19] Gao CY, Xiong HY, Yi D, Chai GJ, Yang XW, Liu L. Study on meteorological factors-based neural network model of malaria [article in Chinese]. *Zhonghua Liu Xing Bing Xue Za Zhi*. 2003;24(9):831-4.

[20] Wen L, Xu DZ, Wang SQ, Li CX, Zhang ZY, Su YQ. Epidemic of malaria in Hainan province and modeling malaria incidence with meteorological parameters [Article in Chinese]. *Chinese Journal of Disease Control and Prevention* 2003;7(6):520-5.

[21] Bi P, Parton KA, Tong S. El Nino-Southern Oscillation and vector-borne diseases in Anhui, China. *Vector Borne Zoonotic Dis*. 2005;5(2):95-100.

[22] Tian L, Bi Y, Ho SC, Liu W, Liang S, Goggins WB, et al. One-year delayed effect of fog on malaria transmission: a time-series analysis in the rain forest area of Mengla County, south-west China. *Malar. J.* 2008;19(7):110.

[23] Huang G, Zhang H, Chen G, Yuan F, Pei S, Hu L, et al. Evaluation of malaria epidemic situation in Tongbai and Dabieshan mountain area in Hubei (Article in Chinese). *Jounral of Tropical Medicine (Gouangzhou).* 2009;9(11):1285-7.

[24] Wang LP, Fang LQ, Xu X, Wang JJ, Ma JQ, Cao WC, et al. Study on the determinants regarding malaria epidemics in Anhui province during 2004-06 [Article in Chinese]. *Zhonghua Liu Xing Bing Xue Za Zhi.* 2009;30(1):38-41.

[25] Li PL, Zhang J, Wang XL, Yang XB, Mao DQ, He YY, et al. Study on the characteristics of major mosquito-borne infectious diseases in Three Gorges Reservoir Area from 1997 to 2008 [Article in Chinese]. *Zhonghua Liu Xing Bing Xue Za Zhi.* 2010;31(1):56-9.

[26] Xiao D, Long Y, Wang S, Fang L, Xu D, Wang G, et al. Spatiotemporal distribution of malaria and the association between its epidemic and climate factors in Hainan, China. *Malaria Journal*. 2010;9(1):185.

[27] Yang G-J, Gao Q, Zhou S-S, Malone JB, McCarroll JC, Tanner M, et al. Mapping and predicting malaria transmission in the People's Republic of China, using integrated biology-driven and statistical models. *Geospatial Health* 2010;5(1):11-22.

[28] Zhang Y, Bi P, Hiller JE. Meteorological variables and malaria in a Chinese temperate city: A twenty-year time-series data analysis. *Environ. Int.* 2010;36(5):439-45.

[29] Zhou SS, Huang F, Wang JJ, Zhang SS, Su YP, Tang LH. Geographical, meteorological and vectorial factors related to malaria re-emergence in Huang-Huai River of central China. *Malaria Journal*. 2010;9(337):doi:10.1186/475-2875-9-337.

[30] Hui FM, Xu B, Chen ZW, Cheng X, Liang L, Huang HB, et al. Spatio-temporal distribution of malaria in Yunnan Province, China. *Am. J. Trop. Med. Hyg.* 2009;81(3):503-9.

[31] Xiao D, Long Y, Wang S, Fang L, Xu D, Wang G, et al. Spatiotemporal distribution of malaria and the association between its epidemic and climate factors in Hainan, China. *Malar. J.* 2010;25(9):185.

[32] Shumway R, stoffer D. *Time series analysis and its applications*. 2nd ed. Now York: Springer Texts in Statistics 2006.

[33] WHO. *Assessing the environmental burden of disease*. [cited 2004 May]; Available from: http://www.who.int/peh/burden/burdenindex.htm.

[34] McMichael A, Campbell-Lendrum D, Kovats S. Annex6.7: Comparative risk assessment of the health effects of climate change. *12th annual meeting of the international society for environmental epidemiology (ISEE);* 2000; 2000.

[35] Gold MR, Stevenson D, Fryback DG. HALYs and QALYs and DALYs, OH MY: similarities and differences in summary measures of population health. *Annual Review of Public Health*. 2002 2002///;23(1):115.

[36] Murray CJL, Acharya AK. Understanding DALYs. *Journal of Health Economics*. 1997 1997/12//;16(6):703-30.

[37] Murray C, Lopez A. *The Global Burden of Disease*. Geneva: World Health Organization, Harvard School of Public Health, World Bank. 1996.

[38] Mathers CD, Bernard C, Iburg KM, Inoue M, Fat DM, Shibuya K, et al. Global Burden of Disease in 2002:data sources, methods and results: *World Health Organization;* 2004.

[39] Mathers C, Vos T, Stevenson C. *The burden of disease and injury in Australia.* Canberra: Australian Institute of Health and Welfare; 1999.

[40] McMichae AJ, Campbell-Lendrum D, Kovats RS, Edwards S, Wilkinson P, Wilson T, et al. Global climate change. *Comparative risk quantification* 2002:1554-649.

[41] CSIRO. *Climate change in Australia*; 2005.

[42] Snow K. Could malaria return to Britain? *Biologist (London).* 2000;47(4):176-80.

[43] Kuhn K, Campbell-Lendrum D, Armstrong B, Davies C. Malaria in Britain: past, present, and future. *Proc. Natl. Acad. Sci. U S A.* 2003;100(17):9997-10001.

[44] Bi P, Zhang Y, Parton KA. Weather Variables and Japanese Encephalitis in the Metropolitan Area of Jinan City, China. *Journal of Infection* 2007; 55:551-556

[45] Woodward A, Hales S, Litidamu N, Phillips D, Martin J. Protecting human health in a changing world: the role of social and economic development. *Bulletin of the World Health Organization.* 2000;78(9):1148-55.

[46] Breman J, Alilio M, Mills A. Conquering the intolerable burden of malaria: what's new, what's needed: a summary. *Am. J .Trop. Med. Hyg.* 2005;71(Suppl 2):1-15.

[47] National Health and Medical Research Council (NHMRC). *Health implications of long term climatic change Canberra:* Australian Government Publishing Service; 1991.

In: Malaria: Etiology, Pathogenesis and Treatments
Editors: A. M. Peterson et al, pp. 215-230
ISBN: 978-1-62100-363-2

Chapter IX

Winning the Fight against Childhood Malaria: The Case for Intermittent Preventive Treatment for Children (IPTc) Combined with Timely Home Treatment - A Case Study from Ghana

Collins K. Ahorlu*
Noguchi Memorial Institute for Medical Research,
University of Ghana, Legon, Ghana.

Abstract (Treatment)

Malaria is estimated to cause between 300 and 500 million clinical cases with about 700,000 to 1.6 million deaths every year, most (about 90%) of these deaths occur in sub-Sahara Africa. Thus, malaria remains a major cause of morbidity and mortality in sub-Sahara Africa. In Ghana malaria accounts for about 32.5% of all Out Patient attendances and about 24.6% of deaths in children under 5 years. The World Health Organization recommended the use of artemisinin based combination therapy (ACT) for the treatment of uncomplicated malaria to provide effective treatment against *P. falciparum* malaria and slow down the spread of drug resistance. Ghana has adopted the use of artesunate + amodiaquine for the treatment of uncomplicated malaria in the country since 2005. Malaria control in Ghana, like elsewhere in sub-Sahara Africa, relies on early diagnosis and prompt treatment of suspected cases and the home is where early recognition and in most cases prompt treatment is initiated. However, the current combination therapy is not widely available for home management as a result of the fear that making these drugs available may lead to abuse and therefore lead to the emergence of Plasmodium falciparum resistance to these drugs. Intermittent preventive treatment (IPT) has now

* Noguchi Memorial Institute for Medical Research, University of Ghana, Box LG581, Legon, Ghana. Email addresses: cahorlu@noguchi.mimcom.org or collins.ahorlu@gmail.com.

been accepted as an important component of the malaria control strategy but has not been implemented in combination with timely home management to measure their impact on malaria prevalence in a target population. Findings reported in this chapter are from a two year implementation of a combined intermittent preventive treatment for children (IPTc) and timely home management of malaria using artesunate + amodiaquine. All children aged six to 60 months received home-based delivery of intermittent preventive treatment using amodiaquine + artesunate, delivered at home by community assistants every four months (six times in 24 months). Malaria parasite prevalence surveys were conducted before the first IPTc and four months after the third and sixth IPTc rounds. Results showed a significant reduction in malaria prevalence from 25% at baseline to 1% at year-two evaluation. At baseline, 13.8% of the children were febrile (axilary temperature of ≥37.50C) compared to 2.0% at year-two-evaluation. The improved access to ACT drugs for the treatment of suspected malaria in children aged six to 60 months could be one of the ways to achieve the Abuja target of getting 60% of under five suspected malaria cases into treatment within 24 hours of symptom onset, which was not achieved by 2005 as was targeted. If policy makers are bold enough to initiate policy to allow adults to participate in IPT at least once or twice in a year, this could further accelerate the reduction in malaria prevalence to a level that will reduce the public health burden of malaria.

Background

Malaria, a vector-borne parasitic infection was first recognized in China about 5,000 years ago with its symptoms being described in other parts of the world for many years (Carter and Mendis 2002). The parasite which causes malaria was noticed in human blood as early as 1880 in Algeria by Laveran but its transmission remained a mystery until 1897 when Ronald Ross established that the malaria parasite is transmitted by mosquitoes (Warrell and Gilles 2002: 1), a discovery which later won him a Nobel Price. The discovery by Ross marked the beginning of research and interventions to control malaria which was at the time present also in Europe and North America (Bruce-Chwatt and Zulueta 1980; Carter and Mendis 2002). Most of the initial control activities centered on vector control, especially larviciding to prevent the breeding of the vector mosquito in water bodies. However, the use of DDT to kill adult mosquitoes which became popular at the beginning of the Second World War was one of the revolutions of malaria control via vector control.

Although, quinine was used for the treatment of malaria, it was not until the discovery of Chloroquine in the 1930s that malaria treatment improved substantially, because chloroquine was safe with very minimal adverse side effects. With all these tools available, malaria eradication was envisioned in the 1950s (Warrell and Gilles 2002:2). This dream of eradicating malaria on the back of DDT against adult mosquitoes, larvicides, and Chloroquine for prophylaxis and treatment, attained major success in Europe and North America, with limited success in the Caribean, parts of Asia and South-Central America, but this was not the case in sub-Sahara Africa (Greenwood et al 2005).

Various factors could be attributed to the failure of the eradication efforts to make impact in sub-Sahara Africa, prominent among them include the ideal climatic condition for sustaining transmission which coincides with the presence of the most efficient of all the mosquito vectors which could sustain transmission even with reduced population coupled with the emergence of drug and insecticide resistance. Moreover, African countries lack both political and financial will to support and sustain the eradication efforts (Killeen et al 2004).

Again, policy makers and disease control officials had virtually eliminated the human factor in transmission from the eradication equation forgetting that human beings are important part of the triad link between the parasite and the mosquito, which is required to sustain transmission. Most control efforts thus far concentrated on how to eliminate the vector mosquito – be it bed net use, indoor residual spraying (IRS) or larviciding, all aimed at 'eliminating' the vector mosquito with very little attention to how to 'eliminate' the parasite vis-à-vis gametocyte from the human population and thereby 'starving' the mosquito of the parasite during blood meal. This is where there is a strong case for IPT in general but IPTc in particular to play a major role in the fight against malaria in Africa.

Malaria is estimated to cause between 200 and 300 million clinical cases with about 700,000 to 1.6 million deaths every year (Hay et al., 2005; Snow et al, 2005; WHO and UNICEF, 2005). About 90% of these deaths are believed to occur in sub-Sahara Africa (WHO 2008, WHO, 2003, Adjuik et al., 2006) where malaria constitute about 10% of the total disease burden (Heggenhougen et al., 2003). The sad aspect of the malaria problem in sub-Saharan Africa is that, the infection is mostly caused by the deadly *Plasmodium falciparum* species of the parasite. Considering the devastating effects of malaria on Africa south of the Sahara, where it is estimated to continue to cause economic loss of more than $2 billion annually (WHO, 2000), Africa leaders together with malaria experts need to be more radical in their control approaches.

According to the Roll Back Malaria programme (RBM, 2002), "malaria has slowed economic growth in African countries by 1.3% per year, the compound effects of which is a gross domestic product level now up to 32% lower than it would have been had malaria been eradicated from Africa in 1960." From all these statistics, one could say that malaria mostly affects those who are poor as well as a cause of poverty, especially in Africa (Carter and Mendis 2002; Sachs and Malaney 2002). Thus, the relationship between malaria and poverty in Africa could be likened to that of the relationship between egg and chicken where one cannot tell which of the two is the outcome of the other. In fact, the global poverty map fits well into the global malaria map and this cannot be a mere coincidence (http://www.earthinstitute.columbia.edu/articles/view/41).

The malaria situation in Ghana is not different from what pertains in most sub-Sahara African countries, where it is the single most important cause of mortality and morbidity especially among children under five years, pregnant women and the very poor. It is estimated that malaria alone causes about 10.6% Disability Adjusted Life Years (DALYs) representing a cost of about 6% of GDP annually in economic burden (Ghana Ministry of Health, 2009). In 2006 malaria accounted for 38.6% of all outpatient clinic visits, 36.9% of all admissions and about 24.6% of all deaths in children under five years of age in Ghana (Ghana Health Service, 2006).In line with WHO recommendation and the observed increasing treatment failure rate of chloroquine, the Ghana National Malaria Control Programme, (GNMCP) has adopted the use of Artesunate + Amodiaquine combinations for the treatment of uncomplicated malaria in the country since January, 2005 (Ghana Ministry of Health, 2009, Koram et al., 2005; Ghana health Service, 2004) later, two other drugs (Artemether + Lumefantrine and Dihydroartemisinin + Piperaquine) were added as alternative first line therapies for use in patients who cannot tolerate the Artesunate + Amodiaquine combination.

Malaria control in Africa and for that matter Ghana relies heavily on early diagnosis and prompt treatment of suspected cases (fevers), however getting 60% of cases, especially children under five years into treatment within 24 hours of symptom onset as declared by African Heads of States in Abuja, continue to be elusive and over five years after the target year of 2005 had come and gone and about ten years since the declaration was made in Abuja (WHO 2000), very little have been achieved. However, the home continue to be where early recognition and in most cases, prompt treatment, is initiated (Ahorlu et al., 2005; Ahorlu et al., 2006; Ahorlu et al., 2009).

Realizing the important role that the home through caretakers could play in the fight against the malaria menace, various initiatives had tried, and continue to incorporate the home into the malaria control venture in an attempt to put the home at the frontline of the battle against malaria, especially in sub-Saharan Africa. These community-level interventions aimed to strengthen the home management of febrile illness suspected to be malaria, especially in children within 24 hours of onset or symptom recognition. Some of these interventions were 'Home Management of Malaria (HMM)' and 'Intermittent Preventive treatment for children (IPTc)' among others. Whiles HMM is based on the principle that malaria is implicated in most fever cases in sub-Sahara African countries, especially in children under five years of age, any fever in a child with no obvious reason to suspect another condition, must be treated as suspected malaria. This principle makes sense within the context of the fact that the *plasmodium falciparum*, the main species in sub-Saharan Africa, could be very lethal and killing its victims, especially children under five years of age within a short time. So, it is better to err on the part of caution than to lose a child. Therefore, in the absence of laboratory services to confirm before treating, it makes sense to treat all fever cases where malaria is suspected as a possible cause. IPTc on the other hand is given to children irrespective of their fever or malaria status at a regular interval to protect the children from malaria infection or at least reduce the severe forms of infections. For instance Kweku et al. (2009) established that a community-based approach of IPTc achieved a higher coverage compared to a facility-based approach. This is an indication that a lot more could be achieved through community involvement in malaria control activities.

Malaria control by prompt and effective treatment remains a challenge, especially in areas where access to timely and effective treatment is a problem in most rural areas in sub-Saharan Africa. The Ghana Health Service for instance, had aimed at treating 55% of under-five febrile malaria cases within 24 hours of symptom onset by 2007, as opposed to the Abuja target of 60% by 2005, but almost four clear years after the expiration of that date (2007), this target is yet to be achieved. It is in these areas that IPTc could become an important component of the malaria control strategy, since it has been demonstrated that IPTi and IPTc reduced incidence or prevalence of malaria and also reduced severe anaemia in the various study populations (Schellenberg et al., 2001; Massaga et al. 2003; Cisse et al., 2006; Dicko et al., 2008; Kweku et al., 2009; Ahorlu et al., 2009).

Results presented in this chapter is an expansion of two previously published papers by the author and his colleagues to demonstrate the potential of the strategy of IPTc delivered at home combined with timely treatment of febrile malaria suspected illness to reduce parasite prevalence and malaria morbidity in children under five years of age. The chapter seeks to emphasize the potential of IPTc in combination with timely home management to achieve the target of getting 55% of children under five into treatment within 24 hours of symptoms onset as projected by malaria control policy makers but was not achieved about four years ago in Ghana (Ahorlu et al., 2009). Thus, the chapter aims at demonstrating how the fight against childhood malaria could be won through community involvement in delivering intermittent preventive treatment for Children (IPTc) combined with timely home management using a case study from Ghana.

Methods

Study Site

The study was conducted at Shime sub-district of the Keta district in the Volta region of Ghana, where Malaria accounts for over 35% of outpatients' clinic attendance in the District (District Annual Report, 2010). The Shime sub-district is one of the four administrative sub-districts recognized by the Ghana Health Service in the Keta District. It is the most deprived area in the district. Electricity supply is limited; it has no secondary school and a very poor road network. During the rainy season, most parts of the area are cut off from the rest of the district. The land is marshy and covered with streams, lagoons and creeks. The entire sub-district has a population of 19,972. However, the study took place in an area with a population of about 8,000. About 99% are Anlo-ewe-speaking people. Their main occupations are farming and fishing.

The area can boast of two health centers and one of them is located within the study area. Almost all the communities in the area have pipe borne water but because of the 'cash and carry system' where residents pay for every bucket of water fetched at the point of fetching, the people continue to use unsafe water from the many water bodies around to complement the safe one. Four out of the 36 communities in the sub-district participated in the study. These communities were selected mainly because of geographical accessibility due to the poor road network within the sub-district upon the advice of the District Director of Health Service (DDHS).

Community Entry and Training of Community Assistants

For a study which depends heavily on community cooperation and participation to succeed, there was a need to have an elaborate community entry plan. The plan involved meetings with the chiefs and elders of the communities to discuss the proposed project and seek for their support and cooperation. After gaining the approval of the chiefs and elders of the communities, it was agreed that a durbar of chiefs and people be organized at each of the four village communities to seek approval and cooperation from the broader community members. At each of these durbars, the project activities, especially drug administration, prevalence surveys (blood sampling) and timely treatments were discussed, questions were asked and answers provided by the research team including the Keta DDHS. Most of the questions were related to why only children under-five years of age were singled out to benefit from the intervention and this was adequately explained, taking the opportunity to let the people know that children under five years of age are the most vulnerable group when it comes to malaria infections and its related deaths. At the durbars, the people were made to select two persons to be trained to deliver the IPTc and timely home management within 24 hours of fever onset. In all, eight persons were selected for training. In one of the villages, four instead of two persons were nominated, so they democratically voted to select the two to be trained without any acrimony. The only requirement for selection was that, the person must be able to read and write so as to be able to keep records during IPTc and timely treatments, especially when the research team is not around. An Assemblyman (an elected local level representative at the district assembly) was selected as a supervisor who visits the four communities on a bicycle. All the community assistants and the supervisor were trained on how to fill all the study forms appropriately, how to weigh the children and record the weight, how to take temperature and record the readings and how to give treatment regimens using the weight-based treatment chart adapted for the study. They were also trained on how to assess a suspected malaria case clinically before making decision to treat or not to treat and how to refer cases, which did not meet the criteria established for suspected malaria in this study, to the health centre and helping them to receive attention at the health centre.

Study Participants

After gaining the support and willingness of the chiefs, elders and the general population to participate in the study, the individual community registers of eligible children aged ≤ 60 months were updated by the trained community assistants to bring them up to date. Beyond the general consent given by the chiefs, elders and people to participate in the study at the durbars, individual consent was sought from each caretaker of a child aged five years or below in the four communities. After gaining consent from caretakers, children aged 6-60 months were enrolled in the study. No caretaker refused to participate. All children (6-60 months old), including those on antiretroviral treatment, were included in the study.

Interventions

Intermittent Preventive Treatment for Children (IPTc)

IPTc was delivered every four months beginning in July 2007 (July and November 2007, March, July and November 2008 and March 2009). The children received 10mg/kg body weight of Amodiaquine (AQ) and 4mg/kg of Artesunate (AS) daily (given as a single dose) over 3 days. All treatments were given under direct observation and children were observed for 5 minutes after drug administration to ensure that they retained the medication. Children who vomited within five minutes after taking the medicines received a repeated full dose. Children were followed up on day 1, 2 and 3 after treatment (the day of treatment was counted as Day 0) with adverse event questionnaire (Ahorlu et al., 2009).

Timely Treatment of Suspected Febrile Malaria in Children

During the four months between IPTc rounds, any child with febrile illness suspected to be malaria by a caretaker was reported to trained community assistants who then evaluated and treated those who met the protocol criteria for suspected febrile malaria illness, which was a child with axillary temperature of $\geq 37.5^{o}$C; whose caretaker reported suspected febrile malaria together with one or more of the following; headache, hot body, weakness, loss of appetite, among others, with no other overtly observed or reported condition. The treatment, just like the IPTc, was the full three-day course of Artesunate and Amodiaquine (Ahorlu et al., 2009). RDT was not used to determine infection status (presence or absence of parasite) before treatment was given and this is a weakness in the study design. However, the clinical evaluation follows the current presumptive diagnosis and treatment as is being done in most rural health facilities in Ghana. It must also be mentioned that due to ethical considerations, community assistants were not allowed to take blood from the children.

The intervention (IPTc combined with timely treatment at home) was evaluated in July 2008, four months after the third round of IPTc and just before the fourth round begins and a second evaluation was done in July 2009, four months after a total of six IPTc rounds in 24 months.

Questionnaire Survey

A simple questionnaire was administered to caretakers during IPTc rounds and prevalence surveys to record febrile illnesses in the seven days prior to those events. That is, caretakers whose children received IPTc at any round and those who participated in the prevalence surveys responded to the questions. Questions asked included: Has your child been well in the past seven days, including now? If no, what is/was wrong with him/her? What was done for the child when you found out that he/she was not well? During the prevalence surveys, however, additional questions were asked about bed net usage.

Sample Size

This was an implementation research which aimed at enrolling every child aged 6 – 60 months, living in the study area, into the study with the consent of their caretakers, mostly parents. However, for the prevalence survey, a sample size of 174 was needed to determine malaria parasite prevalence estimated at 20% in the study population (Kish and Leslie, 1965). At the evaluations however, all available participants at the time were examined. This led to the examination of over 85% of children enrolled into the study at both year-one and year-two evaluations.

Data were analyzed to compare results from baseline to year-one evaluation as well as comparing year-one and year-two evaluations with reference to the baseline results when necessary. All quantitative analyzes were done using Epi Info version 3.4.1.

Laboratory Methods

Prevalence of malaria infection was made with light microscopy using thick and thin blood smears. The thick and thin blood smears were stained with 3% Giemsa for 30 minutes. Parasite density was determined by counting the number of asexual parasites per 200 white blood cells, and calculated per μL assuming a white blood cell count of 8000 cells per μL. Sexual parasite count was done per 1,000 white blood cells. A smear was declared negative if examination of 100 thick-film fields did not reveal the presence of asexual parasites. Quality control was done by allowing a second microscopist to read a random sample of 10% of all slides to confirm the absence or presence of parasites. Haemoglobin concentration was determined from finger pricks using a portable automated Hemocue® photometer (Leo Diagnostics, Sweden) on the field (Ahorlu et al., 2009).

Results

As indicated earlier, this chapter tries to demonstrate that the fight against childhood malaria could be enhanced through the use of IPTc combined with timely home management. This section presents a two year findings from the interventions discussed above. Most of the children received IPTc six times in 24 months. On average, 420 children were seen on each IPTc round, ranging between 413 and 433 per round.

Parasite Prevalence

Malaria parasite prevalence at year-one evaluation was 3.0% (10 out of 357), which further dropped significantly to 1.0% (3 out of 337) at year-two evaluation, a significant reduction of over 60.0%, p<0.001, Fisher exact test). This showed a point parasite prevalence reduction of over 90.0% compare to baseline prevalence rate of 25.3%. There was a significant relationship between febrile status and parasitaemia at year-one evaluation (p<0.001, Fisher exact test) but this was not the case at year-two evaluation, an indication that once parasite prevalence drops in the population, most of the febrile illnesses will no longer be due to malaria infection. Two out of the three parasite positive cases receive IPTc four times and the remaining one received it twice. All the positive infections were *Plasmodium falciparum,* the dominant species in Ghana. Additional clinical and parasitological findings are presented in Table 1.

Anaemia

Anemia was defined in this study as hemoglobin <10 g/dl and trend analysis showed a significant reduction from baseline through to year-two evaluation (p=0.003). Comparing the baseline level of 27.6% to year-two evaluation level of 15.7%, showed about 43.1% reduction in anemia cases in 24 months (Table 1). There was a significant relationship between febrile status and anemia at year-one evaluation (P = 0.01 (Fisher exact test)), but this was not the case at year-two-evaluation. This also indicates that malaria is just a cause of anemia in children aged 6 – 60 months in endemic villages such as our study area, but not the cause, instead other causes such as nutritional and minerals deficiencies may be implicated.

Table 1. Baseline, Year 1 and 2 Evaluation Characteristics, Clinical and Parasitological findings

Variables	Baseline (N = 174)	Evaluation Year 2 (N = 365)
Mean age in months (± std.)	30.5 (16.5) months	38.19 (15.7) months
Sex (% of female)	52.3	50.1
Weight: Mean (± std.)	12.3 (3.5)	12.2 (3.3)
Haemoglobin < 10 g/dl (%)***	48 (27.6)	53 (15.7)
Number (%) febrile ≥ 37.5**	24 (13.8)	8 (2.1)
Parasite prevalence number (%)**	44 (25.3%)	3 (1.0)

± std. = standard deviation. ** P<0.001 and *** P=0.003 (trend analysis).

During the prevalence surveys (baseline and evaluations) a number of febrile illnesses were reported for the children within seven days prior to data collection (Table 2). A trend analysis showed a significant reduction ($p<0.001$). The point prevalence of fever cases showed a reduction of over 85.0% when the baseline level of 42% is compared to the year-two evaluation level of 4.7%. Thus, malaria is a major cause of febrile illness in children under five years of age and as malaria prevalence reduces, febrile illness may also reduce significantly in malaria endemic areas.

Table 2. The distribution of febrile illnesses reported for children within the past seven days prior to the baseline and evaluation prevalence surveys *

Variables	Baseline (N = 174)	Evaluation Year 2 (N = 337)
Chills and Rigors **	18 (10.3)	4 (1.2)
Convulsions	4 (2.3)	0
Diarrhoea **	32 (18.4)	2 (1.2)
Fever / Malaria / Asra **	73 (42.0)	16 (4.7)
Headache **	58 (33.3)	6 (1.8)
Others (Cough, Rashes, Stomach ache etc.) ***	20 (11.5)	16 (4.7)
Vomiting **	20 (11.5)	2 (0.6)

* Sorted in column 1 in alphabetical order. ** $P<0.001$ and *** $P=0.011$ (trend analysis).

Intermittent Preventive Treatment for Children (IPTc)

IPTc was delivered to children aged 6 to 60 months six times (July and November 2007; March, July and November 2008 and March 2009). There have been marginal increases in the number of children at each subsequent treatment round until the fourth, where it dropped marginally from 433 (IPTc3) to 415 (IPTc4), and then increased to 419 (IPTc5) and 421 (IPTc6). The decrease was largely due to some children attaining the age of more than 60 months and were dropped out of the study with a few moving in and out of the communities intermittently. At the time of year-two-evaluation, majority of the children have received all six IPTc doses. A few were lost at various IPTc rounds due mainly to either these children moved out of the study community at one point or the other, or the entry points of participants, since enrolment was prospective and any child who attained the age of six months at any given time was enrolled. However, the number of dropouts at each round was too small for any meaningful comparative analysis to be done on them. During each IPTc round, a number of febrile illnesses were reported by caretakers within the past seven days prior to treatment and trend analysis showed significant reductions in reported fever as the number of IPTc rounds increases (Table 3).

A number of febrile malaria-related illnesses were treated by trained community assistants in between IPTc rounds and trend analysis showed no significant reduction in these reported cases, when analyzed from the first round. However, interviews with caretakers revealed that they were skeptical about the ability of community assistants to manage the febrile illnesses of their children until after the second round of IPTc, so it was decided to perform a second trend analysis starting from the second round of IPTc and this showed a significant reduction in the reported febrile malaria/fever ($p<0.001$) and headache (0.021) reported as the IPTc rounds increased, but this was not the case for chills and rigors, and vomiting (Table 4). An indication that other causes rather than malaria may be responsible for chills and rigors in the children.

Table 3. The distribution of febrile illnesses reported for children within the past seven days prior to each drug administration *

Febrile illness reported in the past seven days prior to drug administration	IPTC1 (N=413)	IPTC2 (N=420)	IPTC3 (N=433)	IPTC4 (N=415)	IPTC5 (N=419)	IPTC6 (N=421)
	Number (%)	Number (%)	Number (%)	Number (%)	Number (%)	Number (%)
Fever / Malaria / *Asra†* **	64 (15.50)	43 (10.20)	11 (2.50)	8 (1.93)	9 (2.15)	7 (1.66)
Headache **	49 (11.90)	39 (9.30)	5 (1.20)	8 (1.93)	11 (2.62)	7 (1.66)
Vomiting **	25 (6.10)	11 (2.60)	1 (0.20)	1 (0.24)	5 (1.19)	2 (0.47)
Chills and Rigors ***	17 (4.10)	10 (2.40)	7 (1.60)	5 (1.20)	6 (1.43)	5 (1.19)
Others (Cough, Rashes, Stomach ache etc.	7 (1.70)	5 (1.20)	9 (2.10)	12 (2.89)	8 (1.91)	10 (2.37)
Convulsions	5 (1.20)	0	0	0	0	0
Diarrhoea	5 (1.20)	1 (0.20)	3 (0.70)	2 (0.48)	2 (0.48)	1 (0.24)

* Sorted in column two in descending order to draw attention to the higher figures reported in that column. ** $P<0.001$ and *** $P=0.002$ (trend analysis).

† *'Asra'* is a local term used collectively to represent fever and/or malaria in the study community.

Table 4. Febrile illnesses treated by community assistants in between IPTC rounds**

Febrile illness treated between TPTC rounds	IPTC1-IPTC2 (N=413)	IPTC2-IPTC3 (N=420)	IPTC3-IPTC4 (N=433)	IPTC4-IPTC5 (N=415)	IPTC5-IPTC6 (N=419)
	Number (%)	Number (%)	Number (%)	Number (%)	Number (%)
Fever/Malaria/*Asra*	5 (1.21)	39 (9.28)	17 (3.93)	13 (3.13)	10 (2.39)
Headache	6 (1.45)	24 (5.71)	17 (3.93)	14 (3.37)	11 (2.62)
Chills and Rigors	4 (0.98)	12 (2.86)	9 (2.08)	11 (2.65)	7 (1.67)
Vomiting	0	4 (0.95)	3 (0.70)	8 (1.93)	4 (0.96)

** Sorted in column three in descending order to draw attention to the higher figures reported in that column.

There was virtually no serious adverse event reported after drug administrations. However, some caretakers reported that their children were weak for about two to four hours after taking the medicines and these were; five (1.21%) IPTc1, four (0.95%) IPTc2, seven (1.65%) IPTc3, four (0.93%) IPTc4, five (1.13%) IPTc5 and five (1.11%) IPTc6. None of these cases warranted any medical intervention. A few caretakers also reported that their children did eat very well after taking the drugs; however this could not be independently verified.

In the 24 months period of the intervention, no caretaker had lost a child, except two infants who died at birth and this was attributed to the absence of a midwife at the community clinic at the time of their birth.

Bed Net Usage

Questions were asked about bed net usage during prevalence surveys and as was expected, about 98.0 % at baseline and 100% at both year-one and year-two evaluations reported that they and their families slept under bed nets the previous night. Comparatively, insecticide-treated net usage has increased significantly from 38.5% at baseline to 60.0% at year one evaluation. This however, increased only marginally from 60.0% at year-one evaluation to 63.0% at year-two evaluation. Comparing baseline level of 38.5% to year-two level of 63.0% however, showed a significant increase of 63.6% in the use of treated bed net in 24 months.

Discussion

This chapter affirmed that childhood malaria-related febrile illnesses could be brought under control by introducing intermittent preventive treatment for children (IPTc) at a regular interval, in this case every four months, combined with timely home management within 24 hours of symptom onset. The main finding was a reduction of over 90.0% in parasite prevalence level in the study population in 24 months (25.0% at baseline and 1.0% at year-two-evaluation). Several studies in IPTi and IPTc interventions measured clinical incidence rather than prevalence and found between 20% and 86.0% reduction with some variations depending on transmission duration and intensity, target population and intervals between treatments (Schellenberg et al., 2001; Massaga et al., 2003; Chandramohan et al, 2005; Cisse et al., 2006; Macete et al, 2006; Chandramohan et al, 2007; Dicko et al., 2008; Kweku et al., 2009; Tagbor et al., 2010) and findings reported in this paper, though measured prevalence, appeared to support the usefulness of IPT intervention in the control of malaria, especially in rural sub-Saharan Africa.

Anemia in children under five years of age, defined as hemoglobin <10g/dl in this study, improved by 55.8% (from 27.6% at baseline to 12.2% at year-two evaluation). This compares well with a recent randomized trial in Tanzania, which showed that IPT given to infants at the time of childhood immunization reduced the incidence of the first episode of malaria and anemia by more than 50.0% during the first year of life (Schellenberg et al., 2001; Massaga et al., 2003).

Malaria-related morbidity in the study population expressed by the presence of fever and other malaria-related signs and symptoms reported has reduced as captured either during prevalence surveys or IPTc administration. Timely treatment of febrile malaria cases in the community did not follow any pattern. However, it could be argued that the community assistants who were on hand to deliver effective treatment in a timely fashion have contributed to the marked reduction in parasitaemia seen during evaluation surveys.

A community randomized trial showed a slightly higher coverage in the community-based delivery arm compared to facility-based arm (Kweku et al., 2009), indicating the importance of local residence in malaria control activities, however, this did not include timely management within 24 hours on symptoms onset and one cannot tell whether the inclusion of timely home treatment will have impacted coverage in the community approach. However, the contributions of trained community assistants in malaria control activities cannot be overemphasized, when well trained, especially to use RDTs to determine infections before giving treatment, they could become a main source of strength in the fight against childhood malaria related febrile illnesses, especially in hard to reach communities in endemic countries. Malaria control programs could be more successful if community assistants could be trained and engaged to deliver IPTc and timely managements to children under five years of age (Ahorlu et al 2011).

Findings reported here present a challenge to the existing practice, especially in most sub-Saharan Africa countries where malaria diagnosis is mostly based on presumption without confirmation. As community interventions or access to treatment increases, this may lead to fewer malaria infections, which may pose the danger of over diagnosis and treatment with expensive drugs of people who do not need it (Ahorlu et al 2011). Control programs should therefore invest in rapid diagnostic test kits where microscopy is not possible. As reported by Zikusooka *et al.* (2008), this may lead to cost savings because artemisinin-based antimalarial drugs are expensive. Goodman *et al.* (1999) also stated that rational use of antimalarials will reduce the potential for emergence of resistance.

The use of IPTc combined with timely home treatment to control malaria was found to reduce malaria prevalence in children aged 6 to 60 months. Although this study cannot determine the contribution of IPTc or timely home treatment to the protection offered to the children because the two interventions were delivered concurrently, the two together in this study offered a major protection against malaria in children, reducing prevalence from 25.0% at baseline to 1.0% at year-two evaluation (twenty-four months of implementation). The question then is, at what point should the provision of IPTc stop? What techniques or methods could be used to mop-up the few parasites that may continue to sustain transmission, because the vector mosquito is known to highly efficient in malaria transmission?

At this point, it may be recommended to reduce the frequency of treatment from every four months to every six months or providing treatment at the beginning of each peak season (two peak seasons in southern Ghana). Either way, the timing must be related to the major peak season in the study area. At certain point, it should be necessary to treat the general population at least once in a year to reduce the circulating parasites in the population such that mosquitoes will have very little or no parasite (gametocyte) to pick during blood meal for transmission.

Findings reported in this chapter indicates that, with consistent efforts, childhood malaria could be put under control such that it may no longer be a major public health problem, especially in sub-Saharan Africa where it is a threat to millions of people. However, to do this will require some bold and firm decisions, especially by African malariologists, malaria program managers and governments to bravely face the odds which militate against scaling up some of these interventions for them to make significant impacts. One such decision should be investing heavily on scaling up IPTc and timely home management of malaria without the fear that it will lead to the emergence of drug-resistant parasites and thereby making the apparently effective ACTs suffer the fate of chloroquine. We believe that when this is done, by the time we lose the current ACT drugs, malaria will have been reduced to such a level that it may no longer pose a public health threat to most African populations.

Africa has been touted as a failed continent or better still, that its leadership had failed, largely because, the leadership of the continent have over the years failed to take bold decisions and be prepared for the consequences but instead, choose to please the rest of the world. A case in point is how malaria was eradicated from parts of Europe and North

America, at the time everybody knew that DDT, the main arsenal used for the fight against malaria, could develop resistance and affect the environment but the leaders of those countries damned the consequences and used it widely and the result today is that those places have been freed from malaria (http://www.pri.org/theworld/?q=node/4288). But when it comes to Africa's turn to use DDT, various arguments were put forward against its use to control malaria and possibly eradicate it, such that DDT was not used extensively in Africa. So if Africans, especially those in sub-Saharan countries will continue to tread cautiously just because they do not want to be criticized, then our leaders would continue to be regarded as failed, because nothing radical can be achieved by conformers, we need transformational leaders who will take well calculated risks to bring malaria under control in Africa. Africa needs leaders who will not hesitate to do the following to bring malaria under control:

i. Scale-up IPTi and IPTc to cover children under 10 years of age. This must be done with the current effective drugs for treating uncomplicated malaria, thus, ACTs.
ii. Scale-up home management of malaria, especially in children under 10 years.
iii. Train community assistants to deliver these interventions together with the use of RDTs.
iv. Continue to promote bed net usage, especially among the children under 10 years of age.
v. Indoor residual spraying must be done but the insecticides being used must be closely monitored and be changed regularly to avoid the emergence of resistance before changing them.
vi. At least, treat the entire population once in a year to reduce the circulating parasite in the population and thereby reducing the chances of mosquitoes picking malaria parasite (gametocyte) during blood meal.

Considering the effect of malaria on Africa's GDP, African governments should move away from waiting for donors to finance their malaria control programs and invest significantly in malaria control activities through budgetary allocations. Let us remember that, malaria is a multi-billion dollar industry and if we want to wait upon those who make living out of that industry to help us control or eradicate malaria, we may be deceiving ourselves. That is why Africa must learn how to solve African problems, and the malaria problem presents an enviable opportunity for African leaders to stand up and be counted. This is our time to make history!

Competing Interests

The author declares that he has no competing interest.

Ethical Review

The Institutional Review Board of the Noguchi Memorial Institute for Medical Research, University of Ghana and the Ethical Review Committee of WHO reviewed and approved the study. Each mother/caretaker was informed of the objectives, methods, anticipated benefits and potential hazards of the study. Caretakers were also informed that they were at liberty to withdraw their children from the study at any time without penalty. They were assured that all information collected during this study would be kept confidential and that in any resulting publication it would not be possible to link the data to individuals in the study.

Acknowledgements

I am grateful to the Keta District Health Administration for collaborating with me on the empirical study presented in this paper. I sincerely thank the Community Assistants who delivered the interventions to the children. Thanks also go to the staffs of the Epidemiology Department, Noguchi Memorial Institute for Medical Research, for their field and laboratory support. Thanks to Mrs. Cynthia Ahorlu for data entry and secretarial support. Many thanks to the chiefs, elders and residents at the study communities, especially all the caretakers and their children for participating in the study, without them there will have been no study. Financial support for this research was provided by the UNDP/World Bank/WHO Special Programme for Research and Training in Tropical Diseases (TDR); however views expressed in this paper do rerpresent that of the donor, they are entirely that of the author.

Reference

Adjuik M, Smith T, Clark S, Todd J, Garrib A, Kinfu Y, Kahn K, Mola M, Ashraf A, Masanja H, Adazu K, Sacarlal J, Alam N, Marra A, Gbangou A, Mwageni E and Binka F. Cause-specific mortality rates in sub-Saharan Africa and Bangladesh. *Bull. World Health Organ.* 2006, 84: 181-188.

Ahorlu CK, Koram KA, Ahorlu C, de Savigny D and Weiss M. Sociocultural determinants of treatment delay for childhood malaria in southern Ghana. *Tropical Medicine and International Health* 2006, 11: 1022 – 1031

Ahorlu CK, Koram KA, Ahorlu C, de Savigny D and Weiss M. Weiss Community concepts of malaria-related illness with and without convulsions in southern Ghana. *Malaria Journal* 2005, 4: 47.

Ahorlu CK, Koram KA, Seakey AK and Weiss MG. Effectiveness of combined intermittent preventive treatment for children and timely home treatment for malaria control. *Malaria Journal* 2009, 8:292.

Bruce-Chwatt, L.J. and Zulueta, J.D (1980). *The rise and fall of malaria in Europe: a historic-epidemiological study*, Oxford, Published on behalf of the Regional Office for Europe of the World Health organization.

Carter, R. and Mendis, K.N. (2002). Evolutionary and historical aspects of the burden of malaria. *Clin. Microbiol. Rev.*, 15 (4): 564-594.

Chandramohan D, Owusu-Agyei S, Carneiro I, Awine T, Amponsa-Achiano K, Mensah N, Jaffar S, Baiden R, Hodgson A, Binka F and Greenwood B. Cluster randomised trial of intermittent preventive treatment for malaria in infants in area of high, seasonal transmission in Ghana. *BMJ* 2005, 331: 727-733.

Chandramohan D, Webster J, Smith L, Awine T, Owusu-Agyei S, Carneiro I. Is the Expanded Programme on Immunisation the most appropriate delivery system for intermittent preventive treatment of malaria in West Africa? *Trop. Med. Int .Health* 2007, 12: 743-50.

Cissé B, Sokhna C, Boulanger D, Milet J, Bâ el H, Richardson K, Hallett R, Sutherland C, Simondon K, Simondon F, Alexander N, Gaye O, Targett G, Lines J, Greenwood B, Trape JF. Seasonal intermittent preventive treatment with artesunate and sulfadoxine-pyrimethamine for prevention of malaria in Senegalese children: a randomised, placebo-controlled, double-blind trial *Lancet* 2006, 367: 659-67.

Dicko A, Sagara I, Sissoko MS, Guindo O, Diallo AI, Kone M, Toure OB, Sacko M and Doumbo OK. Impact of intermittent preventive treatment with sulphadoxine-pyrimethamine targeting the transmission season on the incidence of clinical malaria in children in Mali. *Malaria journal* 2008, 7: 123.

Ghana Health Service Final Draft Antimalarial Drug Policy for Ghana. *Accra*; 2004.

Ghana Ministry of Health (2009). Anti-malaria drug policy for Ghana, *Accra*, Ghana

Goodman CA, Mills AJ. The evidence base on the cost-effectiveness of malaria control measures in Africa. *Health Policy Plan* 1999, 14: 301-12.

Greenwood, B.M., Bojang,K. Whitty, C.J and Targett, G.A (2005). Malaria. *Lancet*, 365 (9469): 1487-98.

Hay, S.I., Guerra, C.A., Tatem, A.J, Atkinson, P.M and Snow, R.M (2005). Urbanization, malaria transmission and disease burden in Africa. *Nat. Rev. Microbiol.*, 3 (1): 81-90.

Heggenhougen, K.H., Hackenthal, V. and Vivek Pramola (2003). *The behavioural and social aspects of malaria and its control*: an introduction and annotated bibliography, WHO, TDR/STR/SEB/vol/03.1.

http://www.earthinstitute.columbia.edu/articles/view/41.

http://www.pri.org/theworld/?q=node/4288.

Killeen, G.F., Seyoum, A and Knols, B.G (2004). Rationalizing historical successes of malaria control in Africa in terms of mosquito resource availability management. *Am. J. Trop. Med. Hyg.,* 71 (2 Suppl). 87-93.

Kish and Leslie. *Survey Sampling*, John Wiley and Sons, NY 1965.

Koram *et al.* Comparative Efficacy of anti malarial drugs including ACTs in the treatment of uncomplicated malaria in young children under 5 in Ghana. *Acta Tropica,* 2005, 95: 194-203.

Kweku M, Webster J, Adjuik M, Abudey S, Greenwood B and Chandramohan D. Options for the Delivery of Intermittent Preventive Treatment for malaria to children: A Community Randomised Trial. *PloS ONE* 2009, 4(9): e7256. Doi:10.1371/journal.pone.0007256.

Macete E, Aide P, Aponte JJ, Sanz S, Mandomando I, Espasa M, Sigauque B, Dobano C, Mbunda S, Dgedge M, Alonso P and Menendez C Intermittent preventive treatment for malaria control adminidtered at the time of routine vaccination in mozambican infants: a randomised, placebo-controlled trial. *J. Infect. Dis.* 2006, 194: 276-285.

Massaga JJ, Kitua AY, Lemnge MM, Akida JA, Malle LN, Ronn AM, Theander TG, and Bygbjerg. Effect of intermittent treatment with amodiaquine on anaemia and malaria fevers in infants in Tanzania: a randomised placebo-control trial. *Lancet* 2003, 361: 1853-1860.

National Malaria Control Programme. *Ghana Health Service Report*. Accra; 2006.

Roll Back Malaria (RBM) (2008). *The Global Action Plan for malaria free world*. Geneva, Roll Back Malaria Partnership.

Roll Mack Malaria (RBM)/WHO (2002). RBM Advocacy Guide, Geneva, *World Health organization.*

Schellenberg D, Menendez C, Kahigwa E, Aponte J, Vidal J, Tanner M, Mshinda H and Alonso P. Intermittent treatment for malaria and anaemia control at time of routine vaccination in Tanzania infants: a randomised, placebo-controlled, double-blind trial. *Lancet* 2001, 357: 1471-1477.

Snow, R.M., Guerra, C.A., Noor, A.M., Myint, H.Y and Hay, S.I (2005). The global distribution of clinical episodes of Plasmodium falciparum malaria. *Nature*, 434 (7030): 214-217.

Tagbor Harry, Cairns Matthew, Nakwa Emmanuel, Browne Edmund, Sarkodie Badu, Counihan Helen, Meek Sylvia and Chandramohan Daniel The clinical impact of combining intermittent preventive treatment with home management of malaria in children aged below 5 years: cluster randomised trial. *Tropical Medicine and International Health* 2010, doi:10.111/j.1365-3156.2010.02699.x.

UNICEF 2001.

Warrell, D.A and Gilles, H.M. (eds.) (2002). *Essential Microbiology*, London, Arnold.

WHO (2003). *The Africa Malaria Report*. Geneva (WHO/CDS/MAL/2003.1093).

WHO (2008). *World Malaria Report. Geneva*, World Health Organization.

WHO and UNICEF (2005). *World Malaria report*. Geneva, World Health Organization and UNICEF.

World Health Organization (WHO) (2000). *The African summit on Roll Back Malaria,* Abuja, Nigeria. Geneva (WHO/CDS/RBM/2000.17).

Zikusooka C.M., McIntyre D. and Banes K.I. Should countries implementing an artemisinin-based combination malaria treatment policy also introduce rapid diagnostic tests? *Malaria Journal* 2008, 7: 176.

In: Malaria: Etiology, Pathogenesis and Treatments
Editors: A. M. Peterson et al, pp. 231-245
ISBN: 978-1-62100-363-2

Chapter X

Natural Acquired Anti- *Plasmodium Falciparum* IgG Antibody Responses in Thai Population

Piyatida Tangteerawatana[1*] and Srisin Khusmith[2**]
[1] Department of Microbiology, Faculty of Medicine, Srinakharinwirot University, Bangkok, Thailand.
[2] Department of Microbiology and Immunology, Faculty of Tropical Medicine, Mahidol University, Bangkok, Thailand.

Abstract

Immunity to malaria has a major role in controlling the disease and its pathogenesis. Naturally acquired antibodies play a crucial role in developing immunity to malaria. Over the past two decades, anti-*Plasmodium falciparum* antibody prevalence to different malaria candidate antigens has been conducted in sera from individuals living in Thailand where malaria is endemic. They were village residents, occupational exposed soldiers, and patients with severe and uncomplicated malaria. Partial seroactivity was observed for anti-immunoglobulin (Ig) G antibodies to ring-infected erythrocyte surface antigens (erythrocyte membrane immunofluorescence [EMIF] whole parasite), Pf332, Pf155/Ring infected erythrocyte surface antigens (RESA), and the repeat region of the circumsporozoite (CS) protein (R32tet32). Prospective studies assessed only the anti-R32tet32 IgG antibody, unable to prevent malaria. Interestingly, all village residents, all occupational exposed soldiers, and all of those with acute falciparum malaria had IgG antibody responses to a late blood stage malaria antigen (whole). Furthermore, significant lowered levels of this antibody were seen in the patients who died, compared to those who recovered. Similar to whole sporozoite IgG antibody responses, significant lowered

[*] Contributor author: Piyatida Tangteerawatana: Department of Microbiology, Faculty of Medicine, Srinakharinwirot University, 114 Sukhumvit 23, Bangkok 10110, Thailand. Phone : 66-02-6491000 ext 4917; Fax : 66-02-6495394, E-mail : piyatida@swu.ac.th.
[**] Reader and co-author.

levels of sporozoite antibodies were observed in cerebral malaria compared to those with acute uncomplicated malaria. The exploration of naturally acquired anti-*P.falciparum* antibody prevalence, and its relation to the past's morbidity and mortality, may provide clue into malaria control strategies, especially vaccination.

Keywords: *P.falciparum*, Antibody, Sporozoite antibodies, Blood stage antibodies, Malaria.

Introduction

Malaria remains a major global public health problem, with transmission occurring throughout Africa, Asia, Oceania, and Latin America, covering over 100 countries. Approximately, 300-500 million clinical cases of malaria occur each year, resulting in 1.5-2.7 million annual deaths (Muentener et al., 1999). In areas of low endemicity, the disease affects all age groups (Gupta et al., 1999); whereas in regions of very high endemicity, the greatest suffering occurs in children less than 5 years of age. Pregnant women, even if previously clinically immune, have a significantly enhanced risk for a pathogenic process that has major effects on their fetus and new born, particularly during the first pregnancy. The intensity of malaria transmission in Thailand is low and seasonal. A retrospective study revealed that severe falciparum malaria in Thailand is mostly characterized by hyperparasitemia and cerebral malaria, with severe anemia being less common (Vannaphan et al., 2005).

Malaria is caused by a protozoa of the phylum *Apicomplexa* Class *Sporozoa*. The family *Plasmodiidae* consists of many species, which have a wide range of vertebrate hosts. Human malaria parasites belong to the genus *Plasmodium*. At least four *Plasmodium* species, namely *P.malariae*, *P.ovale*, *P.vivax*, and *P.falciparum* cause malaria in humans. Falciparum malaria is the most important because of its associated morbidity and mortality. Recently, *P.knowlesi* a simian malaria parasite infecting long-tailed macaques with naturally acquired infections in humans, has been reported in Malaysian Borneo (Singh et al., 2004). To initiate the life cycle, sporozoites inoculated by female anopheline mosquitoes into the human blood stream, invade hepatic cells to establish the liver stage. This stage, commonly called exoerythrocytic schizogony, results in the release of merozoites that invade red cells and establish the erythrocytic stage, responsible for the disease and malaria related deaths. Inducing gametogenesis produces sexual forms, taken up by mosquitoes to ensure the survival of the species.

There are a number of severe complications that are specific to *P.falciparum* infections. In humans, the infection displays a remarkable range of severity, from asymptomatic to severe disease. Most cases of endemic *P.falciparum* malaria remain uncomplicated; yet, some develop a number of severe complications, including cerebral malaria, severe anaemia, and placental malaria. The outcome of an infection and its progression into pathology depend on the specific and dynamic combinations of the host's and parasite's properties. Clinical disease also changes with age, immunity, and transmission rates. Immunity to malaria has a major role in controlling disease and pathogenesis.

The most common clinical manifestation of malaria infection is a non-specific, febrile illness. Typically, the episode may start with non-specific symptoms, usually with an irregularly intermittent fever; accompanied by headache, dizziness, joint pain, malaise, anorexia, nausea, vomiting, diarrhea, and a feeling of chill. Characteristic for almost all episodes are the alterations between fever and fever-free phases, which are the best known symptoms of malaria. In some cases, the spontaneous recovery may even occur without therapy (Beeson and Brown, 2002). In some cases, the disease can progress very rapidly to severe life-threatening malaria, unless appropriate treatment is initiated, and in some cases, despite treatment.

Complicated or severe malaria is a disorder that affects several tissues and organs, characterized by the development of certain clinical findings, including cerebral malaria with: abnormal behavior, impairment of conciousness, seizures, coma or other neurologic abnormalities, severe anaemia, hemoglobinuria, non-cardiogenic pulmonary edema, jaundice, circulatory collapse, acute renal failure, thrombocytopenia, hyperparasitemia, metabolic acidosis, and hypoglycemia (World Health Organization, 2000). A key feature of the biology of *P.falciparum* is its ability to cause infected red blood cells (RBCs) to adhere to the linings of small blood vessels. Such sequestered parasites cause considerable obstruction to tissue perfusion. The cytoadherence mechanical blockage of small blood vessels in the brain causes local cerebral hypoxia and, thus, coma and death. Severe anemia may arise from mechanisms, including acute haemolysis of uninfected RBCs and diserythropoiesis, and nutritional deficiencies. In addition, in severe malaria, there may be marked reductions in the deformability of uninfected RBCs (Dondorp et al., 2000), strongly correlating with acidosis, suggesting that this may be involved in compromising the blood flow through tissues (Miller et al., 2002).

Antibodies are important mediators of acquired immunity to malaria, evidenced by the demonstration that naturally acquired antibodies are associated with protection from symptomatic disease in malaria endemic populations (Cohen et al., 1961; Sabchareon et al., 1991). Although many different types of antibodies are produced by the immune system, only some of these are effective in protecting against malaria. In malaria endemic areas, the rate at which natural immunity develops is dependent on the intensity and stability of exposure to *P. falciparum*, with immunity to severe and mild disease developing more rapidly in areas with higher transmission (Marsh and Kinyanjui, 2006; Gupta et al., 1999). Differences in the acquisition of immunity may influence associations between specific responses and immunity. Furthermore, the prevalence of the major allelic types of specific antigens, and subsequent acquisition of allele-specific immunity, may be different across populations. By exploring the incidence and association between the naturally acquired antibodies which recognize specific candidate antigens, in relation to past clinical outcomes in certain populations living in areas where malaria is endemic, such as, in Thailand, this may help to obtain a greater understanding of naturally acquired immunity to malaria and to contribute to rational vaccine development.

Immunity to Malaria

Naturally acquired immunity to malaria is a slow process and requires repeated parasite exposure to be maintained, and it takes years or decades to develop. The immunity is species, stage, strain, and variants specific (Andrysiak et al., 1986; Fandeur and Chalvet, 1998). Residents in malaria endemic areas frequently have premunition (parasitemia and antibodies (Ab) without symptoms) (Baird et al., 1998). It is rarely sterile, but rather associated with low-grade parasitemias and episodes of clinical disease throughout life (Trape et al., 1994). It is likely that, as acquired immune responses, innate defense mechanisms are of equal importance in controlling malaria.

1. Innate Immunity

Innate immunity is characterized as a non-specific host defense mechanism. The immune cells include: polymorphonuclear (PMN) cells; macrophages; dendritic cells (DCs); natural-killer cells (NK); natural-killer T cells (NKT); gamma/delta (γδ) T cells; and soluble factors, such as interferons and compliment factors contributing to the innate immunity against malaria (Perlmann and Troye-Blomberg, 2002). Recently, it has been recognized that interactions between accessory cells and innate lymphocytes can be bidirectional (Munz et al., 2005). The major role of innate immunity appears to be producing proinflammatory cytokines, such as interleukin (IL)-12 and interferon (IFN)-gamma. The augmented release of IFN-γ stimulates monocytes to secrete tumor necrosis factor (TNF), promoting antiplasmodial properties.

Ligation by pathogens of pattern recognition receptors (PRR) on DC typically causes an activation of the DC. The initial interactions between DC and T cell have important implications for the functional outcome of the T cell response. DCs drive the differentiation of naïve T cells into IFN-γ-secreting Th1 cells, IL-4-secreting Th2 cells, or other subsets, such as IL-10-secreting regulatory T cells. While IL-12 secretion by DCs is crucial to the induction of Th1 cells, the absence of IL-12 is thought to result in a default pathway, leading to the development of Th2 cells (Langenkamp et al., 2000; Shortman and Liu, 2002). Dendritic cells (DCs) are important, both in amplifying the innate immune response and in initiating adaptive immunity and shaping the type of T helper (Th) response. The controversy as to whether DC function is altered may relate to: 1) the parasite virulent; 2) host genetic background; 3) the level of parasitemia, indicating possible difference in antigen dose and/or parasite virulent; 4) whether the DCs were analyzed after a period of maturation in culture or directly *ex vivo* (Stevenson and Urban, 2006).

2. Acquired Immunity

During the infection with *Plasmodium* species in mice and humans, both cell-mediated and antibody-dependent responses are crucial to control the parasitemia.

2.1. Cell Mediated Immunity

Cell mediated immunity (CMI) plays an important role in protective immunity to malaria. Effector components of acquired CMI involve different set of cells, including: T helper (CD4 T cells), T cytotoxic (CTL), and B cells.

CD4 T cells play a central role in regulating *Plasmodium* asexual blood stages immune response via their cytokine production. Sequential production of Th1 and Th2 cytokines is critical for protection (Langhorne et al., 1998; Taylor-Robinson and Phillips, 1994). Of Th1 cytokines, IFN-γ, is the predominant cytokine produced in early acute *P. chabaudi,* as well as

P.falciparum infection; but this cytokine declines as the parasitemia decreases, and is replaced by the Th2 cytokines, IL-4 and IL-10, during the later stages of infection (Tangteerawatana et al., 2007; Taylor-Robinson and Phillips, 1994). IFN-γ, IL4 and IL10 producing CD4 Th cells are important for providing help to B cells, leading to the production of antibodies crucial to the control and elimination of blood stage parasites. Both Th1 and Th2 cells contribute to protective immunity at different times of infection; and the balance of cytokine production between these two subsets could modulate antibody profiles, which, in turn, may alter the final elimination of the parasite and determe the outcome of the disease.

The CD8 T cells represent 30-40% of the T cells in the blood and the secondary lymphoid organs. CD8 T cells recognize antigens in the context of the MHC class I molecule. CD8 T cells have cytolytic granules in their cytoplasm where the pore-forming proteins, perforin, and granzymes reside, mediating thekilling of intracellular microbes or tumor cells (Tschopp and Nabholz, 1990). The target for CD8 CTLs in *Plasmodiam* is thought to be sporozoite antigens, presented by class I MHC molecules on infected liver hepatocytes. In animals, CD8 T cells are critical for eliminating malaria from the liver (Kumar et al., 1988). In humans, a low CD8 CTL response to circumsporozoite proteins was found in acute falciparum malaria (Khusmith et al., 1999). Although CD8 T cells are found in low frequencies in humans, the experiment data implys that they act on the parasite infected hepatocytes *in vivo*. Indeed, MHC class I restricted CD8 T cells in the pre-erythrocytic immunity and contributing to the protection against severe malaria have been reported (Aidoo and Udhayakumar, 2000).

2.2. Antibody Mediated Responses

The mechanisms used by the immune system to fight malaria are not completely understood, although, it is well established that antibodies play a key role in protecting against asexual blood stage malarial parasites (Cohen et al., 1961). In residents of endemic areas, malaria infection induces strong humeral immune responses, involving a production of predominately IgM and IgG but also of other immunoglobulin isotypes (Cohen et al., 1961). A large proportion of this immunoglobulin is non-malaria specific, reflecting polyclonal B cell activation, approximately 5% or more represents species- and stage-specific antibodies reacting with a wide variety of parasite antigens (Cohen et al., 1961). Several lines of evidence from human study supported that the production of parasite-specific antibodies to certain *P. falciparum* antigens may be associated with protection from different phases of malaria infection. Immunoglobulin preparations from immune adults could be used to treat parasitemia in children in West Africa (Cohen et al., 1961). In addition, the passive transfer of antibodies from African immune adults to Gambian children and to adult Thai patients can dramatically reduce parasitemias and clinical symptoms (Bouharoun-Tayoun et al., 1990; Cohen et al., 1961; Sabchareon et al., 1991). Consequently, this suggests the critical role of antibodies in protective immunity against malaria infection by reducing parasitemia and clinical disease.

Although antibodies to *P.falciparum* parasites of all major classes are induced in malaria infected individuals, IgG is the most important in protective immunity. For the study in Thailand, the patients were treated for acute infection with *Plasmodium falciparum* and had been monitored longitudinally over 67 days. The mean maximum anti-sporozoite vaccine antigen (R32tet32) antibody level occurred on day 4. The apparent antibody half-life was 27 days, which is comparable to the half-life of circulating immunoglobulin G in humans (Webster et al., 1987).

Malaria specific antibodies mediate a number of antiparasitic effector functions, either on their own or in collaboration with other effector cells. On their own, antibodies: (1) may neutralize sporozoites and, thus, prevent the sporozoite to enter hepatocytes (Brown et al., 1989); (2) may inhibit the merozoite's invasion into the erythrocyte (Wahlin et al., 1984); (3) may inhibit the transport of nutrients essential to parasite growth (Holder and Freeman, 1984); (4) may inhibit the merozoite release from schizonts (Green et al., 1981); (5) may inhibit cytoadherence and, thus, prevent infected RBC to sequester in the periphery and promote them to be eliminated by the spleen (Newbold et al., 1992); (6) may inhibit the rosetting formation (Carlson et al., 1990); (7) may neutralize the malaria toxin (Schofield et al., 2002). Furthermore, in collaboration with other effector immune cells, antibodies may interact with cells through the Fc receptor and promote phagocyte activation, cytotoxicity, or may co-operate with complement mediated killing (Bouharoun-Tayoun et al., 1990; Giribaldi et al., 2001).

A number of studies have described the associations between the presence of antibodies against certain *P.falciparum* antigens and reduced risk of clinical malaria (Ahlborg et al., 2002; Metzger et al., 2003; Taylor et al., 1998). Target antigens for inducing protective antibodies to the malaria blood stages are those antigens expressed on the surface of infected erythrocytes, possibly located in apical organelles of the merozoites, on the surface of merozoites, or on the infected erythrocytes; all considered as potential vaccine candidates (Bolad and Berzins, 2000). There are a number of candidate proteins derived from different stages of *P.falciparum* that have been determined to be important in the development of humoral immunity, including Pf155/RESA (ring-infected erythrocyte surface antigen) (Siddique et al., 1998), GLURP (glutamate-rich protein) (Theisen et al., 1998), and AMA-1 (apical membrane protein 1) (Amante et al., 1997).

Natural Acquired Anti-*P.Falciparum* IgG Antibody Responses in Thai Population

Due to the potential involvement of antibodies in protective immune responses, several different *Plasmodium falciparum* antigens including pre-erythrocytic stage, asexual and sexual blood stage have been suggested and studied as targets for protective antibodies. It was of interest to review the previous prevalence reports of seroactivity against *P.falciparum* crude and vaccine candidate antigens in individuals residing in areas of different malaria endemicities in Thailand.

1. Anti-*P.Falciparum* IgG

1.1. Sporozoite Antibody

The antibodies to whole *P.falparum* sporozoite antigens and circumsporozoite proteins (CSP) were conducted, testing their reactivity in villager residents, malaria patients, uncomplicated malaria (AM), and cerebral malaria (CM). By using indirect immunofluorescent assay (IFA), the study demonstrated that 33.6 % of people living in an endemic area at Kanchanaburi western Thailand, and 45.2% of patients with acute falciparum malarià admitted to Phra Pokklao Hospital, Chantaburi eastern Thailand had antibodies against the whole sporozoite (Tapchaisri et al., 1983); when investigated patients separately, according to clinical manifestation. Forty-eight percent of CM patients and 49% of AM patients were positive for antibodies against whole *P.falciparum* sporozoites. However, CM patients had significantly lower mean IgG anti-sporozoite titers for *P. falciparum* than did AM patients (*P* less than 0.05), especially when only anti-sporozoite antibody-positive CM and AM patients were compared (*P* less than 0.0005) (Tapchaisri et al., 1985).

The reactivity of circumsporzoite protein (CSP) in repeat and non-repeat region was tested in Thai individuals. R32tet32 contains 32 tandem copies of the tetrapeptide sequence,constituting the immunodominant epitope of the circumsporozoite protein (CSP) (the amino acid sequence MDP (NANP)15NVDP(NANP)15NVDPtet32). Prospective studies showed that 83 % of occupationally exposed soldiers, living at the Thai border at Laos and Cambodia, had an anti-R32tet32 antibody response, occurring during a 10 day interval after the patient's diagnosis of parasitemia (Webster et al., 1988). Similarly, another reported that 70% of Chantaburi Province villages developed antibodies against an epitope in the repeat region of the circumsporozoite (CS) protein, the peptide construct R32tet32 (Wongsrichanalai et al., 1991). These two authors demonstrated that anti-R32tet32 antibody is ill developed under natural conditions and does not appear to protect against developing malaria. These studies, in line with the previous reports, demonstrated that naturally acquired antibodies to sporozoites do not prevent malaria (Hoffman et al., 1987). The prevalence and level of antibodies decreased during the non-transmission wet season, and increased over a 1-2-month transition period. Thus, the CS antibody appeared to reflect the relative population's exposure to the mosquito inoculation of *P. falciparum* sporozoites, and provided a useful measure of malaria transmission dynamics (Webster et al., 1992). Anti-circumsporozoite protein (CSP) antibody responses, demonstrated in individuals resident of malaria endemic areas, are relatively weak and short-lasting when following an immunization with antigens containing repeat sequences (Webster et al., 1988).

Based on the anti-R32tet32 results obtain from an occupationally exposed soldier, the serum sets from 16 men were selected to study the antibodies against the non-repetitive, flanking regions (anti-RLF) of the CS protein. Subjects were assigned to one of three groups based on their antibody responses to the repeat region (anti-R32tet32), observed in association with a microscopically documented case of falciparum malaria: 1) non detectable (n=5); 2) low positive (n=6); 3) modurate-to-high positive (n=5); The study revealed that antibody responses to the repeatless flanking (RLF) regions were observed in all subjects, including five individuals who lacked detectable anti-R32tet32 antibody responses (Brown et al., 1992). The study in human sera from regions of Brazil, Papua New Guinea, and Kenya, in which malaria is endemic, demonstrated that the natural expression of antibody responses to the non-repeat-region-based B-cell epitopes of the CS protein are variable in different populations and increase as a function of the host's age. The antibody pressures, induced by the immunogenic potential of non-repeat-region-based B-cell epitopes, may also contribute to the maintenance of the antigenic diversity of the CS protein (Shi et al., 1993).

1.2. Blood Stage Antibody

The antibodies to asexual blood stage antigens have been determined in Thai endemic areas including: an antibody to whole parasite infected RBCs, glycoprotein (gp) 195, Pf332(2-12)2, or ring infected erythrocyte surface antigens (Pf155/RESA EENV6).

Sera antibodies to acetone fixed thin smears of blood stage *P.falciparum* were investigated in patients admitted to Pra Pokklao Hospital, Chantaburi, eastern Thailand. IFA-IgG antibodies were present in all patients (97). Howere, in patients with the most severe form of the disease, i.e., those who died despite adequate therapy (n=12), antibodies detected in the immunofluorescent antibody test for the blood stage were found at lower levels than in those who recovered (n=85). (Brasseur et al., 1990; Fribourg-Blanc et al., 1985). Sera antibody to glutaraldehyde fixed ring infected erythrocyte surface antigen was also studied in patients sera admitted to Pra Pokklao Hospital. Complicated cerebral malaria (CCM) patients had a significant lower IFA-IgG positive rate and a lower geometric mean reciprocal titre than those of uncomplicated cerebral malaria (UCCM) and non cerebral malaria patient (NCM). (Tharavanij et al., 1988). Similar studies were investigated in patients admitted to Tropical Disease Hospital, Bangkok. The mean ELISA-IgG anti-plasmodial antibodies to the crude blood stage *P.falciparum* tended to be higher in the group with uncomplicated, compared to those with severe disease (Perlmann et al., 2000). The link between morbidity, mortality, and low levels of antibody production suggests that an appropriate immune response to malaria antigens may be required to achieve recovery with drug treatments.

Asexual late blood stages of the *P.falciparum* antibody were studied in rangers and villagers sera at the Thai border at Laos and Cambodia. All of those rangers and villagers had antibodies to asexual late blood stages of *P.falciparum* as described by immunofluorescence assay (IFA), and less than half of those volunteers had anti-Pf155/RESA antibodies [erythrocyte membrane immunofluorescence (EMIF)] (Udomsangpetch et al., 1994). Similar results were obtained for the study by Maneerat et al. (1999) where all endemic residents at Trad Province eastern Thailand develop antibodies to the late blood stages of *P.falciparum,* as determined by IFA; 81% of those volunteers had anti-Pf155/RESA antibodies (EMIF). Furthermore, the sera containing high antibody titres significantly inhibited cytoadherence of *P.falciparum* infected erythrocytes and all the sera variably inhibited rosette formations of parasites (Maneerat et al., 1999). Antibodies preventing cytoadherence and/or rosette formations may prevent the development of cerebral malaria. Thus, antibodies can be involved in anti-disease immunity (Carlson et al., 1990; David et al., 1983)

Concerning seroactivity, IFA-IgG antibodies to malaria late blood stage were present in all patients with cerebral, non-cerebral malaria (Fribourg-Blanc et al., 1985), and malaria residents (Maneerat et al., 1999; Udomsangpetch et al., 1994); whereas ELISA-IgG antibodies to crude extracted *P.falciparum* late blood stage were present in only 22 of 35 patients with uncomplicated malaria and 23 of 35 subjects with severe disease (Perlmann et al., 2000). This suggests that the crude blood stage is more highly immunogenic than crude extract *P.falciparum*. On the other hand IFA is more sensitive than ELISA.

Gp 195 ELISA-IgG in occupationally exposed soldiers, working at the Thai border at Laos and Cambodia were investigated. Eightty-four of 85 men developed positive antibody responses to gp195 during acute falciparum malaria (Brown et al., 1991). The glycoprotein precursor of the major merozoite surface antigen (gp195) is synthesized by trophozoite and schizont stages of the *Plasmodium falciparum* parasite, and has a molecular weight of approximately 195 kDa. This protein is processed at the time of schizont maturation and rupture, producing fragments that are recognized by anti-merozoite antibodies (Brown et al., 1991).

Pf332(2-12)2 and Pf155/RESA (EENV6) were investigated in village residents (ELISA) of Chanthaburi. 43% of residents showed seroactivity to antigen Pf332 repeat sequences, whereas 30% of those showed seroactivity to antigen Pf155/RESA (Iqbal et al., 1993). Pf332 is a giant protein of apparent mol. Wt 2500 kD, exported from the intracellular parasite to the erythrocyte membrane and associated with the membranous cleft (Mattei. D.,71, 1992). The gene has been cloned, in part, and the DNA sequence has revealed repetitive structures coding for 11 degenerated amino acid repeats, rich in glutamic acid (Mattei and Scherf, 1992). A merozoite-derived polypeptide, Pf155, or ring infected erythrocyte surface antigen (RESA) is present in dense granules in the apical region of merozoites (Aikawa et al., 1990). It is released into the parasitophorous vacuole during merozoite invasion and translocated to the inner surface of the RBC membrane. The Pf155/RESA has two regions of tandamly repeated amino acid sequences: EENVEHDA/EENV in the 3' region and DDEHVEEPTVA in the 5' region that contain immunodominant epitopes for B cells (Perlmann et al., 1989). Iqbal et al. show that antibodies reactive with antigen Pf332 repeat sequences are found with high prevalence in individuals resident in malaria endemic areas. The meam antibody concentrations were significantly higher in donors from Liberia, compare with Thai, Madagascar, Gambia and Colombian donors. These observations, regarding to seroreactivities, may reflect the degree of exposure.

Together, partial antibody responses with different seropositives were reported for R32tet32, gp195, Pf332, Pf155/RESA, ring-infected erythrocyte surface antigens (EMIP) and sporozoites (whole) in village residents and malaria patients. The data suggests that inducing B-cell immunological memory of natural infections is not consistent in these endemic areas. This is probably due the complexity of the parasite and the host's genetics. The parasite has epitopes which are immuno-dominant, sub-dominant, variant and conserved. There is evidence showing that children mount a humoral response, predominantly to immuno-dominant variant epitopes on the red cell surface, as well as merozoite surface proteins, leading to strain-specific incomplete immunity. Furthermore, older children and adults respond to multiple variant antigens, as well as conserved epitopes, resulting in long-term protective immunity (Good et al., 2004). However, when adults living in a malaria-endemic country quickly become infected, following a radical cure of malaria, a lack of complete malaria immunity is indicated (Hoffman et al., 1987).

The relationship of the crude anti-*P.falciparum* antigens to the severity of malaria has been investigated. It is of interest that antibodies to both whole infected RBCs (Brasseur et al., 1990; Perlmann et al., 2000; Tharavanij et al., 1988) and whole sporozoites (Tapchaisri et al., 1985) are associated with reducing severity or protecting against mortality and severe forms of the disease. The whole parasite infected RBC generated immunity to a range of parasite antigens. Anti-malaria antibodies against several major malaria antigens are shown to: prevent parasite replication, neutralize parasite toxicity, or inhibit the cytoadherence of infected red cells and, thus, interfere with parasite sequestration. This indicates that the effective acquired immunity of anti-parasite antibodies, as well as anti-disease antibodies, would play significant roles in reducing the morbidity and mortality of the disease. This revelation may suggest that a successful malaria vaccine should contain multiple antigens. Recent studies in human volunteers suggest that an ultra-low dose of malaria parasites (30 *P. falciparum*-infected RBCs) are sufficient to induce protective cellular immune responses

(Pombo et al., 2002). However, it is difficult to grow whole native organisms *in vitro*. A subunit vaccine would be essential in the context that the subunit vaccine would induce immune responses against only those determinants relevant to protection; thus, minimizing the possibility of deleterious responses (Good et al., 2005).

Conclusion

Although malaria is a complex disease, there is accumulating evidence to suggest that an anti-malaria vaccine can be developed successfully (Good et al. 1998, Richie et al., 2002). However, the efficacious human malaria vaccine is still unavailable, and there is an increase in malaria drug resistance. The exploration of the naturally acquired anti-*P.falciparum* antibody prevalence and its relation to morbidity and mortality in the past, such as in the Thai population, may prove valuable for rational vaccine development by providing evidence supporting the target antigens of protective immunity in humans, and to help identify antigens that confer protection from malaria.

References

Ahlborg, N., Haddad, D., Siddique, A. B., Roussilhon, C., Rogier, C., Trape, J. F., Troye-Blomberg, M. and Berzins, K. (2002). Antibody responses to the repetitive Plasmodium falciparum antigen Pf332 in humans naturally primed to the parasite. *Clin. Exp. Immunol.* 129, 318-25.

Aidoo, M. and Udhayakumar, V. (2000). Field studies of cytotoxic T lymphocytes in malaria infections: implications for malaria vaccine development. *Parasitol. Today* 16, 50-6.

Aikawa, M., Torii, M., Sjolander, A., Berzins, K., Perlmann, P. and Miller, L. H. (1990). Pf155/RESA antigen is localized in dense granules of Plasmodium falciparum merozoites. *Exp. Parasitol.* 71, 326-9.

Amante, F. H., Crewther, P. E., Anders, R. F. and Good, M. F. (1997). A cryptic T cell epitope on the apical membrane antigen 1 of Plasmodium chabaudi adami can prime for an anamnestic antibody response: implications for malaria vaccine design. *J. Immunol.* 159, 5535-44.

Andrysiak, P. M., Collins, W. E. and Campbell, G. H. (1986). Stage-specific and species-specific antigens of Plasmodium vivax and Plasmodium ovale defined by monoclonal antibodies. *Infect. Immun.* 54, 609-12.

Baird, J. K. (1998). Age-dependent characteristics of protection v. susceptibility to Plasmodium falciparum. *Ann. Trop. Med. Parasitol.* 92, 367-90.

Beeson, J. G. and Brown, G. V. (2002). Pathogenesis of Plasmodium falciparum malaria: the roles of parasite adhesion and antigenic variation. *Cell Mol. Life Sci* 59, 258-71.

Bolad, A. and Berzins, K. (2000). Antigenic diversity of Plasmodium falciparum and antibody-mediated parasite neutralization. *Scand. J. Immunol.* 52, 233-9.

Bouharoun-Tayoun, H., Attanath, P., Sabchareon, A., Chongsuphajaisiddhi, T. and Druilhe, P. (1990). Antibodies that protect humans against Plasmodium falciparum blood stages do not on their own inhibit parasite growth and invasion in vitro, but act in cooperation with monocytes. *J. Exp. Med.* 172, 1633-41.

Brasseur, P., Ballet, J. J. and Druilhe, P. (1990). Impairment of Plasmodium falciparum-specific antibody response in severe malaria. *J. Clin. Microbiol.* 28, 265-8.

Brown, A. E., Webster, H. K., Gordon, D. M., Permpanich, B. and Gross, M. (1992). Characterization of naturally acquired antibodies to the non-repetitive flanking regions of the circumsporozoite protein of Plasmodium falciparum. *Am. J. Trop. Med. Hyg.* 47, 440-5.

Brown, A. E., Webster, H. K., Lyon, J. A., Thomas, A. W., Permpanich, B. and Gross, M. (1991). Characterization of naturally acquired antibody responses to a recombinant fragment from the N-terminus of Plasmodium falciparum glycoprotein 195. *Am. J. Trop. Med. Hyg.* 45, 567-73.

Brown, A. E., Webster, H. K., Pavanand, K., Permpanich, B., Sookto, P., Sattabongkot, J. and Gingrich, J. B. (1989). Comparison of antibody responses to the circumsporozoite protein repeat region and to intact sporozoites during acute falciparum malaria. *Trans. R. Soc. Trop. Med. Hyg.* 83, 154-7.

Carlson, J., Holmquist, G., Taylor, D. W., Perlmann, P. and Wahlgren, M. (1990). Antibodies to a histidine-rich protein (PfHRP1) disrupt spontaneously formed Plasmodium falciparum erythrocyte rosettes. *Proc. Natl. Acad. Sci. U S A* 87, 2511-5.

Cohen, S., Mc, G. I. and Carrington, S. (1961). Gamma-globulin and acquired immunity to human malaria. *Nature* 192, 733-7.

David, P. H., Hommel, M., Miller, L. H., Udeinya, I. J. and Oligino, L. D. (1983). Parasite sequestration in Plasmodium falciparum malaria: spleen and antibody modulation of cytoadherence of infected erythrocytes. *Proc. Natl. Acad. Sci. U S A* 80, 5075-9.

Dondorp, A. M., Kager, P. A., Vreeken, J. and White, N. J. (2000). Abnormal blood flow and red blood cell deformability in severe malaria. *Parasitol. Today* 16, 228-32.

Fandeur, T. and Chalvet, W. (1998). Variant- and strain-specific immunity in Saimiri infected with Plasmodium falciparum. *Am. J. Trop. Med. Hyg.* 58, 225-31.

Fribourg-Blanc, A., Druilhe, P., Brasseur, P., Rhodes-Feuillette, A., Ballet, J. J. and Tharavanij, S. (1985). Immunological evaluation of cell-mediated and humoral immunity in Thai patients with cerebral and non cerebral Plasmodium falciparum malaria: II. Evolution of serum levels of immunoglobulins, antimalarial antibodies, complement fractions and alpha interferon. *Southeast Asian J. Trop. Med. Public Health* 16, 307-13.

Giribaldi, G., Ulliers, D., Mannu, F., Arese, P. and Turrini, F. (2001). Growth of Plasmodium falciparum induces stage-dependent haemichrome formation, oxidative aggregation of band 3, membrane deposition of complement and antibodies, and phagocytosis of parasitized erythrocytes. *Br. J. Haematol.* 113, 492-9.

Good MF, Kaslow DC, Miller LH. (1998) Pathways and strategies for developing a malaria blood-stage vaccine. *Annu. Rev. Immunol.* 16:57-87.

Good, M. F. (2005). Vaccine-induced immunity to malaria parasites and the need for novel strategies. *Trends Parasitol.* 21, 29-34.

Good, M. F., Stanisic, D., Xu, H., Elliott, S. and Wykes, M. (2004). The immunological challenge to developing a vaccine to the blood stages of malaria parasites. *Immunol. Rev.* 201, 254-67.

Green, T. J., Morhardt, M., Brackett, R. G. and Jacobs, R. L. (1981). Serum inhibition of merozoite dispersal from Plasmodium falciparum schizonts: indicator of immune status. *Infect. Immun.* 31, 1203-8.

Gupta, S., Snow, R. W., Donnelly, C. A., Marsh, K. and Newbold, C. (1999). Immunity to non-cerebral severe malaria is acquired after one or two infections. *Nat. Med.* 5, 340-3.

Hoffman, S. L., Oster, C. N., Plowe, C. V., Woollett, G. R., Beier, J. C., Chulay, J. D., Wirtz, R. A., Hollingdale, M. R. and Mugambi, M. (1987). Naturally acquired antibodies to sporozoites do not prevent malaria: vaccine development implications. *Science* 237, 639-42.

Holder, A. A. and Freeman, R. R. (1984). Protective antigens of rodent and human bloodstage malaria. *Philos. Trans. R. Soc. Lond B. Biol. Sci.* 307, 171-7.

Iqbal, J., Perlmann, P., Greenwood, B. M. and Berzins, K. (1993). Seroreactivity with the Plasmodium falciparum blood stage antigen Pf332 in adults and children from malaria-endemic regions. *Clin. Exp. Immunol.* 94, 68-74.

Khusmith, S., Tangteerawatana, P. and Looareesuwan, S. (1999). Low CD8+ T lymphocyte response to P. falciparum circumsporozoite protein in naturally-exposed malaria endemic populations in Thailand. *Southeast Asian J. Trop. Med. Public Health* 30, 405-11.

Kumar, S., Miller, L. H., Quakyi, I. A., Keister, D. B., Houghten, R. A., Maloy, W. L., Moss, B., Berzofsky, J. A. and Good, M. F. (1988). Cytotoxic T cells specific for the circumsporozoite protein of Plasmodium falciparum. *Nature* 334, 258-60.

Langenkamp, A., Messi, M., Lanzavecchia, A. and Sallusto, F. (2000). Kinetics of dendritic cell activation: impact on priming of TH1, TH2 and nonpolarized T cells. *Nat. Immunol.* 1, 311-6.

Langhorne, J., Cross, C., Seixas, E., Li, C. and von der Weid, T. (1998). A role for B cells in the development of T cell helper function in a malaria infection in mice. *Proc. Natl. Acad. Sci. U S A* 95, 1730-4.

Maneerat, Y., Tiensuwan, M., Siripoon, N., Thaithong, S. and Udomsangpetch, R. (1999). Antiparasite adherence activity in Thai individuals living in a P. falciparum endemic area. *Asian Pac. J. Allergy Immunol.* 17, 23-9.

Marsh, K. and Kinyanjui, S. (2006). Immune effector mechanisms in malaria. *Parasite Immunol.* 28, 51-60.

Mattei, D., Hinterberg, K. and Scherf, A. (1992). Pfl I-I and Pf332: two giant proteins synthesized in erythrocytes infected with Plasmodium falciparum. *Parasitol. Today* 8, 426-8.

Mattei, D. and Scherf, A. (1992). The Pf332 gene of Plasmodium falciparum codes for a giant protein that is translocated from the parasite to the membrane of infected erythrocytes. *Gene* 110, 71-9.

Mazier, D., Nitcheu, J. and Idrissa-Boubou, M. (2000). Cerebral malaria and immunogenetics. *Parasite Immunol.* 22, 613-23.

Metzger, W. G., Okenu, D. M., Cavanagh, D. R., Robinson, J. V., Bojang, K. A., Weiss, H. A., McBride, J. S., Greenwood, B. M. and Conway, D. J. (2003). Serum IgG3 to the Plasmodium falciparum merozoite surface protein 2 is strongly associated with a reduced prospective risk of malaria. *Parasite Immunol.* 25, 307-12.

Miller, L. H., Baruch, D. I., Marsh, K. and Doumbo, O. K. (2002). The pathogenic basis of malaria. *Nature* 415, 673-9.

Muentener, P., Schlagenhauf, P. and Steffen, R. (1999). Imported malaria (1985-95): trends and perspectives. *Bull. World Health Organ* 77, 560-6.

Munz, C., Steinman, R. M. and Fujii, S. (2005). Dendritic cell maturation by innate lymphocytes: coordinated stimulation of innate and adaptive immunity. *J. Exp. Med.* 202, 203-7.

Newbold, C. I., Pinches, R., Roberts, D. J. and Marsh, K. (1992). Plasmodium falciparum: the human agglutinating antibody response to the infected red cell surface is predominantly variant specific. *Exp. Parasitol.* 75, 281-92.

Perlmann, H., Perlmann, P., Berzins, K., Wahlin, B., Troye-Blomberg, M., Hagstedt, M., Andersson, I., Hogh, B., Petersen, E. and Bjorkman, A. (1989). Dissection of the human antibody response to the malaria antigen Pf155/RESA into epitope specific components. *Immunol. Rev.* 112, 115-32.

Perlmann, P., Perlmann, H., Looareesuwan, S., Krudsood, S., Kano, S., Matsumoto, Y., Brittenham, G., Troye-Blomberg, M. and Aikawa, M. (2000). Contrasting functions of IgG and IgE antimalarial antibodies in uncomplicated and severe Plasmodium falciparum malaria. *Am. J. Trop. Med. Hyg.* 62, 373-7.

Perlmann, P. and Troye-Blomberg, M. (2002). Malaria and the immune system in humans. *Chem. Immunol.* 80, 229-42.

Pombo, D. J., Lawrence, G., Hirunpetcharat, C., Rzepczyk, C., Bryden, M., Cloonan, N., Anderson, K., Mahakunkijcharoen, Y., Martin, L. B., Wilson, D. et al. (2002). Immunity to malaria after administration of ultra-low doses of red cells infected with Plasmodium falciparum. *Lancet* 360, 610-7.

Richie TL, Saul A. (2002) Progress and challenges for malaria vaccines. *Nature.* 415(6872), 694-701.

Sabchareon, A., Burnouf, T., Ouattara, D., Attanath, P., Bouharoun-Tayoun, H., Chantavanich, P., Foucault, C., Chongsuphajaisiddhi, T. and Druilhe, P. (1991). Parasitologic and clinical human response to immunoglobulin administration in falciparum malaria. *Am. J. Trop. Med. Hyg.* 45, 297-308.

Schofield, L., Hewitt, M. C., Evans, K., Siomos, M. A. and Seeberger, P. H. (2002). Synthetic GPI as a candidate anti-toxic vaccine in a model of malaria. *Nature* 418, 785-9.

Shi, Y. P., Udhayakumar, V., Alpers, M. P., Povoa, M. M., Oloo, A. J., Ruebush, T. K., 2nd and Lal, A. A. (1993). Natural antibody responses against the non-repeat-sequence-based B-cell epitopes of the Plasmodium falciparum circumsporozoite protein. *Infect. Immun.* 61, 2425-33.

Shortman, K. and Liu, Y. J. (2002). Mouse and human dendritic cell subtypes. *Nat. Rev. Immunol.* 2, 151-61.

Siddique, A. B., Ahlborg, N., Wahlin Flyg, B., Perlmann, P. and Berzins, K. (1998). Antibodies to sequences in a non-repeat region of Plasmodium falciparum antigen Pf155/RESA inhibit either cytoadherence or parasite growth in vitro. *Parasitology* 117 (Pt 3), 209-16.

Singh, B., Kim Sung, L., Matusop, A., Radhakrishnan, A., Shamsul, S. S., Cox-Singh, J., Thomas, A. and Conway, D. J. (2004). A large focus of naturally acquired Plasmodium knowlesi infections in human beings. *Lancet* 363, 1017-24.

Stevenson, M. M. and Urban, B. C. (2006). Antigen presentation and dendritic cell biology in malaria. *Parasite Immunol.* 28, 5-14.

Tangteerawatana, P., Pichyangkul, S., Hayano, M., Kalambaheti, T., Looareesuwan, S., Troye-Blomberg, M. and Khusmith, S. (2007). Relative levels of IL4 and IFN-gamma in complicated malaria: association with IL4 polymorphism and peripheral parasitemia. *Acta Trop.* 101, 258-65.

Tapchaisri, P., Asavanich, A., Limsuwan, S., Tharavanij, S. and Harinasuta, K. T. (1985). Antibodies against malaria sporozoites in patients with acute uncomplicated malaria and patients with cerebral malaria. *Am. J. Trop. Med. Hyg.* 34, 831-6.

Tapchaisri, P., Chomcharn, Y., Poonthong, C., Asavanich, A., Limsuwan, S., Maleevan, O., Tharavanij, S. and Harinasuta, T. (1983). Anti-sporozoite antibodies induced by natural infection. *Am. J. Trop. Med. Hyg.* 32, 1203-8.

Taylor-Robinson, A. W. and Phillips, R. S. (1994). B cells are required for the switch from Th1- to Th2-regulated immune responses to Plasmodium chabaudi chabaudi infection. *Infect. Immun.* 62, 2490-8.

Taylor, R. R., Allen, S. J., Greenwood, B. M. and Riley, E. M. (1998). IgG3 antibodies to Plasmodium falciparum merozoite surface protein 2 (MSP2): increasing prevalence with age and association with clinical immunity to malaria. *Am J Trop Med Hyg* 58, 406-13.

Tharavanij, S., Tapchaisri, P., Mahakunkijcharoen, Y. and Looareesuwan, S. (1988). Antibody against a ring-infected erythrocyte surface antigen in cerebral and non-cerebral malaria patients. *Trans. R. Soc. Trop. Med. Hyg.* 82, 385-8.

Theisen, M., Soe, S., Oeuvray, C., Thomas, A. W., Vuust, J., Danielsen, S., Jepsen, S. and Druilhe, P. (1998). The glutamate-rich protein (GLURP) of Plasmodium falciparum is a target for antibody-dependent monocyte-mediated inhibition of parasite growth in vitro. *Infect. Immun.* 66, 11-7.

Trape, J. F., Rogier, C., Konate, L., Diagne, N., Bouganali, H., Canque, B., Legros, F., Badji, A., Ndiaye, G., Ndiaye, P. et al. (1994). The Dielmo project: a longitudinal study of natural malaria infection and the mechanisms of protective immunity in a community living in a holoendemic area of Senegal. *Am. J. Trop. Med. Hyg.* 51, 123-37.

Tschopp, J. and Nabholz, M. (1990). Perforin-mediated target cell lysis by cytolytic T lymphocytes. *Annu. Rev. Immunol.* 8, 279-302.

Udomsangpetch, R., Troye-Blomberg, M., Brown, A. E., Thaithong, S., Perlmann, P. and Webster, H. K. (1994). Lymphocyte responses to Plasmodium falciparum ring-infected erythrocyte surface antigen (Pf155/RESA) peptides in individuals with naturally acquired Plasmodium falciparum malaria. *Am. J. Trop. Med. Hyg.* 50, 465-71.

Vannaphan, S., Saengnetswang, T., Suwanakut, P., Kllangbuakong, A., Klinnak, W., Rungmatcha, P., Yeamput, C., Tanachartwet, W., Krudsood, S. and Looareesuwan, S. (2005). The epidemiology of patients with severe malaria who died at the Hospital for Tropical Diseases, 1991-2004. *Southeast Asian J. Trop. Med. Public Health* 36, 385-9.

Wahlin, B., Wahlgren, M., Perlmann, H., Berzins, K., Bjorkman, A., Patarroyo, M. E. and Perlmann, P. (1984). Human antibodies to a Mr 155,000 Plasmodium falciparum antigen efficiently inhibit merozoite invasion. *Proc. Natl. Acad. Sci. U S A* 81, 7912-6.

Webster, H. K., Boudreau, E. F., Pang, L. W., Permpanich, B., Sookto, P. and Wirtz, R. A. (1987). Development of immunity in natural Plasmodium falciparum malaria: antibodies to the falciparum sporozoite vaccine 1 antigen (R32tet32). *J. Clin. Microbiol.* 25, 1002-8.

Webster, H. K., Brown, A. E., Chuenchitra, C., Permpanich, B. and Pipithkul, J. (1988). Characterization of antibodies to sporozoites in Plasmodium falciparum malaria and correlation with protection. *J. Clin. Microbiol.* 26, 923-7.

Webster, H. K., Gingrich, J. B., Wongsrichanalai, C., Tulyayon, S., Suvarnamani, A., Sookto, P. and Permpanich, B. (1992). Circumsporozoite antibody as a serologic marker of Plasmodium falciparum transmission. *Am. J. Trop. Med. Hyg.* 47, 489-97.

Wongsrichanalai, C., Webster, H. K., Permpanich, B., Chuanak, N. and Ketrangsri, S. (1991). Naturally acquired circumsporozoite antibodies and their role in protection in endemic falciparum and vivax malaria. *Am. J. Trop. Med. Hyg.* 44, 201-4.

World Health Organization Organization. (2000). Severe and complicated malaria. *Trans. R. Soc. Trop. Med. Hyg.* 94 (Suppl.), 51-90.

In: Malaria: Etiology, Pathogenesis and Treatments
Editors: A. M. Peterson et al, pp. 247-253
ISBN: 978-1-62100-363-2

Chapter XI

The 5th Species Malaria in Human Beings

Viroj Wiwanitkit
Wiwanitkit House, Bangkhae, Bangkok Thailand; visiting professor, Hainan Medical University, China.

Abstract

Malaria is a classical tropical infection. This disease has been known for hundred years. However, it is still the public health problem worldwide. Basically, there are 4 well-known malaria parasite species that cause disease in human beings. However, within the past few years, the newest fifth species was reported. There are many reports on the fifth species of malaria in the present day. In this brief article, the author briefly reviews and presents details of the fifth species malaria.

Introduction

Malaria is a classical tropical mosquito borne infection. This disease has been known for hundred years. Classically, the disease is described as an acute febrile illness with predominant chilling presentation. Malaria can be serious and result in death. It is the disease of the tropical world. Millions of people living in developing countries take risk for getting malaria. Hence, malaria is still the public health problem worldwide.

Microbiologically, malaria is classified as a parasitic disease. The blood parasite in the species of Plasmodium is the pathogen. This is a single cell protozoa that lives in host red blood cell. It is one of the two most common red blood cell parasites (malaria and babesia) that cause infection to many people around the world annually.

Basically, there are 4 well-known malaria parasite species that cause disease in human beings. Those four species are vivax, malariae, ovale and falciparum malaria. However, within the past few years, the newest fifth species was reported. There are many reports on the fifth species of malaria in the present day. In this brief article, the author briefly reviews and presents details of the fifth species malaria.

Discovery of the 5th Species Malaria

The 5th species malaria is an actual new emerging infectious disease. It has just been discovered for a few years. The fifth species of human malaria is *Plasmodium knowlesi*. The first case of this new emerging in infection was reported from Malaysia. It was firstly detected in Borneo Island. After that there are many newly identified cases in nearby area, in particular in the states of Sarawak and Sabah (Malaysian Borneo), and in the Pahang region (peninsular Malaysia) [1]. It is confirmed that the anopheles is the mosquito vector of this new malaria [2]. Focusing on the transmission, it is presently confirmed that it is a zoonosis. Southeast Asian macaques are hosts [3]. The nature of this malaria is very similar to the classical malaria. Singh et al. found that vivax and knowlesi malaria use the Duffy antigen as a receptor to invade human erythrocytes [4 - 5]. By nature, this infection can be fatal and is very difficult in diagnosis [6]. Since this new malaria is morphologically similar to *P. malariae* hence it required molecular diagnosis [6]. Of interest, in a Malaysia report in Lancet, Singh et al reported that "Naturally acquired *P knowlesi* infections, misdiagnosed by microscopy mainly as *P malariae*, accounted for over half of all malaria cases in our study [7]."

For the reason why the monkey malaria jumps across species to human beings, there are many explanations. First, human beings and monkey are very close in phylogenetic consideration. Infection in monkey might cross to human beings. Indeed, many viral diseases including to human immunodeficiency virus is believed to start from monkey. Second, close contact between human beings and monkeys might stimulate the chance for crossing species of the parasite. The close contact between human beings and monkey as pets can be seen in some areas of the world. In Southeast Asia, monkey shows and training schools are available. Thousands of local people have monkeys in their houses.

Endemic Area of he 5th Species Malaria

The endemic area of the 5th species malaria is the tropical world. However, most of the identified cases are from Southeast Asia. There are many factors determining this observation.

1. Southeast Asia is the tropical area.
2. The mosquito vector, anopheles, can be seen in Southeast Asia. Since there are still forests in this area, good habitat for the mosquito vectors can be available.
3. The parasite is believed to circulate mainly within this area.
4. The zoonosis pattern via the monkey is an important determinant the prevalence in human beings. Based on the epidemiological triad, there are three factors to be fulfilled for developing of a disease, human beings or host, agent and environment. In this scenario, human beings and agent live at the same place and same time. The

important environmental determinant is the fact that the monkey, the animal in the zoonosis chain, also live in the same area. Also, many Southeast Asian people, coconut gardeners, feed monkeys in the families as pets for coconut farm work.

5.Since the first case of the 5th species malaria is identified in Southeast Asia, the practitioners in this area might have more concern on this new disease than the others in other parts of the world. At least, many new techniques in malariology are developed in Southeast Asia. It can be said that there are many experts on malaria in Southeast Asia.

It is expected that the 5th species malaria can be seen in other area of the world if all conditions are fulfilled. Indeed, mosquito vectors can be seen in many areas of the world but the monkey might be not available. In cases that there are monkeys, the local people might not live closely to the monkey as seen in case of Southeast Asia.

Case Reports on the 5th Species Malaria

After the first identification of the fifth species malaria in Malaysian Borneo, there are continuous sporadic reported cases. First, many cases are reported from Malaysia [1]. Vythilingam et al. concluded that human knowlesi malaria was occurring in most states of peninsular Malaysia and the main vector was monkey [8].

Focusing on the human cases outside Malaysia, there are many interesting reports.

A. In Asia

1. Thailand

Thailand is a country next to Malaysia. In the Southern Region of Thailand, the culture of local people is very similar to that of the Malaysia. In addition, the climate is very similar. The monkeys can be seen in this area as well. For sure, there are some case reports of knowlesi malaria in Thailand [9]. The first case was reported by Jongwutiwes et al. in 2004 [9]. Putaporntip et al. concluded that 0.57 % of human malaria in Thailand was due to knowlesi malaria [10].

2. Vietnam

Vietnam is another member of Southeast Asian countries. It was reported that knowlesi malaria can be found in central Vietnam [11 - 12]. Of interest, asymptomatic knowlesi malaria infections can also be detected [13].

3. Singapore

Singapore is a small modern island country in Southeast Asia. It lies next to Malaysia. The first case report was a soldier who had undergone training in a forested area in 2007 [14]. Wihtin 2007, there were overall 3 cases of this newly emerged disease in Singapore [15]. However, Jeslyn et al. reported that "the risk of acquiring *P. knowlesi* infection among the general population of Singapore is small as evident from the absence of *P. knowlesi* in peri-domestic monkeys [14]."

4. The Philippines

The Philippines is another tropical island country in Southeast Asia. The new malaria can also be seen in this country. In 2008, the first five cases were reported [16].

5. Myanmar

Although there are limited scientific report from Myanmar there is an interesting report describing that "More than 20% of patients with malaria had *P. knowlesi* infection, which occurred predominantly as a co-infection with either P. falciparum or *P. vivax* [17]."

B. In Europe

1. Spain

There is a case report on knowlesi malaria in traveller [18]. The original site of infection is Malaysia Borneo [18].

2. The Netherlands

The first reported was published by van Hellemond et al [19]. This case is a Malaysian migrant worker [19].

3. Finland

The first reported was published by Kantele et al [20 - 21]. This case is a case of Finnish traveller who visited Malaysia [20 - 21].

4. Sweden

The first reported was published by Bronner et al [22]. This case is a case of Swedish traveller who visited Malaysia [22].

C. USA

The first reported was reported in 2008 [23]. This first case is a traveller to Southeast Asia [23].

Clinical Features of the 5th Species Malaria

The 5th species malaria is a kind of malaria hence the nature of malaria can be seen. The common natures include acute febrile illness, parasitic disease, red blood cell infection and serious. The fever spikes comes at 1-day intervals [1,2, 24]. It is usually misdiagnosed by clinical microscopic evaluation as *P. malariae* in the early phase of the disease [1,2, 24]. Without treatment a serious outcome and fatality can be seen [1,2, 24]. In those serious infection, as high fatality as that of *P. falciparum* infection can be seen. Focusing on treatment, chloroquine can be used in light infections [1,2, 24]. Interesting, more than 90 % of the infection is mild and can use the light infection regimen [25]. However, in serious cases, parenteral therapy with artesunate or quinine is recommended [1,2, 24]. It is interesting that there is no difference in treatment between the new malaria and the others. Hence, this might be the fact that this infection is not discovered for a long time. Wilairatana et al. proposed that "Even with a wrong diagnosis of another malaria species by light microscopy instead of P. knowlesi, the antimalarial drugs given are still effective for treating *P. knowlesi* infection [26]." The prevention is not only mosquito prevention but also avoidance of monkey contact.

Some Facts about the Diagnosis of the 5th Species Malaria

Of interest, there is a question how the actual prevalence of the 5th species malaria in human beings is. Although there is no systematic assessment on the prevalence and there are only case reports in the literature the exact prevalence of the 5th species malaria in human beings might be high. There are many reasons as:

1. The diagnosis of malaria in endemic area is usually based on microscopic diagnosis. This is very difficult to differentiate the new malaria from the old classical malaria species. For sure, many cases can be misdiagnosed to be the classical malaria.
2. The nature of disease is zoonosis. Hence, the simple method for prevention of malaria via mosquito control cannot be successfully implemented for prevention of the new malaria at present.
3. Due to the lack of knowledge and concern among local physician in the endemic area, infected cases can be under diagnosed.

Hence, it is required to promote the knowledge on the 5th species malaria in human beings to the general practitioners. At least, general practitioners in the endemic area have to know the existence of this new disease. In addition, the laboratory technician should also be taught for the natural history and laboratory picture of this new disease. This might help improve the detect of the disease in clinical practice.

Conclusion

The 5th species malaria in human beings is an actual emerging disease that needs urgent concern. This disease is considered zoonosis .There are sporadic reported cases in Asia. It is believed that the actual prevalence of this disease might be high but most cases are misdiagnosed.

References

[1] Sabbatani S, Fiorino S, Manfredi R. The emerging of the fifth malaria parasite (Plasmodium knowlesi): a public health concern? *Braz. J. Infect. Dis*. 2010 May-Jun;14(3):299-309.

[2] Vythilingam I, Tan CH, Asmad M, Chan ST, Lee KS, Singh B.Natural transmission of Plasmodium knowlesi to humans by Anopheles latens in Sarawak, Malaysia. *Trans. R. Soc. Trop. Med. Hyg*. 2006 Nov;100(11):1087-8.

[3] Huang Y, Yang Z, Putaporntip C, Miao M, Wei H, Zou C, Jongwutiwes S, Cui L. Isolation and identification of a South China strain of Plasmodium inui from Macaca fascicularis. *Vet. Parasitol*. 2011 Feb 28;176(1):9-15.

[4] Singh SK, Singh AP, Pandey S, Yazdani SS, Chitnis CE, Sharma A. Definition of structural elements in Plasmodium vivax and P. knowlesi Duffy-binding domains necessary for erythrocyte invasion. *Biochem. J*. 2003 Aug 15;374(Pt 1):193-8.

[5] Singh AP, Puri SK, Chitnis CE. Antibodies raised against receptor-binding domain of Plasmodium knowlesi Duffy binding protein inhibit erythrocyte invasion. *Mol. Biochem. Parasitol*. 2002 Apr 30;121(1):21-31.

[6] Cox-Singh J, Singh B. Knowlesi malaria: newly emergent and of public health importance? *Trends Parasitol*. 2008 Sep;24(9):406-10.

[7] Singh B, Kim Sung L, Matusop A, Radhakrishnan A, Shamsul SS, Cox-Singh J, Thomas A, Conway DJ. A large focus of naturally acquired Plasmodium knowlesi infections in human beings. *Lancet*. 2004 Mar 27;363(9414):1017-24.

[8] Vythilingam I, Noorazian YM, Huat TC, Jiram AI, Yusri YM, Azahari AH, Norparina I, Noorrain A, Lokmanhakim S. Plasmodium knowlesi in humans, macaques and mosquitoes in peninsular Malaysia. *Parasit Vectors*. 2008 Aug 19;1(1):26.

[9] Jongwutiwes S, Putaporntip C, Iwasaki T, Sata T, Kanbara H. Naturally acquired Plasmodium knowlesi malaria in human, Thailand. *Emerg. Infect. Dis*. 2004 Dec;10(12):2211-3.

[10] Putaporntip C, Hongsrimuang T, Seethamchai S, Kobasa T, Limkittikul K, Cui L, Jongwutiwes S. Differential prevalence of Plasmodium infections and cryptic Plasmodium knowlesi malaria in humans in Thailand. *J. Infect. Dis*. 2009 Apr 15;199(8):1143-50.

[11] Van den Eede P, Van HN, Van Overmeir C, Vythilingam I, Duc TN, Hung le X, Manh HN, Anné J, D'Alessandro U, Erhart A. Human Plasmodium knowlesi infections in young children in central Vietnam. *Malar. J*. 2009 Oct 30;8:249.

[12] Cox-Singh J. Knowlesi malaria in Vietnam. *Malar. J*. 2009 Nov 26;8:269.

[13] Van den Eede P, Vythilingam I, Ngo DT, Nguyen VH, Le XH, D'Alessandro U, Erhart A. Plasmodium knowlesi malaria in Vietnam: some clarifications. *Malar. J*. 2010 Jan 18;9:20.

[14] Jeslyn WP, Huat TC, Vernon L, Irene LM, Sung LK, Jarrod LP, Singh B, Ching NL. Molecular Epidemiological Investigation of Plasmodium knowlesi in Humans and Macaques in Singapore. *Vector Borne Zoonotic Dis*. 2011 Feb;11(2):131-5

[15] Lee YC, Tang CS, Ang LW, Han HK, James L, Goh KT. Epidemiological characteristics of imported and locally-acquired malaria in Singapore. *Ann. Acad. Med. Singapore*. 2009 Oct;38(10):840-9.

[16] Luchavez J, Espino F, Curameng P, Espina R, Bell D, Chiodini P, Nolder D, Sutherland C, Lee KS, Singh B. Human Infections with Plasmodium knowlesi, the Philippines. *Emerg .Infect. Dis*. 2008 May;14(5):811-3.

[17] Jiang N, Chang Q, Sun X, Lu H, Yin J, Zhang Z, Wahlgren M, Chen Q. Co-infections with Plasmodium knowlesi and other malaria parasites, Myanmar. *Emerg. Infect. Dis.* 2010 Sep;16(9):1476-8.

[18] Ta TT, Salas A, Ali-Tammam M, Martínez Mdel C, Lanza M, Arroyo E, Rubio JM. First case of detection of Plasmodium knowlesi in Spain by Real Time PCR in a traveller from Southeast Asia. *Malar. J.* 2010 Jul 27;9:219.

[19] van Hellemond JJ, Rutten M, Koelewijn R, Zeeman AM, Verweij JJ, Wismans PJ, Kocken CH, van Genderen PJ. Human Plasmodium knowlesi infection detected by rapid diagnostic tests for malaria. *Emerg. Infect. Dis*. 2009 Sep;15(9):1478-80.

[20] Kantele A, Jokiranta S. Plasmodium knowlesi--the fifth species causing human malaria. *Duodecim.* 2010;126(4):427-34.

[21] Kantele A, Marti H, Felger I, Müller D, Jokiranta TS. Monkey malaria in a European traveler returning from Malaysia. *Emerg. Infect. Dis.* 2008 Sep;14(9):1434-6.

[22] Bronner U, Divis PC, Färnert A, Singh B. Swedish traveller with Plasmodium knowlesi malaria after visiting Malaysian Borneo. *Malar. J.* 2009 Jan 16;8:15.

[23] Mali S, Steele S, Slutsker L, Arguin PM; Centers for Disease Control and Prevention (CDC). Malaria surveillance - United States, 2008. *MMWR Surveill. Summ.* 2010 Jun 25;59(7):1-15

[24] Myrvang B. A fifth plasmodium that can cause malaria. *Tidsskr. Nor. Laegeforen.* 2010 Feb 11;130(3):282-3.

[25] Daneshvar C, Davis TM, Cox-Singh J, Rafa'ee MZ, Zakaria SK, Divis PC, Singh B. Clinical and laboratory features of human Plasmodium knowlesi infection. *Clin. Infect. Dis.* 2009 Sep 15;49(6):852-60.

[26] Wilairatanal P, Krudsood S, Tangpukdee N. Management of Plasmodium knowlesi malaria without PCR confirmation. *Southeast Asian J. Trop. Med. Public Health.* 2010 Jan;41(1):19-21.

In: Malaria: Etiology, Pathogenesis and Treatments
Editors: A. M. Peterson et al, pp. 255-319
ISBN: 978-1-62100-363-2

Chapter XII

The Aetiology, Pathophysiology, Clinical Features and Some Treatment Options of Malaria Fever

Kwabena Nsiah
Department of Biochemistry and Biotechnology, KNUST, Kumasi, Ghana.

Abstract

Malaria fever, caused by four species of Plasmodium, is one of the commonest parasitic diseases plaguing mankind, particularly in the malaria-endemic regions of the world. The most widespread and virulent of the infection is caused by *Plasmodium falciparum*, which is known to affect millions of people annually.This write-up, a compilation of extracts of publications from especially, journals, and books, looks at how the infective protozoan has exploited the use of two hosts, mosquito and man, and while in man, the protozoan's ability to survive in different asexual forms; as hepatic sporozoites and erythrocyte merozoites. Exhibiting structural, biochemical and physiological features of typical Acomplexans, the sporozoites are able to attach to and breach membranes in their invasive journey through the insect-vertebrate hosts. The role of rhoptries and micronemes in the proper orientation of the sporozoite, as well as the further facilitation of the invasion by circumsporozoite protein (CSP) and thrombospondin-related anonymous protein (TRAP) is considered. Both CSP and TRAP are possible candidate proteins for the development of anti-malarial vaccines. While inside the erythrocytes (parasitized erythrocytes), the survival of the parasites depends on their utilization of the host's haemoglobin, which they need to hydrolyse, using a battery of proteases (plasmepsins, falcipain and metalloprotease, falcilysin), followed by detoxification to form haemozoin, the malarial pigment, a biocrystal. The formation of the haemozoin can be the target of attack of some anti-malarial therapies. The parasitisation of the erythrocytes is an adaptive survival strategy for the intruding protozoan, but to the host, it is the harbinger of various pathologies that culminate in a wide array of clinical features attributable to multi-organ failure and even death. Inside the parasitized erythrocytes, some parasite proteins or antigens are secreted to the surface of the erythrocyte membrane. The best characterized of these parasite proteins is PfEMP-

1, a family of proteins encoded by the 'var' genes because each parasite contains many copies of the gene; and by switching expression between the copies, it is able to cause a remarkable degree of antigenic variation, a major ploy for survival. PfEMP-1 plays a key role in the parasite's ability to sequester in the microvasculature of the infected person, and to form rosettes with uninfected erythrocytes. The PfEMP-1 can also bind to a variety of host cell receptors, including CD 36, vCAM, P-selectin, etc. The severity of falciparum infection depends largely on the ability of parasitized erythrocytes to adhere to endothelial cells (ECs) and thus getting sequestered in the capillary network of vital organs such as brain, kidney, lungs and liver. Additionally, adhesion of the parasitised red cells to the ECs causes the activation of ECs, resulting in the over-expression of adhesive molecules and pro-inflammatory cytokines. The pathology of the infection could be ascribed to 'hyperadhesion', and could also be explained based on either the 'mechanical hypothesis', due to hypofusion of tissues, or 'cytokine hypothesis.' The most common complication of falciparum infection is anaemia, in which there could be ineffective erythropoiesis and dyserythropoiesis. Other clinical features are hepatic, renal and pulmonary dysfunctions and cerebral malaria. Attempts at using drugs to break the blood-stage life cycle target some important metabolic processes required for the survival of the parasite. The author and colleagues have shown that in sickle cell anaemia patients with falciparum parasites, the distribution of the reticulocytes is exponential, but in the non-parasitaemic, the distribution is polynomial.

Introduction

Malaria is one of the diseases with the greatest impact on public health worldwide, with around 500 million people suffering the disease and 2-3 million dying each year, especially children under five years in Sub-Saharan Africa (Snow et al, 2005). Malaria primarily affects poor populations in tropical and sub-tropical areas, where the temperature and rainfall are most suitable for the development of the insect vector, Anopheles mosquito (Greenwood et al., 2008).

Due to the high prevalence of malaria in sub-Saharan Africa and parts of Oceania, the relative risks of malaria among travellers are 207.6 and 76.7, respectively (Freedman, 2008). Thus even in the developed world, where the spread of malaria infection has been eliminated, because of travels to endemic areas, there is the problem of imported malaria. International travel permits the importation of *P. falciparum* into countries where the parasite is not endemic. Of the 25–30 million travelers who visit malaria-endemic countries annually, approximately 10,000 return with malaria, often caused by *P. falciparum* (*Muentener et al., 1999; Louton, 2003)*. In the United States, most cases of imported malaria are caused by failure to take appropriate chemoprophylaxis (*Skarbinski et al, 2006)*. There are up to 2000 cases of malaria and 10–20 deaths in the UK each year, making malaria the single most common imported infection among travelers (Smith et al., 2008). However, these figures may seem trivial when set against the global scale of disease, reflected in the 'two worlds of malaria' i.e. in travelers and those living in endemic areas (Wellems and Miller, 2003).

The number of cases of malaria worldwide appears to be growing because of the increasing risk of transmission in areas where malaria control has declined (e.g. India), increasing prevalence of drug-resistant strains of parasites (e.g. chloroquine resistance) and in a relatively few cases, because of increasing international travel (Pasvol, 2005).

Human malaria is caused by one of four Plasmodium species, namely, *P falciparum, P. vivax, P. ovale and P. malariae* (Marsh et al, 1995). Plasmodium parasites are apicomplexans as they belong to the Apicomplexa sub-phylum, characterized by an apical complex of rhoptries, micronemes, dense granules and other organelles specialized for the invasion of host cells (Rogers et al, 1992). All the species of Plasmodium share a general life cycle that alternates between a human host and an insect vector, but they differ by the length of their life cycle, their erythrocyte preferences and their virulence potentiality (Barsoum, 1998). In *P. vivax* malaria, young red blood cells are mainly infected, in *P. malariae*, to the very oldest (McKenzie *et al*, 2001) but in *P. falciparum*, RBCs of all ages are affected, so the infective load and severity of infection are most in the case of *P. falciparum* (Weatherall *et al*, 2002). These age constraints explain why counts of parasitized red cells rarely exceed 25,000 per microlitre with *P. vivax, P. malariae* and *P. ovale*, but may reach 500,000 and beyond with *P. falciparum*, and this partly explains why fatal anaemia occurs in *P. falciparum* infection (Krogstad, 1995). Almost all deaths world-wide are caused by *P. falciparum*, although occasionally, patients die from enlarged spleen during infection with other Plasmodium species (Yagmur *et al*, 2000). *Plasmodium knowlesi* is a fifth species known to cause malaria in man (Cox-Singh et al, 2008).

These five species of malaria parasites are now known to affect humans and differ in their geographic distribution; *Plasmodium falciparum* most common in sub-Saharan Africa and Melanesia (Papua New Guinea and the Solomon Islands); *P. vivax* found mainly in Central and South America, North Africa, the Middle East and within the Indian subcontinent; *P. ovale* found almost exclusively in West Africa; *P. malariae* occurring worldwide, although mainly in Africa and finally *P. knowlesi*, recently documented on the island of Borneo and other parts of Southeast Asia (Cox-Singh et al., 2008).

Because the *Anopheles* mosquito feeds between dusk and dawn, taking proper precautions at this time of day is important. Wearing clothing to cover exposed skin, application of insect repellent-containing DEET (N,N-diethyl-3-methylbenzamide), in concentrations of 20% to 50%, and sleeping in mosquito-proof tents or homes and using bed nets with or without permethrin (an insecticide) all will reduce the risk of contracting malaria (CDC, 2003). Thus, malaria can be prevented by a combination of mosquito-avoidance measures (e.g., mosquito netting, insect repellents, coils and sprays) and chemoprophylactic agents (Boggild et al., 2009).

Though malaria is transmitted predominantly via the bite of female *Anopheles* mosquitos, it can also be transmitted via blood transfusion or organ transplant and through the placenta (Thewing et al., 2007). Other modes of transmission are through bone marrow transplantation, needle stick injuries, and increasingly by the introduction of infected vectors on aircraft (*Muentener, 1999)*. The last named route is called airport malaria, first reported in Europe in 1977 (Rizzo et al., 1989).

The life cycle of *Plasmodium falciparum* is made up of a non-pathogenic, symptomless hepatocytic or pre-erythrocytic stage, followed by a pathogenic red blood cell stage. The parasites show some structural, biochemical and functional adaptive features, which have ensured their continuous survival, despite efforts to get them controlled or eliminated. Features like their complex life cycle in insect-vertebrate hosts, ability to target specific tissues/cells, possession of var genes, expression of various parasite proteins and ability to evade the host immune surveillance, apparently work to the advantage of the parasite.

The variable nature of one of the major parasite proteins, PfEMP1 appears to be in tune with the parasite's strategy of evading the host's immune surveillance, by presenting variable antigenic determinants. These parasite-derived molecules of the red blood cell surface are themselves targets for immunological attack, which the parasites counter with extraordinary capacity for antigenic variation (Kwiatkowski, 2005). By being expressed on the surface of the infected red cells, where they bind to host receptors, sequestering the infected cells, they are protected from spleen-mediated destruction (Kraemer and Smith, 2006).

The retention of the sporozoites in the hepatic sinusoids is possibly mediated by the surface proteins, CSP and TRAP. TRAP is the other protein secreted during gliding in the liver cells (Buscaglia et al, 2003). It belongs to a family of functionally homologous proteins involved in parasite mobility and cell penetration (Kappe et al., 1999).The histidine-rich proteins (HRPs) are also secreted by the parasite; examples are HRP1 and HRP2. HRP1 is one of the major protein components of 'knobs', which are electron-dense structures protruding from the host red cell membrane, important for adhesion of infected red cells (Oh et al, 1997). On the other hand, HRP2 has been implicated as a haem polymerase (Sullivan et al., 1996) that catalyses the formation of haemozoin, the malarial pigment (Choi et al., 1999).

The food vacuole, an equivalent of a mammalian lysosome, is an important organelle of the Plasmodium, formed as some cytoplasmic contents of red cells, especially, haemoglobin, are internalized by the parasite (Goodyear et al, 1997). Within the food vacuole, the malarial parasites need to break down haemoglobin to make room to grow, aside from deriving nutritional benefit (Kwiatkowski, 2005).

A battery of parasitic proteases are known to be involved in the breakdown of haemoglobin; two homologous aspartic proteases, plasmepsin I and II, a cysteine protease, falcipain-2 and a metalloprotease, falcilysin (Rosenthal et al, 1988; Goldberg et al, 1991; Goldberg, 1993). However, the parasite is unable to catabolise the haem liberated (Francis et al, 1997). To protect the parasite membrane against the toxic effects of free haem, this by-product, released from the digested haemoglobin, is detoxified by its polymerization and sequestration as an inert crystalline deposit, called haemozoin (Slater et al, 1991). Both haemoglobin breakdown and detoxification are essential features of parasite biology (Liu et al. 2006). Blocking either process is lethal to the parasite, and can be a therapeutic target against the parasite (Elliot et al, 2008).

Definitely, the parasite is recognized as foreign by the human host, so the appropriate immune response is evoked. There is the more rapid but less specific innate immunity, which is the body's first line of defence, potentially controlling microbes at an early stage by inducing inflammation and fever (Schumann, 2007). When the innate mechanism fails or proves inadequate, then the adaptive or specific immune response, which is slower and time-dependent, becomes operational. When the adaptive immune response is either immature or compromised, the innate immune system constitutes the main defence against infection (Eisen & Michinton, 2003). Antibody formation is an important part of the host adaptive immune response against malaria (Perlmann et al, 1998). Parasite proliferation is associated with the generation of soluble plasmodial antigens (Camus and Hadley, 1985). These antigens may be available for binding by reactive antibodies to form immune complexes, ICs (Mohammed, 1982). ICs can activate complement cascade and stimulate macrophages to produce pro-inflammatory cytokines (Jarvis et al, 1997).

Protective immunity towards malaria develops only after repeated exposure to the falciparum parasite, and it is known to be partly dependent on antibodies towards the variable antigens present at the surface of the infected red cells.

In areas where malaria is holoendemic, people are continuosly infected with the parasite, but the majority of infected adults rarely experience overt disease (Boutlis et al, 2006). People in such areas who experience repeated malaria infections develop a degree of immunity that confers some protection from clinical disease (Marsh, 2002).

Clinical malaria is characterized by high levels of circulating pro-inflammatory cytokines, which are thought to contribute to immunopathy (McCall et al, 2007). The balance between pro- and anti-inflammatory responses is considered critical, for clinical protection. Too little activation of the innate response, results in uninhibited parasite growth, whereas too much activation may cause immunopathy (McCall et al., 2007).

The innate immune response initiates and thus sets the threshold for the immune responses. Toll-like receptors are key receptors involved in the initial activation of the innate immune system, together with other immune signaling pathways, like mannose-binding lectin (MBL), a calcium-dependent (C-type) serum lectin that also plays a significant role in innate immune response. MBL binds microbial surface carbohydrates and mediates opsonophagocytosis directly, or by activation of the lectin complement pathway (Eisen et al, 2003).

Much of the overactive immune responses result from activation of innate immune receptors, such as Toll-like receptors (TLRs), which are critical for pro-inflammatory cytokine production during microbial infection. It is still uncertain which malaria molecule is responsible for activating cytokine production in immune cells. Two proposed molecules are glycosylphosphatidylinositol (GPI) anchor and parasite-derived DNA, bound to haemozoin. These putative 'malarial toxins' have been shown to activate TLR2 and TLR9 respectively (Parroche et al, 2007).

For example, *Plasmodium falciparum* GPI, which is released upon schizont rupture, signals through TLR2 and TLR4 on monocytes to induce TNF production (Zhu et al, 2005). While TNF is known to control parasitaemia, it also induces fever during malaria episodes, and may aggravate cerebral malaria by up-regulating the expression of ICAM-1 and other leucocyte adhesion receptors or brain microvascular endothelial cells (Armah et al, 2005).

To reinforce or supplement the immune response to microbial infections is the genetic make-up of individuals, interacting with some factors in the same environment which sustains and/or promotes the spread of the microbes. The close geographical association between the distribution of malaria and the sickle cell gene supports this concept (Allison et al, 1954). There is therefore, this phenomenon of balanced polymorphism, for which the key exponents were Haldane (1949), Raper (1949), Allison (1957) and Friedman (1970). An individual homozygous for the qualitative structural β^S-haemoglobinopathy, HbS, shows the red cell sickling pathology with its attendant vaso-occlusive crises and plethora of complications. On the other extreme, persons with the wild type haemoglobin, HbAA, never experience any sickling, but such individuals are at the mercy of the ravages of malaria fever. Persons with the sickle cell trait, generally, do not experience sickling; neither do they suffer from serious clinical forms of malaria, though they can be infected. With such a heterozygote advantage, the sickling allele seems to have been preserved in a 'malaria-accommodating' tropical environment.

Reasons given for the heterozygote advantage include selective sickling of parasitized erythrocytes (Luzzato et al, 1970), resulting in their more effective removal by the reticuloendothelial system, inhibition of parasite growth by loss of potassium ions, the lower pH of sickled cells, increased oxidant stress (Friedman et al, 1979) and the greater adherence of the infected red cells to endothelial cells (Kaul et al, 1994).

In addition to the red cell variants, several polymorphisms of mediators of innate immune response have been shown to protect against, or alternatively, predispose to malaria; e.g. mannose-binding lectin, inducible nitric oxide synthase, TNF-α, and interferon receptors (Luty et al, 1998; Cramer et al, 2004).

Three primary pathophysiological events; namely, red blood cell destruction, adhesion of infected RBCs to the capillary veins, especially in the central nervous system, and excessive inflammatory response, underpin the pathophysiology of malaria fever. Plasmodia can be found in the microvasulature of any organ of the host (Udomsangpatch et al, 1997), which reflects the systemic nature of *P. falciparum* malaria. The severity of P. falciparum infection depends largely on the ability of the parasitized red cells to adhere on ECs and sequester in the capillary network of vital organs (eg. brain, lungs, kidneys, liver (van den Heyde et al, 2006).

Two hypotheses for the pathogenesis of malaria have been delineated; the mechanical and cytokine hypotheses (Clark et al, 2006). The roles of cytoadherence, sequestration and rosetting in malaria pathogenesis, as well as the various clinical expressions, are discussed. Possible clinical states are asymptomatic parasitaemia, uncomplicated malaria, then, progressing from mild to severe malaria. Clinical presentations, therefore, range from asymptomatic to multi-organ failure manifestations and death, depending on the following; host factors (age, immunity), parasite factor (plasmodia species) and the geographic location (eg. inoculation rate) (Helbok et al, 2005).

The 2006 treatment guidelines of the WHO list cerebral malaria, metabolic acidosis, severe anemia, and hypoglycemia to be the key common features, together with renal failure and acute pulmonary oedema in adults (WHO, 2006).This report recognizes that the disease manifestation may be different in areas of unstable malaria in much of Asia and Latin America and the remaining parts of the world where malaria is endemic (WHO, 2006).

Malaria in pregnancy is also of importance, by way of its unique pathophysiological processes, together with its exertion of a 'double toll' on the gestating woman and the developing foetus. Of much significance is the sequestration of parasitized erythrocytes to the placenta surface through interactions between PfEMP1 domains and chondroitin sulphate A (Fried and Duffy, 1996; Hviid and Salanti, 2007).

Anaemia, being the most common complication of *P. falciparum* infection (Abdalla *et al*, 1980; Phillips and Pasvol, 1992), is accorded a relatively wide coverage, with respect to the various causes and the consequences.

Due to the morbidities and mortalities associated with malaria, there is global effort to combat the menace posed by the disease and its mosquito vector. Particularly, for the containment of the liver and blood stage parasite forms, various drugs have been used or are being used, with the most potent ones, being of plant origin; eg. quinine, from cinchona plant, and artemisin, from *Artemesia annua*..So far, drugs which have been proven to be effective are those that target some points in the metabolic pathway of the parasite; haemoglobin degradation, heme detoxification, folate biosynthesis and protein synthesis in the parasite apicoplast (Fidock et al, 2004).

The problem of drug resistance to conventional therapies is so huge that it continues to hamper scientific effort of controlling malaria. However, vaccine development offers a viable window of hope, not only for the control, but for the elimination. Unfortunately, the complexity of the malaria parasite, coupled with the lack of evidence of robust infection-induced immunity, has made vaccine development especially difficult. To date, the closest the scientific community has come in looking for an innocuous but effective vaccine is the development of RTS, S vaccine. This vaccine is in the phase III of clinical trials.

Malaria as a Predominantly Tropical Infectious Disease

Malaria is one of the diseases with the greatest impact on public health worldwide, with around 500 million people suffering the disease and 2-3 million dying each year, especially children under five years in Sub-Saharan Africa (Snow et al, 2005). Malaria primarily affects poor populations in tropical and sub-tropical areas, where the temperature and rainfall are most suitable for the development of the insect vector, Anopheles mosquito (Greenwood et al., 2008).

The data in Table 1 provide some laboratory evidence of the prevalence of malaria, in a university community in Ghana, West Africa. The Clinical Analysis Laboratory is run by the Department of Biochemistry and Biotechnology of the Kwame Nkrumah University of Science and Technology, Kumasi. This laboratory is managed by the Medical

Research group of the Department, led by the author, through whose initiative the place was set up in April 2003. The CAn-Lab is a semi-commercial entity, engaged in the carrying out of medical diagnostic tests. It provides reliable diagnostic tests to its clients, either from the university or the surrounding communities.

Table 1. Common tests carried out in the CAn-Lab in 2008

	Jan	**Feb**	**Mar**	**Apr**	**May**	**Jun**	**Jul**	**Aug**	**Sept**	**Oct**	**Nov**	**Dec**
Total no of tests	**246**	**246**	**321**	**365**	**312**	**349**	**299**	**313**	**328**	**433**	**369**	**218**
Mps	20.7	23.2	25.9	21.6	21.5	25.8	25.1	18.5	22.3	25.9	13.6	16.5
Widal	15.9	11.4	12.8	12.1	13.5	15.2	13.0	10.2	12.8	13.9	6.8	6.9
FBS	17.5	12.6	10.0	11.8	10.9	8.0	10.0	9.9	8.2	10.2	11.1	15.6
U/sugar	13.0	9.3	10.3	9.0	8.3	7.2	7.7	7.7	5.2	7.9	8.4	14.2
U/RE	4.9	1.6	1.9	3.0	2.9	0.9	1.3	2.6	2.7	3.4	1.6	2.8
Lipid	1.6	2.4	4.0	2.5	2.9	3.2	3.0	4.2	4.0	6.2	6.5	4.6
Preg T	1.2	2.8	2.5	3.8	2.6	1.4	2.3	1.6	1.8	2.3	1.6	0.0

Mps; malarial parasites, **FBS**; fasting blood sugar, **U/sugar**; urine sugar,
U/RE; urine routine examination; **Preg test**; pregnancy test.

Table 1 shows the major tests carried out in 2008. Throughout the year, the test which was most commonly performed was the blood smear test for malaria, followed by Widal test for typhoid, another infectious disease. For the malaria test, the highest percentage was 25.9, recorded for both March and October, and the lowest was 13.6, in November. Even though the clientele of the laboratory is not large (a maximum of twenty per each working day), the data gives a fair representation of the most common ailments that people take to hospitals, in a typical tropical environment, and malaria tops the list.

The Transmission Cycle for Malaria Infection

The life cycle of *Plasmodium falciparum* is made up of a non-pathogenic, symptomless hepatocytic or pre-erythrocytic stage, followed by a pathogenic red blood cell stage (*Ancsin. & Kisilevsky*, 2004; Marti et al., 2005). The infection begins with the bite of an infectious female Anopheline mosquito that introduces sporozoites into the microvasculature (Rathore et al., 2005). Mosquitoes inject parasites (sporozoites) into the subcutaneous tissue and less frequently directly into the bloodstream; from there, sporozoites travel to the liver (Weatherall et al., 2002).

As infected mosquitoes probe for blood, sporozoites are injected into the skin of the mammalian host and actively move by gliding motility within the dermis to contact and penetrate blood vessels to enter the blood circulation (Amino et al., 2006). Exit from the dermal inoculation site requires that sporozoites traverse cell barriers via breaching the plasma membrane of the host cell (Mota et al., 2001), which is a qualitatively different process from cell invasion. Once in the circulation, sporozoites get confined in the liver, cross the sinusoidal barrier, and productively invade hepatocytes within a vacuole, where they develop into exo-erythrocytic forms, which, when mature, release merozoites that initiate blood stage infection (Coppi et al., 2011).

The sporozoites invade liver cells, where they undergo asexual replication to produce thousands of merozoites, which are able to invade red blood cells (Marti et al, 2005). The asexual cycle within the red blood cell takes 44-48 hours, with subsequent bursting of each infected red cell to release 16-32 merozoites, for re-invasion of new cells: associated with this are the periodic recurring waves of fever (Marti et al, 2005).

The erythrocytic cycle begins with the merozoites' recognition, binding and invasion of red blood cells. Inside the red cells, the parasites go through the ring, trophozoite and schizont stages, to form new merozoites, which are liberated, following red cell lysis, so new red cells are infected (Bannister and Mitchell, 2003).

It is also possible for some merozoites to switch from the asexual replication to a sexual phase, by differentiating into male and female gametes, which are transported to the mosquito's stomach as it ingests a human blood meal (James, 2003). While inside the stomach, the parasite undergoes a series of transformations, female and male gametes cross-fertilise into ookinetes, which traverse the wall of the midgut and develop to form oocysts. The mitotic divisions in the oocyst produce thousands of sporozoites that are released as the oocyst breaks up. The sporozoites travel through the haemolymph to the mosquito salivary glands, ready to be inoculated in a human host the mosquito next feeds on (James, 2003).

Some Structural, Biochemical and Functional Adaptive Features Associated with the Infective Agents

Malaria infection is initiated when the insect vector injects Plasmodium sporozoites into a susceptible vertebrate host. The salivary glands of mosquitoes liberate different soluble components, including antihistamines, vasodilators (bradykinnin), anticoagulants (thrombin), platelet aggregation inhibitors and immunomodulators, which facilitate blood ingestion, and thus contributing to sporozoite survival and ensuring their inoculation (Kappe et al, 2004; Baldacci and Manard, 2004).

Although the molecular mechanisms of invasion are not well understood, ultrastructural studies have revealed a distinct set of steps involving parasite attachment, reorientation, and, ultimately, invasion of the host red blood cell (Chitnis and Blackman, 2000). A number of proteins have been implicated in invasion, but in most cases their precise functions remain unknown. Apical membrane antigen 1 (AMA1), expressed in mature stage parasites is thought to be essential for invasion (Peterson, et al, 1989), and this protein is an important vaccine candidate .

All invasive stages of the Apicomplexa show a common structural organization at their anterior pole called the apical complex (Jensen & Edgar, 1978), which includes a group of secretory organelles known as rhoptries, micronemes and dense granules. The invasion of red blood cells by the merozoite begins with the initial attachment of the parasite and its subsequent reorientation such that its apical end is directed towards the erythrocyte. A moving junction is formed and the parasite pulls itself into the cell, where it stays inside a vacuole that is formed by the host plasma membrane *(Chitnis & Blackman, 2000).* In these apicomplexans, parasite ligands for host-cell receptors are required for their invasion. However, many of the adhesins they require are not displayed statically on the surface of the parasite; instead, they are rather stored in the apically located secretory organelles, the micronemes. Constitutive secretion from these organelles is probably sufficient for gliding motility. However, an enhanced microneme secretion is probably required for invasion. This occurs when Plasmodium sporozoites migrate through cells (*Gantt et al, 2000; Mota et al, 2002).*

The invasive stages of the Apicomplexa also exhibit gliding mobility, a form of substrate-dependent cell locomotion, characterized by the absence of locomotory organelles, like cilia or flagella, and by the absence of any obvious change in cell shape during translocation (King, 1988). One such mechanism involves the use of an actin-myosin motor, present in the parasite's own cytoskeleton to generate the motile force that is required to actively propel the parasite into cells (Leiriae et al, 2002).

During the invasion of the liver and the red cells, the parasites become enclosed within an additional membrane layer, the parasitophorous vacuolar membrane, which acts as a semi permeable barrier between parasite and host, allowing nutrient intake and discharge of parasite-derived factors (Marti et al, 2005). Once the parasite has invaded a new host cell, it resides within the parasitophorous vacuole. In the ring stage intraerythrocytic growth, electron microscopy studies have revealed finger-like projections of the parasitophorous vacuole membrane (Elford et al, 1995). Thus, a major feature of the infected red blood cell cytoplasm is the appearance of densely coated saucer-shaped structures, called Maurer's clefts, that are supposed to serve as transit station or sorting depot for proteins *en route* to the red blood cell membrane; for example, the trafficking of some parasite proteins, like *Plasmodium falciparum* erythrocyte membrane protein1 (PfEMP1) and other exported proteins (Cooke et al, 2004). Several parasite proteins have been shown to be localized in the Maurer's cleft. They are synthesized in the parasite endoplasmic reticulum and then transferred to the cleft (Marti et al. 2005). Subsequently they are transported to the erythrocyte surface. For some authors the Maurer's cleft is a well defined structure continuously supplied with vesicles budding off from the membrane lining the parasitophorous vacuole. Subsequently, vesicles bud off from the cleft and migrate towards the erythrocyte cell surface, with secretion of their contents into the medium and incorporation of some proteins in the erythrocyte plasma membrane (van Ooij C & Haldar, 2007). Maurer's clefts are not found in other species of Plasmodium.

At its developmental stage, the surface of malaria sporozoites is covered by a protein called circumsporozoite protein, CSP (Ozaki et al, 1983; Hollingdale et al, 1984; Nussenzweig & Nussenzweig 1989). CSP plays several roles in the parasite's life, from the time of oocyst development in the mosquito, through the development of the exo-erythrocytic merozoites in the liver (Rathore et al, 2005). Some of the biological functions of CSP include maintenance of species specificity during infection (Rathore et al, 2003), facilitating the passage of sporozoites into the salivary gland of the mosquito (Sidjanski et al,1997) attachment and invasion of liver cells (Cerami et al, 1992), and directly inhibiting protein synthesis in the host cells (Frevert et al, 1998).

In all malaria species the CSP shows a similar structural organization, consisting of a variable central region of repeats and two highly conserved motifs, regions I and II, placed at the amino- and carboxyl-terminal ends of the molecule, respectively. Region I is based on a short five-amino acid motif, KLKQP, which is identical in all malaria parasites so far described in mammals (McCutchan et al., 1990). The central repeat region contains an immunodominant B-cell epitope (Herrington et al, 1987), while the C-terminus contains the TSR or T-cell epitope (Nardin et al, 2000). Vaccines against malaria have been developed, based on structural features of CSP (Herrington et al, 1987; Nardin et al, 2000).

Further studies have shown that another sporozoite protein, thrombospondin-related anonymous protein (TRAP (Rogers et al., 1982; Robson et al., 1992), is required for invasion (Sultan et al., 1997). Although a small amount of TRAP is found on the sporozoite surface, it is found most abundantly in secretory vesicles, micronemes (Rogers et al., 1992a). Upon contact with cells, sporozoites release TRAP onto the apical end of the parasite (Gantt et al., 2000).

There is evidence that sporozoite attachment and invasion of hepatocytes requires the malarial CSP and specifically its region II-plus domain (Cerami et al. 1992). It has also been shown that at least, one of the cell surface ligands for CSP is heparan sulphate (*Pinzon-Ortiz* et al., 2001), and there have been a number of studies suggesting that region II-plus (region II, together with eight downstream residues) serves as the actual heparan sulphate binding site (Ying et al., 1997).

Ancsin and Kisilevsky (2004) argue that even though heparan sulphate is found on all cell surfaces and in the extracellular matrix, the liver heparan sulphate must have unique characteristics for it to act as the principal target molecule for CSP. A study by Lyon et al. (1994), on the structure of rat liver heparan sulphate has shown that, compared with heparan sulphate of other organs, it is more extensively modified and highly sulphated. This is in contrast to endothelial cell heparan sulphate, which is among the most undersulphated heparan sulphate in the body (Lindblom & Fransson, 1990).

In vivo, the heparan sulphate proteoglycans on most cells are not exposed to the circulation, since most organs are behind an endothelial cell barrier that does not permit direct contact with the blood circulation. The sinusoidal lining of the liver, however, is highly fenestrated, and these fenestrations are permanently open, allowing for direct contact between the blood circulation and the underlying hepatocytes and space of Disse (the loose basement membrane between hepatocytes and endothelia). *(Ancsin and Kisilevsky*, 2004)

These findings imply that the degree of glycosaminoglycan chain sulphation and the architecture of the liver sinusoids may account for the selective targeting of CSP of sporozoites to the liver. Studies with recombinant CSP peptides representing portions of CSP, and sporozoites expressing heterologous CSP, suggest that this protein targets sporozoites to both the mammalian liver and the mosquito salivary glands *(Cerami et al., 1992; Frevert et al., 1993)*. The co-receptor on sporozoites for invasion involves, in part, the thrombospondin domains on the circumsporozoite protein and on thrombospondin-related anonymous protein (TRAP). It is these domains that bind specifically to heparin sulphate proteoglycans on hepatocytes in the region in apposition to sinusoidal endothelium and Kuppfer cells (Frevert et al., 1993). The TRAP protein interacts with skeletal proteins in malaria sporozoites (Kappes et al., 1999).

The journey of the sporozoites from mosquito midgut to mammalian liver should be completed in order to establish infection. Although several previous studies have demonstrated that CSP has critical roles in many steps of this journey *(Ménard, 2000; Sinnis & Nardin, 2002),* there has been no unifying hypothesis as to how one protein functions in so many disparate events. In a study by Coppi et al (2011), they explained that different conformations of same protein, could confer on them different functional properties. In this regard, CSP was shown to have two conformational states, an adhesive conformation in which the TSR is exposed and a non-adhesive conformation in which the TSR is masked by the N terminus. The TSR-exposed conformation occurs at the two ends of the sporozoite's life, during sporozoite development and hepatocyte invasion. Between these two spatially and temporally distinct events, the N terminus masks the TSR, a conformation which confers a migratory phenotype upon sporozoites. (Coppi et al, 2011). This is supported by the finding that sporozoite mutants in which the N- terminus is deleted adhere throughout the mosquito hemocoel and cannot exit the mammalian dermis, though they are fully infectious when inoculated intravenously.

The mechanism by which hepatic merozoites reach blood vessels in the liver and escape the host immune system before invading red cells remains unknown. Sturm et al (2006) showed that parasites induce the death and detachment of their host's hepatocytes, followed by the budding of parasite-filled vesicles (merosomes) into the sinusoid lumen. The parasites simultaneously inhibit the exposure of phosphatidylcholine onto the outer leaflet of host plasma membrane, which acts as 'eat me'signal to phagocytes. Thus the hepatocyte-derived merosomes appear to ensure both the migration of parasites into the bloodstream and their protection from host immunity (Sturm et al., 2006). These merosomes have been viewed as aggregates of merozoites, released from the hepatocytes to facilitate their evasion of host antibodies, as the merozoites invade the erythrocytes (Greenwood et al., 2008).

Thus, the *P. falciparum*'s ability to invade both mosquito and vertebrate host, has been ascribed to the sporozoites' use of different invasion mechanisms, involving the participation of yet to be identified parasite proteins (Garcia et al, 2006). Such proteins, when identified and studied, could reveal those involved in invasion, and could be used to develop vaccines for controlling or eradicating the disease (Garcia et al, 2006). So far, the disease has been difficult to control because of the very complex nature of the parasite. The complex life cycle of parasites involves several stages, which probably contributes to its ability to evade immune detection (Ancsin and Kisilevsky, 2004).

PfEMP-1, a protein family encoded by a repertoire of around 60 var-genes per genome, appears at the surface of infected red cells during the trophozoite stage, and the parasite can switch between different variants that are exported to the surface of parasitized red cells in order to evade the host's immune system (Kraemer and Smith, 2006). PfEMP1 binds to a variety of target molecules found on red blood cells, platelets and vascular endothelial cells (Sherman et al, 2003).

The structure of PfEMP1 includes a variable number of two types of adhesive binding domains: Duffy-binding-like (DBL) region and cysteine-rich inter-domain regions (Smith et al, 2001). DBL-1α demonstrates lectin-like properties, causing it to bind primarily to cells bearing A and B blood group oligosaccharides, and to other glycosylated targets, such as the glycoprotein, complement receptor 1, CR1 (or CD 35) and heparin sulphate-like glcosylaminoglycan (Chen et al, 2000). Cysteine-rich interdomain region-1 binds principally to CD 36 (platelet glycoprotein IV), thus targeting platelets and the endothelium (Chen et al, 2000). Herman et al. (2003) describes PfEMP1 as having a large, highly variable ectodomains, consisting of the Duffy binding-like, DBL, and cysteine-rich interdomain regions, CIDR), which are known to interact with a number of cellular host receptors such as CD36, ICAM-1. CSA, PECAM, E-selectin, vCAM and others. The N-terminal of the DBL-1α has the highest degree of sequence conservation among all domains of PfEMP1 (Flick and Chen, 2004), and it is responsible for binding to host receptors on both red cells and endothelial cells (Rowe et al, 1997). This domain has a key role to play in parasite sequestration in the microvasulature (Vogt et al, 2002), and contributes to severity of disease (Pathirana et al, 2005).

The diversity within the PfEMP1 gene family is extensive, and numerous *var* genes appear in the parasite population. Although each parasite expresses a single *var* gene (Chen et al., 1998). this can change at a rate of up to 2% per generation (Roberts et al., 1992). The variable nature of PfEMP1 appears to be in tune with the parasite's strategy of evading the host's immune surveillance, by presenting variable antigenic determinants. These parasite-derived molecules of the red blood cell surface are themselves targets for immunological attack, which the parasites counter with extraordinary capacity for antigenic variation (Kwiatkowski, 2005). In addition, the propensity to sequestration, enables the parasite adhere to the microvasculature, preventing their being taken to the spleen for the reticuloendothelial system to remove them from circulation. In the midst of the infection, antibodies that recognize PfEMP1 and other parasite proteins are produced (Miller et al, 2002). By being expressed on the surface of the infected red cells, where they bind to host receptors, sequestering the infected cells, they are protected from spleen-mediated destruction (Kraemer and Smith, 2006). Apart from the sequestration protecting the parasites, it prolongs the infection (Higgins, 2008).

The *P. falciparum* adhesion process is comparable to adhesion of leukocytes, where most parasites first tether, then roll, before becoming firmly adherent (Cooke et al., 1994). Most host receptors are involved with tethering and rolling but are unable to support firm adhesion under flow on their own (Ho & White, 1999; Rogerson et al., 1997). Binding to these host receptors is important, as it significantly increases adhesion that may allow the parasite to efficiently bind to endothelium of various organs (Yipp et al., 2000). Only two receptors, CD36 and chondroitin sulfate A (CSA), provide stable stationary adherence (Ho & White, 1999; Rogerson et al., 1997).

Parasite entry into erythrocytes is key to the establishment of blood stage infection and thus is central to both acute and severe malaria. Entry is a complex, dynamic process Dvorak et al., 1975; Gilson & Crabb, 2009). The invading merozoite stage must orient such that its apical end containing specialized secretory organelle, containing micronemes, rhoptries and dense granules, is pointed at the erythrocyte. Interaction of the merozoite with the erythrocyte leads to the formation of a parasite-host cell junction. Invagination of the erythrocyte bilayer then results in engulfment of the parasite and establishment of the intracellular "ring-stage" parasite surrounded by a vacuolar membrane (Bannister et al., 2000). Several pieces of evidence show that these multiple steps of entry are mediated by parasite proteins that reside on the surface of the merozoite, its apical organelles and adhere to erythrocytes (Chitnis, 2000; Cowman & Crabb, 2002). Several hundred parasite proteins bearing a "host-targeting" (HT) or plasmodial export element (PEXEL) are also predicted to be exported to the erythrocyte during the terminal steps of invasion (or early vacuole formation) as well as intracellular parasite proliferation (Hiller et al., 2004).

The histidine-rich proteins (HRPs) are also secreted by the parasite: these include HRP1 Kilejian et al, 1986) and HRP2 (Panton et al, 1989). Plasmodium falciparum HRP1 is one of the major protein components of 'knobs', which are electron-dense structures protruding from the host red cell membrane, important for adhesion of infected red cells (Oh et al, 1997). Other adhesive protein families that have been identified in the erythrocyte knobs in addition to the histidine-rich protein2 are rifins (Kyes et al., 1999), rosettins (Helmby et al., 1993), and others. Most of these are also variable proteins of importance in the host-parasite relationship, but their relative pathogenetic significance seems to be less prominent than that of the PfEMP-1.

HRP2 has been implicated as a haem polymerase (Sullivan et al., 1996) that catalyses the formation of haemozoin (Choi et al., 1999). HRP2 is a 30 kD water-soluble protein, localized in the parasite food vacuole and on the red cell membrane, exclusively produced by *P. falciparum*, and because HRP-2 is eventually excreted in blood and accumulates in correlation to diseases severity (Desakorn et al, 1996), it has been used as one of the rapid diagnostic tests (RDTs). Other parasite proteins, aldolase and lactate dehydrogenase, glycolytic enzymes, have also been exploited in the development of the RDTs. Of the three parasite enzymes used for the RDTs, the one found most abundantly in the blood is HRP-2; the difference in relative abundance may be caused by a rate of clearance that is highest for pLDH antigens (*Iqbal* et al., 2004). HRP-2 antigens have been shown to clear more slowly from the blood, as they may persist for up to 2 weeks, even after malaria is cured in the patient (*Mayxay* et al., 2001; *Iqbal* et al., 2004).

Parasites that have replicated inside a vacuole need to exit from both the vacuole and the cell, whereas those in the cytoplasm only need to escape from the cell itself. In *Plasmodium* merozoites, distinct proteases are involved in leaving the vacuole and the cell *(Salmon et al, 2001; Wickham et al, 2003).*

Parasite Food Vacuole Events; Haemoglobin to Haemozoin Transformation

During the blood stages of its life cycle, *Plasmodium* is inside a cell in which haemoglobin is extremely abundant, and this serves as the main source of amino acids for the parasite (Francis et al, 1997). As the parasite matures, it develops a special organelle, called the cytostome, an invagination of the parasite plasma membrane, for the uptake of host cytoplasm *(Goldberg, 1993).* As the parasite progresses within the host, from immature ring stage to the trophozoite stage and then to the replicating schizont stage, quite a substantial amount of haemoglobin from the red blood cell cytosol are internalized (Goodyear et al, 1997) to form a food vacuole, within which the internalized haemoglobin is digested. In addition, *Plasmodium* (in the erythrocytic stages) and other apicomplexan parasites, have been shown to render the parasitophorous vacuole membrane freely permeable to small cytosolic molecules through the introduction of high-capacity channels or pores *(Desai et al, 1993; Desai & Rosenberg, 1997).*

The developing parasite depends on the host's haemoglobin as a source of amino acids and iron (Francis et al, 1997). The malarial parasites need to break down haemoglobin to make room to grow, aside from any nutritional benefit they may derive from this (Kwiatkowski, 2005). The parasite is able to digest about 75% of the host cell haemoglobin, but is unable to catabolise the haem liberated (Francis et al, 1997). To protect the parasite membrane against the toxic effects of free haem, the haem moiety released from the digested haemoglobin is detoxified by its polymerization and sequestration as an inert crystalline deposit called haemozoin, or malaria pigment (Slater et al, 1991).

In the vacuole of P falciparum, several proteases have been identified to be involved in the process of breaking down haemoglobin. After being endocytosed to the acidic food vacuole, haemoglobin is degraded by four parasite proteases, proposed to act in a semi-ordered manner (Goldberg et al, 1991; Goldberg, 1993). Two homologous aspartic proteases, plasmepsin I and II initiate the degradation by cleaving the haemoglobin in a highly conserved hinge region (Goldberg et al, 1993). A cysteine protease, falcipain-2 and a metalloprotease, falcilysin, act further downstream, breaking the haemoprotein to small peptides (Rosenthal et al, 1988). Falcipain cysteine proteases play important roles in hemoglobin degradation, both directly and as activators of plasmepsin hemoglobinases (Sijwali et al., 2006). The parasite is also able to degrade the haem in the presence of GSH, which is present in millimolar concentrations in blood cells and parasite compartments (Atamna and Ginsburg, 1995). About 30-50% of free haem is detoxified by polymerization at the trophozoite stage (Wood and Eton, 1993), and the remainder is detoxified by GSH-dependent degradation. The two degradation processes of free haem are initiated by haem-HRP2 and haem-GSH complex formation, respectively. Antimalarials such as chloroquine, and quinine also bind to the free haem and inhibits its degradation.

Alternatively, the haem can be broken down non-enzymatically (Loria et al 1999). Non-enzymatic catabolism of haem liberates iron and generates hydrogen peroxide (Atamna and

Ginsberg, 1993). The formation of haemozoin is also associated with peroxidation of lipids and proteins in the digestive vacuole (Schwarzer et al, 2003). The high concentrations of haemozoin and the acidic pH in the digestive vacuole favour unspecific haem-catalysed lipid peroxidation, leading to a complex array of oxygenated products (Schwarzer et al, 2003). Both haemoglobin breakdown and detoxification are essential features of parasite biology (Liu et al. 2006). Blocking either process is lethal to the parasite, and can be a therapeutic target against the parasite (Elliot et al, 2008).

Host Immunity to Malaria Infection

Protective immunity towards malaria develops only after repeated exposure to the falciparum parasite, and it is known to be partly dependent on antibodies towards the variable antigens present at the surface of the infected red cells (Hommel et al, 1983; Marsh and Howard, 1986; Snow et al., 1997). Antibody formation is an important part of the host immune response against malaria (Perlmann et al, 1998). Parasite proliferation is associated with the generation of soluble plasmodial antigens (Camus and Hadley, 1985). These antigens may be available for binding by reactive antibodies to form immune complexes, ICs (Mohammed, 1982). ICs can activate complement cascade and stimulate macrophages to produce pro-inflammatory cytokines (Jarvis et al, 1997).

Another form of the immune response is seen as the asexual schizonts differentiate in the hepatocytes, and antigens specific to the liver stage are formed (Holder, 1999). It has been proposed that these antigens, together with those brought in with the invading sporozoite, are in part processed by the host cell and presented on the surface in combination with class 1 major histocompatibility complex (MHC). This presentation can lead to recognition by cytotoxic T-lymphocytes and killing of the infected cell, or stimulation of T cells to produce cytokines such as γ-interferon that can lead ultimately to the death of the intracellular parasite (Holder, 1999) Potentially any parasite protein expressed by the liver stage could stimulate the host immune system and lead to parasite killing at this stage.

Many intracellular parasites, like the Plasmodium and viruses can be cleared within days or weeks by the adaptive cytotoxic immune response that involves expansion of CD8 T cells (Rouzine & McKenzie, 2003). The infected hepatocyte may present parasite-derived peptides on MHC molecules to both $CD4^+$ and $CD8^+$ T cells (*Plebanski, M. & Hill, 2000*), thereby initiating specific adaptive immune responses. These cells both kill infected cells and impede virus replication with soluble cytokines. In murine models of vaccination with attenuated sporozoites, $CD8^+$ T cells, probably through the secretion of IFN-γ (*Renggli, 1997*), initiate a cascade of events ending with the destruction of intrahepatic parasites (*Ferreira et al., 1986*). Because red blood cells do not express the critical molecule MHC-1 on their surface, the blood-stage malaria parasites cannot induce the CD8 T cell response and, even though the response is induced by other infected tissues, such as liver, are probably not vulnerable to its cytotoxic action (Rouzine & McKenzie, 2003). Fortunately, *Plasmodium*-infected red blood cells seem to induce innate immune responses that slow the growth of early blood-stage infections; so far, the best known of these involve inflammatory cytokines (Kwiatkowski, 1989; Richards, 1997).

The adaptive or specific immune response is slower and time-dependent. In contrast, there is the more rapid but less specific innate immunity, which is the body's first line of defence, potentially controlling microbes at an early stage by inducing inflammation and fever (Schumann, 2007). Clonal expansion of lymphocytes, in response to infection is absolutely necessary for the generation of an efficient immune response in adaptive immunity. However, it takes three to five days for sufficient numbers of clones to be produced and to differentiate into effector cells, which allows more than enough time for most pathogens to damage the host (Medzhitov & Jaheway, 2000). In contrast, the effector mechanisms of innate immunity, which include antimicrobial peptides, phagocytes, and the alternative complement pathway, are activated immediately after infection and rapidly control the replication of the infecting pathogen (Medzhitov & Jaheway, 2000). For this reason, containing the infection until the lymphocytes can begin to deal with it has long been considered the main function of innate immunity.

Among innate immune cells, splenic marginal zone B (MZB) lymphocytes (Zandvoort & Timens, 2002) are strategically located to respond to blood-borne microorganisms and viruses and to play an important role in host defence (Zandvoort & Timens, 2002; Pillai et al., 2005). Upon antigen encounter, MZB cells swiftly produce large quantities of IgM antibodies that mediate protection at early stages of infection (Oliver et al., 1999). Apart from their ability to produce antibodies, MZB cells also affect the T cell response. For instance, they can migrate into the splenic follicles to deliver immune complexes to follicular dendritic cells (DC), a mechanism that is crucial for the initiation of the adaptive immune response (Cinamon et al., 2008)

Clinical malaria is characterized by high levels of circulating pro-inflammatory cytokines, which are thought to contribute to immunopathy (McCall et al, 2007). The balance between pro- and anti-inflammatory responses is considered critical, for clinical protection. Too little activation of the innate response, results in uninhibited parasite growth, whereas too much activation may cause immunopathy (McCall et al., 2007).

Studies from various laboratories have demonstrated that proinflammatory responses, including the production of TNF-α (Miller et al, 2002), IFNγ, IL-12, and reactive oxygen and nitrogen intermediates by the innate immune system in response to microbes are critical for killing the pathogenic organisms (Hunt and Grau, 2003; Stevenson & Riley, 2004). The inflammatory cytokines can also control infection by promoting macrophage phagocytosis and by complement activation (*Gasque, 2004; Amarante-Paffaro* et al., 2004). In addition, the innate immune response is critical in determining the nature of adaptive immune responses, *i.e.* the specificity of the adaptive immunity against pathogens depends on the pattern of early cytokine expression (Stevenson & Riley, 2004).

When the adaptive immune response is either immature or compromised, the innate immune system constitutes the main defence against infection (Eisen & Michinton, 2003). The innate immune response initiates and thus sets the threshold for the immune responses. Toll-like receptors are key receptors involved in the initial activation of the innate immune system,. together with other immune signaling pathways. Mannose-binding lectin (MBL) is a calcium-dependent (C-type) serum lectin that also plays a significant role in innate immune response. MBL binds microbial surface carbohydrates and mediates opsonophagocytosis directly, or by activation of the lectin complement pathway (Eisen et al, 2003).

The best characterized molecules of malarial antigens is the PfEMP1. Antibody formation is a prominent part of the host immune response against malaria (Perlmann et al,

1998). Parasite proliferation is associated with the generation of soluble plasmodial antigens (Camus and Hadley, 1985). These antigens may be available for binding by reactive antibodies to form immune complexes (Mohammed, 1982). Immune complexes can activate the complement cascade and stimulate macrophages to produce pro-inflammatory cytokines (Jarvis et al, 1997), which can contribute to the pathogenesis of severe malaria (Abdalla et al, 1983). Circulating immune complexes have been found to be common during malarial infection. The clinical manifestations of malaria can be caused by exaggerated host immune response to the falciparum rather than the sole presence of blood parasites (Franklin et al., 2011).

Much of the overactive immune responses result from activation of innate immune receptors such as Toll-like receptors (TLRs), which are critical for pro-inflammatory cytokine production during microbial infection. Research has shown that the innate immune responses to various microbial pathogens are mediated by the TLRs, a family of signal transducing proteins (Takeda and Akira, 2004). It is still uncertain which malaria molecule is responsible for activating cytokine production in immune cells. Two proposed molecules are glycosylphosphatidylinositol (GPI) anchor and parasite-derived DNA, bound to haemozoin. These putative 'malarial toxins' have been shown to activate TLR2 and TLR9 respectively (Parroche et al, 2007).

For example, *Plasmodium falciparum* GPI, which is released upon schizont rupture, signals through TLR2 and TLR4 on monocytes to induce TNF production (Zhu et al, 2005). TLRs are receptors of the innate immune system that recognize a variety of microbial products such as lipopolysaccharides from Gram negative bacteria (Medzhitov, 2001), molecules derived from protozoan parasites, including *Plasmodium falciparum* (Parroche et al, 2007). Together with the intracellular nod-like receptors (NLRs), TLRs are key recognition molecules (Kawai and Akira, 2005). Infected red cells may induce TNF release from monocytes through cytoadherence interactions, or through release of parasite-derived factors, like GPI (Zhu et al, 2005). Furthermore, the *P. falciparum* GPI-induced proinflammatory responses in macrophages, have been proven to proceed through the recognition of mainly TLR2 and to a lesser extent through TLR4, and the cell signaling involves the activation of MAPK-, ERK-, p38-, JNK-, and NF-κB-signaling pathways (*Krishnegowda*.et al., 2005).

While TNF is known to control parasitaemia, it also induces fever during malaria episodes, and may aggravate cerebral malaria by up-regulating the expression of ICAM-1 and other leucocyte adhesion receptors or brain microvascular endothelial cells (Armah et al, 2005).

Since the TLRs are essential for initiating innate immune responses, they are required for early parasite control, except that they may also aggravate the pathophysiology (Gazinelli et al, 2004). Reduced GPI responsiveness may cause severe malaria due to both inadequate innate responses at disease onset and insufficient stimulation of adaptive or specific immunity during preceding infections (Mockenhaupt et al, 2005). Common TLR4 mutations in African children increase the risk of severe malaria (Mockenhaupt et al, 2005).Inhibiting activation of TLRs or other nucleic acid-sensing TLRs by antibodies, peptides or small molecules will provide a better clinical outcome by preventing the excessive production of inflammatory mediators, as seen in malaria (McCall et al, 2007).

Engagement of most of the TLRs triggers a signaling pathway leading to the translocation of transcription factor, NF-κB into the nucleus, followed by the subsequent release of pro-inflammatory cytokines (Schumann, 2007). Apart from other activities, many of these factors induce the activation of the inducible cyclooxygenase-2 (COX-2), which up-regulates prostaglandin synthesis, changing the set-point of the thermoregulatory centre of the host, leading to fever (Ball et al, 2004). Malaria causes pro-inflammatory priming of innate immune responses (McCall et al, 2007), resulting in an immunological state that is notably enhanced. Such a 'primed' immune response could be expected to prevent super infection with bacteria or viruses and might be crucial for host survival.

In areas where malaria is holoendemic, people are continuosly infected with the parasite, but the majority of infected adults rarely experience overt disease (Boutlis et al, 2006). People in such areas who experience repeated malaria infections develop a degree of immunity that confers some protection from clinical disease (Marsh, 2002). . Even after many exposures, humans are not refractory to malaria parasites but develop clinical immunity that prevents symptomatic disease (Weatherall et al., 2002). This type of immunity limits disease and, although the individual may harbor low numbers of parasites, they do not develop into a symptomatic infection (Snow & Marsh, 1998). Until the age of approximately six months, children are protected from malaria by maternal antibodies, and as maternal protection wanes, susceptibility to clinical disease and mortality increase greatly (Crawley, 2004).

The role of anti-PfEMP1 antibodies in protection from pathogenic infections is highlighted again in placental malaria. Exposure to parasites that sequester in the placenta during pregnancy induces strain-transcending immunity that blocks adhesion of infected erythrocytes to CSA and may protect the mother and foetus from placental malaria in subsequent pregnancies (Fried et al., 1998).

Some patients with imported malaria may be expected to have some degree of immunity. Factors associated with immunity include, residence in a malaria-endemic area, previous infection with malaria and ethnicity (Jennings et al, 2006). It is commonly believed that immunity to malaria is lost once an individual moves away from a malaria-endemic area, making previously immune persons develop high risk of severe disease, should they become re-infected (Marsh, 2002). But it is also evident that previously immune individuals, although they do become sick, have significantly lower parasite densities and a lower risk of severe and fatal outcomes than comparable, previously naive persons (Straik and Riley, 2004).

In highland areas, prolonged periods of low or no exposure to infective mosquitoes during the dry season presumably results in the reduction in the number of parasites that become established in the liver. This may in turn, lead to diminished antigen-specific immunity to pre-erythrocytic and blood-stage *P. falciparum*, with increased susceptibility to malaria infection when transmission rates rise during the rainy season (John et al, 2000). In such highland areas above 1600 m, low temperatures inhospitable to the malaria vector and parasite lead to very low malaria transmission for much of the year *Minakawa* et al, 2002). In the absence of repeated exposure, development of immune responses to malaria is delayed or may wane (John et al., 2000), and older children and adults are susceptible to clinical malaria (Hay et al, 2002).

Marsh (2002) contended that there is no marker that has been reliably shown to correlate with immunity to malaria, though he conceded there are some inherent resistance traits such as sickle cell trait and other haemoglobinopathies, known to be associated with protection against severe disease. Day and colleagues (1999) were also not sure of what precisely constitutes immunity to malaria. What they were certain of was that however immunity is defined, it is mediated in part by pro-inflammatory and anti-inflammatory cytokines, and there is evidence that these cytokines have prognostic role. High serum concntrations of TNF-α and IL-10 are associated with higher parasite counts and more severe symptoms (May et al, 2000).

Balanced Polymorphism; The Survival Advantage for Malaria

The association between β-thalassemia and resistance to malaria was first proposed by Haldane in 1949 and became known as the "malaria hypothesis". Subsequently, varying degrees of evidence emerged that demonstrated a relative resistance to malaria by numerous hereditary red cell disorders including other haemoglobinopathies, membrane protein disorders and enzyme deficiencies, as well as blood group polymorphisms. That the sickle cell trait has some survival advantage was suggested by Raper (1949), who was the first to speculate that the sickle cell trait was linked to a survival advantage for some adverse tropical condition, and Mackey and Viralelli (1954), suggested this factor might be malaria. The close geographical association between the distribution of malaria and the sickle cell gene supported this concept (Allison et al, 1954).

There is a considerable body of evidence that demonstrates a co-evolutionary relationship between P. falciparum and humans (Williams, 2006; Weatherall et al., 2008). The host evolves new genetic determinants, which decrease susceptibility to infection, while the pathogen in turn, evolves virulence factors, resulting in ongoing adaptations in host and pathogen fitness. Using the sickle cell trait as an example, malaria has selected for the abnormal β-hemoglobin gene (HbS) in the host, but so far there have been no counteractive adaptations identified in the parasite. In addition, the disorder decreases the fitness of the uninfected host. This trade-off in a population leads to a balanced polymorphism (Haldane, 1949) and explains the high allele frequencies of disorders like sickle cell disease, thalassemia and G6PD deficiency. It has been observed that a recessive condition could remain prevalent because the heterozygote enjoys some unrelated health advantage, such as being resistant to an infectious disease (Lewis, 2003). Studies have shown that AS children with parasitemia are 50–90% less likely to progress to mild or severe malaria (Aidoo et al., 2002; May et al., 2007), and AS children who do develop severe malaria are less likely to die from the disease (Olumese et al., 1991). Although sickle trait does not seem to protect children against infection by *P. falciparum* parasites, AS children generally have lower parasite densities than AA children during episodes of asymptomatic infection and symptomatic malaria (Allison, 1954; Aidoo et al., 2002; May et al., 2007).

Evolutionary selection by malaria is remarkable in two respects (Kwiatkowski, 2005). Firstly, the selective pressure is very strong, accounting for why the HbS allele has risen to high frequencies in areas of malaria endemicity, despite the fatal consequences for the homozygous. Secondly, different populations have developed independent evolutionary responses.

There were some conflicting results on the protective effect of the sickle cell trait, as this effect was found to be overridden by the role of acquired immunity. Examination of young children confirmed that there were lower parasite rates and densities (Gilles et al, 1967). As a child ages, the protective effect of HbAS increases, implying that the sickling trait enhances, or acts in synergy with the acquired immune response (Weatherall et al, 2005). It is now accepted that the sickle cell trait offers protection at a critical period of early childhood, between the time of loss of passively acquired immunity to the time of development of active immunity (Allison 1957). The mechanism behind this is uncertain, but probable factors suggested are selective sickling of parasitized erythrocytes (Luzzato et al, 1970), resulting in their more effective removal by the reticuloendothelial system, inhibition of parasite growth by loss of potassium ions, the lower pH of sickled cells (Friedman et al, 1979) and the greater adherence of the infected red cells to endothelial cells (Kaul et al, 1994).

Other investigators have suggested that sickle trait promotes enhanced phagocytosis of ring-infected erythrocytes by splenic macrophages. Ayi *et al.* (2004) reported that these parasitized AS erythrocytes were ingested by macrophages more readily than their AA counterparts and proposed that enhanced phagocytosis of ring-parasitized AS erythrocytes in the spleen helps to lower parasite densities in AS children. Parasite-induced sickling of AS erythrocytes (Luzzato et al., 1970), reduced invasion and impaired development of parasites in AS erythrocytes at low-oxygen tension (Pasvol et al., 1978), and enhanced phagocytosis of ring-parasitized AS erythrocytes (Ayi et al., 2004); all might contribute to the increased removal of parasites by the spleen and reduce parasite densities in AS children. Protection has also been attributed to defective invasion or growth of the parasite in the mutant red blood cells (Friedman, 1979), while other studies found normal invasion and growth (Luzi et al, 1990). Increased osmotic resistance, enhanced oxidant radical production due to unpaired globin chains, increased sickling, ionic imbalances and membrane rigidity, have been suggested as possible causes of the impaired growth of the parasites in the mutant red blood cells (Serjeantson et al, 1977; Roth et al, 1978; Weatherall, 1997; Greene, 1993).

HbC has also been reported to alter the display of PfEMP1 in infected red blood cells, thereby reducing the strength of their adherence to host tissue (Fairhurst et al, 2005). The influence of HbC is to modulate the consequences of the bonding between parasitized red cells and host cells. The modulation may tone down the pathways of inflammation that have an important role in symptoms and severe clinical presentations of the disease.

Indeed, multiple human erythrocyte mutations associated with a survival advantage in *P. falciparum* infection are thought to have been developed (Cserti and Dzik, 2007). One of these involves the structural haemoglobinopathies, of which HbS and Hb C are examples. Others are quantitative haemoglobinopathies (eg. the thalassaemias), membrane mutations (spherocytosis, ellipsocytosis, ovalocytosis) and enzymopathies (glucose-6-phosphate dehydrogenase deficiency) (Serjeantson et al, 1977; Roth et al, 1978; Weatherall, 1997; Greene, 1993; Kwiatkowski, 2005).

The erythrocyte membrane protein that has been implicated in malaria resistance in ovalocytosis is an anion exchanger known as ‘band-3 protein’, encoded by SCC4A1 gene. A 27 base pair deletion in this gene results in a form of ovalocytosis, which has been shown to be protective against malaria infection and against cerebral malaria (Allen et al, 1999).

Different populations have developed independent evolutionary responses to malaria; a phenomenon that is seen at both global and local levels (Kwiatkowski, 2005). The most common global example is seen in the beta-globin gene, in which three different coding single nucleotide polymorphisms, are reported to confer protection against malaria; Glu 6 Val (HbS), Glu 6 Lys (HbC) and Glu 26 Lys (HbE). HbS is common in Africa, but is rare in South East Asia, whereas the opposite is the case for the HbE allele.

At the local level, the Dogon people of Mali, in contrast to their other West African counterparts, are noted to have a much lower frequency of HbS, as compared to HbC (Agarwal et al, 2000). These differences in the geographic distributions of the various alleles lend support to the proposal that different populations have evolved different genetic variants for protection against malaria (Kwiatkowski, 2005).

In addition to the red cell variants, several polymorphisms of mediators of innate immune response have been shown to protect against, or alternatively, predispose to malaria; e.g. mannose-binding lectin, inducible nitric oxide synthase, TNF-α, interferon receptors (Luty et al, 1998; Cramer et al, 2004).

The reason why severe malarial anaemia occurs more commonly very early in life is still unclear, though it has been suggested that a possible factor could be the inability of the young children to maintain IL-10 production in response to inflammatory processes (Nussenblatt, 2001). The high frequency of severe malarial anaemia and the particularly high erythropoietin responses in very early life, sheds some light on the pathophysiology of severe anaemia in early childhood, as well as clinical and therapeutic implications (Nussblant et al, 2001). Erythropoietin has been shown to cross the blood-brain barrier and protects against experimental brain damage and acts in other tissues as tissue-protective cytokines (Ghezzi and Brines, 2004). Epo is required for sustained proliferation and differentiation of erythroid cells (Casals-Pascual et al, 2008). Some studies have revealed high levels of epo in African children with severe anaemia (Casals-Pascual et al (2006). Malaria appears to increase epo concentrations up to 30-fold higher than those found in anaemia not associated with acute malaria infection (Casals-Pascual et al (2006).

Pathophysiology and Pathogenesis of Malaria

Serious sequealae can result from three primary pathophysiological events; namely, red blood cell destruction, adhesion of infected RBCs to the capillary veins, especially in the central nervous system; and excessive pro-inflammatory response. The third factor is responsible for symptoms such as rigours, chills, spiking fever, sweating, vasodilation and hypoglycaemia (Clark et al, 2006). The initial pro-inflammatory response during malaria appears to play a critical role in the development of cerebral malaria, anaemia and death (Kwiatkowski et al, 1990).

Plasmodia can be found in the microvasulature of any organ of the host (Udomsangpatch et al, 1997), which reflects the systemic nature of *P. falciparum* malaria. Different organ systems are usually simultaneously affected to different extents, ranging from mild dysfunction at the sub-clinical level to complete organ failure, triggered by both sequestration of a critical parasite biomass in small vessels and tissue hypoxia (Helbok et al, 2005). High parasite burden results in cytokine activation, hypofusion and tissue hypoxia (White, 2002). Pathophysiologic and pathologic features of severe falciparum malaria include sequestration, cytoadherence, rosette formation and reduced red cell deformability (White, 2002).

The severity of P. falciparum infection depends largely on the ability of the parasitized red cells to adhere on ECs and sequester in the capillary network of vital organs (eg. brain, lungs, kidneys, liver (van den Heyde et al, 2006). The mature parasites avoid the spleen by sequestering in capillaries and microvenules in the various organs. Moreover, activation of

ECs results in an over-expression of different mediators, such as adhesion molecules ("hyperadhesion" phenomenon), pro-inflammatory cytokines, coagulation factors, which contribute to the pathology (van den Heyde et al, 2006).

Two hypotheses for the pathogenesis of malaria have been delineated; the mechanical and cytokine hypotheses (Clark et al, 2006). The former hypothesis espouses the concept of insufficient oxygen delivery to vital organs, while in the latter, excessive release of pro-inflammatory cytokines, serves as driving force for disease and death. Both host-derived and pathogen-derived molecules have been proposed as the cytokine-inducing 'malaria toxin' (Parroche et al, 2007). Genetic variation affecting the activity of certain cytokine genes may produce individuals with a more exaggerated or prolonged inflammatory response (Duff, 2006). One of the many actions of the cytokines responsible for systemic inflammation is to disable oxidative phosphorylation within mitochondria (Clark et al, 2006). This is reflected in the hyperlactacidaemia, commonly seen in severe malaria. An additional pathway through which the inflammatory cytokines reduce oxygen consumption is through the formation of peroxynitrite, a product of the reaction of nitic oxide (from action of cytokine-induced nitric oxide synthase, iNOS) and superoxide (Clark et al, 2006).

P. falciparum adhesion to human ECs can specifically trigger pro-inflammatory gene expression (Tripathi et al, 2009), oxidative stress and caspases activation (Pino et al, 2003), further leading to perturbation of the endothelial barrier integrity (Taoufiq et al,

2008) Subsequent to adhesion, the release of soluble parasite proteins and their accumulation in the vasculature may cause cytokine recruitment and endothelial cell destruction (Clark and Cowden, 2003). Cytokines are intercellular signal molecules that coordinate the host's inflammatory response to injury. The inflammatory response is usually tightly controlled, so the response is commensurate with the challenge, eradicating pathogens and repairing damaged tissues (Duff, 2006). However, inflammation is also an important component in the pathogenesis of many chronic diseases (Duff, 2006). For example, cytokines have been identified as key mediators in rheumatoid arthritis (di Giovine et al, 1988), asthma (Sousa et al, (1996) and diabetes (Arnush et al, 1998). Cytokines with pyrogenic activity are secreted from phagocytes, circulate and alter temperature regulatory systems in pre-optic areas within the hypothalamus (Parroche et al, 2007).

Parasite sequestration is exacerbated by cytokine-mediated up-regulation of host endothelial receptors that bind to parasitized erythrocytes (eg. ICAM-1, vCAM). Cytokines such as TNF-α and interferon-γ suppress haematopoiesis and enhance uptake of non-infected red blood cells (Young, 1995), contributing to the anaemia. Parasitized erythrocytes are avidly phagocytosed by circulating and resident phagocytes (Facer and Brown, 1981), and ingested haemozoin inhibits important cellular functions (Schwarzer et al, 1998); upsets the production of several cytokines (Achyangkul et al, 1994), and appears to play a role in immunodepression (Schwarzer et al, 1998). When phagocytosed by monocytes, the haemozoin-laden monocytes were unable to repeat phagocytosis to produce oxidative burst (Schwarzer et al, 1992), to kill ingested bacteria (Fiori et al, 1993). Low levels of cytokines may be beneficial, but high levels are found to be harmful, contributing to placental dysfunction, suppression of erythropoiesis, inhibition of gluconeogenesis and increased cytoadherence (McGee et al, 1992)

Several studies show that excessive production of proinflammatory mediators results in systemic and organ-related pathological conditions (Kwiatkowski et al., 1990; Hommel, 1993; Takeda et al., 2003; Hunt & Grau, 2003). Malaria-infected individuals have been shown to produce high levels of TNF-α and IFN-γ and nitric oxide, which are associated with fever, cerebral and other forms of malaria (Kwiatkowski et al., 1990; Hommel, 1993; Takeda et al., 2003; Hunt & Grau, 2003). Adherence of the parasite-infected erythrocytes to the microvascular capillaries of various organs and in the dermal tissues potentially promotes pathogenesis because of the high parasite burden and severe proinflammatory responses in localized areas, leading to endothelial damage and organ dysfunction (Hommel, 1993). In addition, up-regulation of endothelial cell adhesion molecules in response to TNF-α potentially augments the adherence, aggravating the destruction of the endothelia and causing organ-related pathological conditions (Schofield et al., 1996).

GPIs have been proposed as the dominant parasite factors responsible for malaria pathogenesis. Later studies have shown that the GPIs of *P. falciparum* can induce the expression of iNOS, up-regulate the expression of intracellular adhesion molecule 1 (ICAM-1), vascular cell adhesion molecule 1 (vCAM-1), and E-selectin in endothelial cells, implicating these processes in malaria pathogenesis (Schofield et al., 1996). Erythrocytes infected with mature malaria parasites (trophozoites and schizonts), form rosettes by binding to uninfected RBCs via complement receptor 1 (CR1), on the surface of the erythrocytes (Rowe et al, 1997).

Rosetting, the spontaneous binding of infected erythrocytes to uninfected erythrocytes, is mediated by the parasite ligand PfEMP1 on the surface of the infected erythrocytes (Rowe et al, 1997), binding to a variety of uninfected erythrocyte receptors, including CR1, which is an immune regulatory protein found on erythrocytes and a variety of leucocytes (Cockburn et al, 2004). Its functions include control of complement activation and the clearance of opsonised immune complexes from circulation (Ahearn and Fearon, 1989; Cockburn et al, 2004). Rosetting contributes to the pathogenesis of severe malaria, so it it is a parasite virulence factor towards the host, but to the parasite itself, rosette formation may enhance its growth and survival, leading to hyperparasitaemia (Rowe et al, 2002).

CR1 levels vary between 50-1,200 per cell (Ahearn et al, 1989; Rowe et al, 2002). In Caucascians, there are polymorphisms of RBC CR1, which comprises low and high CR1 expression haplotypes (Cockburn et al, 2004). As the number of CR1 on RBCs increases, so does the tendency to form rosettes (Rowe et al, 1997). There is strong indirect evidence from human genetic epidemiological studies, supporting the pathogenic role for rosetting. Human RBC polymorphisms of rosetting receptors that reduce the ability of *P. falciparum* to form rosettes, such as CR1 deficiency (Rowe et al., 1997) and blood group O (Carlson et al., 1994) confer protection against severe malaria (*Cockburn* et al, 2004; Rowe et al, 2007). These polymorphisms have a specific effect on rosetting and do not influence total parasite burdens (*Cockburn* et al, 2004; Rowe et al, 2007).

Carlson et al. (1992; 1994), in their studies showed that rosetting parasites show a preference for erythrocytes with either A or B blood group antigens, and form larger, stronger rosettes with cells of the preferred type compared with group O cells. The preference for the A antigen is particularly common (*Udomsangpetch et al., 1993)*, and direct binding of the parasite rosetting ligand PfEMP1 to the A antigen has been demonstrated (Chen et al., 2000). The mechanism through which binding to A antigen (and rosetting in general) might lead to lower haemoglobin levels is unclear. One possibility is that parasite-induced damage of the uninfected erythrocytes in rosettes could occur, including the formation of oxidative products such as 4-hydroxynonenal *Skorokhod et al., 2007)*, that could lead to the phagocytic clearance of uninfected cells and so contribute to anemia (Doumbo et al, 2009). If rosettes in group A patients are larger (i.e., contain more uninfected erythrocytes per rosette than in B and O patients) this could lead to greater clearance of uninfected erythrocytes and account for the relationship with haemoglobin level.

Compounds that reverse rosetting *in vitro*, may have potential as adjunctive therapies for severe malaria (Vogt et al., 2006). Rosette-disrupting therapies that relieve or prevent microvascular obstruction have potential to ameliorate the symptoms of severe malaria. Heparin has been shown to reverse rosetting in a subset of rosetting isolates (Carlson et al., 1992; Rowe et al., 1994).

The pathogenesis of malaria is best understood for *P. falciparum* infection. Falciparum malaria is an acute febrile illness characterised by fever, chills, headache, anaemia and splenomegaly, which responds promptly to appropriate antimalarial therapy. Untreated, the patient will either die in the acute attack (occurs in less than 5% of patients) or survive with almost no development of immunity against the next infection unless the one has been exposed to years of repeated challenge (Ho and White, 1999).

Several factors contribute to the severity of clinical disease. In severe malaria, release of oxygen free radicals and a variety of pro-inflammatory cytokines can lead to increased vascular permeability, leakage of colloid from intravascular space, pathologic vasodilation, and myocardial depression, with ultimate hypovolaemia and impaired organ perfusion (Kavishe *et al*, 2006). In children with malaria, lipid peroxidation in blood plasma and red cells is increased, while red cell antioxidants like GSH, catalase and tocopherol are lower in malaria patients than in control subjects (Becker *et al*, 2004). The intracellular parasite digestion of haemoglobin, releases free ferroprotoporphyrin or haem, which in the presence of oxygen, oxidises to ferriprotoporphyrin or haemin (Kavishe *et al*, 2006). This process produces superoxide, which dismutates to hydrogen peroxide and oxygen. Several studies have shown that an increase in oxidative stress in parasitised RBCs offers an advantage to parasite clearance than worsening the pathology (Deharo *et al*, 2003).

Glutathione (GSH) is an antioxidant, needed for the growth of the malarial parasites (Ferreira *et al*, 2004), and it is also required for maintaining the redox state of the host cell. Altered redox state of the host cells, especially the endothelial cells may exacerbate disease complications, for example, by enhancing endothelial damage, brain inflammation and development of cerebral malaria. Oxidative stress can also increase oxidative damage of red cell membrane, reducing the deformability of the cells, and ultimately inducing removal and massive destruction of red cells by macrophages, leading to increased severity of anaemia, occlusion of microvasculature, cerebral pathology (hypoxia) and cardiac failure seen in falciparum malaria (Becker *et al*, 2004).

Erythropoietin is known to provide neuroprotective effect, as it is known to prevent neuronal apoptosis (Siren et al, 2001) and down-regulate inflammatory response in the brain (Villa et al, 2003). The specific mechanisms responsible for increased levels of erythropoietin in patients with acute anaemia include hypoxia, hypoglycaemia and oxidant stress (Idro et al, 2005). These three conditions have been shown to induce the expression of hypoxia-inducible transcription factor, which up-regulates the production of erythropoietin and other hypoxia-related proteins (Fandrey et al, 1997). Activation of vascular endothelial growth factor (VEGF) has also been reported in patients with cerebral malaria (Denninger et al, 2003). VEGF, an angiogenic factor, is associated with poor outcome in cerebral malaria, as it could contribute to the pathophysiolgy of cerebral malaria by increasing the permeability of the blood brain barrier (Zhang et al, 2000).

Antibodies can damage tissue. During type III hypersensitivity reactions as defined by Coombs and Gell (1963), immune complexes deposit in tissue and activate phagocytic cells and complement. Immune complexes play a role in chronic inflammatory diseases such as rheumatoid arthritis (Firestein, 2003) Malaria has been associated with circulating immune complexes (Adam et al., 1981), and immunoglobulin and parasite antigen depositions have been observed in the basement membrane of endothelial cells during cerebral malaria (Oo et al., 1987) and in that of trophoblast during placental malaria (Maeno et al., 1993).

Clinical Presentation

The definitive diagnosis of falciparum malaria is made by the examination of a blood film, although in high transmission areas, the presence of parasites in the blood does not equate with the patient being ill with malaria. The gold standard for diagnosis is light microscopy of Giemsa-stained thick and thin smears. The thick smear is more sensitive for diagnosing malaria, whereas the thin smear is done for species identification and quantification of parasite burden. Other diagnostic modalities, including fluorescent microscopy and polymerase chain reaction-based testing, are available but not routinely used (Griffith et al., 2007).

Reliance on clinical diagnosis of malaria has been shown to have a specificity of 42% when a combination of fever, splenomegaly, and nail-bed pallor was used, and a specificity of 21% when fever alone was used (Redd et al., 1996). Some infections with symptoms similar to malaria are influenza, dengue fever, viral encephalitis, febrile gastroenteritis, lobar pneumonia, meningitis, septicaemia, rickettsial infections, leptospirosis, and urinary tract infections (Long, 2009).

Immunosuppression often accompanies severe malaria. Secondary bacterial infection (septicaemia, bacterial pneumonia, urinary tract infections or meningitis) can therefore occur early in severe malaria and lead to shock and multiorgan failure (Berkley et al., 1999). Common organisms include pneumococci, salmonella, *Escherichia coli* and other Gram-negative organisms. Fever blisters ('cold sores') due to *Herpes simplex* are a common accompaniment of malarial infection (Pasvol, 2005).

Asymptomatic carriage is the norm in some areas owing to the protective effect of the immune system (Baird, 1998). Without diagnostic acumen, there will be failure to treat life-threatening conditions, errorneous diagnosis and treatment, and dissipation of resources (Breman et al, 2007). However, in Africa, most infections are treated presumptively on the basis of symptoms, rather than a positive blood smear test (Biritwum et al, 2000). Some persons are at special risk of developing malaria. These include those with no immunity against malaria; for example infants and unexposed persons and persons who have lost the acquired immunity, like pregnant women, the elderly and people who have left an area of transmission (Breman et al, 2001). In fact, children under the age of five are the most vulnerable to malaria morbidity and mortality due to their immune-naive status (Breman et al, 2001). Until the age of approximately six months, children are protected from malaria by maternal antibodies (Crawley, 2004).

Infection with *P. falciparum* has a wide spectrum of infestations that are roughly classified into three clinical groups: asymptomatic infection, mild malaria and severe malaria.

In malaria-endemic areas, a significant proportion of children harbour parasites without presenting signs of clinical malaria, and are considered as asymptomatic cases (Greenwood, 1987). Clinical presentation, therefore, varies from asymptomatic to multi-organ failure manifestations and death, depending on the following; host factors (age, immunity), parasite factor (plasmodia species) and the geographic location (eg. inoculation rate) (Helbok et al, 2005).

Uncomplicated and Complicated Malaria

In children, uncomplicated malaria usually presents as fever, and non-specific symptoms, such as vomiting, and/or diarrhoea, a clinical picture that resembles that of other childhood infectious diseases (Greenword et al, 2008). Mild or uncomplicated malaria is usually not lethal, whereas severe or complicated malaria has a mortality rate of 20 to 30% (White, 2008). Severe malaria has been defined as a parasite load greater than 5%, end organ damage, severe anaemia, or hypoglycaemia, requiring parenteral therapy with quinidine plus tetracycline, doxycycline, or clindamycin in the United States (Griffith et al., 2007). In clinical practice, any patient with suspected malaria who demonstrates complicated disease, i.e. prostration, any impairment of consciousness, convulsions or any manifestation of shock, decreased urinary output, respiratory distress or abnormal bleeding, should be treated with parenteral rather than oral drugs (Pasvol, 2005). Moreover, some patients because of nausea or vomiting, induced by either disease or drug(s), are unable to take oral drugs and require parenteral treatment (Pasvol, 2005).

In adults, severe malaria is characterized by multi-organ failure, including renal failure. This is uncommon in children with severe malaria, who usually present with prostration, respiratory distress and/or cerebral malaria (Greeword et al, 2008).

High parasite burdens combined with the unique ability of infected erythrocytes to adhere to host endothelium contribute to microvascular occlusion, metabolic derangement and acidosis, which lead to the manifestations of severe malaria (acute respiratory distress syndrome, renal insufficiency and cerebral malaria) (Cooke *et al,* 2000). It is known that host glucose is the main energy source for asexual stages of *P. falciparum* and that the more mature form of the parasite consumes up to 70 to 80 times the amount of glucose required by uninfected erythrocytes *in vitro (Sherman, 1988): this can contribute to hypoglycaemia,* a common complication of the primary disease. The increased glucose uptake by the parasite aside, there could be decreased glycogen stores from anorexia, depletion of glucose stores because of starvation or malnutrition, malabsorption of glucose due to decreased splanchnic blood flow and cytokine-induced impairment of gluconeogenesis (Association of.Physicians, 2009). In addition, treatment with quinine causes a hyperinsulinaemic effect, further driving the blood sugar down (Griffith et al., 2007).

Hepatic Dysfunction

There has been tremendous increase in the knowledge of hepatocyte dysfunction occurring in malaria; hence more cases are being reported from different parts of world.

Many of such reports on malarial hepatopathy, are from Asian countries, especially from India (WHO, 2000). The majority of the cases have either isolated infection with *P. falciparum* (Anand et al, 1992; Kochar et al., 2003; Devarbhavi et al., 2005) or a mixed infection with both *P. falciparum and P. vivax* .(Joshi et al., 1986) The extent of liver involvement varies from a minimal abnormality in liver function tests to hepatic encephalopathy. (Joshi et al., 1986; Ayyub et al., 2000).

There is a wide variation in reported cases of jaundice in malaria. In a study of 732 patients with falciparum malaria in an endemic area, jaundice occurred in 5.3% of the patients (Anand et al., 1992). Mehta *et al* (1989), in a study of 425 cases of falciparum malaria have also reported jaundice in only 2.58%. Murthy et al. (1998), found jaundice in 62% of patients with falciparum malaria. Wilairatana et al. (1994), from Thailand, reported an incidence of jaundice in 32% of falciparum malaria although the bilirubin was predominantly unconjugated. In children, Bag et al. found 'hepatitis' in 8% children with complicated falciparum malaria (Bag et al, 1994).

Some possible reasons for such a wide variation in reports of jaundice could include endemic versus epidemic areas, age group, vivax versus falciparum/mixed infection and analyzing only complicated cases where the incidence is higher (Anand & Puri, 2005). A study from Thailand has suggested that pre-existing helminth infections are associated with protection from malaria-related acute renal failure and jaundice by influencing sequestration (Nacher et al., 2001). Another possible factor could be associated viral hepatitis, which could also be endemic (Bansal et al., 2002). Underlying chronic liver disease due to hepatitis B virus has been reported to be a risk factor for severe malarial infection and their coexistence may result in exaggerated hepatocyte dysfunction (Anand & Puri, 2005).

Jaundice can result from either severe haemolysis or hepatic involvement. The rupture of hepatocytes during the primary schizogony results in cellular damage but this does not result in significant hepatic dysfunction (Anand & Puri, 2005). Severe infestation of the red blood cells by *P. falciparum* and resultant haemolysis results in the rising bilirubin (Kochar et al., 2003)

In an Indian study by Joshi et al. (1986), involving nine patients with acute liver failure due to Plasmodium falciparum liver injury, admitted to a Liver Unit, blood film examination showed P. falciparum alone in seven and along with P. vivax in the remaining two patients. The liver was palpable in all the patients, and eight had splenomegaly. Investigations revealed mild to moderate abnormality in liver function tests. All were negative for the markers of acute infection due to hepatitis A and B viruses. Liver histology, which was identical in all eight patients where liver biopsy was done, showed centrizonal necrosis and hyperplastic Kupffer cells loaded with malarial pigment. All the patients recovered with specific anti-malarial and supportive treatment. The study by Joshi et al. (1986) showed that malaria due to P. *falciparum* may present as jaundice and encephalopathy.

"Malarial hepatitis" is a term commonly used to describe hepatocytic dysfunction in severe and complicated malaria; however, actual inflammation of the liver parenchyma is almost never seen as the hepatic dysfunction has been suggested to be due to the failure of bilirubin excretion, as a result of heavy parasitaemia, endotoxaemia, ischaemia, acidosis or a combination of some or all of these factors (Anand & Puri, 2005).Malarial hepatitis is characterized by a rise in serum bilirubin along with the rise in serum alanine transaminase levels to more than three times the upper limit of normal (Anand et al., 1992). This should be in the absence of evidence of exposure to hepatotoxic drugs and absence of clinical or serological evidence of viral hepatitis.

According to the WHO, jaundice is one of the cardinal manifestations of severe malaria. It results from the intravascular haemolysis of parasitized erythrocytes, hepatic dysfunction and possibly an element of microangiopathic haemolysis associated with disseminated intravascular coagulation (WHO, 2000). The changes in liver may result from alteration in blood flow through the organ as parasitized red blood cells adhere to endothelial cells, blocking the sinusoids and obstructing the intrahepatic blood flow. The histopathological changes reported in the malaria patients include hepatocyte necrosis, cholestasis, bile stasis, granulomatous lesions and malarial nodules. The bile stasis is due to impairment of bilirubin transport because of reticulo-endothelial blockage and disturbance of hepatocyte microvilli (Anand et al., 1992; Srivastava et al., 1996; Premaratna et al., 2001).

Intravascular haemolysis of parasitized and non-parasitized red blood cells has been considered as an important factor in the cause of mild to moderate jaundice, but then, the bilirubin is predominantly unconjugated and its levels do not rise very high (Kochar et al., 2003). Haemolysis significantly contributes to the rising bilirubin in severe malarial infection. The parasite, especially *P. falciparum,* infects a large number of red cells which are then destroyed in the spleen, resulting in haemolytic anaemia. This is characterized by elevated serum bilirubin (dominant unconjugated fraction), without any significant elevation of the liver enzymes.

However, from the study of Kochar et al. (2003), they found cases of conjugated hyperbilirubinaemia. Hepatic bilirubin excretion involves the secretion of conjugated pigment across the canalicular membrane. This rate-limiting step in bilirubin excretion is an active, energy-dependent transport process (Seymour et al., 1967). When large amounts of bilirubin saturate the secretory apparatus, there is regurgitation of conjugated bilirubin from the liver cells in the plasma. The effect of parasitaemia on hepatocytes in experimental *P. berghi* infection in mice showed a 30–40% decrease in hepatic cytochrome P-450 and associated monooxygenase activity (Taliaferro *& Mulligan, 1937)*. Similar effect on bilirubin excretion may be responsible for conjugated hyperbilirubinaemia.

Furthermore, liver function abnormalities have been reported with administration of anti-malarial drugs, like mefloquine (Gotsman et al., 2000), amodiaquine (Raymond et al., 1989) and pyrimethamine sulfadoxine combination (Meier et al., 1990). Most of the literature available on hepatic dysfunction due to antimalarial drugs is with long-term prophylactic administration of these drugs (Bhalla et al., 2006).

Hyperactive Malaria Splenomegaly

In malarial infection, the spleen plays a critical role in clearance of parasitised RBCs and immunity against blood-stage parasites (*Engwerda* et al., 2005). The spleen is the major site of elimination of parasitised RBCs via erythro-phagocytosis, elaboration of protective immune mechanisms, and hypersensitivity reaction manifesting as splenic enlargement (*Engwerda* et al., 2005). It is worth noting that splenomegaly is generally, not an uncommon finding in Africa (Adekile et al, 1991). In an age- and sex-matched study comparing 310

Nigerians and 100 US patients with SCD-SS, the Nigerians had a higher prevalence of persistent splenomegaly compared with the Americans (Adekile et al, 1991).

It is believed that malaria is a contributing factor to the syndrome of persistent splenomegaly, which is found in the general population in malaria-endemic regions. Previously referred to as tropical splenomegaly syndrome, it is now known as hyperactive malarial splenomegaly (HMS), a condition which is the most frequent cause of massive splenomegaly in areas with a stable transmission of malaria (Crane, 1986). Hyperactive malaria splenomegaly may result from aberrant immunologic response to malaria antigens after repeated infections, resulting in hypertrophy, sometimes associated with secondary hypersplenism (Fakunle, 1981; Bates et al, 1991). In HMS, there is an abnormal response to recurrent malaria infection, as a result of defective regulation of T suppressor cells (Bradley et al., 1996; Vinetz et al, 1998). The interaction of repeated malarial infection and unknown host factors results in the production of cytotoxic Ig M antisuppressor lymphocyte (CD8+) antibodies. This causes inhibition of suppressor T cells, which normally regulate IgM production (Hoffman et al., 1984). This leads to uninhibited B cell production of IgM and the formation of cryoglobulins (IgM aggregates and immune complexes). Hyperreactive malarial splenomegaly is marked by elevated levels of IgM and antimalarial antibodies (De Cock et al., 1986), and total serum immunoglobulin levels (Logie et al., 1973) and immune complex deposition (Maeno et al., 1993). The need to clear these macromolecular aggregates stimulates the reticuloendothelial system, resulting in hyperplasia. This causes the progressive and massive enlargement of the spleen and hepatomegaly.

The massively enlarged spleen shows dilated sinusoids lined with reticulum cells showing marked erythrophagocytosis and lymphocytic infiltration of the pulp. Liver exhibits sinusoidal dilatation, infiltration with lymphocytes and hyperplasia of the Kupffer's cells with phagocytosis of cellular debris and red cells.Histology of spleen would show normal white pulp but congested red pulp with polyclonal plasma cells (Chim et al., 2004). In a study on the mechanism of splenic macrophage hyperplasia, the number of splenic macrophages in *P. berghei*–infected mice dramatically increased within 4 days after infection (Wyler et al., 1977). On the basis of this study, Wyler et al. found that most of the increase in splenic macrophages during acute phase do not appear to derive from local proliferation and suggested that splenic macrophages presumably increase as a result of "trapping" of blood monocytes (Wyler et al., 1977).

The prognosis of hyperactive malaria is poor, with a mortality of 50% in endemic areas, which could rise to 85%, in the presence of severe splenomegaly (Crane, 1986).

Respiratory Distress

One of the complications, usually found in adults is malaria-associated acute lung injury and its more severe form, malaria-associated acute respiratory distress syndrome (Schofield & Grau, 2005). Respiratory distress is manifested by rapid laboured breathing, sometimes abnormal in rhythm (Marsh et al., 1995). Tachypnea may be the result of respiratory compensation for a profound metabolic acidosis as occurs in the majority of cases, or perhaps the result of secondary lung infection due to the immunosuppression that may accompany acute disease (Association of Physicians, 2009).

As a matter of fact, metabolic acidosis is a prominent determinant of survival and directly leads to respiratory distress (Taylor et al., 1993). In most cases, this is predominantly (but not exclusively) a lactic acidosis (English et al., 1996a). Children with severe malaria have multiple causes of lactic acidosis, from increased production by parasites, through direct stimulation by cytokines, to decreased clearance by the liver. However, the most important by far is likely to be the combined effects of several factors in reducing oxygen delivery to tissues (English et al., 1997).

Between 9 and 21% of adult patients with severe malaria suffer from non-cardiogenic pulmonary oedema, although this is rarely observed in children (Taylor and White, 2002; Mohan et al., 2008). Malaria-associated acute respiratory distress syndrome is also frequently observed in pregnant women with severe malaria and is often associated with other complications, including cerebral malaria (Van den Steen et al., 2010).

Plasmodium falciparum infection causes respiratory symptoms that resemble influenza-like illness. The pulmonary oedema is accompanied by intra-alveolar hyaline membranes and proteinaceous debris, associated with malaria antigens. Pulmonary oedema is associated with high parasitaemia and often lead to the respiratory distress syndrome (Punyagupta et al, 1974). Pulmonary oedema may be the consequence of hypoalbuminaemia, iatrogenic fluid overload or direct alveolar capillary damage produced by parasites and neutrophils, leading to vascular occlusion, resulting in the acute respiratory distress (Maguire et al., 2005). Profound hypoalbuminaemia, could be as a result of the catabolic effects of the acute infection, potentiating the leak of fluid into the alveolae (Association of Physicians, 2009). Infected erythrocytes are observed to sequester onto the endothelium in small capillaries and larger blood vessels in the lung (Corbett et al., 1989), but less massively, compared with the sequestration of infected erythrocytes in the brain of patients with cerebral malaria. Furthermore, mononuclear cells as well as polymorphonuclear granulocytes are found to sequester in pulmonary vessels (MacPherson et al., 1985; Valecha et al, 2009).

In malaria caused by *Plasmodium vivax*, pulmonary oedema usually has a relatively good prognosis (Tan et al., 2008), although lethal cases have been reported (Valecha et al., 2009). However, a higher mortality rate, (up to 80%) is associated with the acute respiratory distress syndrome, caused by the more prevalent *Plasmodium falciparum* (Taylor and White, 2002; Mohan et al., 2008). This syndrome often occurs during or even after antimalarial treatment, and is aggravated by fluid overload (Charoenpan et al., 1990).

Renal Disorder

Clinically significant renal involvement is associated with infections by *Plasmodium falciparum* and *P.malariae* (Naqvi et al., 2003). The latter can cause an immune complex-mediated glomerular disease, leading to nephrotic syndrome. The clinical spectrum of renal involvement in falciparum malaria, has been said to vary widely (Sitprija, 1988). Some report urinary sediment abnormalities, mild proteinuria, fluid and electrolyte changes and acute renal failure (ARF) (Boonpucknavig and Sitprija, 1979). Acute renal failure is associated with falciparum malaria in Southeast Asia, India, and sub-Saharan Africa (Barsoum, 2000). ARF occurs in 1–5% of native patients in endemic areas (Sheehy & Reba, 1967; Prakash et al.,

1996), yet it is much more frequent in non-immune Europeans; reported figures usually are 25 to 30% (Barsoum, 2000).

The onset of ARF is usually within 4-7 days after the appearance of fever, and the duration ranges from a few days to several weeks, and may be oliguric or non-oliguric (Boonpucknavig and Sitprija, 1979). ARF is commonly observed in patients with heavy parasitaemia or intravascular haemolysis, with or without G6PD deficiency (Boonpucknavig and Sitprija, 1979). In a study in eastern India (Mishra et al., 2007) many deaths were recorded in cerebral malaria patients, either because of ARF alone (9.75%) or in combination with other serious complications (26.82%). An increasing trend of ARF has been recorded (Nitya et al., 2001), which may be caused by the inappropriate use of drugs, resulting in direct nephrotoxicity, hemolysis (Mishra & Mohanty, 2001), or severe jaundice (*Suvanapha* et al., 1992).

Two mechanisms have been suggested to be involved in the pathogenesis of ARF in falciparum malaria; impaired microcirculation (ischaemia) due to parasitised erythrocytes and non-specific effects of infection (Sitprija, 1988). The latter include hypovolaemia, intravascular haemolysis, disseminated intravasular coagulation, endotoxinaemia and cholestatic jaundice (Prakash et al., 1998). The pathophysiologic changes that are known to occur during the acute phase of renal failure are conditions like, dehydration, hypotension, hyponatraemia, a reduced circulating blood volume due to generalised vasodilation and disseminated intravascular coagulation (Barsoum, 1998).

Parasitised red cells have decreased deformability, which results in sluggish flow in the microcirculation. Ischaemic acute tubular necrosis (ATN) is by far the most common pathology resulting from hypovolaemia, peripheral pooling of blood, blockage of microcirculation by parasitized red blood cells (Naqvi et al., 2003). Haemodynamic and oxygen transport studies have shown evidence of reduced renal blood flow and oxygen delivery (Day et al., 1997), and features of acute renal tubular necrosis have been identified in a histopathological study of malaria-associated acute renal failure (Stone et al., 1972). The histologic picture in malarial ARF shows a variable mixture of acute tubular necrosis (ATN), interstitial nephritis, and glomerulonephritis (Taylor et al., 1993). ATN is the most consistent histologic finding. Tubular changes include cloudy swelling, hemosiderin granular deposits, and variable degrees of cell necrosis. The tubular lumen often contains hemoglobin casts. The interstitium is oedematous with a moderate to dense mononuclear cellular infiltration, and the venules may show clumps of parasitized erythrocytes. Malaria antigens can be detected in renal tubular epithelial cells in association with red cell casts. Progression to renal failure can also occur in some patients with falciparum malaria admitted in intensive care units (Krishnan and Karnad, 2003). There can be elevated creatinine levels which become normalized in surviving children given standard management, including fluid administration, suggesting that hypovolaemia (leading to reversible impairment of renal perfusion) was involved. Elevated urea and creatinine could be attributed to dehydration (English et al., 1997). However, raised plasma creatinine was an independent predictor of mortality. A study of children in Papua New Guinea (Day et al., 2000), and studies in Vietnamese adults have shown that base deficit was the best correlate with a fatal outcome, with serum creatinine and lactate accounting for most of the variation in serum base deficit (Marsh et al., 1995). Rust-tinged urine is associated with hyperbilirubinaemia caused by red cell destruction (Devarbhavi et al, 2005).

Severe jaundice is seen in some falciparum malaria patients, with cholestatic jaundice and acute renal failure (Mahakur et al., 1983). Other studies report that massive intravascular hemolysis is the main mechanism behind ARF (Chugh et al., 1977; Mahakur et al., 1983). Generally, in falciparum malaria, haemolytic jaundice predominates, and the jaundice could be severe in cases of ARF associated with oliguria. Very severe hyperbilirubinaemia may be due to intrahepatic cholestasis (Dash et al., 1994). In several studies, both direct and indirect bilirubin, together with bile acid have been implicated in the pathogenesis of malarial ARF (Odel et al., 1967; Baum et al., 1969; Aoyagi & Lowenstern, 1969).

Rhabdomyolysis is another uncommon way of inducing renal failure in malaria infection. The diagnosis is based on high serum level of muscular enzymes, Creatine Phosphokinase and clinical symptoms like myalgias (Reynaud et al., 2005). Only a few publications are available about rhabdomyolysis and *P. falciparum* infection (*Knodel & Moore, 1993; Allo et al., 1997)*. The mechanism postulated to explain rhabdomyolysis is the sequestration of parasitized erythrocytes in striated muscle capillaries, inducing microcirculatory obstruction. *Plasmodium falciparum* may also induce myositis with myoglobinuria (*Sinniah & Lye, 2000)*. This mechanism may explain the muscle pain experienced by some patients and the high level of creatine phosphokinase.

Prognosis of ARF is favourable in patients who have early and frequent dialysis, but prognosis is poor when multiple organs are involved, especially when acute respiratory failure is present. The association of impaired renal function with liver dysfunction has been noted, and may well represent common pathology (Sitprija, 1988). Visceral organ dysfunction presumably results from the sequestration of erythrocytes containing inactive forms of the parasite in microcirculation and their local metabolic, ischaemic and toxic effects (Sitprija, 1988).

Malaria in Pregnancy (Placental Malaria)

In pregnant women, malaria may result in foetal growth restriction, pre-term delivery or foetal loss. These may be due to the accumulation of falciparum-infected red cells in the proteoglycan matrix of the placental intervillous spaces (Wellems et al, 2009). Inflammation caused by parasitized red cells in the placenta is associated with blockage of blood flow to the foetus (Dorman et al, 2002), accounting for foetal death, intrauterine growth restriction, miscarriage and premature delivery (Dorman et al, 2002).

Pregnant women are particularly susceptible to malaria as the placenta provides a new target for the adhesion of the infected red blood cells. These erythrocytes are sequestered to the placenta surface through interactions between PfEMP1 domains and chondroitin sulphate A (Fried and Duffy, 1996; Hviid and Salanti, 2007). Parasite-infected cells in the placenta express variant surface antigens (VSAs), mainly the variant surface antigens of chondroitin sulphate protein (Breman et al, 2007). The lack of immunity to these VSAs results in the placental pathology.

Women in their first pregnancy more commonly experience placental malaria because of their expression of forms of PfEMP1 that bind placental chondroitin sulphate A, which are antigenically new to the immune systems, compared with women who have been previously pregnant (Fried and Duffy, 1996). Antiadhesion antibodies, which limit the accumulation of parasites in the placenta appear in pregnant women from Africa and Asia, who have been pregnant in previous occasions, but not in those with first-time pregnancies (Fried et al, 1998). Women become resistant to placental malaria over successive pregnancies as they acquire antibodies that inhibit the binding of placental parasites to chondroitin sulfate A (Fried et al., 1998). Such antibodies are associated with a decreased risk of placental malaria and increased birthweight and gestational age of the newborn (Duffy and Fried, 2003). First time mothers with active pacental malaria have elevated levels of total IgG and IgM (Logie et al., 1973), but these do not inhibit the binding of placental parasites (Fried et al., 1998) and this latter observation may explain the slow clearance of parasites from these women (Brabin & Rogerson, 2001). In women without specific immunity, phagocytic cells may play a more prominent role in clearing parasites (Graham, 1938). The maternal compartment of the placenta has also been reckoned to contain macrophages with strong phagocytic activity, which has been correlated with the frequency of severe maternal anemia (Rogerson et al., 2003).

Cerebral Malaria

Cerebral malaria (CM) is the most common complication of *P. falciparum* infection, which may result in severe complications (*Newton & Krishna,* 1998), including long-term neurologic impairment *(Boivin,* 2002), multi-organ failures (*Kochar et al., 2002)*, and high mortality rates *Shukla* et al., 1995), in the absence of prompt diagnosis and appropriate treatment. It is universally fatal if not treated promptly, and 20% of adults who receive adequate treatment still die (Warrel et al, 1990). Fever is a characteristic feature of *P. falciparum* infection (*Newton & Krishna,* 1998), yet a significant proportion of CM patients (20%) were afebrile on admission, probably because of self-medication with anti-malarial/anti-pyretic drugs by the patient before admission (*Takshande et al., 2006).*

The pathogenesis of cerebral malaria is not completely understood, and the factors involved in the development of the neurological sequelae remain unclear. In the central nervous system, it has been hypothesized that activation of the cerebral endothelial cells causes disruption of the blood-brain barrier that could result in the perturbation of brain parenchyma by parasite proteins (Brown et al, 1999). Rosette formation can be linked to the development of cerebral malaria, as they are noted to cause plugging of cerebral capillaries, interfering with cerebral blood flow. Rosetting reduces blood flow, promotes cytoadherence to endothelium, enhances anaerobic glycolysis and reduces pH (Weatherall et al, 2002). Unbridled cytoadherence-rosetting-sequestration, results in poor tissue perfusion, organ dysfunction, anaerobic glycolysis in tissues and lactic acidosis (Weatherall et al, 2002). The clinical course of cerebral malaria is characterized by diffuse, potentially reversible encephalopathy associated with fits and loss of consciousness (Turner, 1997; Idro et al, 2005).

Red blood cell CR1 has been implicated in the pathogenesis of severe malarial anaemia (Waitumbi et al, 2000) and cerebral malaria (Rowe et al, 1997). CR1 deficiency is claimed to protect against severe disease by reducing rosette-mediated microvascular obstruction (Cockburn et al, 2004)

Anaemia due to Plasmodium Infection

Anaemia is the most common complication of *P. falciparum* infection (Abdalla *et al*, 1980; Phillips and Pasvol, 1992), and is particularly severe in children and pregnant women living in endemic areas (Lavez et al, 2005). Relatively little is known about the specific pathophysiology of malarial anaemia (Menedez *et al*, 2000). Severe malarial anaemia is defined as Hb concentration less than 5g/dl in the presence of falciparum asexual parasitaemia, but in the absence of any other or additional cause of anaemia (English, 2000). A striking haematologic feature of severe malarial anaemia is the development of life-threatening haemolytic anaemia, with inadequate reticulocyte response (Srichaikul et al, 1967; Abdalla et al, 1980). The abnormality of erythroid development is rapidly reversed by effective anti-malarial therapy, and reticulocyte count peaks after one week (Srichaikul et al, 1967). A low reticulocyte count in the face of severe haemolysis is one of the characteristic features of severe malarial anaemia in humans, non-human primates and rodents (Roberts *et* al, 2005).

Barnwell (2005) also observed impaired reticulocytosis, which was attributed to malfunctioning bone marrow. Although the cause is not certain, pro-inflammatory cytokines, particularly TNF-α have been thought to be the major cause of bone marrow dysfunction (Clark and Chaudhri, 1988). Chang and Stevenson (2004) have suggested parasite factors (haemozoin, toxins), pro-inflammatory cytokines and a non-optimal response to erythropoietin, to affect the erythrocytic precursors to cause dyserythropoiesis.

Erythropoiesis is the process by which erythroid progenitors proliferate and differentiate into non-nucleated reticulocytes in the bone marrow (Robson & Weatherall, 2009). The inadequate erythropoiesis in malaria is not due to the deficient erythropoietin production (Chang & Stevenson, 2004). Rather, emerging evidence suggests the involvement of cytokines and other mediators of inflammation (such as hemozoin). This is not entirely unexpected since cytokines are known to play a role in the maturation of erythroid of cells (Chasis and Mohandas, 2008).

Dyserythropoiesis or morphologically and/or functionally abnormal production of erythrocytes, coincides with reduced reticulocytosis, indicating functional disruption of the output from the bone marrow (Abdalla, 1980). Additionally, Casals-Pascual *et al* (2006) have reported that haemozoin directly inhibits erythropoiesis, independently from TNF-□, and that haemozoin and TNF-α have additive effect on the development of erythroid cells.

Several studies have indicated that *P falciparum*–induced anemia is associated principally with the destruction of unparasitised red cells (Abdallah et al., 1980; Philip & Pasvol, 1992; Looaresuwan et al, 1991). and is exacerbated by defects in erythropoiesis (Abdallah et al., 1980; Wickramansingh and Abdalla, 2000). Extravascular haemolysis of both infected and uninfected red cells occurs in hyperparasitaemic *P falciparum* infections and is thought to result from destruction by the "pitting" of parasites by macrophages in the spleen, decreasing the deformability of these cells (Philip & Pasvol, 1992; Wickramansingh and Abdalla, 2000).

One possibility for the decreased deformability of uninfected red cells is inferred from its extremely strong correlation with acidosis, suggesting that the acidosis may play a major role in compromising tissue blood flow. Patients with malaria are often dehydrated and relatively hypovolaemic (English et al., 1996a), potentially exacerbating microvascular obstruction by reducing perfusion pressure. RBC destruction is also an inevitable part of malaria, and anaemia further compromises oxygen delivery (Miller et al., 2002).

Hosts respond to *P falciparum* infection by increasing the proliferation and activity of macrophages responsible for the phagocytosis of infected red cells and apparently normal uninfected cells (Philip & Pasvol, 1992). This phagocytosis may occur directly through membrane modifications, or it may be mediated by opsonizing antibodies. IgG and complement C3 have been detected on erythrocytes from malaria patients with severe anaemia (Facer and Brown, 1981; Waitumbi et al, 2000; Ekvall, 2003).

From the foregoing, immune complex-mediated haemolysis has been suggested as another contributory factor to malarial anaemia in some populations (Robson and Weatherall, 2009). Observations supporting this are that some patients with malaria develop a positive direct Coombs' antiglobulin test. Furthermore, red cell sensitization is usually associated with C3, or can occur with IgG alone or combinations of C3, C4 and IgG. Recent data suggest that it is not just host proteins on the surface of uninfected red cells that result in haemolysis. Immunoglobulin-antigen complexes containing the *P. falciparum* ring surface protein (RSP-2) have been reported (Robson and Weatherall, 2009). Soon after merozoites have infected a red cell, RSP-2 is expressed on the cell surface and may play a role in adhesion to endothelial cells. This protein is also found on the surfaces of uninfected red cells and erythroblasts in bone marrow from patients infected by *P. falciparum*, suggesting a role for RSP-2 in the development of anaemia (Layez et al., 2005).

According to Barnwell (2006), in most severe malarial anaemia, intravascular haemolysis is not apparent, and destruction of uninfected red cells is more than ten-fold greater than any lysis caused by parasitisation. Moreover, mathematical modeling of haematologic data from experimental human *P. falciparum* infections (Jakeman et al. 1999) as well as analysis of clinical data from endemic areas (Price et al. 2001) has suggested that up to twelve uninfected red cells are lost for every infected red cell, supporting the point that the destruction of red cells following parasitisation, cannot account for the degree of anaemia seen in malaria infection, implying that the destruction of the uninfected red cells is the major cause of haemoglobin loss (Ekvall, 2003).

According to Collins et al. (2003), severe anaemia does not occur as a result of destruction of infected RBCs *per se*, because for every infected RBC destroyed, approximately 32 non-infected RBCs are removed from circulation. Greenwood et al. (1991) saw it as a mystery, the fact that even though the red cell is the primary target of the malaria parasites, severe anaemia is seen in a small proportion of malaria cases.

The biological activity of haemozoin is very high, as it catalyses the formation of free radicals through repeated redox cycles, initiated by Fe^{2+} (Arese and Schwarzer, 1997). Intracellular or membrane-bound haemozoin in contact with erythroid cells causes cellular dysfunction and oxidative damage (Casals-Pascual et al. 2006).

Though it can be reiterated that the pathogenesis of malarial anaemia includes intravascular haemolysis, extravascular clearance of parasitised and non-parasitised erythrocytes and bone marrow dysfunction, the relative contributions of these factors are not understood yet (Roberts et al. 2005). In a study involving Thai patients, Looareesuwan et al. (1987) reported that malarial anaemia was partly caused by the loss of both infected and uninfected red cells, which were destroyed by haemolysis or phagocytosis.

The rigidification of the membranes of infected and uninfected red cells was seen as another important factor in the destruction of these cells through the spleen (Dondorp et al.

1999; 2000). Parasitised cells have increased osmotic fragility and reduced deformability, and the clearance rate of these cells from the circulation is proportional to the severity of infection and the degree of splenomegaly (Looareesuwan et al. 1991). Indeed, it is well documented that survival of uninfected red cells is significantly reduced (Abdalla et al. 1980, 1983; Waitumbi et al. 2000). Although the causes of the decreased life span of the red cells are unclear, increased haemolysis secondary to erythrophagocytosis mediated by immunoglobulins and complement has been reported (Abdalla et al. 1983; Waitumbi *et al*, 2001). According to Abdalla (1988), the presence of circulating monocytes containing phagocytosed uninfected red cells suggests that during malaria infection, uninfected red cells develop lesions that activate monocytes to capture and engulf them. The nature of the lesion that triggers red cell phagocytosis is not clear, but Waitumbi et al. (2001) and Newton et al. (1997), suspected the deposition of antibody on the surface of the red cells. However, the red cell surface antigen has not been consistently observed in all studies (Facer et al. 1980).

IgG may be deposited on the surface of RBCs in patients with falciparum infection through several mechanisms. During the infection, reactive oxygen species are produced owing to the effect of TNF-α or other cytokines (Jakobsen et al, 1995). Another possibility is that the uninfected red blood cells are seen as senescent cells, and are thus removed (Omodeo-Salé et al. 2003). This study showed that the falciparum parasite induces biochemical modifications in the membrane of both infected and uninfected red cells, mimicking the physiologic cell aging process. These effects were thought to have been produced by falciparum-induced oxidative stress.

Changes induced by the falciparum parasite on the properties of infected red blood cells include increase in phospholipids content due to high biosynthetic activity (Jain, 1988), necessary for membrane biogenesis, and essential to parasite survival. Oxidative stress increases with age in erythrocytes, and it is intensified by falciparum infection. This is manifested as increased endogenous thiobarbituric-reactive substances in older red cells, indicative of higher level of peroxidation in aged cells (Ando et al. 1995). Membrane damage is increased in infected red cells, shown by lower unsaturation index and modified phospholipids pattern, whereby phosphatidylserine and phosphatidylcholine are markedly decreased (Omodeo-Salé et al. 2003). Oxidative stress induced by falciparum might contribute to the loss of phosphatidylserine by changing the transbilayer organization of the membrane phospholipids, and enhancing phosphatidylserine exposure on the outer surface. Alterations in the organization of phospholipids have been shown to compromise membrane integrity, leading to early haemolysis or reticulo-endothelial clearance (Allen et al. 1988) or phagocytosis (Boas et al. 1998).

Hypersplenism is also considered to contribute to the early anaemia of acute malaria through sequestering of red blood cells. The persistent, often worsening anaemia, seen weeks after clearance of parasitaemia could be through phagocytosis of both parasitised and non-parasitised red cells by a hyperactive reticuloendothelial system (Dondorp *et al*, 1999; Menendez *et al*, 2000). Malaria can also cause anaemia of inflammation (Clark and Chaudri, 1988).

Recently, one of the causes of malarial anaemia, has been linked to the production of hepcidin, in response to some cytokines. IL6 induces hepcidin expression, which is a master regulator of iron trafficking, leading to decreased iron availability for erythropoiesis (Weiss, 2008). As part of the acute phase response, the peptide hepcidin is synthesized and released by hepatocytes resulting in increased serum ferritin and a reduction of bio-available iron.

Hepcidin binds to the iron exporter ferroportin, which is expressed on the surface of macrophages, resulting in the internalization of the complex and its degradation (Nemeth & Ganz, 2006). Hence, iron is retained by macrophages, rather than being released into the circulation, bound to transferrin and transported to the bone marrow or spleen where it can be re-cycled in erythropoiesis. Hepcidin is clearly implicated in the anaemia of inflammation or chronic disease (Weiss, 2008). It is not yet clear the extent of the role of hepcidin in malarial anaemia. During the acute phase of malaria infection the serum iron level rapidly decreases and iron is sequestered in the marrow. Serum ferritin levels are high mimicking what is seen in other acute infections (Robson & Weatherall, 2009).

In a study in which hepcidin expression in anaemic Tanzanian children with febrile *P. falciparum* malaria with high parasite densities was compared with malaria-naïve Dutch volunteers who were experimentally infected with *P. falciparum*, hepcidin concentrations were increased in both groups and associated with profound disturbances in iron homeostasis (de Mast et al., 2009). This study, which was an experimental human malaria model showed that even a mild increase in serum hepcidin, induces hypoferraemia and a steep fall in the haemoglobin content of reticulocytes, which is suggestive of impaired iron incorporation in haemoglobin (de Mast et al., 2009).

In malaria-endemic settings of sub-Saharan Africa, age patterns of anaemia show a peak between 1 and 5 years (Crawley, 2004). The effect of malaria parasitaemia on anaemia has been shown to decrease with age (Stoltsfus *et al*, 2000). In a study by Cramer *et al* (2004) on Ghanaian children with severe malaria, severe anaemia was the most predominant, followed by prostration and respiratory distress, which confirmed previous findings in highly endemic areas (WHO, 2000).

In another Ghanaian study involving sickle cell patients, it has been shown that for those patients with falciparum parasites, the distribution of reticulocytes was exponential, while a polynomial distribution was seen in the non-parasitaemic (Nsiah et al, 2010). A mathematical model, based on categorical reticulocyte levels and their frequencies, was derived. The exponential distribution of the parasitaemics shows the fluctuations in the retic counts of this group was not much. For the non-parasitaemics, the polynomial pattern showed that frequency does not diminish completely to zero.The physiological explanation is that in the case of the parasitaemic, due to some parasite factors which can act to impair erythropoiesis, low retic counts occur at a higher frequency. On the other hand, in the non-parasitaemic (assuming there are no other confounding factors), due to effective erythropoiesis, it is more likely for higher levels of reticulocytes to be seen.

Drug Therapies

The Global Malaria Eradication Programme was launched in 1955 by the WHO, based on two approaches; the use of chloroquine for drug therapy and the use of DDT for the control of the vector. Haemoglobin degradation, haem detoxification, folate biosynthesis and protein synthesis in the parasite apicoplast, are effective targets for therapeutic intervention in malaria (Fidock et al, 2004). Whilst the majority of cases of malaria worldwide are mild and can be treated with oral drugs, a minority, mainly because of delays in diagnosis or treatment, may develop complicated, life-threatening disease requiring parenteral therapy (Pasvol, 2005). In clinical practice, any patient with suspected malaria who demonstrates complicated disease, i.e. prostration, any impairment of consciousness, convulsions or any manifestation of shock, decreased urinary output, respiratory distress or abnormal bleeding should be treated with parenteral rather than oral drugs (Pasvol, 2005).

Antifolate antimalarial drugs act by inhibiting the parasite enzyme, dihydrofolate reductase (Hutchings et al, 1952). This enzyme catalyses the NADPH-dependent reduction of dihydrofolate to tetrahdrofolate, an essential cofactor in *de novo* synthesis of nucleotides. Although the action of these drugs is many times more potent for the enzyme of *Plasmodium* spp. than for that of mammals, overdosing can cause megaloblastic anemia in humans (*Fleming et al., 1974).* At the appropriate dosing, these drugs prevent malarial haemolysis, reducing demand for folate and preventing megaloblastic anaemia (Fleming, 1989).

Pyrimethamine inhibits parasite growth by binding to the enzyme dihydrofolate reductase, which exists in *Plasmodium falciparum* and other protozoa (Ferone and Roland, 1980). Pyrimethamine and sulphadoxine act synergistically to inhibit two enzymes important in the biosynthesis of folic acid by the parasite, dihydrofolate reductase (DHFR) and dihydropteroate synthetase (DHPS) (Hopkins Sibley et al, 2001).

The 8-aminoquinolines, like primaquine and taferoquine, target the liver stage parasites, while the 4-aminoquinolines (eg. chloroquine, amodiaquine and quinolinemethanols, including quinine, mefloquine, concentrate within the parasite food vacuole. Some drugs attack the parasite electon transport system, like Atovaquone, an inhibitor of the mitochondrial cytochrome bc1 complex (Bairs, 2005).

Chloroquine acts by preventing the polymerization of toxic haem released during the proteolysis of haemoglobin in the food vacuole of the parasite (Slater, 1993; Dorn et al, 1995). It is thought to kill parasites by inhibiting the process of crystallization necessary to detoxify ferriprotophyrin IX, (FPIX) into haemozoin (Sullivan et al, 1993). Chloroquine (CQ) inhibits the breakdown of FPIX, released after the proteolysis, causing a build-up of free FPIX and/or CQ-FPIX complex that may ultimately kill (Slater, 1993; Dorn et al, 1995). A quinoline-haem complex is incorporated into the growing polymer to terminate chain extension, blocking further polymerization. The weak base CQ, accumulates in the acidic food vacuole, binding to the FPIX (Chou et al, 1980). Thus the food vacuole of the parasite is the target of action of the quinoline antimalarials (Bray et al, 2005).The FPIX is potentially toxic due to its pro-oxidant and lytic activities (Companale et al, 2003).

Currently, Artemisinin combination therapies (ACTs) are the recommended first-line treatment for uncomplicated *Plasmodium falciparum* malaria in endemic regions (WHO, 2006). Artemisinin is a sesquiterpene lactone with a 1,2,4-trioxane heterocyclic core that incorporates a peroxide bridge or linkage that is essential for its activity (Meshnick, 2002). The artemisinins contain pharmacophoric peroxide bond that undergoes reductive activation by haem released by the parasitic haemoglobin digestion (Francis et al, 1998).The irreversible redox reaction between antimalarial peroxide and FPIX, produces carbon-centred radicals or carbocations that alkylate haem (Meshnick et al, 1991), and proteins (Asaramahasakida et al, 1994).

There is evidence that artemisinins are activated inside the parasite by ring opening, which generates radical intermediates that react with susceptible parasite targets (Meshnick, 2002; O'Neill et al., 2010). However, the origin and nature of the artemisinin activator is not clear. Some studies point to haemoglobin-derived haem or ferrous iron, or other host or parasite-derived iron sources (O'Nell & Posner, 2010), suggesting that parasite uptake and hydrolysis of haemoglobin is necessary for artemisinin activity. Artemisinin is highly potent against haemoglobin-digesting stages of malaria parasites (O'Neill et al., 2010) and against other hemoglobin-degrading pathogens such as Schistosoma species (Klayman, 1985), but it is much less potent against other pathogens (Kaiser et al., 2007). This suggests that hemoglobin digestion plays a critical role in the mechanism of action of this drug class (Klonis et al., 2011).

The artemisin antimalarials are produced semi-synthetically from extracts of *Artemesia annua* or sweet wormwood, also called qinghao in Chinese (Klayman, 1985). The primary extract from the plant is chemically converted into several active derivatives, like artesunate, artemether and dihydro-artemisinin, which are able to act rapidly against both the parasites' asexual and sexual stages (Sutherland et al, 2005). As monotherapies, artemisin derivatives are effective for the treatment of uncomplicated malaria, but because of their rapid clearance in plasma, complete cure requires a longer treatment (up to 7 days). This raises concern about their potential of inducing drug resistance. It is to prevent such a resistance that the artemisin combination therapies (ACTs) were developed. These involve the simultaneous administration of two or three antimalarials, each with a distinct mechanism against the parasite. The WHO first endorsed ACTs for the treatment of malaria in 2004 and recommended a switch to ACTs as first-line treatment of malaria in 2006. However, due to high cost, some patients may use artemisinin monotherapies, which are cheaper than ACTs but could accelerate the development of resistance, as reported by Jambou et al in 2005.

The clinical effectiveness of the artemisinin derivatives depends on their following features; rapid onset of action and activity against all the erythrocytic stages of the parasite. One of their disadvantages is, having short *in vivo* half lives, requiring a three-day treatment regimen in combination with longer-acting antimalarials to maximize cure rate (Ridley (2002). The artemisin derivatives act rapidly against the asexual blood stage parasites to alleviate symptoms, while having the additional effect of killing gametocytes and so decreasing parasite transmission. The effect of the longer-acting partner is to continue decreasing the parasite biomass after the artemisinin derivative has fallen below therapeutic levels (Greenword et al, 2008). The fluctuations in the supplies of these drugs is another disadvantage, as their isolation from plants is the only practical means of obtaining them (Kindermans et al, 2007). ACT treatment failure has been reported in some places, an indication that resistance to these drugs is emerging (Dondorp, et al, 2010)

Drug resistance continues to threaten conventional therapies. Point mutations in the DHFR and DHPS genes confer resistance to pyrimethamine and sulphadoxine, respectively, with decreasing in vitro P. falciparum susceptibility related to the number of mutations in each gene (Triglia et al, 1997). The emergence and spread of resistance strains has also rendered CQ ineffective in many malaria-endemic regions. The activity of CQ depends on a high level of accumulation within the malarial parasite, and drug resistance arises from reduced drug accumulation (Bray et al, 1999), due to the mutation of Plasmodium falciparum CQ-resistance transporter (PfCRT). However, the mechanism behind the cause of the resistance is uncertain (Ginsburg and Stein, 1991)

Factors that contribute to drug resistance are drug pharmacokinetics (Hastings et al, 2002), overusage of drugs (Simpson et al, 2000), cross resistance between drugs (Iyer et al, 2001), inadequate treatment through inappropriate prescription, non-compliance (Simpson et al, 2000).The best approach for slowing the development of drug resistance is optimal treatment of individuals after the development of clinical symptoms and subsequent confirmation of malaria (Gatton et al, 2004).

Vaccine Development for Malaria Infection

The concept that vaccination may be a useful tool to control the disease is based on a number of observations. Individuals continually exposed to infection by the parasitic protozoan responsible do eventually develop immunity to the disease, and passive immunization with antibody from immune donors can have a dramatic effect on blood stage parasitemia (Cohen et al., 1961). Furthermore, inoculation of live attenuated parasites can protect naive volunteers against infection (Clyde et al., 1973), and immunization with whole killed organisms can protect in animal models (Mitchell et al., 1975).

The complete protection generated by vaccination with radiation-attenuated sporozoites in animal models and in humans (*Nussenzweig* 1967; *Edelman, et al., 1993)* supports the feasibility of a pre-erythrocytic vaccine. Such a vaccine could eliminate, or reduce to a sub-clinical level, the number of parasites that emerge from infected hepatocytes to initiate the red cell phase of the life cycle that is responsible for the clinical manifestations of malaria (Miller et al., 2002). There is consensus that a highly effective malaria vaccine would require a combination of key antigens and/or epitopes from different stages of the life cycle and that induction of both humoral and cellular immunity is required for optimal efficacy (Hoffman, 1996) Merozoite antigens are a major focus of vaccine development, in which immunization generally aims to induce antibodies that inhibit invasion and subsequent replication (Fowkes et al., 2010). Antibodies to merozoite antigens are also believed to be important in mediating acquired immunity (Boyle et al., 2010).

Though vaccines offer the most cost-effective strategy for preventing infectious diseases, the development of a highly effective vaccine is yet to be accomplished. The complexity of the malaria parasite, coupled with the lack of evidence of robust infection-induced immunity, has made vaccine development especially difficult (McGregor, 1974). The most successful vaccines against infectious diseases work by mimicking natural immunity to elicit long-lasting antibody responses (Robinson and Amara, 2006). McGregor (1974) raised the issue that humoral immunity to malaria is incomplete and does not eradicate all parasites or provide protection against future challenge. Vaccines are known to be successful against diseases in which natural infections lead to long-lasting immunity, but in malaria, natural immunity is slow to develop and is incomplete, even after years of continuous exposure (McGregor et al, 2006).

To date, the majority of pre-erythrocytic stage vaccines have been based on the structure of CSP (Nassenzweigh et al, 1967), the predominant surface antigen on sporozoites. The most advanced and moderately effective malaria vaccine with the greatest potential of being licensed is RTS, S, which relies on the administration of a complex construct made up of the central repeat and C-terminus of CSP, fused to the hepatitis B virus surface antigen (HBsAg) and the free HBsAg (Bejon et al, 2008). Through antibody and cell-mediated responses, this vaccine targets the pre-erythrocytic stage, and through multiple clinical trials, has shown efficacy rates ranging from 30-66%, and 30% effectiveness against clinical malaria in children aged 1-4 years (Aponte et al, 2007). There is the need to develop vaccines that target blood-stage malaria parasites.

Malarial proteases are attractive antimalarial targets for vaccine development, because of their crucial role in parasite development, especially in the process of host erythrocyte rupture/invasion and haemoglobin degradation (Rosenthal, 2001).

Conclusion

This write-up has highlighted the structural, physiological and biochemical features of the Plasmodium parasite that has enabled it survive two-prong attacks from man; first, from immune responses (both innate and adaptive), and second, from man's technological advancement through the development of anti-malarial drugs for systemic pharmacological control or insecticides for external vector control. Being Acomplexans, the Plasmodium falciparum, though a tiny protozoan, is endowed with various features that enable it succeed in the invasion of insect-man hosts.

The success of the Plasmodium, of course, is at the expense of man, especially in malaria-endemic regions. This is borne out from the high morbidities and mortalities associated with the infection. The persitance of the parasites, high multiplication rates, cytoadherence, sequestration, rosetting, utilization of host glucose; all these contribute to the pathology of the parasite's biological and biochemical features. Even in some cases, the immune response of man which should have overcome the infective agent, rather gets haywire, turning inimical to man. For example, the production of anti-inflammatory and pro-inflammatory cytokines, is tilted towards pro-inflammation and pro-oxidation, conditions that cause damage to tissues and organs. The damage caused results in the various clinical states, which have been explained. To curtail or slow down the pathology and the attendant morbid clinical features, pharmcological intervenions have been evolved, targeting some strategic points of the parasite's metabolic machinery. But here too, the versality of the protozoan has swung into action, manifesting in the development of resistance against anti-malarial drugs, to the extent that the current first-line drug, artemisin, which held a lot of promise, is now under the 'resitance-development' albatross of falciparum.

What remains man's hope of conquering the parasite is the developmentof vaccines, for which RTS, S appears to be the trail blazer. However, more scientific, financial social and political efforts aere required, for the ultimate to be achieved.

References

Abdalla, S.H. (1988) Peripheral blood and bone marrow leucocytes in Gambian children with malaria: numerical changes and evaluation of phagocytosis. *Ann Trop Paediatr. 8*:250

Abdalla, S.H., Kasili, F.G., Wertherall, D.J. (1983). The Coomb's antiglobulin test in Kenyans. *Trans R Soc Trop Med Hyg. 77*:99-102

Abdalla, S.H., Weatherall, D.J., Wickvanasinghe, S.N. and Hughes M. (1980). The anaemia of P. falciparum malaria. *Br J Haematol. 46*:171-183

Achyangkul S Sangkrai P Webster HK (1994). Plasmodium falciparum pigment induces monocytes to release high levels of TNF-α and IL-1β. *Am J Trop Med Hyg. 51*:430-435

Adam, C., Geniteau, M., Gougerot-Pocidalo, M., Verroust, P., Lebras, J., Gibert, C., Morel-Maroger, L. (1981). Cryoglobulins, circulating immune complexes, and complement activation in cerebral malaria. *Infect Immun. 31*: 530-535

Agarwal A , Guindo, A., Cissoko, Y., Taylor, J.G., Coulibaly, D., Koné, A.,Kayentao, K., Djimde, A., Plowe, C.V. Doumbo, O., Wellems, T.E., Diallo, D, (2000*)*. Hemoglobin C associated with protection from severe malaria in the Dogon of Mali, a West African population with a low prevalence of hemoglobin S. *Blood 96:*2358–2363

Ahearn,J.M. & Fearon, D.T. (1989).Structure and function of the complement receptors, CR1 (CD 35) and CR2 (CD21). *Adv Immunol. 46*:183-219

Aidoo, M. Terlouw, D.J., Kolczak, M.S., McElroy, P.D., ter Kuile, F.O., Kariuki, S., Nahlen, B.L., Lal, A.A., Venkatachalam Udhayakumar, V. *(*2002*)*. Protective effects of the sickle cell gene against malaria morbidity and mortality. Lancet 359*:*1311–1312.

Aikawa, M., Yoshida, N., Nussenzweig, R. S., Nussenzweig, V. (1981) *Trans. R. Soc. Trop. Med. Hyg. 126:*2494–2495

Albrecht, L. Moll, K. Normark, J., Chen, Q., Wahlgren, M. (2011) Var gene transcription and PfEMP1 expression in the resetting and cytoadherence of Plasmodium falciparum clone, FCR3S1.2. *Malaria J. 10*:17

Allen, T.M., Williamson, P. and Schlegel, R.A. (1988). Phosphatidylserine as a determinant of reticuloendothelial recognition of liposome models of the erythrocyte surface. *Proc Natl Acad Sci USA*. 85:8067-8071

Allison, A.C. (1957). Parasitological reviews. Malaria in carriers of sickle-cell trait and in newborn children. Exp Parasitol. 6:418-447

Allo, J.C., Vincent, F., Barboteu, M., Schlemer, B. (1997).Falciparum malaria: an infectious cause of rhabdomyolysis and acute renal failure. Nephrol Dial Transpl *12:2033–2034*

Al-Yaman, F., Genton, B., Mokela, D., Raiko, A., Kati, S., Regerson, S., Reeder, J., Aipers, M. (1995). Human cerebral malaria: lack of significant association between resetting and disease severity. *Trans R Soc Trop Med Hyg. 89*:55-58

Amarante-Paffaro, A., Queiroz, G. S., Correa, S. T., Spira, B, and Bevilacqua, E. (2004). Phagocytosis as a potential mechanism for microbial defense of mouse placental trophoblast cells. Reproduction *128: 207-218*

Amino, R., Giovannini, D., Thiberge, S., Gueirard, P., Boisson, B., Dubremetz, J.F., Prévost, M.C., Ishino, T., Yuda, M., Ménard, R. (2008). Host cell traversal is important for progression of the malaria parasite through the dermis to the liver. Cell Host Microbe. *3:*88–96.

Amino, R., Thiberge, S., Martin, B., Celli, S. Shorte, S., Frischknecht, F., Ménard, R. (2006). Quantitative imaging of *Plasmodium* transmission from mosquito to mammal. *Nat. Med. 12:*220–224

Anand, A.C. and Puri, P. (2005). Jaundice in malaria. *J Gastroenerol. Hepatol. 20*:1322-1332

Anand, A.C., Ramji, C., Narula, A.S., Singh, W. (1992). Malarial hepatitis: A heterogeneous syndrome? *Natl Med J India. 5*:59-62

Ancsin, J. B. & Kisilevsky, R. (2004). Significance for malarial sporozoite attachment to hepatocytes. *J Biol Chem. 279*:21824-21832

Ando, K., Beppu, M., Kikugawa, K. (1995). Evidence of accumulation of lipid hydroperoxides during the aging of human red blood cells in the circulation. *Biol Pharm Bull. 18*:659-663

Aoyagi, T. & Lowenstern, L.M. (1969). Effect of bile acid renal ischemia on renal function. *J Lab Clin Med. 71*:686-690

Aponte, J.J. Aide, P., Renom, M., Mandomando, I., Bassat, Q., Sacarlal, J., Nelia Manaca, M., Lafuente, S., Barbosa, A., Leach, A., Lievens, M., Vekemans, J., Sigauque, B., Dubois, M-C., Demoitié, M-A., Sillman, M., Savarese, B., McNeil, J.G., Macete, E., Ripley Ballou, W., Cohen, J., Pedro, Alonso, L.P. (2007). Safety of the RTS,S/AS02D candidate malaria vaccine in infants living in a highly endemic area of Mozambique: a double blind randomised controlled phase I/IIb trial). *Lancet 370*:1543-1551

Arese, P. and Schwarzer, E. (1997) Malarial pigment (haemozoin) a very active 'inert' substance..*Ann Trop Med Parasitol. 91*:501-516

Armah, H Wiredu, E.K., Dodoo, A.K., Adjei, A.A., Tettey, Y., Gyasi, R. (2005) Cytokines molecules expression in the brain in human cerebral malaria. *Int J Environ Res Public Health. 2*:123-131

Arnush, M., Hetmeier, M.R. Scarim, A.L., Marino, M.H., Manning, P.T. Corbett, J.A. (1998).IL-1 produced and released endogenously within human islets inhibits beta cell function. *J Clin Invest. 102*:516-526

Asaramahasakida. W., Ittarat, I., Pu, J.M., Ziffer, H., Meshnick, S.R. (1994). Action of antimalarial endoperoxides with specific parasite proteins. *Antimicrob Agents Chemother. 38:*1854-1858

Association of Physicians (2009). New developments in the management of malaria in adults. *QJM. 102*:685-693

Atamna, H. & Ginsberg, H. (1993). Origin of reactive oxygen species in erythrocytes infected with Plasmodium falciparum. *Mol Biochem Parasitol. 61*:231-242

Ayi, K. , Turrini, F. , Piga, A. , Arese, P. (2004). Enhanced phagocytosis of ring-parasitized mutant erythrocytes: A common mechanism that may explain protection against falciparum malaria in sickle trait and beta-thalassemia trait. Blood 104*:*3364–3371

Ayyub, M., Barlas, S., Lubbad, E. (2000). Usefulness of exchange transfusion in acute liver failure due to severe falciparum malaria. *Am J Gastroenterol. 95*:802-4

Bag, S., Samal, G.C., Deep, N., Patra, U.C., Nayak, M., Mehar, L.K. (1994). Complicated falciparum malaria. *Indian Pediatr. 31*:821-825.

Baird, J.K. (1998). Age-dependent characteristics of protection versus susceptibility to Plasmodium falciparum. Ann Trop Med Parasitol. 92:367-390

Baird, J.K. (2005). Effectiveness of antimalarial drugs. *New Engl J Med. 352*:1565-1577

Baldacci, P. & Manard, R. (2004). The elusive malaria sporozoite in the mammalian host. *Mol Parasitol. 54*:298-306

Ball, H.J., McDonald, H.G., McGregor, S.S., Hurt, N.H. (2004). Cyclooxygenase-2 in the pathogenesis of murine cerebral malaria. *J Infect Dis. 189*:751-758

Bannister, L. & Mitchell, G. (2003). The ins, outs and roundabouts of malaria. *Trends Parasitol. 19*:209-213

Bannister, L.H., Hopkins, J.M., Fowler, R.E., Krishna, S., Mitchell, G.H. (2000). A brief illustrated guide to the ultrastructure of Plasmodium falciparum asexual blood stages. *Parasitol Today.16*:427–43

Bansal, R., Kadhiravan, T., Aggarwal, P., Handa. R., Biswas, A., Wali, J.P. (2002). *Plasmodium vivax* and hepatitis E co-infection-A rare cause of malarial jaundice. *Indian J Gastroenterol. 21*:207-8.

Barnwell, J.W. (2006). [Comment] Malaria: death and disappearing erythrocytes. *Blood 107*:854-856

Barsoum, R.S. (2000). Malarial acute renal failure. *JASN. 11*: 2147-2154

Barsoum, R.S. (1998). Malarial nephropathies. Nephrol Dial Transpl *20*:1588-1597

Barsoum, R.S., Sitprija, V. (1996). Tropical nephrology. In: *Diseases of the Kidney*, 6th Ed., edited by Schrier RW, Gottaschalk CW, Boston, Little, Brown & Co. pp2221 -2268

Baum, M., Sterling, G,A. Dawson, J.L. (1969). Further study into obstructive jaundice and ischaemic renal disease. *Br Med J. 2*:229-232

Becker, K., Tilley, L., Vennerstrom, J.L., Roberts, D., Rogerson, S., Ginsburg, H. (2004). Oxidative stress in malaria parasite-infected erythrocytes: host-parasite interactions. *Int J Parasitol. 34:*163-189

*Bedu-Addo G. & Bates, I. (*2002). *Causes of massive splenomegaly in Ghana.* Lancet *360: 449–454*

Berkley, J.*, Mwarumba, S., Bramham, K. et al. (1999). Bacteraemia complicating severe malaria in children.* Trans R Soc Trop Med Hyg. *93:*283*–286*

Bhalla, A., Suri, V., Singh, V. (2006) [Review] Malarial hepatopathy. *J Postgrad Med. 52*:315-320

*Boivin, M.J. (*2002). *Effects of early cerebral* malaria *on cognitive ability in Senegalese children.* J Dev Behav Pediatr. *23:* 353*–364.*

Bejon, P. Lusingu,J.,Olotu,A., Leach, A.,Lievens,M.,Vekemans,J., Mshamu, S., Lang T., Gould, J., Dubois, M-C. et al (2008).Efficacy of RTS,S/AS01E vaccine against malaria in children 5 to 17 months of age. *New Engl J Med. 359*:2521-2532

Biritwum, R.D., Wellbeck, J., Barnish, G. (2000). Incidence and management of malaria in two communities of different socio-economic levels in Accra, Ghana, *Ann Trop Med Parasitol. 94*:771-778

Boas, F.E., Forman, L., Beutler, E. (1998). Phosphatidylserine exposure and red cell viability in red cell aging and hemolytic anemia. *Proc Natl Acad Sci USA. 95*:3077-3081

Boggild, A.K., Page, A.V., Keystone, J.S., Morris, A.M., W. Conrad Liles, W.C. (2009). Delay in diagnosis: malaria in a returning traveller. *CMAJ. 180:*

Boonpucknavig, U. & Sitprija, V. (1979). Renal disease in acute Plasmodium falciparum infection in man. *Kidney Int. 16*:44-52

Boutlis, C.S., Yeo, T.W., Anstey, N.M. (2006). Malaria tolerance- For whom the cell tolls? *Trends Parasitol. 22*:371-377

Boyle, M.J., Richards, J.S., Gilson, P.R., Chai, W., Beeson, J.G. *(2010).* Interactions with heparin-like molecules during erythrocyte invasion by *Plasmodium falciparum* merozoites. *Blood 115:*4559*–*4568

Brabin, B. J., Rogerson, S.J. (2001). The epidemiology and outcomes of maternal malaria. P. E. Duffy, P.E.., Jr, & M. Fried, M., Jr, (eds). *Malaria in Pregnancy: Deadly Parasite, Susceptible Host* pp 27-52. Taylor and Francis, London

Bradley, D., Newbold, C.I., Warrell, D.A. (1996). Malaria. In Oxford Textbook of Medicine, vol 1 (eds Weatherall, D.J., Ledingham, J.G.G., Warrell, D.A. pp 835-868, Oxford University Press, Oxford.

Bray, P.G., Janneh, O., Raynes, K.J., Mungthin, M., Ginsburg, H., Ward, S.A. (1999). Cellular uptake of chloroquine is dependent on binding to ferroprotophyrin IX and is independent of NHE activity in Plasmodium falciparum. *J Cell Biol. 145*:363-376

Bray, P.G., Ward, S.A., O'Neill, P.M. (2005). Quinine and artemisinin: chemistry, biology and history. *Curr Top Microbiol Immunol. 295*:3-38

Breman, J.G., Alilio, M.S., White, N.J. (2007). Defining and defeating the intolerable burden of malaria III. Progress and perspectives. *Am J Trop Med Hyg. 77 (6Suppl)*: vi-xi

Breman, J.G. Egan, A., Keusch, G.T. (2001). The intolerable burden of malaria: a new look at the numbers. *Am J Trop Med Hyg. 64 (suppl 1-2)*:iv

Brown, H., Hien, T.T., Day, N., Mai, N.T., Chuong, L.V., Chau, T.T., Loc, P.P., Phu, N.H., Bethell, D., Farrar, J., Gatter, K., White, N., Turner, G. (1999) Evidence of blood-brain barrier dysfunction in human cerebral malaria. *Neuropathol Appl Neurobiol. 25*:331-340

Buscalglia, C.A., Coppers, I., Itol, W.G., Nussenzweig, V. (2003) Sites of interaction between aldolase and TSP-related anonymous protein in Plasmodium. *Mol Biol Cell. 14*:4947-4957

Camus, D. & Hadley, T.J. (1985) A Plasmodium falciparum antigen that binds to host erythrocytes and merozoites. *Science. 230*:553-556

*Carlson, J., Ekre, H.P., Helmby, H., Gysin, J., Greenwood, B.M., Wahlgren, M. (*1992). *Disruption of Plasmodium falciparum erythrocyte rosettes by standard heparin and heparin devoid of anticoagulant activity.* Am J Trop Med Hyg *46: 595–602*

Carlson, J., Nash, G.B., Gabutti, V., al-Yaman,F., Wahlgren, M. (1994). Natural protection against severe malaria due to impaired rosette formation. *Blood 84*:3909-3914

Casals-Pascual C., Idro, R., Gicheru, N., Gwer, S., Kitsao, B., Gitau, E., Mwakesi, R., Roberts, D.J., Newton, C.R.J.C. (2008). High levels of erythropoietin are associated with protection against neurological sequelae in African children with cerebral malaria. *Proc Natl Acad Sci. USA. 105*:2634-2639.

Casals-Pasual, C., Kai, D., Newton, C.R.J.C., Peshu, N. and Roberts, D.J. (2006) Thrombocytopenia in falciparum malaria is associated with high concentrations of IL-10. *Am J Trop Med Hyg*. 75:434-436

Centers for Disease Control and Prevention. *Health Information for International Travel, 2003-2004. Atlanta: U.S. Department of Health and Human Services, Public Health Service; 2003*

Cerami, C., Frevert, U., Sinnis, P., Takacs, B., Clavjo, P., Santos, M.J., Nussenzweig, V. (1992). The basolateral domain of the hepatocyte plasma membrane bears receptors for the circumsporozoite protein of Plasmodium falciparum sporozoites. *Cell. 70*:1021-1033

Chang, K.H. & Stevenson, M.M. (2004). Malarial anaemia: mechanisms and implications of insufficient erythropoiesis during blood-stage malaria. *Int J Parasitol. 34*:1501-1516

Charoenpan, P., Indraprasit, S., Kiatboonsri, S., Suvachittanont, O., Tanomsup, S. (1990). Pulmonary edema in severe falciparum malaria: hemodynamic study and clinicophysiologic correlation. *Chest 97*:1190–1197

Chasis, J.A. & Mohandas, N. (2008). Erythroblastic islands: niches for erythropoiesis. *Blood. 112*:470–478

Chen, Q, Fernandez, V., Sundström, A., Schlichtherle, M., Datta, S., Hagblom P., Wahlgren, M (1998). Developmental selection of *var* gene expression in *Plasmodium falciparum. Nature. 394*:392–395

*Chen, Q., Heddini, A., Barragan, A., Fernandez, V., Pearce, S.F., Wahlgren, M. (*2000a). *The semiconserved head structure of Plasmodium falciparum erythrocyte membrane protein 1 mediates binding to multiple independent host receptors.* J Exp Med. *192: 1–10*

Chen, Q, Schlichtherle M, Wahlgren, M. (2000). Molecular aspects of severe malaria. *Clin Microbiol Rev. 13*:439-450

Chim, C.S., Wong, S.S., Lam, C.C., Chan, K.W. (2004). Concurrent hyperreactive malarial splenomegaly and quartan malarial nephropathy - Plasmodium malariae revisited. *Haematologica. 89*:ECR21

Chitnis, C. E. & Blackman, M. J. (2000). Host cell invasion by malaria parasites. *Parasitol. Today* 16:411-415

Chitnis, C.E. (2001). Molecular insights into receptors used by malaria parasites for erythrocyte invasion. *Curr Opin Hematol.8*:85–91

Choi, C.Y.H., Cerda, J.F.,Chu, H-A., Babcock, G.T. Marletta, M.A. (1999). Spectroscopic characterization of the heme-binding sites of histidine-rich protein 2. *Biochem. 38*:16916-16924

Chou, A.C., Chevli, R., Fitch, C.D. (1980). Ferriprotophyrin IX fulfills the criteria for identification as the chloroquin receptor of malaria parasites. *Biochem. 19*:1543-1549

Chug, K.S., Singhal, P.C., Sharma, B.K. (1977). Acute renal failure due to intravascular hemolysis in North Indian patients. Am J Med Sci. 274:134-146

Cinamon, G., M. A. Zachariah, O. M. Lam, F. W. Foss, Jr, J. G. Cyster. 2008. Follicular shuttling of marginal zone B cells facilitates antigen transport. Nat. Immunol. *9: 54-62*

Clark, I.H., Budd, A.C., Alleva, L.M, Cowden, W.B. (2006) Human malarial disease is a consequence of inflammatory cytokine release. *Malaria J. 5*:85

Clark, I.A. & Chaudhri, G. (1988). Tumor necrosis factor may contribute to the anaemia of malaria by causing dyserythropoiesis and erythrophagocytosis. *Br J Haematol. 70*:99-103

Clark, I.H. & Cowden, W.B. (2003). The pathophysiology of falciparum malaria. *Pharmacol Ther. 99*:221-260

Clyde, D.F., Most, H., McCarthy, V.C., Vanderberg, J.P. (1973). Immunisation of man against sporozite-induced falciparum malaria. Am J Med Sci. 266:169-177

Cockburn, I.A., Mackinnon, M.J., O'Donnel, A., Allen, S.J., Moulds, J.M., Baisor, M., Bockarie, M. Reeder, J.C., Rowe, J.A. (2004). A human complement receptor 1 polymorphism that reduces Plasmodium falciparum rosetting confers protection against malaria. *Proc Natl Acad Sci. USA 101*:272-277

Cohen, S., McGregor, I.A., Carrington, S.C. (1961). Lancet (London) 192:733-737

Collins, W.E., Jeffery, G.M., Roberts, J.M. (2003). A retrospective examination of anemia during infection of humans with Plasmodium vivax. *Am J Trop Med Hyg. 64*:406-412

Coppi,, A., Natarajan, R., Pradel, G., . Bennett, B. L., James, E. R., Roggero, M. A., Corradin, G., Persson, C., Tewari, R., Sinnis, P. (2011). The malaria circumsporozoite protein has two functional domains, each with distinct roles as sporozoites journey from mosquito to mammalian host. *J Exp Med. 208*:341-356

Corbett, C.E., Duarte, M.I., Lancellotti, C.L., Silva, M.A., Andrade, H.F. Jr. (1989). Cytoadherence in human falciparum malaria as a cause of respiratory distress. *J Trop Med Hyg 92*:112–120

Companale, N., Michel, C., Daubenberger, C.A., Wehlam, D.A., Gorman, J.J., Noris, N., Becker, K., Tilley, L. (2003). Identification and characterization of the heme-interacting proteins in the malaria parasite, Plasmodium falciparum. *J Biol Chem. 278*:27354-27361

Cooke, B.M., Berendt, A.R., Craig., A.G., MacGregor, J. Newbold C.I., Nash, G.B. (1994). Rolling and stationary cytoadhesion of red blood cells parasitized by *Plasmodium falciparum*: separate roles for ICAM-1, CD36 and thrombospondin. Br J Haematol.. 87:162–170

Cooke, B.M., Wahlgren, M., Coppel, R.L. (2000). Falciparum malaria sticking up, standing out and out-standing *Parasitol Today. 16*:416-420

Cooke, B.M., Lingelbach, K., Bannister, L., Tilley, L. (2004). Protein trafficking in Plasmodium falciparum-infested red blood cells. *Trends Parasitol. 20*:581-589

Cowman, A.F., Crabb, B.S. (2002). The Plasmodium falciparum genome—a blueprint for erythrocyte invasion. *Science. 298*:126–128

Cox-Singh, J., Davis, T.M.E., Lee, K-S., Shamsul, S.S.G., Matusop, A., Ratnam, S., Rahman, H.A., Conway, D.J.,Singh, B. (2008). Plasmodium knowlesi in humans is widely distributed and potentially life threatening. *Clin Infect Dis. 46*:165-171

Crane, G.G. (1986). Hyperactive malaria splenomegaly (tropical splenomegaly syndrome). *Parasitol Today. 3*:4-9

Cramer, J.P., Mockenhaupt, F.P., Ehrhardt, S.,Burkhardt, J., Otchwemah, R.N., Dietz, E., Gellert S., Bienzle, U. (2004) *iNOS* promoter variants and severe malaria in Ghanaian children (pages 1074–1080). *Trop Med Int Health. 9*:1074-1080

Crawley, J. (2004). The malaria burden: clinical and epidemiological impact. *Am J Trop Med Hyg. 71*:25-34

Cserti, C.M., Dzik, W.H. (2007) The ABO blood group system in Plasmodium falciparum malaria. *Blood. 110*:2250-2258

Dash, S.C., Bhuyan, U.N., Bunyan, A. et al., (1994). Falciparum malaria complicating cholestatic jaundice and acute renal failure. *J Assoc Phys Ind. 42*:101-102

Day, N.P., Hien, T.T., Schollaardt, T., Loc, P.P., Chuong, L.V., Chau, T.T., Mai, N.T., Phu, N.H., Sinh, D.X., White, N.J., Ho, M. (1999) The prognostic and pathophysiologic role of pro- and anti-inflammatory cytokines in severe malaria. *J Infect Dis. 180*:1288-1297

Day, N.P., Nguyen, H.P., Pham, P.L. (1997). Renal disease. II. Malaria and acute renal failure. J R Coll Physicians Lond. *31:*146*–148.*

Day N, Phu N, Mai N, Chau T, Loc P, Chuong L, Sinh D, Holloway P, Hien T, White N. (2002). The pathophysiology and prognostic significance of acidosis in severe adult malaria. Crit Care Med *2000; 28:1833–1840*

De Cock, K. M., Hodgen, AN., Jupp, R.A., Slavin, B., Siongok, T.K., Rees, P.H., Lucas, S.B. (1986). Immunoglobin M and malarial antibody levels in hyper-reactive malarial splenomegaly. *J. Trop Med Hyg. 89*:119-121

Deharo, E., Barkan, D., Kruglink, M., Golenser, J., Ginsburg, H. (2003). Potentiation of the antimalarial action of chloroquine in rodent malaria by drugs known to reduce cellular glutathione levels. *Biochem Pharmacol. 66*:809-817

Denninger, M.H., Winkler, S., Kremsner, P.G., Meyermann, R., Schluesner, H.J. (2003). Angiogenic proteins in the brains of patients who died with cerebral malaria. *J Neuroimmunol. 142*:101-111

Desai, M.R., Terlouw, D.J., Kwena, A.M., Phillips-Howard, P.A., Kariuki, S.K., Wannmuehler, K.A., Odhacha, A., Hawley, W.A., Shi, Y.P., Nahlem, B.L., Terkuite, F.O. (2005) Factors associated with hemoglobin concentrations in pre-school children in western Kenya: Cross-sectional studies. *Am J Trop Med Hyg. 72*:47-59

Desai, S.A, Krogstad, D.J., McCleskey, E.W. (1993). A nutrient-permeable channel on the intraerythrocytic malaria parasite. Nature ***362***: 643–646

Desai, S.A. & Rosenberg, R.L. (1997) Pore size of the malaria parasite's nutrient channel. Proc Natl Acad Sci USA. ***94***: 2045–2049

Desakorn, V., Silamut, K., Angus, B., Sahassamuda, D., Chotivamich, K., Suntharasamai, P., Simpson, J., White, N.J. (1997) Semi-quantitative measurement of Plasmodium falciparum antigen PfHRP-2, in blood and plasma. *Trans R Soc Trop Med Hyg. 91*:479-483

Devarbhavi, H., Alvares, J.F., Kumar, K.S. (2005). Severe falciparum malaria simulating fulminant hepatic failure. *Mayo Clinic Proc. 80*:355-358

Dondorp, A.M. Angus, B.J., Chotivanich, K., Silamut, K., Ruangveerayuth, R., Hardeman, M.R., Kager, P.A., Vreeken, J. and White, N.J. Red blood cell deformability as a predictor of anemia in severe falciparum malaria. (1999). *Am J Trop Med Hyg. 60*:733-737

Dondorp. A.M., Yeung, S., White, L., Nguon, C., Day, N.P.J., Socheat, D., von Seidlen, L. (2010). Artemisinin resistance: current status and scenarios for containment. *Nat Rev Microbiol. 8*:272-280

Dondorp, A.M., Kager, P.A., Vreeken, J. and White, N.J. (2000) Abnormal blood flow and red blood cell deformability in severe malaria. *Parasitol Today 16*:228-232

Dorman, E.K., Shulman, C.E., Kingdom, J., Bulmer, J.N., Mwendwa, J., Peshu, N., Marsh, K. (2002) Impaired uteroplacental blood flow in pregnancies complicated by falciparum malaria. *Ultrasound Obstet Gynecol. 19*:165-170

Dorn, A. Stoffel, R., Matile, H., Bubendorf, A., Ridley, R.G. (1995). Malarial haemozoin/β-haematin supports haem polymerization in the absence of protein. *Nature 374*:269-271

Doumbo, O. K., Thera, M. A., . Koné, A. K., Raza, A. Tempest, L. J. . Lyke, K. E., Plowe, C. V., Rowe J. A. (2009). High Levels of *Plasmodium falciparum* rosetting in all clinical forms of severe malaria in African Children. *Am J Trop Med Hyg. 81:* 987-*993*

Duff, G.W. (2006) Evidence for genetic variation as a factor in maintaining health. *Am J Clin Nutr. 83*:431S-435S

Duffy, P. E., Fried, M. (2003). Antibodies that inhibit *Plasmodium falciparum* adhesion to chondroitin sulfate A are associated with increased birth weight and the gestational age of newborns. *Infect. Immun.* 71: 6620-6623

Dvorak, J.A., Miller, L.H., Whitehouse, W.C., Shiroishi, T. (1975). Invasion of erythrocytes by malaria merozoites. *Science. 187*:748–750

Edelman, R., Hoffman, S. L., Davis, J. R., Beier, M., Sztein, M. B., Losonsky, G., Herrington, D. A., Eddy, H. A., Hollingdale, M. R., Gordon, D. M., et al. (1993). J. Infect. Dis. 168 :1066-*1070*

Eisen, D.P. & Michinton, R.M. (2003). Impact of mannose-binding lectin on susceptibility to infectious diseases. *J Infect Dis. 37*:1496-1505

Ekvall, H. (2003). Malaria and anemia. *Curr Opin Hematol. 10*:108-114

Elliot, D.A., McIntosh, M.T., Hosgood, H.D. III, Chen, S., Zhang, G., Baevova, P., Joiner, K.A. (2008). Four resistant pathways of hemoglobin uptake in the malaria parasite Plasmodium falciparum. *Proc Natl Acad Sci.USA. 105*:2463-2468

Elford, B.C & Cowan, G.M., Ferguson, D.J. (1995). Parasite-regulated membrane transport procedures and metabolic control in malaria-infected erythrocytes. *Biochem J. 308*:361-374

English, M. (2000) Life-threatening severe malarial anaemia. *Trans R Soc Trop Med Hyg. 94*:585-588

English M, Waruiru, C., Amukoye, E., Murphy, S., Crawley, J., Mwangi, I., Peshu, N., Marsh, K. (1996a). Deep breathing in children with severe malaria: indicator of metabolic acidosis and poor outcome. *Am J Trop Med Hyg. 55*:521–524.

English M, Sauerwein, R., Waruiru, C., Mosobo, M., Obiero, J., Lowe, B., Marsh, K. (1997). Acidosis in severe childhood malaria. *Q J Med. 90*:263–270

English, M., Waruiru, C., Lightowler, C., Murphy, S.A., Kirigha, G., Marsh, K. (1996). Hyponatraemia and dehydration in severe malaria. *Arch Dis Child 1996*; *74*:*201*–5.

Engwerda, C.R., Beattie, L., Amante, F.H. (*2005)*. The importance of the spleen in malaria. *Trends Parasitol 21*: *75*–80

Facer, C.A. & Brown, J. (1981). Monocytes erythrophagocytosis in falciparum malaria. *Lancet i*:897-898

Facer, C.A., Bray, R.S. and Brown, J. (1980). Direct Coombs antiglobulin reaction in Gambian children with Plasmodium falciparum malaria, I: incidence and class specificity. *Clin Exp Immunol. 35*:119- 127

Fairhurst, R.M., Baruch, D.I., Brittain, N.J., Ostera, G.R., Wallach, J.S., Hoang, H.L., Haton, K., Guindo, A., Makobongo, M.O. Schwartz, O.M., Tounkara, A., Doumbo, O.K., et al. (2005). Abnormal display of PfEMP21 on erythrocytes containing HbC may protect against malaria. *Nature 435*:1117-1121

Fakunle, Y.M. (1981). Tropical splenomegaly, part 1: tropical Africa. *Clin Haematol. 10*:963-975

Fandrey, J., Frede, S., Ehleben, W., Porwol, T., Acker, H., Jelkmann, W. (1997). 496Cobalt chloride and desferrioxamine antagonize the inhibition of erythropoietin production by reactive oxygen species. *Kidney Int 51*: 492-496

Ferone R & Roland S. (1980). Dihydrofolate reductase: thymidylate synthase, a bifunctional polypeptide from Crithidia fasciculate. *Proc Natl Acad Sci. USA. 77*:5802-5806.

Ferreira, A., Schofield, L., Enea, V., Schellekens, H., van-der-Meide, P., Collins, W. E., Nussenzweig, R. S. & Nussenzweig, V. (*1986*) *Science 232 , 881*-884

Fidock, D.A., Rosenthal, P.J., Craft, S.L., Brun, R., Nwaka, S. (2004). Antimalarial drug discovery: efficacy controls for compound screening. *Nat Rev Drug Discov. 3*:509-520

Fiori, P.L., Rappeli, P, Mirkarimi, S.N. Ginsburg, H., Cappucinelli, P., Turrini, F. (1993). Reduced microbicidal and anti-tumor activities of human monocytes after ingestion of Plasmodium falciparum-infected red blood cells..*Parasite Immunol. 15*:647-655

Firestein, G. S. (2003). Evolving concepts of rheumatoid arthritis. *Nature 423*: 356-361

Fleming, A.F. (*1989)*. Tropical obstetrics and gynaecology. 1. Anaemia in pregnancy in tropical Africa. *Trans R Soc Trop Med Hyg 83*: *441*–448

Fleming, A.F., Warrell, D.A., Dickmeiss, H. (*1974)*. Letter: Co-trimoxazole and the blood. *Lancet 2*: *284*–285.

Flick, K. & Chen, Q. (2004). Var genes, PfEMP1 and the human host. *Mol Biochem Parasitol. 134*:3-9

Fowkes, F.J., Richards, J.S., Simpson, J.A., Beeson, J.G. *(*2010*)*. The relationship between anti-merozoite antibodies and incidence of *Plasmodium falciparum* malaria: A systematic review and meta-analysis. *PLoS Med 7:*e1000218

Francis, S.E. Sullivan, D.J., Goldberg, D.E. (1997). Hemoglobin metabolism in the malaria parasite Plasmodium falciparum. *Ann Rev Micribiol. 51*:97-123

Franklin, B.S., Ishizaka, S.T., Lamphier, M., Gusovsky, F., Hansen, H., Rose, J., Zheng, W., Ataide, M.A., de Oliveira, R.B., Golenbock, D.T., Gazzinelli, R.T. (2011) Therapeutical targets of nucleic acid-sensing Toll-like receptors prevents experimental cerebral malaria. *Proc Natl Acad Sci. USA. 108*:3689-3694

Freedma, D.O. (2008) *Malaria prevention in short-term travelers.* N Engl J Med *359:*603–*12.*

Frevert, U., Gehinski, M.R., Hugel, F.U., Allon, M., Schreier, H., Smulevitch, S., Shakibaei, M., Clavijo, P. (1998). *EMBO J. 17*:3816-3826

Frevert, U., Sinnis, P., Cerami, C., Shreffler, W., Takacs, B., and Nussenzweig, V. *(*1993*).* Malaria circumsporozoite protein binds to heparan sulfate proteoglycans associated with the surface membrane of hepatocytes. *J. Exp. Med.* 177*,* 1287–*1298*

Fried, M. and Duffy, P.E. (1996). Adherence of Plasmodium falciparum to chondroitin sulphate A in the human placenta. Science. 212:1502-1504

Fried, M. Nosten, F., Brockman, A., Brabin, B.J., Duffy, P.E. (1998), Maternal antibodies block malaria. *Nature 395*:851-852

Friedman, M.J. (1979) Oxidant damage mediates variant red cell resistance to malaria. *Nature 280*:245-247

Gantt, S., Persson, C., Rose, K., Birkett, A. J., Abagyan, R., Nussenzweig, V. (2000). Antibodies against thrombospondin-related anonymous protein do not inhibit *Plasmodium* sporozoite infectivity in vivo. *Infect. Immun. 68*: 3667-3673

Garcia, J.E., Puentes, A., Patarroyo, M.E. (2006) Developmental Biology of sporozoite-host interactions in Plasmodium falciparum malaria: Implications for vaccine design. *Clin Microbiol Rev. 19*:686-707

Gasque, P. (2004). Complement: a unique innate immune sensor for danger signals Mol. Immunol. *41:*1089-*1098*

Gazinelli, R.T., Ropert, C., Campos, M.A. (2004). Role of toll/interleukin-1 receptor signaling pathway in host resistance and pathogenesis during infection with protozoan parasites. *Immunol Rev. 201*:9-25

Gell, P.G.H., Coombs, R.R.A. (1963). *Clinical Aspects of Immunology* pp 317-337. Blackwell, Oxford

Ghezzi, P. & Brines, M. (2004) Erythropoietin as an anti-apoptotic tissue-protective cytokine. *Cell Death Differ. 11*:S37-S44

Gilles, H.M., Fletcher, K.A., Hendrikse, R.G., Reddy, S., Allen, N. (1967) Glucose-6-phosphate dehydrogenase deficiency, sickling and malaria in African children in south western Nigeria. *Lancet. i*:138-140

Gilson, P.R. & Crabb, B.S..(2009). Morphology and kinetics of the three distinct phases of red blood cell invasion by Plasmodium falciparum merozoites. *Int J Parasitol. 39*:91–96

di Giovine, F.S., Nuki, G., Duff, G.W. (1988). Tissue necrotic factor in synovial exudates. *Ann Rheum Dis. 47*:768-772

Ginsburg, H. & Stein, W.D. (1991) Kinetic modeling of chloroquine uptake by malaria-infected erythrocytes. *Biochem Pharmacol. 41*:63-70

Goldberg, D.E. (1993) Haemoglobin degradation in Plasmodium-infected red blood cells. *Semin Cell Biol. 4*:355-361

Goldberg, D.E., Slater, A.F.G., Beavis, R., Chavit, B., Cerami, A. and Henderson, G.B. (1991) Hemoglobin degradation in the human malaria pathogen Plasmodium falciparum: a catabolic pathway initiated by a specific aspartic protease. *J. Exp. Med.* 173:961-969

Goodyear, I.D., Pouvelle, B., Schneider, T.G., Trelka, D.P., Taraschi, T.F. (1997) Characterisation of macromolecular transport pathways in malaria-infected erythrocytes. *Mol Biochem Parasitol.* 87:18-28

Gotsman, I., Azaz-Livshits, T., Fridlender, Z., Muszkat, M., Ben-Chetrit, E. (2000). Mefloquine-induced acute hepatitis. *Pharmocotherapy* 20:1517-1519

Garnham, P. C. C. (1938). The placenta in malaria with special reference to reticulo-endothelial immunity. *Trans R. Soc. Trop. Med. Hyg. 32*:13–22

Greene, LS (1993) G6PD deficiency as protection against falciparum malaria: an epidemiologic critique of population and experimental studies. *Year Phys Anthropol. 30*:153-178

Greenwood, B.M. (1987). Asymptomatic malaria infection: do they matter? *Parasitol Today 3*: 206-214

Greenwood, B., Marsh, K. & Snow, R. (1991). Why do some African children develop severe anemia? *Parasitol Today. 7*:277-281

Greenwood BM, Fidock DA, Kyle DE, Koppe SHI, Alonso PL, Collins FH, Duff PE (2008) Malaria, progress, perils and prospects for eradication. *J Clin Invest. 118*:1266-1276

Griffith, K.S., Lewis, L.S., Mali, S., Parise, M.E. (2007). Treatment of malaria in the United States: a systematic review. *JAMA.297:*2264-2277

Haldane, J.B.S. (1949). The rate of mutation of human genes. Proceedings of the VIII international congress of genetics. *Hereditas. 35*:267-73.

Hastings, I.M., Watkins, W.M., White, N.J. (2002). The evolution of drug-resistant malaria: the role of drug elimination half-life. *Phil Trans R Soc London B Biol Sci. 357*:505-519

Hay, S.I., Noor, A.M., Simba, M., Busolo, M., Guyatt, H.L., Ochola, S.A., Snow, R.W. (2002). Clinical epidemiology of malaria in the highlands of western Kenya. Emerg Infect Dis *8: 543–548.*

Helbok, K., Dent, W., Nacher, M., Kackner, P., Treeprasertsuk, S., Krudsoods, S., Wilairatana, P., Silacharmroon, U., Looareesuwan, S., Schmutzzhard, E. (2005). The use of the multiorgan-dysfunction score to discriminate different levels of severity in severe and complicated Plasmodium falciparum malaria. *Am J Trop Med Hyg. 72*:150-154

Helmby, H., Cavelier, L., Pettersson, U., Wahlgren, M. (1993). Rosetting: *Plasmodium falciparum* -infected erythrocytes express unique strain-specific antigens on their surface. *Infect Immun 61*:284 -288

Herrington, D.A., Clyde, D.F., Lasonsky, G., Cortesia, M., Murphy, J.R., Davis, J. Baqar, S., Felix, A.M., Heimer, E.P., Giellssen, D. et al (1987). Safety and immunogenicity in man of a synthetic peptide malaria vaccine against Plasmodium falciparum sporozoites. *Nature 328*:257-259

van den Heyde, H.C., Nolan, J., Combes, V., Gramaglia, I., Grau, G.E. (2006). A unified hypothesis for the genesis of cerebral malaria: sequestration, inflammation and hemostasis leading to microcirculatory dysfunction. *Trends Parasitol. 22*:503-508

Higgins, M.K. (2008). The structure of chondroitin sulphate-binding domain important in placental malaria. *J Biol Chem. 283*:21842-21846

Hiller, N.L., Bhattacharjee, S., van Ooij, C., et al. (2004). A host-targeting signal in virulence proteins reveals a secretome in malarial infection. *Science. 306*:1934–1937

Ho, M. & White, N.J. (1999). Molecular mechanisms of cytoadherence in malaria. *Am J Physiol. 276*:C1231–C1242

Hoffman, S. L. *(*1996*).* Malaria Vaccine Development: A Multi-immune Response Approach. Am. Soc. Microbiol. Washington, DC *pp* 1–12

Hoffman, S.L., Piessens, W.F., Ratiwayanto, S., Hussein, P.R., Kurniawan, L. Piessens, P.W., Campbell, J.R., Marwoto, H.A. (1984). Reduction of suppressor T lymphocytes in the tropical splenomegaly syndrome. *N Engl J Med. 310*: 337-341

Holder, A.A. (1999). Malaria vaccines. *Proc Natl Acad Sci. USA. 96*:1167-1169

Hollingdale, M.R., Nardin, E.H., Thoravanji, S., Schwarz, A.L., Nussenzweig, R.S. (1984) Inhibition of entry of Plasmodium falciparum P. vivax sporozoites into cultured cells: an in vivo assay of protective antibodies. *J Immunol. 132*:909-913

Holt, G.D., Pangburn, M.K., Ginsburg, V. (1990). Properdin binds to sulfatide [Gal(3-SO_4)beta 1-1 Cer] and has a sequence homology with other proteins that bind sulfated glycoconjugates. *J. Biol. Chem. 1990 265*: 2852-2855

Hommel, M., David, P.H., Oligino, L.D. (1983). Surface alterations of erythrocytes in Plasmodium falciparum. Antigenic variation, antigenic diversity, and the role of the spleen. *J Exp Med. 157*:1137-1148

Hopkins Sibley, C., Hyde, J.E., Sims, P.F., Plowe, C.V., Kublin, J.G., Mbenu, E.K., Cowman, E.F., Winstanley, P.A., Watkins, W.M., Nzila, A.M. (2001). P-sulfadoxine resistance in Plasmodium falciparum: what next? *Trends Parasitol. 17*:582-588

Hunt, N., and Grau, G. E. (2003), Cytokines: accelerators and brakes in the pathogenesis of cerebral malaria. Trends Immunol. *24, 491-499*

Hutchings, G.H., Falco, E.A., Vanderweff, H., Russell, P., Elion, G.B. (1952). Antagonists of nucleic acid derivatives: 2,4-diaminopyrimidines. *J Biol Chem. 199*:43-56

Hviid, L. & Salanti, A. (2007). VAR2CSP and protective immunity against pregnancy-related Plasmodium falciparum malaria. *Parasitol. 134*:1871-1876

Idro, R., Jenkins, N.E., Newton, C.R. (2005). Pathogenesis, clinical features, and neurological outcome of cerebral malaria. *Lancet Neurology 4*:827

Iqbal, J., Siddique, A., Jameel, M., Hira, P.R. (*2004*). Persistent histidine-rich protein 2, parasite lactate dehydrogenase, and pan-*malaria*l antigen reactivity after clearance of Plasmodium falciparum monoinfection. *J Clin Microbiol 42*: *4237*–4241

Iyer, J.K., Milhotts, W.K., Cortese, J.I., Kublin, J.G., Plowe, C.V. (2001). Plasmodium falciparum cross-resistance between trimethoprim and pyrimethamine. Lancet. 358:1066-1067

Jakobsen, P.H., Bate, C.A.W., Taverne, J., Playfair, J.H. (1995) Malaria: toxins, cytokines and disease. *Parasite Immunol. 17*:223-231

Jain, S.K. (1988). Evidence for membrane lipid peroxidation during the in vivo aging of human erythrocytes. *Biochim Biophys Acta. 937*:205-210

Jakeman, G.N., Saul, A., Hogarth, W.L. and Collins, W.E. (1999) Anaemia of acute malaria infection in non-immune patients primarily results from destruction of uninfected erythrocytes. *Parasitol. 119*:127-133

Jambou R, Legrand E, Nimug M, Khim N, Lim P, Volney B, Ekala MT, Bouchier C, Esterre P, Fandeur T, Mercereau-Puijalon O. (2005). Resistance of Plasmodium falciparum field isolates to in vitro artemether and point mutations of the SERCA-type PfATPase 6. *Lancet 366*:1960-1963

James, A.H. (2003) Blocking malaria parasite invasion of mosquito salivary glands. J *Exp Biol. 206*:3817-3821

Jarvis, J.N., Wang, W., Moore, H.T., Zhao, I. Xu, C. (1997) In vitro induction of pro-inflammatory cytokine secretion by juvenile rheumatoid arthritis synovial fluid immune complexes. *Arthritis Rheum. 40*:2039-2046

Jensen, J.B. & Edgar, S.A. (1978). Fine structure of penetration of cultured cells by Isospora canis sporozoites. *J Protozool. 25*:169-173

John, C.C., Sumba, P.O., Ouma, J.H., Nahlem, B.L., King, C.L., Kazura, J.W. (2000) Cytokine responses to Plasmodium falciparum liver-stage antigen 1 vary in rainy and dry seasons in highland Kenya. *Infect Immun. 68*:5198-5204

Joshi, Y.K., Tandon, B.N., Acharya, S.K., Babu, S., Tandon, M. (1986). Acute hepatic failure due to Plasmodium falciparum liver injury. Liver. 198

Kaiser, M., Wittlin, S., Nehrbass-Stuedli, A., Dong, Y., Wang, X., Hemphill, A., Matile, H., Brun,[1], R., Jonathan L. Vennerstrom, J.L (2007). Peroxide bond-dependent antiplasmodial specificity of artemisinin and OZ277 (RBx11160) *Antimicrob Agents Chemother 51:*2991–2993

Kappe, S., Bruderer, T., Gantt, S., Fujoka, H., Nussenzweig, V. (2004) Plasmodium sporozoite molecular biology. Annu Rev Cell Dev Biol. 20:29-59

Kappe, S., Bruderer, T., Gantt, S., Fujoka, H., Nussenzweig, V., Menard, R. (1999) Conservation of a gliding motility and cell invasion machinery in apicomplexan parasites. J Cell Biol. 147:937-943

Kaul, D.K., Chen, D., Zhan, J. (1994). adhesion of sickle cells to vascular endothelium is critically dependent on changes in density and shape of red cells. *Blood. 83*:3006-3017

Kavishe, R.A. Koenderink, J.B., McCall, M.B.B. Peters, W.H.M., Mulder, B., Cornelus C. Hermsen, C.C., Sauerwein, R.W., Russel, F.G.M., van den Ven, A.J.A.M. (2006). Severe Plasmodium falciparum malaria in Cameroun: Associated with Glutathione S-transferase M1 null genotype. *Am J Trop Med Hyg.75*:827-829

Kawai, T., Akira, S. (2005). Pathogen recognition with Toll-like receptors. *Curr Opin Immunol. 17*:338-344

Kharazani, A., Jepsen, S., Anderson, B.J. (1987). Generation of reactive oxygen radicals by human phagocytic cellsactivated by Plasmodium falciparum. *Scand. J Immunol. 25*:335-341

Kilejian, A., Sharma, Y.D., Karoui, H., Naslund, L. (1986) Histidine-rich domain of the knob protein of the human malaria parasite Plasmodium falciparum. *Proc Natl Acad Sci.USA. 83*:7938-7941

Kindermans, J.M., Pilley, J., Olliaro, P., Gomes, M. (2007). Ensuring sustained ACT production and reliable artemisin supply. *Malaria J. 6*:125

King, C.A. (1988). Cell motility of sporozoan protozoa. Parasitol Today. 4:315-319

Klayman, D.L. (1985). Qinghaosu (artemisinin): an antimalarial drug from China. *Science. 228*:1049-1055

Klonis, N., Crespo-Ortiz, M.P., Bottova, I., Abu-Bakar, N., Kenny, S., Rosenthal, P.J. Tilley, L. (2011),. Artemisinin activity against *Plasmodium falciparum* requires hemoglobin uptake and digestion. *Proc Natl Acad Sci. USA. 108*:11405-11410

Kochar, D.K., Agarwal, P., Kochar, S.K Jain, R., Rawat, N., . Pokharna, R.K , Kachhawa, S., T. Srivastava, T. (2003). Hepatocyte dysfunction and hepatic encephalopathy in *Plasmodium falciparum* malaria. *QJM. 96 (7): 505-*

Kochar, D.K., Shubhakaran, K., Kumawat, B.L., Kochar, S.K., Halwai, M., Makkar, R.K., Joshi, A. *(2002)*. Cerebral *malaria* in Indian adults: a prospective study of 441 patients from Bikaner, north-west India. *J Assoc Physicians India 50*: *234*–241.

Knodel, J.P.& Moore, G.E. (1993). Rhabdomyolysis malaria. *N Eng J Med. 329*:*1206*–1207

Kraemer, S.M. and Smith J.D. (2006) A family affair: var genes, PfEMP1 binding, and malaria disease. *Curr Opin Microbiol. 9*:374-380

Krishnan, A. & Karnad, D.R. (2003). Severe falciparum malaria: an important cause of multiple organ failure in Indian Intensive Care Unit. *Crit Care Med. 31*:2278-2284

Krishnegowda, G., Hajjar, A. M., Zhu J. Z., Douglass, E. J., Uematsu, S., Akira, S., Wood, A. S., and Gowda, D. C. (2005) induction of proinflammatory responses in macrophages by the glycosylphosphatidylinositols of *plasmodium falciparum*: cell signaling receptors, glycosylphosphatidylinositol (gpi) structural requirement, and regulation of gpi activity. *J. Biol. Chem.* 280: 8606-8616

Krogstad, D.J. (1995) Principles and Practice of Infectious Diseases. In: Mancell, G.L., Bennett, J.E. and Dolin, R. (eds.), Churchill Livingstone, New York, pp 2415-2427

Kwiatkowski, D., Cannon, J.G., Maigue, K.R., Cerami, A., Dinarello, C.A. *(*1989*)*. Clin Exp Immunol 77*:*361–366

Kwiatkowski, D.P. (2005) How malaria has affected the human genome and what human genetics can teach us about malaria. The Am J Hum Genet. 77:171-192

Kwiatkowski, D.P, Sambou, I., Twumasi, P., Greenwood, B.M., Hill, A.V.S. Manogue, K.R. Cerami, A., Castracane, J., D.R. Brewster, D.R. (1990). TNF concentration in fatal cerebral, non-fatal cerebral, and uncomplicated Plasmodium falciparum malaria. *Lancet. 236*:1201

Kyes, S., Horrocks, P., Newbold, C. (2001) Antigenic variation at the infected red cell surface in malaria. *Annu Rev Microbiol. 55*:673-707

Kyes, S.A., Rowe, J.A., Kriek, N., Newbold, C.I. (1999). Rifins: A second family of clonally variant proteins expressed on the surface of red cells infected with *Plasmodium falciparum. Proc Natl Acad Sci USA.*96 : 9333-9338,1999

Layez, C., Nogueira, P., Combes, V., Costa, F.T.M., Juhan-Vague, I., Pereira da Silva, L.H., Gysin, I. (2005). *Plasmodium falciparum* rhoptry protein RSP2 triggers destruction of the erythroid lineage. *Blood. 106*:3632-3638

Lawler, J. & Hynes, R.O. (1986) The structure of human thrombospondin, an adhesive glycoprotein with multiple calcium-binding sites and homologies with several different proteins. *J Cell Biol.* 103:1635-1648

Leiriae, P., Rodrigues, C.D., Albuquerque, S.S., Mota, M.M. (2002). Survival of protozoan intracellular parasites in host cells. *EMBO Reports* 5:1142-1147

Lewis, R. (2003) Human Genetics, 5th ed., pp 286-293, McGraw Hill, Boston.

Lindblom, A. & Fransson, L. A. (1990). Endothelial heparan sulphate: Compositional analysis and comparison of chains from different proteoglycan populations *Glycoconj. J. 7:545–562.*

Liu, J., Istvan, E.S., Gluzman, I.Y., Gross, J., Goldberg, D.E. (2006). Plasmodium falciparum ensures its amino acid supply with multiple acquisition pathways and redundant proteolytic enzyme systems. *Proc Natl Acad Sci.USA. 103*:8840-8845

Logie, D. E., McGregor, I.A., Rowe, D.S., Billewicz, W.Z. (1973). Plasma immunoglobulin concentrations in mothers and newborn children with special reference to placental malaria: studies in the Gambia, Nigeria, and Switzerland. *Bull W HO. 49*: 547-554

Long, E.G. (2009). Requrements for diagnosis of malaria at different levels of the laboratory network in Africa. *Am J Clin Pathol. 131*:858-860

Looaresuwan, S., Davis, T.M., Supanaranond, W., Desahorn, V., Silamut, K., Krishna, S. et al (1991) Erythrocyte survival in severe falciparum malaria. *Acta Trop. 48*:263-270

Looareesuwan, S., Ho, M., Wattanagoon, Y., White, N.J., Warrell, D.A., Bunnag, D., Harinasuta, T. and Wyler, D.J. (1987). Dynamic alterations in splenic function in falciparum malaria. *N Engl J Med. 317*:675-679

Loria, P, Miller S, Foley M, Tilley L (1999) Inhibition of the peroxidation degradation of haem as the basis of action of chloroquin and other quinoline antimalarials. *Biochem J. 339*:363-370

*Loutan, L. (*2003). *Malaria: Still a threat to travellers.* Int J Antimicrob Agents *21: 158–163.*

Luty, A.J., Kun, J.F., Kremsner, P.G. (1998). Mannose-binding lectin plasma levels and gene polymorphisms in *plasmodium falciparum* malaria *J Infect Dis. 178*:1221-1224

Luzzato, L, Nwachuku-Jerratt, E.S., Reddy S. (1970). Increased sickling in parasitized erythrocytes as mechanism of resistance against malaria in sickle-cell trait. *Lancet. i*:319-321

Luzzi, G.A., Torii, M., Aikawa, M., Pasvol, G. (1990) Unrestricted growth of Plasmodium falciparum in microcytic erythrocytes in iron deficiency and thalassaemia. *Br J Haematol. 74*:519-524

Lyon M., Deakin J. A., Gallagher J. T. (1994) Liver heparan sulphate structure. A novel molecular design. *J Biol Chem. 269:11208–11215.*

Mackey, J.P. & Vivarelli, F. (1954). Sickle-cell anaemia. *BMJ. i*:276

Mahakur, A.C., Pandar, S.N., Nanda, B.K. et al. (1983). Malarial acute renal failure. *J Assoc Phys Ind. 31*:633-636

Marsh, K. (2002) Immunity of Malaria. Warrel D.A., Giles, H.M. (eds). Essential Malariology, 4th ed., London; Arnold, pp 252-267

MacPherson, G.G., Warrell, M.J., White, N.J., Looareesuwan, S., Warrell, D.A. (1985) Human cerebral malaria: a quantitative ultrastructural analysis of parasitized erythrocyte sequestration. *Am J Pathol. 119*:385–401

Maeno, Y., R. Steketee, W., Nagatake, T., Tegoshi, T., Desowitz, R.S., Wirima, J.J., Aikawa, M. (1993). Immunoglobulin complex deposits in *Plasmodium falciparum*-infected placentas from Malawi and Papua New Guinea. *Am. J. Trop. Med. Hyg. 49*: 574-580

Maguire, G.P., Handojo, T., Pain, M.C. et al. (2005). Lung injury in uncomplicated and severe falciparum malaria: a longitudinal study in papua, Indonesia. *J Infect Dis. 192:*1966-74.

Marsh, K. & Howard, R.J. (1986). Antigens induced on erythrocytes by Plasmodium falciparum: expression of diverse and conserved determinants. *Science. 23*:150-153

Marsh, K., Forster, D., Waruiru, C., Mwangi, I., Winstanley, M., Marsh, V., Newton, C., Winstanley, P., Warn, P., Peshu, N., Pasvol, G., Snow, R. (1995). Indicators of life-threatening malaria in African children. *N Engl J Med. 332*:1399-1404

Marti M, Baron J, Rug M, Tilley L, Cowman AF (2005) Signal-mediated export of proteins from the malaria parasite to the host erythrocyte. J Cell Biol 171:587-592 de Mast, Q., van Dongen-Lases, E.C., Swinkels, D.W., Nieman, A.E., Roestenberg, M., Druilhe, P., et al. (2009). Mild increases in serum hepcidin and interleukin-6 concentrations impair iron incorporation in haemoglobin during an experimental human malaria infection. *Br J Haematol. 145* 6: 657–64

May, J., Lell, B., Luty, A.J., Meyer, C.G., Kremsner, P.G. (2000) Plasma IL-10, tissue necrosis factor (TNF)-alpha ratio is associated with TNF promoter variants and predicts malarial complications. *J Infect Dis.* 182:1570-1573

May, J. et al., (2007). Hemoglobin variants and disease manifestations in severe falciparum malaria. *J Am Med Assoc 297:*2220–2226.

Mayxay, M., Pukrittayakamee, S., Chotivanich, K., Looareesuwan, S., White, N.J. (*2001).* Persistence of Plasmodium falciparum HRP-2 in successfully treated acute falciparum *malaria. Trans R Soc Trop Med Hyg 95*: *179–*182

McCall, M.B.B., Netea, M.G., Hensen, C.C., Jensen, T., Jacobs, L., Golenbock, D., van der Ven, A.J.A.M., Sanerwein, R.W. (2007). Plasmodium falciparum infection causes proinflammatory priming of human TLR responses. *J Immunol. 179*:162-171

McCutchan, T. F., Kissinger, J. C., Touray, M. G., Rogers, M. J., Li, J., Sullivan M., Braga E. M., Krettli A. U., Miller L. H. (1990) Comparison of circumsporozoite proteins from avian and mammalian malarias: biological and phylogenetic implications. *Proc. Natl. Acad. Sci. U. S. A.* 93*:*11889–11894

McGee James, O.D., Isaacson, P.G., Wright, W.A. (1992). *Pathology of Tropical Infections: Oxford Textbook of Pathology, volume 26*, pp 2191-2194

McGregor, I.A. (1974). Mechanisms of acquired immunity and epidemiological patterns of antibody responses in malaria in man. *Bull World Health Org. 50*:259-266

McGregor et al (2006) Live attenuated B pertussis as a single-dose nasal vaccine against whooping cough. *PLoS Pathog. 2*:e65

McKenzie, F.E., Jeffery, G.M., Collins, W.E. (*2002).* Plasmodium vivax blood-stage dynamics. *J Parasitol 88*: *521–*535

Medzhitov, R., & Jaheway, C. Jr. (2000). Innate immunity. *New Engl J Med.* 343:338-344

Mehta, S.R., Naidu, G., Chandar, V., Singh, I.P., Johri, S., Ahuja, R.C. (1989). Falciparum malaria: Present day problems: An experience with 425 cases. *J Assoc Physics India. 37*:264-267

Meier, P., Schmid, M., Staubi, M. (1990*). Acute hepatitis following administration of fansidar*. Schweiz Med Wochenschr. 120:221-225.

Ménard, R.(2000). The journey of the malaria sporozoite through its hosts: two parasite proteins lead the way. *Microbes Infect.* 2*:*633–642

Menendez, C., Fleming, A.F., Alonso, P.L. (2000). Malaria-related anaemia. *Parasitol Today. 16*:469-476

Meshnick, S.R. *(*2002*).* Artemisinin: Mechanisms of action, resistance and toxicity. *Int J Parasitol 32:*1655–1660

Meshnick SR, Thomas A, Ran ZA, Xu C-M, Pan H-X (1994). Artemisinin (qinghaosu): the role of intercellular hemin in its mechanism of antimalarial action. *Mol Biochem Parasitol. 49*:181-190.

Miller, L.H., Baruch, D.I., Marsh, K., Doumbo, O.K. (2002). The pathogenic basis of malaria. *Nature 415*:673-679

Minakawa, N., Sonye, G., Mogi, M., Githeko, A., Yan, G. (2002). The effects of climatic factors on the distribution and abundance of malaria vectors in Kenya. *J Med Entomol 39:833*–841

Mishra, S.K. & Mohanty, S. (*2001).* Clinical presentations of severe and complicated *malaria* in India. *J Indian Acad Clin Med 2*: *125*–127.

Mishra, S.K., Mohanty, S., Satpathy, S.K., Mohapatra, D.N. (*2007).* Cerebral *malaria* in adults - a description of 526 cases admitted to Ispat General Hospital in Rourkela, India. *Ann Trop Med Parasitol 101*: *187*–193.

Mitchell, G.H., Butcher, G.A., Cohen, S.(1975). Merozoite vaccination against Plasmodium knowlesi malaria. *Immunol. 29*:387-407

Mockenhaupt, F. P., Cramer, J P., Lutz H, Miriam S.S., Eckert, J., Oh, N-R Otchwemah, R. N., Dietz, E., Ehrhardt, S., Schröder, N. W. J., Bienzle, U., Schumann, R. R. (2006). Toll-like receptor (TLR) polymorphisms in African children: Common *TLR-4* variants predispose to severe malaria. *Proc Natl Acad Sci.USA. 103*:177-182

Mohammed, I. (1982) The role of immune complexes in human malaria and some of its implications. *J Infect. 4*:97-104

Mohan, A., Sharma, S.K., Bollineni, S. (2008). Acute lung injury and acute respiratory distress syndrome in malaria. *J Vector Borne Dis 45*:179–193

Mohanty, D., Marwaha, N., Ghosh, K., Sharma, S., Garewal, G., Shah, S., Devi, S. Das, K.C. (1988) Functional and ultrastructural changes of platelets in malarial infection. Trans R Soc Trop Med Hyg. 82:369-375

Mohanty, N., Satpathy, S.K. and Nanda, P. (2004). Hepathopathy in complicated falciparum malaria report from eastern India. *Trans R Soc Trop Med Hyg. 98*:753-754

Molyneux, M.E., Looaresuwan, S., Menzies, I.S. et al (1989). Reduced hepatic flow and intestinal malabsorption in severe falciparum malaria. Am J Trop Med Hyg. 40:470-476

Mota, M.M., Hafalla, J.C., Rodriguez, A. (2002) Migration through host cells activates *Plasmodium sporozoites* for infection. Nat Med ***8***: 1318–1322

*Muentener, P., Schlagenhauf, P., Steffen, R. (*1999*). Imported malaria (1985–95): Trends and perspectives.* Bull World Health Organ *77:*560*–566.*

*Mukherjee, A.P., White, J.C., Lau, K.S. (*1971). *Falciparum* malaria *associated with jaundice, renal failure and anaemia.* Trans R Soc Trop Med Hyg *65: 808–814*

Murthy, G.L., Sahay, R.K., Sreenivas, D.V., Sundaram, C., Shantaram, V. (1998). Hepatitis in falciparum malaria. *Trop Gastroenterol. 19*:152-154

Nacher M, Singhasivanon P, Silachamroon U *et al. (2001).* Helminth infections are associated with protection from malaria-related acute renal failure and jaundice in Thailand. *Am. J. Trop. Med. Hyg. 65:* 834*–836*

Naqvi, R., Ahmad, E., Akhtar, F., Naqvi A., Rizvi, A. (2003). Outcome in severe acute renal failure associated with malaria. *Nephrol. Dial. Transplant. (2003) 18*): 1820-1823

Nardin, E. H. Oliveira, G. A., Calvo-Calle, J. M. Castro, Z. R., Nussenzweig, R. S., Schmeckpeper, B., Hall, B. F., Diggs, C., Bodison, S. Edelman, R. (2000). Synthetic Malaria Peptide Vaccine Elicits High Levels of Antibodies in Vaccinees of Defined HLA Genotypes. *J Infect Dis. 182*: 1486-1496

Nemeth, E. & Ganz, T. (2006). Regulation of iron metabolism by hepcidin. *Annu Rev Nutr. 26*:323-42

Newton, C.R. & Krishna, S. (*1998*). Severe falciparum *malaria* in children: current understanding of pathophysiology and supportive treatment. *Ann Trop Med Parasitol 79*: *1*–53.

Newton, C.R.J.C., Warn, P.A., Winstanley, P.A., Peshu, N., Snow, R.W., Pavol, G. and Marsh, K. (1997) Severe anaemia in children living in a malaria endemic area of Kenya. *Trop Med Int Health. 2*: 165-178

Nitya, N., Aggarwal, H., Sharma, M., Singh, M. (*2001*). Systemic manifestations of *malaria*. *J Indian Acad Clin Med 2*: *189*–194.

Norman, J., Nilsson, D., Ribacke U., Winter, G., Moll, K., Wheelock, C.E., Bayarugaba, J., Kironde, F., Egwang, T.G., Cheng, Q., Anderson, B., Wahlgren M. (2007). PfEMP1DBL-1alpha amino acid motifs in severe disease states of Plasmodium falciparum. *Proc Natl Acad Sci. USA.40*:15835-15840

Nsiah, K., Dzogbefia, V. P. Ansong, D., Boateng, H., Ocloo, D., Osei-Frempong, E., Kena Frempong, N., Osei Akoto, A. (2010). The incidence of malaria and the comparison of hematological and biochemical indices of Plasmodium falciparum-parasitemic and aparasitemic sickle cell disease (SCD) patients. *Int J Lab Hematol*. 32: e197-e207

Nussenblatt, V., Mukasa, G., Metzger, A., Ndeezi, G., Garrett, E., Semba, R.D. (2001) *Clin Diagn Lab Immunol*. 8:1164-1170

Nussenzweig V., Nussenzweig R.S. (1989). Rationale for the development of engineered sporozoite malaria vaccine. *Adv. Immun. 45:*283–334.

Nussenzweigh, R.S., Vanderberg, J., Most, H., Orton, C. (1967) Protective immunity produced by the injection of X-irradiated sporozoites of Plasmodium berghei. *Nature 216*:160-162

Odel, G.B., Natzschka, J.C., Storey, G.N.B. (1967). Bilirubin nephropathy in the Gunn strain rat. *Am J Physiol. 221*:931-935

Oh, S. S., Chishti, A. H.; Palek, J., Liu, S-C. (1997). Erythrocyte membrane alteration in Plasmodium falciparum sequestration. *Current Opin Hematol. 4*:148-154, 1997

Oliver, A. M., F. Martin, J. F. Kearney. (*1999*). IgMhighCD21high lymphocytes enriched in the splenic marginal zone generate effector cells more rapidly than the bulk of follicular B cells. *J Immunol. 162*: *7198*-7207

*Olumese, P.E. et al., (*1997*)*. The clinical manifestations of cerebral malaria among Nigerian children with the sickle cell trait. *Ann Trop Paediatr 17:*141–145.

Omodeo-Salé, F., Motti, A., Basilico, N., Parapiki, S., Olliaro, P. and Taramelli, D. (2003) Accelerated senescence of human erythrocytes cultured with Plasmodium falciparum. *Blood 102*:705-711

O'Neill, P.M., Barton, V.E., Ward, S.A. *(*2010*)*. The molecular mechanism of action of artemisinin. The debate continues. *Molecules 15:*1705–1721.

O'Neill, P.M. & Posner, G.H. *(*2004*)*. A medicinal chemistry perspective on artemisinin and related endoperoxides. *J Med Chem 47:*2945–2964

Oo, M. M., Aikawa, M., Than, T., Aye, T.M., Myint, P.T., Igarashi, I., Schoene, W.C/. (1987). Human cerebral malaria: a pathological study. *J Neuropathol Exp Neurol. 46*: 223-231

van Ooij C, Haldar K (2007). Protein export from Plasmodium parasites. *Cell Microbiol* 9*:*573-582

Ozaki, L.S., Svec, P., Nussenzweig, R.S., Nussenzweig, V., Godson, G.N. (1983) Structure of the plasmodium knowlesi gene coding for the circumsporozoite protein..*Cell. 34*:815-822

Pagola, S., Stephens, P.W., Bohle, D.S., Kosar, A.D., Madsen, S.K. (2000) The structure of malaria pigment β-haematin. *Nature. 404*:307-310.

Panton, L.J., McPhie, P., Maloy, W.L., Wellems, T.E., Taylor, D.W. and Russell J. Howard, R.J. (1989). Purification and partial characterization of an unusual protein of *Plasmodium falciparum:* histidine-rich protein II. *Molec Biochem Parasitol. 35*:149-160

Parroche, P., Lauw, F.N., Goutaguy, N., Latz, E., Monks, B.G., Visintin, A., Halmen, K.A., Lamphier, M., Olivier, M., Bartholomeu, D.C., Gazzinelli, R.T., Golenbock, D.T. (2007) Malaria hemozoin is immunologically inert but radically enhances innate responses by presenting malaria DNA to Toll-like receptor 9. *Proc Natl Acad Sci. USA. 104*:1919-1924

Pasvol G. (2005). The treatment of complicated and severe malaria. *Br Med Bull. 75-76*: 29-47

Pathirana, S.L., Alles, H.K., Bandara, S., Phone-Kyaw, M., Perera, MK., Wickremasinghe, A.R., Mendis, K.N., Handunetti, S.M. (2005) ABO-blood-group types and protection against severe Plasmodium falciparum malaria. *Ann Trop Med Parasitol.* 99:119-124

Perlmann, P., Perlman, H., Berzins, K., Troge-Blamberg, M. (1998) Selected problems of malaria blood stage immunity. *Tokai J Exp Clin Med.* 23:55-62

Peterson, M. G.,. Marshall, V. M Smythe, J. A. Crewther, P. E.. Lew, A. Silva, A Anders, R. F., Kemp, D. J. (1989). Integral membrane protein located in the apical complex of Plasmodium falciparum. *Mol. Cell. Biol. 9*:3151-3154.

Phillips, R.E. Pasvol, G. (1992) Anaemia of Plasmodium falciparum. Baillieres Clin Haematol. 5:315-320

*Pillai, S., A. Cariappa, S. T. Moran. (*2005). *Marginal zone B cells.* Annu Rev Immunol. *23: 161-196*

Pino, P., Vouldoukis, I., Dugas, N., Hassani-Loppion, G., Dugas, B., Mazier, D. (2003) Redox-dependent apoptosis in human endothelial cells after adhesion of Plasmodium falciparum-infected erythrocytes. *Ann N Y Acad Sci.* 1010:582-586

Pinzon-Ortiz, C., Friedman, J., Esko, J., and Sinnis, P. (2001) The binding of the circumsporozoite protein to cell surface heparan sulfate proteoglycans is required for *Plasmodium* sporozoite attachment to target cells *J. Biol. Chem.* 2001 276: 26784-26791 276, 26784–26791

Plebanski, M. & Hill, A. V. (2000). The immunology of malaria infection. *Curr. Opin. Immunol.* 12 :437-441

Premaratna, R., Gunatilake, A.K., Desilva, N.R., Tilakaratney, Fonreka, M.M., Desilva, H.J. (2001). Severe hepatic dysfunction associated with falciparum malaria. *Southeast Asian J Trop Med Public Health. 32*:*70*–72.

Price, R.N., Simpson, J.A., Nosten, F., Luxemburger, C., Hkirjaroen, L., ter Kuile, F., Chongsuphajnisiddhi, T. and White, N.J. (2001) Factors contributing to anemia after uncomplicated falciparum malaria *Am J Trop Med Hyg*. 65:614-622

Punyagupta, S., Srichnikul, T., Nitinayanat, P., Petchclai, B. (1974). Acute pulmonary insufficiency in falciparum malaria: summary of 12 cases with evidence of disseminated intravascular coagulation. *Am J Trop Med Hyg. 23*:551-559

Raper, A.B. (1949). The incidence of sicklaemia. E AfrMed J. 26:281-282

Rathore, D., Hrstka, S.C.L., Sacci, J.B. Jr., de la Vega, P., Linhardt, R.J., Kumar, S., McCutchan, T.F. (2003). Molecular mechanism of host specificity in *plasmodium falciparum* infection: role of circumsporozoite protein. *J Biol Chem*. 278:40905-40910

Rathore, D., Sacci, J. B., de la Vega, P., McCutchan T. F. (2002). Binding and invasion of liver cells by *Plasmodium falciparum* sporozoites: essential involvement of the amino terminus of circumsporozoite protein. *J. Biol. Chem. 277*:7092-7098

Rathore, D., Nagarkatti, R., Jani, D., Chattopadhay, R., de la Vega, P., Kumar, S., McCutchan, T.F. (2005) An immunologically cryptic epitope of Plasmodium falciparum CSP facilitates liver cell recognition and induces protective antibodies that block liver invasion. *J Biol Chem. 280*:20524-20529

Raymond, J.M., Dumas, F., Baldit, C., Couzigou, P., Beraud, C., Amouretti, M. (1989). Fatal acute hepatitis due to amodiaquine. *J Clin Gastroenterol. 11*:602-603

Redd, S.C., Kazembe, P.N., Luby, S.P. et al. (1996). Clinical algorithm for treatment of *Plasmodium falciparum* malaria in children. *Lancet.347:*223–227

Renggli, J., Hahne, M., Matile, H., Betschart, B., Tschopp, J. & Corradin, G. (*1997*) *Parasite Immunol. 19 , 145*-148

Reynaud, F., Mallet, L., Lyon, A., Rodolfo, J.C. (2005). Rhabdomyolysis and acute renal failure in *Plasmodium falciparum* malaria. *Nephrol Dial Transpl 20:847*

Richards, A.L. *(*1997*).* Tumour Necrosis Factor and Associated Cytokines in the host's response to malaria. *Int J Parasitol 27:*1251–1263

Ridley RG (2002) Medical need, scientific opportunity and the drive for international drugs. *Nature 415*:686-693

Rizzo, F., Morandi, N., Riccio, G., Ghiazza, G., Garavelli, P. (1989). Unusual transmission of falciparum malaria in Italy. *Lancet. 1*:*555*–556

Roberts, D.J., Casals-Pascula, C., Weatherall, D.J. (2005). The clinical, pathophysiological features of malarial anaemia. *Curr Top Microbial Immunol. 295*:137-167

Roberts, D.J., Craig, A., Berendt, A.R., Pinches, R., Nash, G., Marsh, K. Newbold, C.I. (1992). Rapid switching to multiple antigenic and adhesive phenotypes in malaria. *Nature. 357*:689–692

Robinson, H.L. & Amara, R.R. (2005). T cell vaccines for malarial infections. *Nat Med. 113*:525-532

Robson, K.J., Hall, J.R., Jennings, M.W., Harris, T.J., Marsh, K., Newbold, C.I., Tate, V.E., Weatherall, D.J. (1988). A highly conserved amino-acid sequence in thrombospondin, properdin and in proteins from sporozoites and blood stage of human malarial parasite. *Nature 335*:79-82

Robson, K.J.H. & Weatherall, D.J. (2009). Malarial anemia and STAT6. *Haematologica. 94*:157-159.

Rogers W. O., Rogers M. D., Hedstrom R. C., Hoffman S. L. (1992). Characterization of the gene encoding sporozoite surface protein 2, a protective *Plasmodium yoelii* sporozoite antigen. *Mol Biochem Parasitol. 53:*45–52

Rogers W. O., Malik A., Mellouk S., Nakamura K., Rogers M. D., Szarfman A., Gordon D. M., Nussler A., Aikawa M., Hoffman S. L.*(1992a)* Characterization of Plasmodium falciparum sporozoite surface protein 2. *Proc. Natl. Acad. Sci. U. S. A 89:*9176–9180

Rogerson, S.J., Novakovic, S., Cooke, B.M., Brown, G.V. (1997). *Plasmodium falciparum*-infected erythrocytes adhere to the proteoglycan thrombomodulin in static and flow-based systems. *Exp Parasitol. 86*:8–18

Rogerson, S.J., Pollina, E., Getachew, A., Tadesse, E., Lema, V.M., Molyneux, M.E (2003). Placental monocyte infiltrates in response to *Plasmodium falciparum* malaria infection and their association with adverse pregnancy outcomes. *Am J Trop Med Hyg. 68*: 115-119

Rosenthal, P. J. (2001). Protease inhibitors, *In* P. J. Rosenthal (ed.), *Antimalarial chemotherapy: mechanisms of action, resistance, and new directions in drug discovery.* pp. 325-345. Humana Press, Totawa, NJ.

Rosenthal, P.J., Mckerrow, J.H., Aikawa, M., Nagasawa, H. and Henderson, G.B. (1988) A malarial cysteine proteinase is necessary for hemoglobin degradation in Plasmodium falciparum. *J Clin Invest.82*:1560-1566

Roth, E.F., Friedman, M.J., Ueda, Y., Tellez, I., Trager, W. Nagel, R.L. (1978) Sickling rates of human AS cells infected in vitro with Plasmodium falciparum malaria. *Science. 202*:650-652

Rouzine, I.M. & McKenzie, F.E. (2003). Link between immune response and parasite synchronization in malaria. *Proc Natl Acad Sci. USA*. 100:3473-3478

Rowe, A., Obeiro, J., Newbold, C.I., Marsh, K. (2002). Positive correlation between rosetting and parasitemia in Plasmodium falciparum clinical isolates. *Am J Trop Med Hyg.* 66:458-460

Rowe, J.A., Handel, I.G., Thera. M.A., Deans, A.M., Lyke. K.E., Kone, A., Diallo, D.A., Raza, A., Kai, O., Marsh, K., Plowe, C.V., Doumbo, O.K., Moulds, J.M. (*2007*). Blood group O protects against severe Plasmodium falciparum *malaria* through the mechanism of reduced rosetting. *Proc Natl Acad Sci USA 104*: *17471*–17476

Rowe, J.A., Moulds, J.M., Newbold, C.I., Miller, L.H. (1997). Plasmodium falciparum rosetting mediated by a parasite-variant erythrocyte membrane protein. *Nature 388*:292-295

Rowe, J.A., Raza, A., Diallo, D.A., Baby, M., Poudiougo, B., Coulibaly, D., Cockburn, I.A., Middleton, J., Lyke, K.E., Plowe, C.V., Doumbo, O.K., Moulds, J.M. *(2002). Genes Immun. 3*:497-500

Schofield, L. & Grau, G.E. (2005). Immunological processes in malaria pathogenesis. *Nat Rev Immunol. 5*:722–735

Schumann, R.R. (2007) Malarial fever: hemozoin is involved but toll-free. *Proc Natl Acad Sci. USA. 104*:61743-61744

Schwarzer E, Alessio M, Ulliers D, Arese P. (1998). Phagocytosis of malarial pigment, haemozoin, impairs the expression of major histocompatibility complex class II antigen, CD54 and CD 11c in human monocytes. *Infect Immun. 66*:1601-1606

Schwarzer E, Alessio M, Ulliers D, Giribaldi G, Ginsberg H, Arese P. (1992) Impairment of macrophage functions after ingestion of Plasmodium falciparum-infected erythrocytes or isolated malarial pigment. *J Exp Med. 176*:1033-1041

Schwarzer, E., Kuhn, H., Valante, E. and Arese, P. (2003) Malaria-parasitized erythrocytes and hemozoin nonenzymatically generate large amounts of hydroxyl fatty acids that inhibit monocyte functions. *Blood* 101:722-728

Sejeantson, S, Bryson K, Amato D, Babona D (1977) Malaria and hereditary ovalocytosis. *Human Genet.* 37:161-167

Seymour, R., Reycraft, D.W., Hano, J.E., Barry, W. (1967). The liver in malaria. Arch Path. *83:271–277.*

Sheehy, T.W. & Reba, R.C. (1967). Complications of falciparum malaria and their treatment. *Ann Int Med. 66*: *807*–809

Sherman, I.W. (*1988)*. Mechanisms of molecular trafficking in malaria. *Parasitol 96*: *S57–*S81

Sherman, I.W., Edo, S., Winograd, E. (2003) Cytoadherence and sesquestration in Plasmodium falciparum: defining the ties that bind. *Microbes Infect.*5:897-909

Shukla, M.M., Singh, N., Singh, M.P., Tejwani, B.M., Srivastava, D.K., Sharma, V.P. (*1995)*. Cerebral *malaria* in Jabalpur, India. *Indian J Malariol 32*: *70–*75.

Sidjanski, S.P., Vanderberg, J.P., Sinnis, P. (1997). Anopheles stephensi salivary glands bear receptors for region I of the circumsporozoite protein of Plasmodium falciparum. *Mol Biochem Parasitol.* 90:33-41

Sijwali, P.S., Koo, J., Singh, N., Rosenthal, P.J. *(2006).* Gene disruptions demonstrate independent roles for the four falcipain cysteine proteases of *Plasmodium falciparum. Mol Biochem Parasitol 150:*96–106

Simpson, JA, Watkins ER, Price, RN, Aarons, L, Kyle, DE, White NJ (2000) Mefloquine pharmacokinetic models: implications for dosing and resistance. *Antimirob Agents Chemotherap.* 44:3414-3424

Sinniah, R. & Lye, W (2000). Acute renal failure from myoglobinuria secondary to myositis from severe falciparum malaria. *Am J Nephrol. 20*: *339–*343

Sinnis, P.& Nardin, E. (2002). Sporozoite antigens: biology and immunology of the circumsporozoite protein and thrombospondin related anonymous protein. *In Malaria Immunology*. P. Perlmann, M. Troye-Blomberg, editors. S. Karger AG, Basel, Switzerland. 70–96

Sirén, A-L., Fratelli, M., Brines, M., Goemans, C., Casagrande, S., Lewczuk, P., Keenan, S., Gleiter, C., Pasquali, C., Capobianco, A,.Mennini, T., Heumann, R., Cerami, A., Ehrenreich, H., Ghezzi, P. (2001). Erythropoietin prevents neuronal apoptosis after cerebral ischemia and metabolic stress *Proc Natl Acad Sci USA. 2001 98:* 4044-4049

Sitprija, V. (1988). Nephropathy in falciparum malaria. *Kidney Int. 34*:867-877

Skarbinski J, James EM, Causer LM, Barber AM, Mali S, Nguyen-Dinh P, Roberts JM, Parise ME, Slutsker L, Newman RD, *2006. Malaria* surveillance—United States, 2004. *MMWR Surveill Summ 55*: *23–*37.

Skorokhod, A., Schwarzer, E., Gremo, G., Arese, P. (*2007*). HNE produced by the *malaria* parasite Plasmodium falciparum generates HNE-protein adducts and decreases erythrocyte deformability. *Redox Rep 12*: *73–*75

Smith, A.D., Bradley, D.J., Smith V. et al. (2008). Imported malaria and high risk groups: observational study using UK surveillance data 1987-2006. *BMJ. 337:*a120.

Smith JD, Gannain B, Baruch DI, Kyes S (2001) Decoding the language of var genes and Plasmodium falciparum sequestration. *Trends Parasitol.* 17:538-545

Snow, R.W., Gnerra, C.A., Noor, A.M., Myint, H.Y., Hay, S.I. (2005) The global distribution of clinical episodes of Plasmodium falciparum malaria. Nature. 434:214-217

Snow, R.W. & Marsh, K. (1998). New insights into the epidemiology of malaria relevant for disease control. *Br Med Bull. 54*:293–309

Snow, R.W., Omumbo, J., Lowe, B., Molyneux, C., Obiero, J., Palmer, A., Weber, M., Pinder, M., Nahlen, B., Obonyo, C.. Newbold, C., Gupta, S, Marsh, K. (1997). Relation between severe malaria morbidity in children and level of Plasmodium falciparum transmission in Africa. *Lancet 349*:1650-1654

Slater, A.F.G., Swiggard, W.J., Orton, B.R. et al. (1991) An iron-carboxylate bond links the heme units of malaria pigment. *Proc Natl Acad Sci USA. 88*:325-329

Sousa, A.R., Lane, S.J., Nakhosteen, J.A., Lee, T.H., Poston, R.N. (1996) Expression of interleukin-1 beta and IL-1-receptor antagonist (IL-1a) on asthmatic bronchial epithelium. *Am J Respir Crit Care Med. 154*:1061-1066

Srichaikul, T., Panikbutr, N. and Jeumtrakul, P. (1967) Bone-marrow changes in human malaria. *Ann Trop Med Parasitol. 61*:40-51

Srivastava, A., Khanduri, A., Lakhtakia, S., Pandey, R. (1996). Falciparum malaria with acute liver failure. *Trop Gastroenterol. 17*:*172*–174.

Stoltzfus, R.J., Chwaya, H.M., Montresor, A., Albonico, M., Savioli, L. and Tielsch, J.M. (2000) Malaria, hookworms and recent fever are related to anemia and iron status indicators in 0- to 5-y old Zanzibari children and these relationships change with age. *J Nutr. 130*:1724-1733

Straik, S. & Riley, E.M. (2004) Does malaria suffer from lack of memory? Immunol Rev. 201:268-290

Stone, W.J., Hanchett, J.E., Knepshield, J.H. (1972). Acute renal insufficiency due to falciparum malaria: Review of 42 cases. *Arch Intern Med. 129*:*620*–627

Sturm, A., Amino, R., van de Sand, C., Regen, T., Retzlaff, S., Rennenberg, A., Krueger, A., Pollok, J.M., Menard, R. and Heussler, V.T. (2006) Manipulation of host hepatocytes by the malaria parasite for delivery into liver sinusoids. *Science. 313*:1287-1290

Sullivan, D.J., Gluzman, I.Y., Goldberg, D.E. (1996). Plasmodium hemozoin formation mediated by histidine-rich proteins. *Science. 271*:219-222

Sultan A. A., Thathy V., Frevert U., Robson K. J. H., Crisanti A., Nussenzweig V., Nussenzweig R. S., Menard, R.(1997). TRAP is necessary for gliding motility and infectivity of Plasmodium sporozoites. *Cell 90:*511–522

Sutherland, C.J., Ord, R., Dunyo, S., Jawara, M., Drakeley, C.J., Alexander, N., Coleman, R., Pinder, M., Walraven, G., Target, C.H. (2005) Reduction of malaria transmission to Anophelous mosquitoes with a six-dose regimen of co-arthemeter. *PLoS Medicine. 2*: e92

Suvanapha, R., Sitprija, V., van Ypersele de Strihou C. *(1992).* Acute *renal* failure in the tropics and hantavirus disease. Cameron S, Davison AM, Grunfeld JP, Kerr D, Ritz E, eds. *Oxford Textbook of Clinical Nephrology, First Edition.* Oxford: Oxford University Press, 1124–1146.

Takeda, K. & Akira, S. (2004) Microbial recognition by toll-like receptors. *J Dermatol Sci. 34*:73-82

Takshande, A.,, Vilhekar, K., Jain, M, Atkari, S. *(2006).* Clinicohematological profile of cerebral *malaria* in a rural hospital. *J Indian Acad Clin Med 7*: *308*–312

Taliaferro, W.H., Mulligan, H.W. (1937). The histopathology of malaria with special reference to the function and origin of the macrophages in defence. *Indian M Res Mem. 39*:1

Tan, L.K., Yacoub, S., Scott, S., Bhagani, S., Jacobs, M. (2008). Acute lung injury and other serious complications of Plasmodium vivax malaria. Lancet Infect Dis *8:449–454*

Taoufiq, Z., Gay, F., Balvaryos, J., Ciceron, L., Tefit, M., Lechat, P., Mazier, D. (2008) Rho kinase inhibition in severe malaria: thwarting parasite-induced collateral damage to endothelia. *J Infect Dis. 197*:1062-1073

Taylor, T.E., Borgstein, A., Molyneux, M.E. (1993). Acid-base status in paediatric Plasmodium falciparum malaria. *Q J Med 1993*; *86*:*99*–109.

Taylor, W.R. & White, N.J. (2002). Malaria and the lung. *Clin Chest Med.* 23:457–468

Thewing, J., Skarbinski, J., Newman, R.D., et al., (2007). Malaria surveillance-United States, 2005. *MMWR Surveill Summ. 56(6):23-38*

Triglia, T Menting JG, Wilson, C Cowman AF (1997) Mutations of dihydropteroate synthetase are responsible for sulfore and sulfonamide resistance in Plasmodium falciparum. *Proc Natl Acad Sci USA. 94*:13944-13949

Tripathi, A.K., Sha, W., Shulaev, V., Stins, M.S., Sullivan, D.J. Jr. (2009) Plasmodium falciparum erythrocytes induce NF-kappaB regulated inflammatory pathways in human cerebral endothelium. *Blood 114*:4243-4252

Turner, G. (1997) Cerebral malaria. *Brain Pathol. 7*:569-582

Udomsangpetch, R., Reinhardt, P.H., Scollaardt, T., Elliot, J.F., Kubes, P., Ho, M. (1997) Promiscuity of clinial Plasmodium falciparum isolates for multiple adhesive molecules under flow conditions. *J Immunol. 158*:4358-4364

Udomsangpetch, R., Todd, J., Carlson, J., Greenwood, B.M. (*1993)*. The effects of hemoglobin genotype and ABO blood group on the formation of rosettes by Plasmodium falciparum-infected red blood cells. *Am J Trop Med Hyg. 48*: *149*–153

Valecha, N., Pinto, R.G., Turner, G.D., Kumar, A., Rodrigues, S., Dubhashi, N.G., Rodrigues, E., Banaulikar, S.S., Singh, R., Dash, A.P., *et al.* Histopathology of fatal respiratory distress caused by *Plasmodium vivax* malaria. *Am J Trop Med Hyg 81*:758–762

Van den Steen, P.E., Geurts, N, Deroost, K., Van Aelst, I., Verhenne, S., Heremans, H. Damme, J. V., Opdenakker, G. (2010). Immunopathology and Dexamethasone Therapy in a New Model for Malaria-associated Acute Respiratory Distress Syndrome *Am J Respir Crit Care Med. 181*:957-968

Villa P Bigini, P., Mennini, T., Agnello D., Laragione, T.,Cagnoto, A., Viviani, B., Marinovich, M., Cerami, A., Coleman, T.R., Brines M., Ghezzi, P. (2003) Erythropoietin selectively attenuates cytokine production and inflammation in cerebral ischaemia by targeting neuronal apoptosis. *J Exp Med. 198*:971-975

Vinetz, J.M., Li, J., MacCutchan, T.F., Kaslow, D.C. (1998). Malarial infection in a 74-year-old Greek woman with splenomegaly. *New Engl J.Med. 338*:367-371

Vogt, A.M., Barragan, A., Chen, Q., Kironde, F., Spillmann, D., Wahlgren, M. (2003) Heparan sulphate on endothelial cells mediatethe binding of Plasmodium-infected erythrocytes via the DBL-1-aipha domain of PfEMP1. *Blood. 101*:2405-2411

Vogt, A.M., Pettersson, F., Moll, K., Jonsson, C., Normark, J., Ribacke, U., Egwang. T.G., Ekre, H.P., Spillmann, D., Chen, Q., Wahlgren, M. (*2006*). Release of sequestered *malaria* parasites upon injection of a glycosaminoglycan. *PLoS Pathog 2*: *e100*

Waitumbi, J.N., Opollo, M.O., Muga, R.O., Misore, A.O.,Stoute, J.A. (2000). Red cell surface changes and erythrophagocytosis in children with severe Plasmodium falciparum anemia in *Blood 95*:1481-1496

Weatherall, DJ (1997) Thalassemia and malaria, revisited *Ann Trop Med Parasitol. 91*:885-890

Weatherall, D.J. (2008). Genetic variation and susceptibility to infection: the red cell and malaria. *Br J Haematol.141*:276-286

Weatherall, D.J., Miller, L.H., Baruch, D.I., Marsh, K., Doumbo, O.K., Casals-Pascual, C., Roberts, D.J. (2002). Malaria and the Red Cell. *Hematology*, 35 - 57.

Weatherall, M.W., Higgs, D.R., Weiss, H., Weatherall, D.J., Sejeant, G.R. (2005) Phenotype/genotype relationships in sickle cell disease: a pilot twin study. *Clin Lab Haematol. 27*:384-390

Weiss G. (2008). Iron metabolism in the anemia of chronic disease. *Biochim Biophys Acta.* Aug 22 Epub

Wellems, T.E. & Miller, L.H. (2003). Two worlds of malaria. *N Engl J Med 349:*1496-8.

White, N.J. (2002) Malaria. In: Cook, G., Zumla, A. (eds.) Manson's Tropical Diseases. Philadelphia: WB Saunders, pp 1205-1297

White, N.J. Qinghaosu (artemisinin): the price of success. *Science. 320*:330–334

Wilairatana, P., Looareesuwan, S., Charoenlarp, P. (1994). Liver profile changes and complications in jaundiced patients with falciparum malaria. *Trop Med Parasitol. 45*:298-302

Williams, T.N. (2006). Human red blood cell polymorphisms and malaria. *Curr Opin Microbiol. 9*:388-394

World Health Organisation (2006). *Guidelines for the treatment of malaria* (WHO, Geneva)

World Health Organisation (2000). WHO Communicable Disease Cluster. Severe falciparum malaria. Trans Roy Soc Med Hyg. *94(Suppl.):*1*–90.*

Wyler D, Gallin J, (*1977*).. Spleen-derived mononuclear cell chemotactic factor in malaria infections: a possible mechanism for splenic macrophage accumulation. *J Immunol 118*: *478*–484.

Yagmur, Y., Kara, I.H., Aldemir, M., Buyukbayram, H., Tacyildiz, I.H. and Keles, C. (2000) Spontaneous rupture of malaria spleen: two case reports and review of literature. *Crit Care 4*: 309-313

Ying, P., Shakibaei, M., Patankar, M. S., Clavijo, P., Beavis, R. C., Clark, G. F., Frevert, U. (*1997*) *The Malaria circumsporozoite protein: interaction of the conserved regions I and II-plus with heparin-like oligosaccharides in heparan sulfate. Exp. Parasitol. 85*, *168*–182

Yipp BG, et al. (2000). Synergism of multiple adhesion molecules in mediating cytoadherence of *Plasmodium falciparum*-infected erythrocytes to microvascular endothelial cells under flow. *Blood. 96*:2292–2298

Yoshida, N., Nussenzweig, R. S., Potocnjak, P., Nussenzweig, V., Aikawa M. (1980). *Science 207:71–73.*

Young, N.S. (1995) Aplastic anaemia. Lancet. 346:228-232

Zandvoort, A.& Timens, W. (*2002).* The dual function of the splenic marginal zone: essential for initiation of anti-TI-2 responses but also vital in the general first-line defense against blood-borne antigens. *Clin Exp Immunol. 130*: *4*-11

Zheng, L., Jiang, Q., Zhang, R., Davies, K., Powers, C., van Bruggen, N., Chopp, M. (2000) VEGF enhances angiogenesis and promotes blood-brain barrier leakage in the ischemic brain. *J Clin Invest. 106*:829-838

Zhu, J., Krishnegowada, G., Gowda, D.C.(2005). Induction of proinflammatory responses in macrophages by the glycosylphosphatidylinositols of *Plasmodium falciparum*: the requirement of extracellular signal-regulated kinase, p38, c-jun N-terminal kinase and nNF-κB pathways for the expression of proinflammatory cytokines and nitric oxide. *J Biol Chem. 280*:8606-8616

In: Malaria: Etiology, Pathogenesis and Treatments
Editors: A. M. Peterson et al, pp. 321-337

ISBN: 978-1-62100-363-2

Chapter XIII

The Nature of the Malaria Paroxysm

Filiberto Malagón
Laboratorio de Malariologia, Departamento de Microbiología y Parasitologia, Facultad de Medicina, Universidad Nacional Autonoma de Mexico.

Abstract

This study attempts the reconstruction of the most characteristic clinical picture of the acute phase of malaria, the malarial paroxysm, describing the elements that participate on the part of the parasite and the host, the way they become integrated, and how they function to produce the classical clinical manifestations of what we call malaria.

Introduction

Malaria is a parasitic disease and one of the most important transmissible diseases in the world, principally located in the tropics and secondarily in temperate regions. Today five species of malaria parasites are considered the etiologic agents of the disease all of them belong to the genus *Plasmodium*: *P. falciparum*, *P. vivax*, *P. malariae*, *P. ovale,* and *P. knowlesi*. The first four species coming in its origin from African apes from whom the infection was inherited to humans, the fifth species, a parasite previously considered to be confined to monkeys in South East Asia, has been found infecting humans during the last decade, as much frequently as to be regarded a new *Plasmodium* species infecting humans. [1-4].

Fever is an adaptive brain response to local and systemic inflammation and, it is almost universally present among vertebrates [5]. One of the most significant clinical manifestations of malaria is the sadden rise of fever of limited duration and periodic repetition, commonly associated to other symptoms such as headache, myalgias, arthralgias, fatigue, gastrointestinal symptoms and in severe cases with involvement of lungs, kidney and central nervous system.

The malarious paroxysm, however, is identified with the febrile syndrome that is present during the acute period of the malaria infection.
Thanks to the characteristic periodicity of the fever it has been possible to trace the presence of malaria since the early written manuscripts of human kind, such as the Ebert's papyrus in the ancient Egypt, and the Hippocrates manuscripts in the ancient Greece [6, 7]. In modern times fever was, and still is, the reference to identify potential malaria infected individuals in the clinical and epidemiological studies, as well as in the malaria control campaigns.

The first names to refer to those malarial or febrile paroxysms were coined by Hippocrates who making reference to its periodic character described and called them as the "tertian" and the "quartan" fevers, to name those fevers that repeated each third or fourth day which he associated, since then, with patients living in marshy and unhealthy places [8]. One can see that malaria is a disease clinically defined without knowing the etiological agent. Once Laveran discovered the causal agent of malaria, associations were made between stages of the parasites development in the patient's blood and its clinical manifestations. Later, in 1889 Golgi found that there were two kinds of tertian fevers, both with different clinical manifestations and blood parasites with different morphology. Guided by these findings he divided the tertian fevers into benign and malign (this last also called aestivo-autumnal malaria). As the benign tertian malaria was associated to a parasite morphologically different to that causing the malignant tertian malaria, the first was named *Plasmodium vivax* and the second *Plasmodium falciparum*. It was also recognized, that the malarial paroxysm was associated with the end of the parasites reproduction in erythrocytes i.e. with the end of the parasite erythrocytic schizogony [9,10,11]. In this way, a paroxysm is in fact the host response to a stage of the parasite's development in blood, which takes the shape of a periodic event in the fashion of a circadian rhythm, with the parasite performing as the clock. It is, at this point (the very end of the XIX century), that this disease commences to be associated with the products of the host-parasite interactions.

Today, knowledge has reached the point so as to make possible to identify the elements, and trace the processes that participate in the genesis of clinical signals that identify the malaria paroxysm. The description of these events chain with an attempt to interpret what they signify is the aim of this chapter.

The Parasite and the Host

The infective form of the human malaria parasites, under natural forms of transmission, is the sporozoite if transmission is produced by the mosquito bite, or the merozoite as well as other blood stages, if transmission is carried out through placental blood, from mother to fetus. Sporozoites are deposited into the small blood vessels of the skin by the infected mosquito when biting, and by this via reach the liver cells where reproduction takes place. In congenital malaria, infected pregnant women transmit her malaria parasites to her product by trans-placental transmission. It is well known that hepatocytes invasion by the sporozoites and the resulting lysis of these cells, does not produce clinical signs nor detectable pathological changes, and that total pathology and symptomatology in malaria is the consequence of the parasite invasion of erythrocytes. These circulating cells are the parasite host cells where malaria parasites reproduce in a cycling fashion erythrocyte to erythrocyte, before the manifestation of clinical signals appear to make patent the presence of the parasite [12].

From the five *Plasmodium* species that infect man, two species (*P. vivax* and *P. ovale*) have bi-circadian erythrocytic cycles of reproduction whose end marks the 48h periodicity of the febrile paroxysms. *P. falciparum* has a periodicity of 36 to 48h, while *P. malariae* shows tri-circadian cycles, producing paroxysms each 72h. Finally *P. knowlesi* the last of the human species consider has a circadian cycle with paroxysms every 24h. These periods of time mark the beginning and the end of the malaria parasites reproduction in the erythrocyte i.e. since the merozoites invasion of a new erythrocyte up to the final stage of the schizont, when the erythrocyte disrupts and a new generation of merozoites is released into the blood stream, for each merozoite to repeat the invasion of a new erythrocyte to recycle processes and times in the way of a biological clock [13], see fig 1.

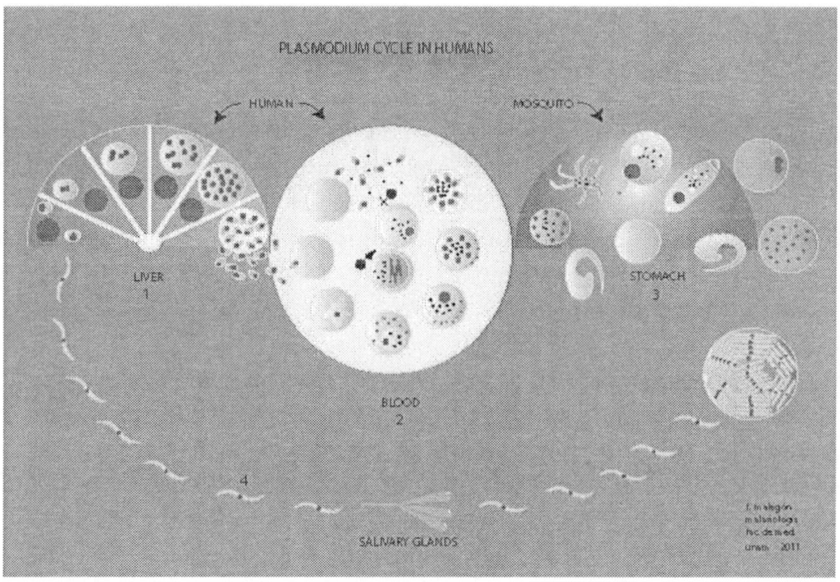

Figure 1. Life cycle of malaria parasites in humans. 1, shows the liver with cells infected by sporozoites, in the first liver cell (from left to right) a couple of parasites are seen, to remember that in relapsing species some sporozoites growth into schizonts immediately, while others remain dormants. The other cells show different stages of exoerythrocytic development with hepatic merozoites release at the end 2, represents the inside of a blood vessel and shows a whole erythrocytic cycle starting with the erythrocyte invasion of hepatic merozoites, followed for the different asexual stages: trophozoites, schizonts, segmenters, free erythrocytic merozoites, and the immature sexual cells. 3, shows stages of the parasite developing in the mosquito stomach: exflagelation of microgametocyte, fecundation of macrogametocyte, resulting ooquinete, and development of oocyst with production and release of sporozoites 4, salivary glands ejecting sporozoites when biting a new host.

Malaria Paroxysm Initiated by a Toxin

The end of the *Plasmodium* reproduction in erythrocytes signals the beginning of the febrile paroxysm. This coincidence, between the end of the malaria parasites erythrocytic schizogony and the commence of the paroxysm clinical signs, has made thought that the infected erythrocyte rupture and the release of merozoites was responsible of the paroxysm initiation. This coincidence, make to think that a toxin was responsible of the paroxysm and that this toxin would be present in the residual products of the parasite which has accumulated into the cytoplasms of the schizont and of the infected erythrocyte, as products of the metabolic processes of growth, reproduction and differentiation of the new parasites, and released at the moment of the erythrocyte rupture. Such a toxin, however, has proved very difficult to identify. Brown proposed in 1912 that malaria pigment (hemozoin) released by the parasite during erythrocyte rupture is the parasite toxin involved in the paroxysm set up, he experimentally reproduced chills and fever in a rabbit inoculated with malarial pigment [14]. In 1969 Maegrith published an interesting paper in which he described what he believed to be a toxin present in the serum of malaria-infected animals, capable to produce alterations in hepatocytes. He described it as a compound of low molecular weight, of less than 1000 Kd, with little nitrogen, but he could not recognize if such compound was synthetized by the parasite or the host [15]. In 1989 Ian Clark [16] called the attention on the similitude of the clinical features between the endotoxic shock developed in mice suffering bacteremia and mice infected with lethal strains of malaria parasites, and suggested that a substance similar to LPS (lipopolysaccharide) of gram negative bacteria could be involved in the malaria clinical expression, inducing the production of TNF alpha (tumor necrosis factor), which then would explain the clinical similarities between these two entities. At that time the plasmodia were not suspected to be TNF alpha producers, condition reserved mainly to gram negative bacteria, or to be more precise, specifically to the LPS of its cellular wall of which the lipidic component (lipid A) is the biologically active compound [17]. However, LPS is not a constituent of malaria parasites.

In 1990, Taverne and colleges [18] found that human and rodent *Plasmodium* possessed exoantigens which induced macrophages to produce TNF alpha and that those exoantigens have a glycolipid nature. Finally, the compound glycosylphosphatidylinositol (GPI) was incriminated as the causal molecule that activated the paroxysmal process. The toxin (GPI) was present in the malaria parasite membrane; however, the same compound is also widely distributed as normal component of many if not all membranes of human cells. The erythrocytes themselves contain that compound embedded in their membrane lipidic bilayer [19, 20]. At first it was difficult to understand that a molecule present in both parasites and host cells were a toxin, however if we look at some features of this molecule one can accept the toxic activity of that molecule. Firstly, GPI is a trans-membrane glycolipid molecule that is present in the membranes of all eukaryotic cells, more abundant in membranes of protozoa than in other cells [21], and its main function is to anchor certain proteins on the cellular surface. Not all GPIs have an equal molecular construction, because different species or cellular types differ widely in fatty acyl/alkyl and sugar residual substituents, variations that confer structural diversity to GPIs and with it different properties with a wide range of biological activities [22]. GPI of the malaria host cells is different to that of the parasite which, when isolated, purified and put in contact with macrophages, make them to produce TNF alpha [23]. In 1994 Gerold first identified GPI in the blood stage of P. falciparum, and later they were found in all malaria stages of development, including those of the mosquito vector [24].

Activation of Macrophages

Schizogony is the asexual process through which the malaria parasites reproduce in their mammal's host cells. In this process the parasite stage under reproduction (the schizont) synthetize and divide its chromatin in the number of pieces necessary to produce its brood, without chromatin organizing into chromosomes. In the end of the process the schizont is an intraerythrocytic sac containing certain number of nuclei, in which each nuclei develop its own membrane and organelles, and in the process each new parasite englobes a portion of the mother cell cytoplasm. When schizogony comes to an end, the segmenter as it is called, is just a sac inside another sac (the almost empty erythrocyte), full of new young parasites, fitted (with their apical complex) to invade cells, but together with them there is malaria pigment, residual cytoplasm of the segmenter, and accumulated metabolites as byproducts of the processes that make up the new generation of merozoites. Together with the rupture of the erythrocyte and schizont membranes, at the end of the erythrocytic cycle, all retained contents are liberated to the circulating plasma, including merozoites. The GPI molecules are then in the merozoites membrane and in the free membrane remnants of the disintegrated schizont. As this process occurs macrophages [25] are activated by any of the freed compounds or particles, including the merozoites themselves, however, activation is mainly triggered by parasite GPI and pigment. Commencement of activation occur when parasite GPI, free or associated to SMP1 (surface merozoite protein 1), links mainly to TLR2 a macrophage membrane receptor of GPI and as result of its activation macrophages start to produce proinflammatory cytokines which include: TNF alpha, interferon gamma, IL1, IL6 IL12 and nitric oxide, all of it corresponding to an early macrophage unspecific defense response of innate immunity to restrict expansion and damage of the parasite.

The synthesis of these lymphokines probably occur in chain, in which the TNF alpha primarily secreted induce the synthesis of IL-1 and this one induces the production of IL-6, as it happens when the macrophages are stimulated with LPS [26].

The phylogenetic predecessor of TNF is probably a defense molecule present in an earthworm (*Eisenia foetida*) that seems unrelated to the TNF of vertebrates, although with functional homology to TNF [27]. However, with no doubt the *Drosophila* TNF called Eiger share a common origin with the vertebrate TNF family [28].

In vertebrates TNF is predominantly produced by macrophages upon the proper stimulus, although monocytes and lymphocytes may also produce it. In humans TNF is encoded in chromosome 6, in a cluster with the genes encoding lymphotoxin a and b, two cytokines structurally related to TNF. Soluble forms of these molecules and their receptors are present in plasma at high concentrations in malaria sufferers [29].

TNF is not a single molecule but a superfamily of compounds which together with their receptors, form a web of signaling pathways with many functions in the innate and adaptive immunesystem. The TNF superfamily comprehend more than 20 receptor-ligand systems, among which the following are included: TNF, Lymphotoxin a (LTa), LTb and others. Among TNFs two types can be distinguish one that is present in membrane as a trans membrane glycoprotein and the soluble TNF that is free in the plasma. Both TNFs have their own receptors, the Membrane TNF is thought to predominantly activate the receptor TNFR2, while soluble TNF activates TNFR1. The latter being the predominantly expressed while TNFR2 is expressed mainly in endothelial cells [30].

All proinflammatory molecules above mentioned including TNF alpha, and other cytokines participate in inflammatory processes, TNF alpha possesses 55 to 75 Kd receptors in membranes of almost all cells of the organism. Cells that take up TNF in its membrane receptors generate a response which may differ among cells of different tissues, in the case of skeletal muscle cells, for instance, they synthetize and liberate prostaglandins, while TNF alpha stimulated adipocytes inhibits the fat synthesis from plasma triglycerides.

Subjects infected by malaria parasites have high Levels of TNF in their plasma and it correlates with the degree of parasitemia and the gravity of clinical signals [31, 32]. In the same way TNF soluble receptors (sTNF-R55 and sTNF-R75) are at high concentration in plasma of people infected by *Plasmodium falciparum* [33].

When to Talk About Fever or Hyperthermia

Humans maintained under basal conditions keep their body temperature oscillating through a band of 37° +/- 0.5° C. The brain is in charge to regulate and maintain this temperature through the thermoregulatory centers located in the hypothalamus supraoptic and paraventricular nuclei. Neurons from these nuclei are monitoring body temperature and adjust it through physiological changes to the 37°C reference temperature, when needed, sending effector signals to stimulate or inhibit heat generation or heat dissolution. Thermoregulatory neurons reference temperature is the one that determine the temperature at which the body has to be maintained and neurons function in consequence.

Under normal physiological conditions, drastic changes in body temperature can be observed with no changes in reference temperature, as it usually happens in athletes practicing intense exercises. The runners of 100 plane meters may reach temperatures of 40°C or more, but restoration of body basal temperature is fast and they only require some minutes, because there has not being reference temperature modification, which is maintained at 37°+/-0.5°C. It is worth to remember that under these circumstances fever does not exist, instead it is a state of hyperthermia [34].

In pathologic conditions, however, neurons reference temperature is altered and such alteration may be produced for several molecules, mostly by prostaglandins. It is believed that prostaglandin E2 (PGE2) is produced in the preoptical area vessels of the brain itself and is responsible of moving up the reference temperature and thus generates fever, [35, 36]**. It is** essential for fever induction that PGE2, whatever it is produce, enters in contact with the thermoregulatory neurons expressing EP3 receptors on its membrane [37], once activated, EP3 expresses by changing up the neurons reference temperature, to set it above 37.5°C, and then keeping it high while the stimulus that generate prostaglandins persists. Thus, when body temperature gets above 37.5°C by change of reference temperature of the thermoregulatory neurons, it is a truth fever.

The Paroxysm in Malaria

As above said, when the malaria parasites in blood are in the final schizont stage and ruptures, the compounds, particles and new parasites released produce the activation of macrophages, which in turn liberate TNF and other proinflammatory cytokines that initiate a chain or network of responses that build malaria disease. TNF acts on vascular endothelium cells activating the production of prostaglandins, among other things, which in turn are legated to receptors of thermoregulatory neurons, which respond changing the reference temperature from 37.5ºC to 40ºC, for instance. At the moment of change, the neurons of the hypothalamic thermoregulatory centers are registering a body temperature of 37ºC, while the mandatory reference temperature is now of 40ºC. Body temperature does not match with the reference temperature thus, the neurons reading is, "body temperature is cold", because it has to be at 40ºC and it is just at 37ºC. Therefore, the response is the activation of the supraoptic nuclei that activates when body temperature is below the reference temperature. Neurons generate thermoeffector signals, in two directions, to raise body temperature at the level marked by the reference temperature, one to retain the existing heat and the other to generate more heat. The signals that allow retaining heath, act on peripheral blood vessels nervous terminals producing constriction of blood vessels. The diminished volume of circulating blood produces less blood irrigation of the skin, that clinically is manifested as teguments paleness, and have the effect of diminishing the loss of heat by radiation and convection, while other signals act on respiratory centers to produce hypoventilation to diminish the lost of heat by evaporation, that clinically is observed as diminished respiration rate and superficial breathing.

From the signals that generate heat, apart of some increase in the general metabolism through the endocrine system, mainly by the activity of the thyroid gland, all skeletal muscles of the organism become the principal heat producers. At this step, striated muscles that normally are voluntarily activated, turn uncontrollable; yaw muscles show rhythmic contractions that make teeth to chatter, muscles of limbs and trunk increase its normal tension or fall in tremor or shivering, while piloerection, also called chicken skin or hair-erection is the result of skin hair muscles contraction. All this muscle activity produces a metabolic increase of muscle masses, resulting in fast heath production. During fever the striated muscle expresses a free protein, the UCP3 (uncoupling protein 3) that can covert intracellular ATP (adenosine triphosphate) into heat, allowing that muscle masses act as heat generators [5].

At this stage of the malarial paroxysm, the patient experiment a very intense cold, some times accompanied of pain on lumbar region or a sensation of pain on all body, hair included, with also headache, nausea, vomiting and diarrhea. Temperature rise and reach the febrile state, although the patient may continue to feel cold, if body temperature has not match the reference temperature. In fact it is probable that no human pathology exists that cause as much intense coldness sensation as malaria. As body temperature rise cold sensation disappear, until body temperature match reference temperature of the thermoregulatory neurons (in our example, 40ºC). Febrile temperature remains as long as the parasites persist stimulating macrophages and endothelium cells of blood vessels, with production of TNF and prostaglandins. Fever continues for several hours, some times up to ten.

When production of TNF-prostaglandins return to their normal levels, reference temperature automatically return to its normal value of 37+-0.5ºC, although, in cases of severe malaria, after a paroxysm, temperature may stay little below normal, for some time. At the moment when the normal reference temperature return, the body temperature registered by the thermoregulatory neurons is 40ºC, thus again reference and body temperature does not match. Mandatory reference temperature turn now to be 37ºC, while temperature detected by the neurons is 40ºC, so now the neuron readings is: "it is too hot", thus neurons from the paraventricular nuclei are activated and effector signals are sent in two directions, one to interrupt heat production and the other to dissipate the existing heat.

In response to the neuron signals, general metabolism is reduced, skeletal muscle is relaxed, now peripheral vessels are dilated, the skin become hot and red and heat is lost by radiation, there is hyperventilation and heat is released by evaporation with the exhaled hot air coming from the lungs, finally, the patient release heat dramatically through diaphoresis, abundant sweat cover all body surface, the patient ends exhausted and usually fall sleep. When the patient wake up he or she is still weak but usually strong enough to follow their quotidian activities until the paroxysm repeats 24, 36, 48 or 72 hours later, depending on the species of *Plasmodium* that infect them, see fig 2.

Classically the temperature charts of malaria patients register a double peak fever with periodicity of 36 to 48 h in the case of *P. falciparum* infection, just one peak fever of less duration with periodicity of 48h in *P. vivax* infection, that is similar for *P. ovale* and fevers of one peak but with periodicity of 72h in the case of *P. malariae* infections. Synchronicity of the paroxysms usually does not occurs during the early phase of the infection, some days of infection may has to pass to see the typical periodicity.

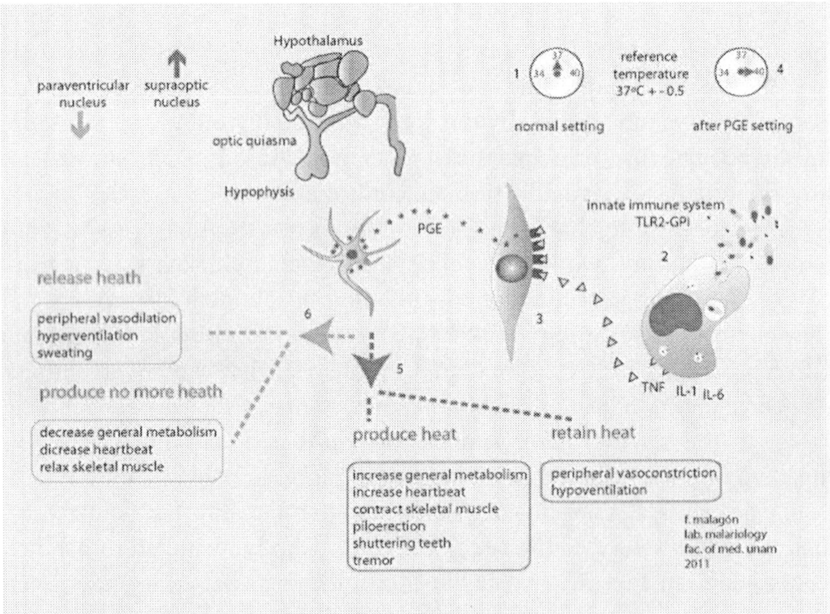

Figure 2. Malaria aparoxysm. 1, shows the normal setting of the reference temperature in thermoregulatory neurons before paroxism. 2, merozoites are just released in plasma at the end of schizogony, and a macrophage links on parasites glycosylphosphatidylinositol (GPI) through its toll-like receptors (TLR2), and is activated to respond with secretion of TNF and other interleukins. 3, shows an endothelial cell catching tumor necrosis factor (TNF) on its receptors, and responding with production of prostaglandins (PGE). 4. The stimulus of PGE on the thermoregulatory neurons change the reference temperature to 40°C (example). 5, neurons of the supraoptic nuclei send effector signals to produce and retain heat in order to rise body heat to match the new reference temperature; as result, 40°C fever is established and maintained as long as the PGEs are being produced. When PGE secretion comes to an end, reference temperature return to normal, and now thermoregulatory neurons of the paraventricular nuclei are activated and effector signals are send to produce no more heat and release the excessive heat, to match the now normal reference temperature of 37°C.

Latency and Relapses

After Laveran discovery of the malaria parasites in 1880 [38] and the discovery of malaria transmission by Anopheles mosquitoes by Grassi and Bignami [39] and Ross [40], when the complete life cycle of the malaria parasites seemed to be known, two main questions remained to be answered, the first was, where the parasite go and stay during the 12 or more days of prepatent period, after sporozoites are inoculated by the mosquito?, and the second, where the parasites are during the weeks, months or even years of latency infection after primary attack in infections that present relapses?. The answer to the first question arrived more than 40 years later when professor Garnham discovered that sporozoites are hidden inside hepatocytes to develop an exoerythrocytic cycle in the liver [41], before the parasite invade erythrocytes. Professor Garnham did special emphasis on the existence of the exoerythrocytic cycle, to explain relapses, proposing that from all the hepatic merozoites released some of them went to circulating blood and start erythrocytic invasion while others turn again to reinvade liver cells. When mechanisms of defense eliminated the circulating parasites, and the erythrocytic cycle disappeared,, the cycle hepatocyte-hepatocyte would keep the parasite going on in the liver, he thought, but with no parasites in circulating blood. Later research, however, did not demonstrate the existence of an exoerythocytic cycle, so with time he agreed on the nonexistence of the hepatic cycle.

The answer to the second question had to wait another 40 years when the Krotoskis, the same professor Garnham and others found in 1980, [42, 43] that from the sporozoites introduced by the mosquito some developed into exoerythrocytic schizonts in the liver, at once, while the others remained inside hepatocytes as round metabolically arrested cells, some times with the appearance of a bird's eye, that they called hypnozoites. At last, professor Garnham had not been very much mistaken, parasites instead of multiplying in the liver and producing a cycle liver-liver, they remain dormant inside the liver cells and awake to reassume its asexual development when, probably, a signal arrives.

If malaria infection is left to its own natural expression, i.e. with no treatment, without reinfections, and in absence of complications, as time pass the paroxysms become less severe and of shorter duration, until finally they disappear in approximately six months or less in *P. falciparum* infections, and in less time in *P. malariae*. Although, the symptoms disappear the parasites may be circulating in blood in very low number and for a variable period of time, as in the case of *P. malariae* infections in which parasites may be circulating in blood in asymptomatic individuals during 30 or 40 years and, after this lapse, clinical symptoms can be present again when conditions are given for a recrudescence to occur [44]. However, In *P. vivax* and *P. ovale* infections when left to evolve freely (with no treatment) after certain number of episodes (three to five or more) the paroxysms disappear, and the infection enters into a clinical and parasitological phase of latency in which the patient seem to be clinically cured and no circulating parasites in blood may be demonstrated. However, after some weeks or months the infection relapses, with reappearance of paroxysmal clinical symptoms and parasites in blood. In relation to relapses in *P. knowlesi* no information is available on what is the expression of this species in human infections.

The *Plasmodium* species involved in these latency-relapse events, are those species that posses a metabolically arrested or sleeping or dormant stage when infecting the liver, called hypnozoite. The relapsing species are *P. vivax* and *P. ovale*. It has been thought that in these species during transmission, the mosquito deliver, most times, two type of sporozoites, one that directly develop into asexual forms that reproduce as a liver schizont, which release hepatic merozoites to initiate the erythrocytic cycle in blood. In this type of sporozoites about 12 days have to pass between the time of the mosquito inoculation and the release of hepatic merozoites to blood. The second type of sporozoites inoculated by the mosquito bite, once it has invaded the hepatocytes become a round small cell with central nucleus, already mention above, the hypnozoite (sleeping parasite). However, No one knows what is the signal the hypnozoite is waiting to awake and proceeds its growth, development and differentiation. Awaking sporozoites mark the end of latent infection, and the beginning of a relapse that start with growth and reproduction of the parasite in the hepatocyte that was already inhabiting, with the release of merozoites and the reinfection of erythrocytes in blood and reinstallation of malaria paroxysms, until a new latent period is installed again.

The number of latent periods as well as the time duration of each one is unpredictable, however, as latent periods proceed, it can be expected that each new relapse would present malarial paroxysms of less clinical severity and with reduced paroxysmal events, until finally it disappear in the term of one to five years, in most cases.

There exist in nature the presence of *P. vivax* strains without the two expected types of sporozoites transmitted for the mosquito in which the total population of sporozoites developing in the mosquito, seems to be of the second type i.e. hypnozoites. These *P. vivax* strains were classically described in the past to occur in temperate countries such as in Holland (the Dutch strain), in north Russia and Siberia (hibernans strain) in north USA (the San Elisabeth strain) [45] and probably also present in North and Central China [46], and Korea [47]. These strains were called strains of longue incubation period because after they enter in their host's liver cells, they remain dormant for 253 to 381 days. It was observed that these parasites were transmitted by the mosquito during the summer, but the infected hosts did not manifest the blood infection, nor either clinical signs until the arrival of the spring, just when mosquito vectors awake of the winter hibernation and are ready to transmit malaria. In these cases malaria parasites remain dormant in hypnozoite stage since they arrive to the liver after mosquito bite, thus the subjects are infected but asymptomatic, because the parasite is metabolically in arrest.

When attending a patient infected with *P. vivax*, a treatment with drugs acting solely against blood forms, may produce an artificial latent period, which later ends with a relapse, because schizonticidal drugs does not kill hypnozoites. These experiences may lead to confusion if failure of the treatment is interpreted as resistance of the parasite against the drug.

Chronic Malaria

There are, however, some malaria patients whose clinical manifestations seem to persist despite they receive proper treatment and, there are reasonable arguments to be secure that reinfections are not occurring. In these cases, which some call "chronic malaria", the patients apparently cured present a diminished clinical picture from time to time, which is difficult to recognize as a malarial paroxysm and practically endures for all their life. The frequency at which these paroxysm-like are observed is different in each patient, and is non periodic, its variability in time is quite unpredictable, they may have one or more events per year or even one each several years. Some times the febrile accesses and associated symptoms are linked to stress, intense physical work, exposition to heath sources, changes of temperature or changes of altitude. All patients have had a story of malaria infection some time in the past, and relate their present symptoms with those they suffered during the past malaria infection (their malaria paroxysms) that in opinion of the patient never disappeared, they just changed the temporality of its emergence, duration and severity. Another constant is the absence of parasites in their blood, as demonstrated by microscopic studies, however, an antimalaric treatment usually relieve or ameliorate their symptoms.

The Non Specificity of the Malarial Response

The story started with the publication of Beutler and coworkers in 1985 when they reported cachexia in rabbits inoculated with *Trypanosoma* , which died with a minimal parasitemia and extreme hypertriglyceridemia because of the loss of lipoprotein lipase activity. The same deficiency was noted in mice upon the administration of LPS of *Escherichia coli*. It was also shown that macrophages responded to stimulus of bacterial endotoxins and protozoal products, liberating a monokine that suppress the activity of lipoprotein lipase. This monokine was purified and called cachectin for the cachexia it produced when administered to animals [48]. Years later, cachectin was rediscover by others and named it tumor necrosis factor or TNF, which is the today accepted name.

In 1989 Chokri observed that TNF, LPS or interferon caused regression and necrosis of solid tumors of mice. Labeled activated macrophages and LPS were traced and it was found that macrophages localized in the periphery of the tumor while LPS was mostly observed in the liver, although with some slow accumulation in the center of the tumor [49]. Later Dumont showed the antitumoral properties of TNF released by activated macrophages in a human model [50]. Oncologists were enthusiastic because these experiences opened the perspective of a successful treatment of cancer, thus many trials of recombinant human TNF were performed on terminal cancer patients [51, 52, 53, 54]. These assays gave us the opportunity to observe the variety of side effects produce just for the sole application of TNF in absence of any infectious disease, to my surprise the patients not just presented fever, but fatigue, chills, headache, anorexia, nausea, vomiting, diarrhea, leucopenia, triglyceridemia, thrombocytopenia, splenomegaly and involvement of lungs, kidney and central nervous system, depending of the doses received. Practically all clinical manifestations present in malaria are also present in subjects without malaria but being exposed to different doses of recombinant TNF, which reproduce, just in my own opinion, a malaria infection without malaria parasites, see fig 2. It is not difficult to understand now, why almost all responses of the host to the malaria parasites are unspecific, see fig 3.

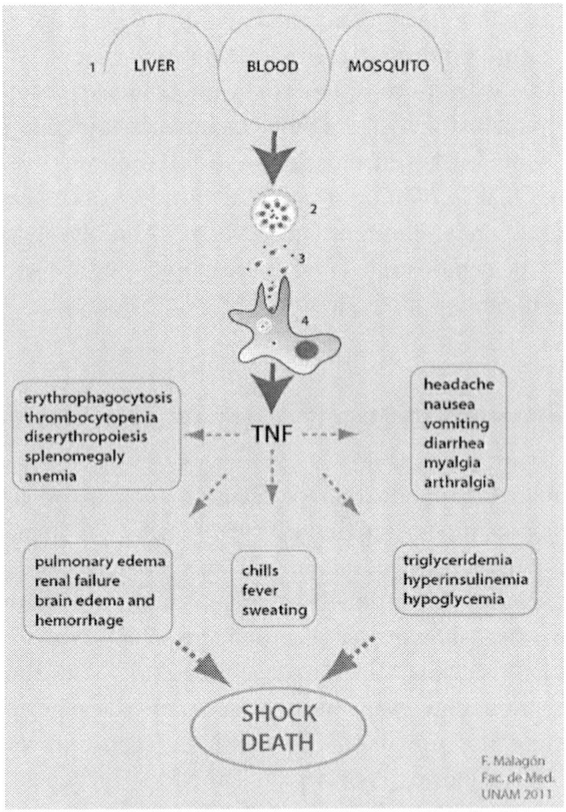

Figure 3. Symptoms and clinical signs in malaria. The response of the host to malaria parasites, by the activation of macrophages and release of inflammatory cytokines, produce a chain reaction that involve the whole human body functions, and whose severity may vary from host to host, from benign to fatal outcome if complicated. 1, is the malaria life cycle. 2, is a segmenter developing in an erythrocyte. 3, are merozoites, pigment and parasite-erythrocytes debris. 4, is a macrophage phagocyting merozoites, pigment and cellular debris, getting activated in the process to produce TNF which commence the cascade of events that produce physiological and pathological changes with the clinical manifestations enlisted. As described in main text, in absence of the malaria parasites a clinical frame with some or many of the clinical elements shown in this diagram can be reproduce with the sole inoculation of TNF.

Reflections

It is familiar to all physicians that inflammation is the central process of almost all insult be mechanical, chemical, biological, psychological, or even social. When a microbe enter in contact with the living cells of the skin, our cells spread information of the microbe presence, leukocytes and macrophages attend the call and aggregate around the microbe site, interaction between microbes and cells deliver local compounds that produce changes on vessels to increase blood volume on the fight site, the skin become red (erythema), and hot, permeability of the local vessels change and plasma pass to intercellular spaces, skin infected site increase in size (edema), granulocytes release their lethal granules and everything around is destroy (necrosis), the same granulocytes, skin cells and microbes die producing their remains a dense white or yellowish material call pus, all debris are taken out by macrophages and or are exuded, and the lesion is repaired and a mark or scar is left. This picture with multiple variants can be expect to be reproduced wherever an inflammation take place.

In malaria as in other diseases in which the offending microbe is not localized but circulate in blood, the parasite become ubiquitous because they follow the blood through all the vessels network and due that there are almost no places in the organism where blood do not run, the parasite and their products are everywhere and enter in contact with the endothelial layer of all vessels in the organism producing systemic inflammation on vessels of all the body, whose clinical expression may produce signals in any organ, system or tissue. This explain why malaria diagnoses is so difficult, because each patient may express the infection in different organs and any single organ may be involved.

Although malarial paroxysm usually comes together with headache, nausea, vomiting, diarrhea, myalgias, arthralgias and fatigue, the fever syndrome, i.e. all signs and symptoms associated to fever, are the central components of malaria paroxysm in acute malaria, as clinically has been seen. Now it is clear that malaria is a network of cellular responses result of interactions among all cells, tissues, and organs that compose our organism. It is also clear that paroxysm is a response of the brain thermoregulatory centers as result of the organic chain responses induced by malaria parasites and executed by the host.

According to Kluger, fever is a phenomenon of adaptive response so generalized in nature, that it seems to be already present in Protista of the genus *Paramecium* [55]. The fever conform a part of the struggle against infections and other organic aggressions. This function of protection seems to be accomplished when fever is moderate, because it stimulates the organic defensive responses. However, an uncontrolled inflammatory response may induce to high fever and other potentially dangerous effects on the vascular system of different organs that may lead patients to death. In severe *P. falciparum* malaria, the damages produced by the response to the parasite, are explained through an over expression of responses normally useful, mediated by inflammatory cytokines mainly TNF, IL1, IL6 e IL12 [56, 57, 58].

Discussion above exposed makes evident that in a strict sense the disease we know as malaria, is not directly produced by the parasites of the genus *Plasmodium*, the role that this parasites perform in disease genesis is that of an inducer, i.e. the parasites convey with them molecules that induce responses on the hosts cells, and these responses are those that generate the most varied clinical manifestations present in malaria, regardless they are benign or malign. One may correctly appreciate that malaria parasites are only inducers of a disease that we attributed to them, but the disease itself is the product of the cellular response of the infected individual. In other terms, in malaria we themselves generate our disease, our malaria, and eventually our death.

The emerging image coming out from this analysis would seem to confine those host-parasite responses just to *Plasmodium* like an exclusive event of the malaria parasites. However, the disease seems to be the current coin to pay the process of adaptation, i.e., to pay the right to continue alive when external agents invade us and also when internal misbalances ends with our functional harmony. In my opinion, the building of diseases and death with our own cellular components would be the most complete and final expression of life, and therefore the most generalized.

Conclusion

It is an assay that reconstructs the chain of physiological processes and its clinical expressions that make up the malarial paroxysm.

The analysis of the paroxysmal components allowed finding that the physiological and pathological changes occurring during the process, are not a direct effect of the parasite on the host but a response of the host to the parasite. In this process the parasite play the role of an inducer agent that turn on a chain of responses of the host that make up the disease, i.e. the parasite is inductor of a disease created by the host himself.

The chain of host responses induced by malaria parasites point towards a very general and unspecific process in which the role of inductor may be occupied for other transmissible and infectious agents.

References

[1] Singh B, Sung LK, Matusop Asmad, Radhakrishnan A, Shamsul SSG, Cox-Singh J, Thomas A, Conway DJ. A large focus of naturally acquired *Plasmodium knowlesi* infections in human beings. *Lancet* 2004;363:1017-1024

[2] White NJ. *Plasmodium knowlesi*: the fifth human malaria parasite. *Clin Infect Dis* 2008;46:172-173

[3] Bronner U, Divis PCS, Färnert A and Singh B. Swedish traveller with *Plasmodium knowlesi* malaria after visiting Malaysian Borneo. *Malaria J* 2009; 8:15

[4] Ta Tang TH, Salas A, Tammam MA, Martines MC, Lanza M, Arroyo E, Rubio JM. First case of detection of *Plasmodium knowlesi* in Spain by real time PCR in a traveller from South East Asia. Malaria J 2010;9:219

[5] Saper CB. Neurobiological basis of fever. *Ann NY Ac Sc* 1998;856:90-94.

[6] Garnham PCC. Malaria parasites and other haemosporidia. Oxford, UK: Blackwell Scientific Publications;1966

[7] Cox FEG. History of human Parasitology. *Clin Microbiol Rev* 2002;15:595-612.

[8] Cunhaa ChB & Cunhab BA. Brief history of the clinical diagnosis of malaria: from Hippocrates to Osler. *J Vector Borne Dis* 2008;45:194–199

[9] Golgi C. On the cycle of development of malarial parasites in tertian fever: differential diagnosis between the intracellular malarial parasites in tertian and quartan fever [in Italian]. Extracts reprinted in: Kean, B. H., Mott, K. E. and Russell, A. J. (Eds.) Tropical Medicine and parasitology: classic investigations. Vol. 1 Cornell University Press, Ithaca 1978. *Arch. Sci. Med.* (Torino*)* 1889;13:173–196

[10] Garnham PCC. Reflections on Laveran, Marchiafava, Golgi, koch and Danilewsky after sixty years. *Trans Roy Soc Trop Med Hyg* 1967;61:753-764

[11] Cox FEG. History of the discovery of the malaria parasites and their vectors. *Parasites & Vectors* 2010;3:5

[12] Bruce-Chwatt LJ. Essential Malariology. William Heinemann Medical Books, London, 1980

[13] Anonymous. Biological rhythms in malaria. *Lancet* 1969;1:403-404

[14] Brown WH. Malarial pigment (hematina) as a factor in the production of the malarial paroxysm. *J Exp Med*, 1912;15:579-597

[15] Maegraith BG. Is there a malaria toxin? *J Gen Microbiol* 1969;59:11-12

[16] Clark IA, Chaudhri G. Malaria pathology. in: Stevenson MM, editor. Malaria: host responses to infection. Boca ratón FL. CRC Press; 1989

[17] Galanos C, Luderitz O, Rietschel ET, Westphal O, Brade H, Brade L, et al. Synthetic and natural *Escherichia coli* free lipid A express identical endotoxic activities. *Eur J Biochem* 1985;148:1-5

[18] Taverne J, Bate CAW, and Playfair JHL. Malaria exoantigens induce TNF, are toxic and are blocked by T-independent antibody. *Immunol Lett* 1990;25:207-212

[19] Kipps TJ. The cluster of diferentiation (CD) antigens. In: Ernest Beutler, editor. Williams Hematology. Fifth edition. NY, USA: McGrawHill; 1995

[20] Palek J. The red cell membrane. In: Ernest Beutler, editor. Williams Hematology. Fifth edition. NY, USA: McGrawHill; 1995

[21] Arrighia RBG, Fayeb I. *Plasmodium falciparum* GPI toxin: A common foe for man and mosquito. *Acta Tropica* 2010;114:162–165

[22] Gowda DC. Structure and activity of glycosylphosphatidylinositol anchors of *Plasmodium falciparum. Microbes and Infection* 2002; 4:983–990

[23] Ramachandra S. Naik RS, Branch OH, Woods AS, Vijaykumar M, Perkins DJ, Nahlen BL, Altaf A. Lal AA, Cotter RJ, Costello CE, Ockenhouse CF, Davidson EA, and Gowda DC. Glycosylphosphatidylinositol Anchors of *Plasmodium falciparum*: Molecular Characterization and Naturally Elicited Antibody Response That May Provide Immunity to Malaria Pathogenesis. *J Exp Med* 2000; 192:1563-1575

[24] Gerold P, Dieckmann-Schuppert A, and Schwarz RT. Glycosylphosphatidylinositols synthesized by asexual erythrocytic stages of the malarial parasite, *Plasmodium falciparum*. *J Biol Chem* 1994;269:2597-2606

[25] Gordon S. The macrophage: Past, present and future. Eur. *J. Immunol.* 2007;37: S9–17.

[26] Dantzer R, Bluthe R-M, Gheusi G, Cremona S, Laye S, Parnet P, et al. Molecular basis of sickness behavior. *Ann NY Ac Sc* 1998; 856:132-138

[27] Beschin A, Bilej M, Brys L, Torreele E, Lucas R, Magez S, De Baetselier P. Convergent evolution of cytokines. *Nature* 1999;400:627-628

[28] Collette Y, Gilles A, Pontarotti P and Olive D. A co-evolution perspective of the TNFSF and TNFRSF families in the immune system. *Trends Immunol* 2003;24:387-394

[29] Körner H, McMorran B, Schlüter D, Fromm P. The role of TNF in parasitic diseases: Still more questions than answers. *Inter J Parasitol* 2010;40: 879–888

[30] Randall LM, Engwerda CR. TNF family members and malaria: Old observations, new insights and future directions. *Exp Parasitol* 2010;126:326–331

[31] Grau GE, Terrie A, Taylor TE, Molyneux ME, Wirima JJ, Vassalli P, et al. Tumor necrosis factor and disease severity in children with falciparum malaria. *N Engl J Med* 1989;320:1586-1591

[32] Kwiatkowski D, Hill AVS, Sambou I, Twumasi P, Castracane J, Manogue K R, et al. TNF concentration in fatal cerebral, non-fatal cerebral, and uncomplicated Plasmodium falciparum malaria. *Lancet* 1990;33:1201-1204

[33] Deloron P, Lombard PR, Ringwald P, Wallon M, Niyongabo T, Aubry P, et al. Plasma levels of TNFα soluble receptors corelate with outcome in human falciparum malaria. *Eur Cytokine Netw* 1994;5: 331-336

[34] Roth J, Christoph Rummel Ch, Barth SW, Gerstberger R, Hubschle T. Molecular Aspects of Fever and Hyperthermia. *Neurol Clin* 2006;24:421–439

[35] Matsumura K, Cao Ch, Wuatanabe Y. Possible role of cyclooxygenase-2 in the brain vasculature in febrile response. *Ann NY Ac Sc* 1997;813:302-306

[36] Nakamura K, Matsumura K, Kaneko T, Kobayashi S, Katoh H, and Negishi M. The rostral raphe pallidus nucleus mediates pyrogenic transmission from the preoptic area. *J Neurosci* 2002; *22*:4600–4610

[37] Narumiya S and Furuyashiki T. Fever, inflammation, pain and beyond: prostanoid receptor research during these 25 years. *FASEB J* 2011;25:813-818

[38] Laveran A. Note sur un noveau parasite trouvé dans le sang de plusieurs malades atteints de fièvre palustre. *Bull Acad Méd Paris* 1880;9:1235-1236

[39] Grassi, B., Bignami A, and Bastienelli G. *Ulteriori richerche sul ciclo dei parassiti malarici umani nel corpo del zanzarone.* (Nota preliminare.) Atti *R Accad Lincei* 1989;5(Ser. 8):21-28.

[40] Ross R. The role of the mosquito in the evolution of the malaria parasite. *Lancet* 1898; ii:489

[41] Garnham PCC. Exoerythrocyticc schizogony in malaria. *Trop Dis Bull* 1948;45:831-844

[42] Krotoski WA, Krotoski DM, Garnham PCC, Bray RS, Killick-Kendrick R, Draper CC, Targett GAT, Guy MW. Relapses in primate malaria: discovery of two populations of exoerythrocytic stages. Preliminary note. *Brit Med J* 1980;1:153–154

[43] Cogswell FB. The hypnozoite and relapse in primate malaria. *Clin Microbiol Rev,* 1992;5:26-35

[44] Collins WE, Jeffery GM. Plasmodium malariae: parasite and disease. *Clin Microbiol Rev* 2007;20:579–592

[45] Garnham PCC, Bray RS, Bruce-Chwat LJ, Draper CC, Killick-Kendrick R, Sergiev PG, Tiburskaja NA, Shute PG, & Maryon M. A strain of *Plasmodium vivax* characterized by prolonged incubation: morphological and biological characteristics. *Bull. WHO* 1975;52:21-32

[46] Yang B. Experimental and field studies on some biological characteristics of *Plasmodium vivax* isolated from tropical and temperate zones of China. *Chin Med J* 1996;109:266-71

[47] Moona KT, Kimb YK, Koc DH, Inho Parkd I, Shine DC, Kim C. Recurrence rate of vivax malaria in the Republic of Korea. *Trans Roy Soc Trop Med Hyg* 2009;103:1245—1249

[48] Beutler B, Mahoney J, Le Trang N,Pekala P, and Cerami A. Purification of cachectin, a lipoprotein lipase suppressing hormone secreted by endotoxin induced RAW 264.7 cells. *J. Exp. Med.* 1985;161:984-995

[49] Chokri M, Freudenberg M, Galanos C, Poindron P, Bartholeyns J. Antitumoral effects of lipopolysaccharides, tumor necrosis factor, interferon and activated macrophages: synergism and tissue distribution. *Anticancer Res* 1989; 9:1185-1190

[50] Dumont S, Mabondzo A, Hartmann D, Gilgenkrantz JL, Kessler R, Poindron P, Bartholeyns J. Study of the dependence of human monocytes and macrophages

antitumoral properties upon TNF-alpha expression or release. *Anticancer Res* 1990;10:949-954

[51] Jakubowski AA, Casper ES, Gabrilove JL, Templeton M-A, Sherwing SA, and Oettgen HF. Phase I trial of intramuscularly administered tumor necrosis factor in patients with advanced cancer. *J clin Oncol* 1989;7:298-303

[52] Creagan ET, Kovach JS, Moertel CG, Frytak S, Kvols LK. A phase I clinical trial of recombinant human tumor necrosis factor. *Cancer* 1988;62:2467-2471

[53] Spriggs DR, Sherman ML, Michie H, Arthur CA, Imamura K, Wilmore D, Frei III E and Kufe DW. Recombinant human tumor necrosis factor administered as a 24-hour intravenous infusion. A phase I and pharmacologic study. *J Natl Cancer Inst* 1988;80:1039-1044

[54] Sherman ML, Spriggs DR, Arthur KA, Imamura K, Frei E and Kufe DW. Recombinant human tumor necrosis factor administered as a five-day continuous infusión in cancer patients: phase I toxicity and effects on lipid metabolismo. *J Clin Oncol* 1988;6:344-350

[55] Kluger MJ, Kozak W, Conn CA, Leon LR, Soszynski. Role of fever in disease. *Ann NY Ac Sc* 1998; 856:224-233

[56] Clark IA, Cowden WB. The pathophysiology of falciparum malaria. *Pharmacol Ther* 2003;99:221-260

[57] Gimenez F, Barraud de Langerie S, Fernandez C, Pino P, Mazier D. Tumor necrosis factor alpha in the pathogenesis of cerebral malaria. *Cell Mol Life Sci* 2003;60:1623-1635

[58] Manish R, Tripathy R, Das BK. Plasma glucose and tumor necrosis factor-alpha in adult patients with severe falciparum malaria. *Trop Med Int Health* 2003;8: 125-128.

In: Malaria: Etiology, Pathogenesis and Treatments
Editors: A. M. Peterson et al, pp. 339-361

ISBN: 978-1-62100-363-2

Chapter XIV

Haemoglobinopathies: Natural Selection at Work Against *Plasmodium Falciparum* Malaria

Benno Kreuels[a*] and Federica Verra[b*]

[a] Section for Tropical Medicine, 1st Medical Department, University Medical Centre Hamburg-Eppendorf, Hamburg, Germany.

[b] Department of Immunology and Infection, Faculty of Infectious and Tropical Diseases, London School of Hygiene and Tropical Medicine, London, UK.

Abstract

Malaria continues to exert a strong selective pressure on humans resulting in genetic adaptations, such as haemoglobin structural variants (HbS, HbC, and HbE) and haemoglobin production disorders (α and β thalassaemias), which have reached high frequencies in populations exposed to malaria. Epidemiological studies have confirmed and expanded the hypothesis, originally formulated by Haldane on the basis of the geographical distribution of thalassaemia, that these adaptive traits have been maintained at such high frequency despite their fitness cost due to a selective advantage offered by protection against *Plasmodium falciparum* malaria. Moreover, there is evidence that this protection may vary according to the *P. falciparum* transmission intensity, which modulates the level of selective pressure, thus of the advantage conferred, and ultimately the frequency and dynamics of these adaptive traits in human populations. However, the mechanisms by which protection against malaria infection and disease is achieved in carriers of these traits remain elusive. In addition, clinical epidemiological studies have indicated that homozygote carriers of HbS may paradoxically be at a higher risk of severe malaria when infected with *P. falciparum*, thus emphasizing the importance of prompt and adequate treatment.

We aim to evaluate the current state of the art in relation to malaria pathogenesis with a particular focus on new insights into the biological mechanisms underlying the

* Corresponding authors: b.kreuels@uke.de; federica.verra@lshtm.ac.uk

protection exerted by such genetic adaptations. Understanding these mechanisms in individuals carrying adaptive traits may unravel important clues as to what is necessary to induce protection against malaria, and may thus be of relevance for future vaccine design.

Keywords: *Plasmodium falciparum* malaria, haemoglobinopathies, genetic polymorphism, immuno-epidemiology, pathogenesis, protection.

Introduction

Malaria, a disease caused by protozoan parasites of the genus *Plasmodium* and transmitted by Anopheline mosquitoes, remains a huge burden for human populations living in tropical areas, where approximately 1 million deaths are recorded each year, with the heaviest toll paid by children in sub-Saharan Africa (Guerra, Gikandi et al. 2008). Four distinct species are traditionally recognized as human malaria parasites: *Plasmodium falciparum*, *P. malariae*, *P. ovale* and *P. vivax*, amongst which *P. falciparum* is the most lethal accounting for the majority of deaths. Furthermore, a recent large focus of naturally acquired infections in humans with *P. knowlesi*, a simian malaria parasite infecting long-tailed macaques monkeys, has been described in Malaysian Borneo and elsewhere in South-east Asia (Singh, Kim Sung et al. 2004; Lee, Divis et al. 2011). Moreover, recent reports of *P. falciparum* from different species of primates in the African continent (Liu, Li et al. 2010; Prugnolle, Durand et al. 2010) suggest that the host specificity may not be as strict as previously assumed and raise the possibility of a more diverse zoonotic reservoir available to *P. falciparum*. Despite enormous efforts the development of an effective vaccine is yet to be accomplished. Compared to that of other infectious diseases the pathogenesis of malaria represents an extreme challenge to vaccine development due to the complex host-parasite interactions. The coevolution between malaria parasites and humans has resulted in an arms race, whereby each organism has evolved elaborate strategies, with signatures of selection exerted by the human host on the *Plasmodium* genome, and by malaria selective pressure on humans. Environmental factors, transmission intensity, increasing parasite drug resistance, mosquito population dynamics, and varied genetic backgrounds of the host confer additional complexity to the disease (Mackinnon and Marsh 2010): unravelling such host and parasite factors, and the interactions between them, will be crucial for understanding the basis of innate and acquired protective immunity, and to develop new tools in malaria control.

The genetic basis of some important haemoglobin disorders was discovered in the middle of the last century, when the biological paradox of the high frequency of these deleterious mutations in some populations was first observed. Thalassaemia, causing microcytic anaemia in many areas of the Mediterranean, was one example: the British evolutionary biologist JBS Haldane proposed in 1949 that the mutant allele reached and maintained its high frequency not by means of an exceptionally high mutation rate, but rather as a consequence of the selective advantage against *P. falciparum* malaria, whose distribution largely overlaps with that of thalassaemia. Haldane's hypothesis stated that the disadvantage of the mutant homozygous state would have been counterbalanced by an advantage of the heterozygous state (Haldane 1949). A few years later in the case of a structural variant of the haemoglobin, HbS, it was observed that despite the heavy genetic load of sickle cell disease, a severe haemolytic and vaso-occlusive syndrome suffered by HbSS homozygotes, HbAS heterozygotes are healthy and are protected from severe forms of malaria, resulting in a balanced polymorphism whereby the advantage of protection experienced by HbAS heterozygotes balances the disadvantage associated with HbSS homozygosity (Allison 1954). The aim of this article is to give an updated overview of common haemoglobinopathies and haemoglobin production disorders, which have been shown to confer protection against *P. falciparum* malaria, with a particular focus on recent insights into the biological mechanisms underlying such protection.

Malaria Parasite Life Cycle and Clinical Manifestations

The life cycle of the malaria parasite in the human host can be divided into a pre-erythocytic and an erythrocytic phase. The pre-erythrocytic phase includes the injection into the bloodstream of the invasive stage known as sporozoite, during the Anopheline mosquito blood meal, and their asexual multiplication in the host target cells, the hepatocytes. This phase is asymptomatic and corresponds to the pre-clinical incubation period of 7-21 days. Merozoite stage parasites then infect the erythrocytes where asexual multiplication continues. The rupturing of the erythrocytes with the release of parasite derived toxins into the bloodstream is the main cause of fever and one of the causes of malarial anaemia. Gametocytes, the initial sexual stage of *Plasmodium*, become infectious for mosquitoes after a maturation process. Mosquitoes ingest mature gametocytes whilst feeding, thereby allowing completion of the parasite life cycle; within the mosquito female and male gametocytes differentiate into female and male gametes, undergo fertilization and meiosis ultimately developing into sporozoites.

Infected erythrocytes containing parasites in later stages of development become less deformable and are therefore filtered in the spleen (Buffet, Safeukui et al. 2011). However, in the case of *P. falciparum*, the parasite modifies the surface of the erythrocyte, inducing its adherence to the endothelium of microvasculature and thereby avoiding passage through the spleen. Different parasites can bind to varied host receptors on endothelial and blood cells with different affinity and specificity, and this variability is believed to affect the tissue distribution of parasites and the pathogenesis of malaria (Newbold, Craig et al. 1997; Newbold 1999). The *P. falciparum* Erythrocyte Membrane Protein 1 (PfEMP1) is the crucial molecule on the surface of the infected erythrocyte binding to various receptors (Baruch, Pasloske et al. 1995). The outcome of infection with *P. falciparum* depends on the interplay of host and parasite factors. Clinical disease is modulated by age, immunity and transmission intensity, and ranges from uncomplicated malaria (UM) whose main symptoms are a variable combination of fever, chills and sweats, headache, vomiting, watery diarrhoea, anaemia, jaundice, and splenomegaly to complicated disease. In children convulsions, coughing and rapid shallow breathing are also relatively common symptoms. The most common complications of malaria infection, defined as severe malaria, are severe malarial anaemia (SMA), cerebral malaria (CM) and respiratory distress (Marsh, Forster et al. 1995). SMA is defined by low haemoglobin levels (less than 5g/dl) and/or haematocrit less than 15% packed cell volume. CM entails neurological involvement, with manifestations that can vary from prostration to impaired consciousness and deep coma. Finally respiratory distress is the most apparent clinical manifestation of metabolic acidosis. Despite therapy, mortality rates for severe malaria in children can range from 1% in patients with only severe anaemia (7% in CM, and 24% in respiratory distress [metabolic acidosis]) to 35% in patients with all three complications (Maitland and Marsh 2004). This heavy toll of disease exerted on humans by malaria parasites has been the driving force for the selection of haemoglobinopathies and other genetic adaptive traits which confer protection against severe malaria. The level of protection offered by each adaptive trait against different manifestations of mild and severe malaria has been shown to differ. A number of possible mechanisms by which protection is conferred have been proposed; some suggesting a direct effect on the parasite life cycle, others suggesting an influence of the genetic traits on the immune response and on the development of host immunity.

Malaria Immunity

Immunity to *P. falciparum* malaria infection and disease is acquired after repeated episodes. In the first few infections the inflammation triggered by innate effector mechanisms may be severe and lead to death, as observed in malaria endemic areas in younger children. The kinetics of malaria infection indicate that innate responses are essential in the initial phase of parasite replication in order to control the first wave of parasitaemia; thus, the host can elicit specific adaptive immune responses to clear the infection (reviewed by Stevenson and Riley 2004). With age, and further exposure to malaria, individuals acquire the ability to control the extent and outcome of infection more effectively, and older children and adults develop nearly complete protection against severe illness and death. However, sterile immunity is never achieved, and adults continue to be susceptible to low density parasite infection (reviewed by Langhorne, Ndungu et al. 2008).

As the development of immunity depends on exposure, acquired immunity is gained at a faster pace where transmission intensity is higher: in these areas the brunt of malaria deaths occur in infants whereas in areas of moderate transmission the risk of death affects mainly children up to the age of five years, and in areas of low transmission the ability to limit severe disease and death is not established until the early teens or later (Snow, Omumbo et al. 1997).

This gradient of acquisition of immunity to severe malaria, mild disease and uncomplicated parasite infection suggests that distinct mechanisms and different arms of humoral and cellular immunity are involved in the development of protective immunity.

Following primary infection, the first interaction between malaria parasites and the effector molecules of acquired immunity occurs during the pre-erythrocytic stage following the inoculation of sporozoites into the blood stream, when antibodies can act via opsonisation to clear invasive forms of the parasite before they reach the liver (Schofield, Villaquiran et al. 1987; Nussenzweig and Nussenzweig 1989), and by blocking the invasion of hepatocytes (Pasquetto, Fidock et al. 1997). The major malaria vaccine candidate that is currently being tested in the field is based on the circumsporozoite protein (CSP), the most abundant protein on the sporozoite surface, which is involved in binding to hepatocytes. However, the evidence that antibodies against sporozoites correlate with protection against infection or disease remains controversial (reviewed by Marsh and Kinyanjui 2006).

It has recently been demonstrated that $CD8^+$ T-cell priming in a pre-erythrocytic vaccine animal model occurs primarily in lymph nodes, and not in the liver or other secondary lymphoid tissues (Chakravarty, Cockburn et al. 2007). Sporozoites were observed not only in the liver but, importantly, also retained in the dermis for long periods and in the draining lymph nodes where they were presumably processed and presented by antigen presenting cells such as dendritic cells to naïve $CD8^+$ T cells; these specific CD8+ T cells then migrated to the liver, where they eliminated parasitised hepatocytes. Activated $CD8^+$ T cells produce IFN-γ while monocytes and dendritic cells produce IL-12. IL-12 also induces IFN-γ production in Natural Killer cells in a positive feedback loop (Riley, Wahl et al. 2006). IFN-γ activates NO synthase, and induces the L-arginine dependent NO pathway, responsible for the elimination of infected hepatocytes or intrahepatocyte schizonts via cytotoxicity, or cellular mediated inhibition of parasite growth (reviewed by Good and Doolan 1999). Nevertheless, the remarkably short time to re-infection in adults with detectable blood stage parasites suggests that immunity against the pre-erythrocytic stage is not particularly effective (reviewed by Marsh and Kinyanjui 2006).

Invasion of erythrocytes is the crucial step in malaria pathogenesis and therefore the most likely target of protective immune responses. The first evidence of the importance of antibodies was gathered by the passive transfer of protection to naive recipients via sera from immune subjects (Cohen, Mc et al. 1961). Different mechanisms can contribute to protection against blood stage infection mediated by antibodies: opsonisation of merozoites for uptake through Fc receptors and/or complement receptors on phagocytes, blocking invasion of erythrocytes, complement-mediated lysis of infected erythrocytes, opsonisation of infected erythrocytes for phagocytosis and/or inhibition of adherence of infected erythrocytes to the endothelium, and neutralisation of malaria toxins. Furthermore, cytophilic antibodies (IgG1 and IgG3 subclasses in humans) can act together with monocytes in Antibody Dependent Cellular Inhibition (ADCI) and killing of infected erythrocytes (Bouharoun-Tayoun, Attanath et al. 1990). The relative contributions of each of these mechanisms remain debated (reviewed by Langhorne, Ndungu et al. 2008). The identification of immunological correlates of protection in different epidemiological settings has not always given a consistent result; however, there is a general consensus on the idea that antibodies directed against many antigens on the merozoite and on the surface of infected erythrocytes, or those released during merozoite invasion, can confer protection. Recent evidence supports the notion that not only the levels but also the diversity of the antibody response as well as the fine specificity of antibodies are key elements in the development of protective immunity (Gray, Corran et al. 2007; Osier, Fegan et al. 2008).

Variant surface Antigens (VSA), including PfEMP1, are considered one of the main targets of protective IgG in malaria (Bull, Lowe et al. 1998; Nielsen, Staalsoe et al. 2002). Parasites responsible for clinical disease have been observed to express VSA to which the patient has no pre-existing antibodies, thus it is assumed that an individual needs to acquire antibodies of diverse specificity in order to control the many diverse parasite variants occurring within each infection (Marsh and Howard 1986; Bull, Lowe et al. 1998; Giha, Staalsoe et al. 1999). The intrinsic nature of the *var* multigene family (encoding for PfEMP1) - which entails the capacity of each parasite clone to switch from one variant to another during the same infection (antigenic variation) - together with the high degree of variation in the expression of *var* genes is consistent with the slow acquisition of immunity (Su, Heatwole et al. 1995; Scherf, Hernandez-Rivas et al. 1998). Differences in VSA expressed during severe malaria (VSA_{SM}) and uncomplicated malaria (VSA_{UM}) have been observed (Bull, Kortok et al. 2000). This may relate to particular characteristics of certain VSA, which bind more efficiently to specific endothelial receptors than others, and appear to be more conserved due to functional constraints (VSA group A). These more frequently recognised VSA_{SM} are associated with severe malaria in individuals with little pre-existing immunity, whereas (VSA_{UM}) that bind less efficiently and are more rarely recognised are associated with uncomplicated malaria and asymptomatic infection in semi-immune individuals. These findings fit well with the observation that protection against severe and life threatening disease precedes immunity to uncomplicated malaria and asymptomatic infection (Hviid 2005).

Haemoglobin Structural Variants and Their Impact on Malaria Susceptibility

Haemoglobin comprises four globin chains: fetal haemoglobin (HbF) has two α and two γ chains ($\alpha_2\gamma_2$), whereas adult haemoglobin (HbA) has two α and two β chains ($\alpha_2\beta_2$). Genes in the α-globin and β-globin gene clusters, respectively on chromosomes 16 and 11, control globin chain production.

Hundreds of haemoglobin gene variants occur at low prevalence worldwide (Chui, Hardison et al. 1998); however, only three haemoglobin structural variants are observed at polymorphic frequencies[25]: HbS (β6Glu→Val), HbC (β6Glu→Lys), and HbE (β26Glu→Lys).

HbS – Sickle Cell Trait and Sickle Cell Disease

HbS, described for the first time by Herrick in 1910 (Herrick 1910), who reported the peculiar sickle-shaped erythrocytes found in a patient of African origin, is widespread in all malaria endemic areas, and common in sub-Saharan Africa with carrier frequencies for HbS ranging from 15-20% up to 40% in some areas of east Africa (Livingstone 1967). Haplotype analysis suggests that the β^S mutation may have occurred at least twice, once in Africa and once in either the Middle East or India (Flint, Harding et al. 1993). Within Africa the presence of the same mutation on different haplotypes (Senegal, Benin, Cameroon, CAR) may be explained by multiple independent origins (Chebloune, Pagnier et al. 1988). The initial evidence of protection against malaria came from the observation that HbAS individuals were less likely to be parasitaemic (Allison 1954). Results of case-control studies have shown HbAS conferring >70% protection against different forms of severe malaria, and up to 60% protection against all forms of clinical malaria (Allison 1954; Hill, Allsopp et al. 1991; Aidoo, Terlouw et al. 2002). A longitudinal study in Mali demonstrated a significant delay in the first episode of malaria in HbAS children under 10 years (Crompton, Traore et al.

[25] frequency at which the simultaneous occurrence of two or more genetic variants in the same locality can not be explained only by recurrent mutation or immigration.

2008). A recent report demonstrated a significant reduction in stunting as a result of a reduced incidence of uncomplicated malaria episodes and moderate anaemia in HbAS children (Kreuels, Ehrhardt et al. 2009). To date, there is convincing epidemiological evidence that HbAS protects against all manifestations of complicated malaria, as well as uncomplicated malaria, moderate anaemia and high density parasitaemia, but not against infection itself.

In contrast to heterozygotes (HbAS), who are generally asymptomatic, homozygotes (HbSS) suffer from sickle cell disease. The clinical presentation of sickle cell disease is complex and is affected by several concurrent factors, including the α-globin status and levels of HbF. Sickle cell disease can have a better prognosis with an increased proportion of HbF, which is genetically determined and differs according to the β-globin haplotype (Labie, Pagnier et al. 1985; Nagel, Fabry et al. 1985; Oner, Dimovski et al. 1992). Additional genetic variation has been recently described by fine mapping of modulatory genes which influence HbF levels (Galanrneau 2010). This complexity is reflected by clinical variation in the prevalence of anaemia, pain, stroke, leg ulcers, pulmonary hypertension, osteonecrosis and hepatobiliary complications (Steinberg 2009). Moreover, hydroxyurea, the main treatment used to prevent sickle cell disease complications and reduce mortality, has variable efficacy, which may also be explained by genetic variation.

Several studies (Okuonghae, Nwankwo et al. 1992; Aluoch 1997; Komba, Makani et al. 2009) investigating the impact of sickle cell disease on the clinical presentation of malaria found a lower prevalence of malaria infection and a lower parasite density in HbSS individuals. However, a study in Tanzania found that, while parasitemia prevalence may be lower, these individuals are at higher risk of both severe anaemia and death when hospitalized due to malaria (Makani, Komba et al. 2010), thus emphasizing the importance of prompt and adequate treatment.

Haemoglobin C, a West African Haemoglobinopathy

Studies performed in West Africa (Agarwal, Guindo et al. 2000; Modiano, Luoni et al. 2001; Rihet, Flori et al. 2004; May, Evans et al. 2007) recently demonstrated the protective value of the HbC allele, which appears to be restricted to this area and have emerged only once in Africa (Livingstone 1967). A case control study conducted in Burkina Faso where HbC reaches its highest allele frequency (~0.13) conclusively demonstrated approximately 90% protection against clinical malaria in homozygotes and 30% in heterozygotes (Modiano, Luoni et al. 2001). This observation suggested a recessive selection model, as higher protection is conferred by the homozygote state consistent with the epi-unicentric geographic distribution of the HbC allele in West Africa, and with the observation that the HbC allele is much older than the sympatric HbS Benin mutation (Modiano, Bancone et al. 2008). Furthermore, this adaptive trait seems to provide a selective advantage not only to the host (due to protection against clinical malaria) but also to the parasite, as HbCC individuals seem to have a higher gametocyte density and are more infectious for mosquitoes (Gouagna, Bancone et al. 2010). Contrasting results on the protective value of the HbC allele were previously reported in a study from Mali (Guinet, Diallo et al. 1997), which showed no evidence of protection of HbAC heterozygotes against severe and uncomplicated malaria, possibly the result of a lack of statistical power. In 2004, studies from Ghana (Mockenhaupt, Ehrhardt et al. 2004) and Burkina Faso (Rihet, Flori et al. 2004) confirmed the protection conferred by the HbC allele against both mild and severe malaria. More recently a case-control study in Ghana showed that the protective role of HbC may be confined to cerebral malaria (May, Evans et al. 2007). This is further supported by data from a longitudinal cohort study showing no protection conferred by HbAC against mild clinical malaria or asymptomatic parasitemia (Kreuels, Kreuzberg et al. 2010). In contrast to the convincing information on the protection offered by HbAS, the data on HbAC seem less clear. While there is good evidence for a protective effect against severe (cerebral) malaria, conflicting results on uncomplicated malaria and parasitaemia may be due to differences in age of participants and transmission intensity between studies.

While individuals with HbAC, similar to those with HbAS, do not suffer from pathological manifestations due to the mutation itself, the homozygous HbCC state, differently from HbSS, is characterized by mild haematological symptoms (Roberts, Harris et al. 2004). An intermediate condition is present in the compound heterozygous HbCS state (reviewed by Nagel, Fabry et al. 2003). This raises questions regarding the dynamics between the alleles in areas where both are present. A second non-African haplotype carrying the β^C mutation has been described in Thailand (Sanchaisuriya, Fucharoen et al. 2001) suggesting the possibility of a multi-centric origin also for this haemoglobin variant outside Africa.

Proposed Mechanisms of Protection Conferred by HbS and HbC

Despite the robust epidemiological evidence that these mutations confer protection against malaria the mechanisms by which protection is exerted remain debated for both haemoglobin variants HbC and HbS. Several, not mutually exclusive, mechanisms have been proposed to explain the protection conferred by HbC and HbS.

An "immunological hypothesis" was initially proposed by Ringelhann et al., who demonstrated a higher survival rate in carriers of HbAS and HbAC, but a higher rate of low density parasitaemia, indicating a better immunological defense against the deleterious effects of *P. falciparum* infection with persistent parasitaemia stimulating antibody production (Ringelhann, Hathorn et al. 1976). This was supported by a study carried out in Nigeria where a normal humoral immunity in sickle cell disease was reported (Storey, Fleming et al. 1979). Conversely evidence of a reduced humoral, but increased cell mediated, immune response to *P. falciparum* antigens in HbAS individuals has been reported (Le Hesran 1999). Enhanced immune recognition of variant surface antigens (VSA) was initially observed in HbAS individuals by Marsh et al., (Marsh, Otoo et al. 1989) and further demonstrated in a study showing that the presence of the HbAS genotype was associated with enhanced recognition of two randomly selected clinical isolates amongst Gabonese children (Cabrera, Cot et al. 2005). A cohort study in Kenya showed that the protective effect of HbAS against clinical malaria increased from age 2 to age 10, lending further support to the hypothesis of an accelerated acquisition of immunity against mild clinical malaria in HbAS (Williams, Mwangi et al. 2005a). Recently, an abnormal display of *Pf*EMP1, causing a drastic reduction of this molecule on the surface of infected HbAC and HbCC erythrocytes (Fairhurst, Fujioka et al.

2003; Fairhurst, Baruch et al. 2005), therefore entailing reduced cytoadhesion and impaired rosetting *in vitro,* was reported. On this basis it has been proposed that HbC-dependent protection against severe malaria might be attributed to the reduced *Pf*EMP1-mediated adherence of parasitized erythrocytes in the microvasculature. The importance of this finding is supported by the results of a case-control study in Ghana (May, Evans et al. 2007), where the protective effect of HbAC against severe malaria was confined to cerebral malaria, which is mediated by adherence of infected erythrocytes to the capillaries in the brain. Furthermore, impaired cytoadherence of infected HbAS erythrocytes has been recently demonstrated, providing for the first time a convergence in the possible mechanism of protection conferred by both haemoglobin variants (Cholera, Brittain et al. 2008). A study carried out in Burkina Faso (Verra, Simpore et al. 2007) showed that HbC or HbS carriage was associated with higher levels of antibodies against VSA and various malaria antigens in a low transmission urban area, although no differences were detected in a high transmission rural area. In both contexts the response against tetanus toxoid was not influenced by the β-globin genotype, indicating that HbS and HbC may specifically influence the immune response to malaria, rather than overall immune function. The enhanced immune reactivity to malaria antigens in both HbC and HbS carriers supports the hypothesis that the protection against malaria of these adaptive genotypes might be at least partially mediated by acquired immunity against malaria (Verra, Simpore et al. 2007). Intriguingly, another study in Burkina Faso suggests an epistatic interaction between HbC and genes involved in the activation of NK cells (Atkinson, Barbier et al. 2011), further supporting modification of the immune response to malaria by HbC.

In contrast, other proposed hypotheses of protection rely on mechanistic features of the altered erythrocytes rather than an immune-mediated mechanism, including the inhibition of parasite development inside erythrocytes (Friedman, Roth et al. 1979), enhanced phagocytosis of ring infected erythrocytes (Ayi, Turrini et al. 2004), and prolonged retention of HbF (Pasvol, Weatherall et al. 1977). It has recently been suggested that the mechanism of protection conferred by HbS may be due to a higher filtration rate of infected erythrocytes in the spleen caused by an increased stiffness of these altered erythrocytes compared to normal erythrocytes (Buffet, Safeukui et al. 2011). Accelerated clearance of infected erythrocytes carrying the sickle cell trait has also been associated with premature expression of apoptotic markers (Lang, Kasinathan et al. 2009), which is consistent with previous observations of enhanced phagocytosis (Ayi, Turrini et al. 2004). These mechanisms support the idea that some innate condition related to the altered erythrocytes mediates the protection afforded by HbS. In addition, a mechanism which confers tolerance to malaria infection in HbS has recently been proposed based on the heme oxygenase-1 (HO-1, encoded by the *Hmox1* gene). HO-1 expression is induced in haematopoietic cells by free heme, which is released from haemoglobin more rapidly in HbS, and becomes cytotoxic. This enzyme counterbalances the deleterious effect of free heme by degrading it to biliverdin, iron and carbon monoxide; the carbon monoxide prevents further accumulation of free heme after *P. falciparum* infection in mice carrying the HbS mutation with a specific protective effect against cerebral malaria (Ferreira, Marguti et al. 2011). This study did not support the consistent observation of reduced parasite density in HbAS heterozygotes in humans, which raises questions as to the application of findings from experimental rodent malaria to human malaria (Rosenthal 2011).

A microsatellite polymorphism[26], in the promoter region of *Hmox1* has been investigated in CM patients in Myanmar showing a significant association between the homozygotes of the short allele and CM (Takeda, Kikuchi et al. 2005). A cohort study of children in Angola has revealed the occurrence of a haplotype, which determines increased *Hmox1* mRNA expression in peripheral blood cells, associated with increased risk of CM in this population (Sambo, Trovoada et al. 2010). Further investigations of *Hmox1* variants should address its possible involvement in the protection and/or susceptibility to malaria in humans conferred by haemoglobinopathies such as HbS, which causes chronic haemolysis, and would therefore benefit from an accessory genetic factor compensating for the increased free heme typically associated with this condition.

There is good *in vitro* and epidemiological data that both HbS and HbC influence the host immune response to malaria and some convincing evidence of innate mechanisms of protection. It remains unclear, however, whether the mechanisms of protection are the same for HbS and HbC. Some epidemiological data indicate that the protection offered by HbS may be due to an innate mechanism, while the immunological hypothesis may be more important in HbC. A study in Ghana found that carriers of HbAS were protected against uncomplicated malaria and had lower parasite densities at 3-24 months, an age where immunity has not yet developed, (Kreuels, Kreuzberg et al. 2010), while the same study showed no protective effect for HbAC. In addition, a study including children from the age of 6 months onwards (Mockenhaupt, Ehrhardt et al. 2004) showed a protective effect of HbAC only against severe malaria, while another study, including children aged 6 years and older (Rihet, Flori et al. 2004), showed a protective effect of HbAC against both severe and uncomplicated malaria. These results support an involvement of HbC in the acquisition of immunity, possibly by a quicker acquisition of antibodies against Variant surface Antigens (VSA), including PfEMP1.

HbE, a Non African Haemoglobinopathy

HbE is probably the most common haemoglobin variant in the world, and although its distribution is limited to South-east Asia, with highest frequency reaching 55% in Laos, Cambodia and Thailand (Flatz 1967), there is evidence for multiple origins of this mutation (Antonarakis, Orkin et al. 1982). Heterozygous carriers are asymptomatic whereas HbEE homozygotes have a mild anaemia due to the less efficient production of this haemoglobin variant (Olivieri, Muraca et al. 2008) resulting in a molecule more susceptible to oxidative stress. The concomitant occurrence of HbE with other erythrocyte disorders such as thalassaemias, particularly given the high frequency of these traits in South-east Asia, may result in a more severe condition. A large survey of haemoglobinopathies in Thailand did not observe any selective advantage conferred by HbE against *P. falciparum* infection (Kruatrachue, Bhaibulaya et al. 1969). However, epidemiological evidence of protection was established by a case control study in Thailand showing that HbE confers protection against severe malaria only (Hutagalung, Wilairatana et al. 1999; Chotivanich, Udomsangpetch et al. 2002). I*n vitro* experiments have provided evidence of impairment of parasite growth in

[26] A microsatellite polymorphism presents allelic variants which differ for the number of nucleotide repeats.

HbEE erythrocytes (Nagel, Raventos-Suarez et al. 1981) or of no inhibition of parasite development (Santiyanont and Wilairat 1981). However, studies using normal and HbE erythrocytes showed reduced invasion of HbAE compared to normal HbAA and HbEE erythrocytes at high parasitemia, suggesting an explanation for the epidemiological observation of protection restricted to severe malaria since the reduced invasion is limited to a subpopulation of all erythrocytes, thus, only relevant when the parasite density is high.

Haemoglobin Production Disorders: α- and β-Thalassaemia

Thalassaemias together with haemoglobin structural variants, with their high prevalence and distribution in malaria endemic areas, provide the most compelling evidence of genetic factors controlling the susceptibility of an infectious disease in humans (Haldane 1949; Flint, Hill et al. 1986; Weatherall 1987). Thalassaemias are the most common haemoglobin variants causing reduced synthesis or abrogation of globin chains.

Both α and β chains can be affected, determining two major varieties of disorders: α-and β-thalassaemia. The normal α globin genotype (αα/αα) can be altered in several ways, leading to different clinical syndromes. The deletion of both linked *HbA* genes is referred to as α^0-thalassaemia (––/αα heterozygote; ––/–– homozygote), whereas the deletion or inactivation by point mutations of only one of the pair of genes leads to α^+-thalassaemia (–α/αα heterozygote; –α/–α homozygote), the most common monogenic disease in the world population. The clinical presentation is determined by the number of functional genes, which determines the level of functional α globin chains. While α^+-thalassaemia heterozygotes (–α/αα) are usually asymptomatic, homozygotes (–α/–α) and α^0-thalassaemia heterozygotes (––/αα) have mild anaemia with microcytic, hypochromic erythrocytes. The combination of α^0 and α^+-thalassaemia entailing the loss of three out of four α globin loci (––/–α) results in a more severe phenotype known as haemoglobin H disease. The marked impairment of α globin chain production in this case leads to an accumulation of excess β globin chains. The free β chains are soluble enough to form the homotetrameric HbH ($\beta_2\beta_2$) giving the disease its name. HbH is not functional for oxygen transport and is relatively insoluble causing a chronic haemolytic anaemia associated with leg ulcers, pulmonary hypertension, osteonecrosis and hepatobiliary complications. Since α globin chains are needed for the production of fetal haemoglobin, individuals with HbH disease are symptomatic at birth, with neonatal jaundice and anaemia. In homozygotes α^0 thalassaemia (––/––; Hb Bart's hydrops fetalis syndrome), due to a complete loss of α globin chains, only homoetrameric Hb Bart's (γ_4) and HbH (β_4) are produced, usually leading to death in utero.

Similarly β-thalassaemia synthesis can be completely (β^0) or partially (β^+) abrogated leading to different clinical syndromes. However, interestingly, this is rarely due to deletions, but rather due to mutations affecting the promoter region of *HbB*, either causing a premature termination, or altering the correct splicing. Clinically, β-thalassaemia can be classified as β-thalassaemia minor (β/β^+,β/β^0), which is usually asymptomatic but can lead to mild anaemia; β-thalassaemia intermedia (mainly corresponding to β^+/β^0), causing a moderate anaemia with blood transfusions often necessary, and β-thalassaemia major (β^0/β^0), which leads to severe chronic anaemia and requires regular blood transfusion. In addition to the effects of severe anaemia, individuals with β-thalassaemia major suffer from chronic haemolysis due to the precipitation of excess α globin chains, a massive expansion of bone marrow progenitors and organ damage due to transfusional iron overload. In contrast to severe α-thalassaemia, newborns with β-thalassaemia are asymptomatic and the full clinical picture only develops as HbF production declines in the first months of life. The clinical presentation of β-thalassaemia is extremely varied and does not necessarily correspond to a certain genotype. For example, the excess of α globin chains may be reduced by concomitant α-thalassaemia and, as mentioned above, similar symptoms may also be caused by HbE with a reduced production of β globin chains. A number of additional genetic modifiers of β-thalassaemia have been identified (reviewed by Thein 2005).

α-and β-Thalassaemias and Their Impact on Malaria Susceptibility

As mentioned above, Haldane proposed his malaria hypothesis on balancing selection in 1949 after noting the overlapping geographical distribution of the thalassaemias and *P. falciparum* malaria. The distribution of α-and β-thalassaemias overlaps, and both forms occur throughout sub-Saharan Africa and the Mediterranean region, the Middle East, the Indian subcontinent and South-East Asia.

A case control study carried out in Papua New Guinea demonstrated that α^+-thalassaemia confers protection against severe malaria in both genotypes; furthermore, this study provided evidence for protection against infections other than malaria (Allen, O'Donnell et al. 1997). However, in line with other malaria protective genes, α^+-thalassaemia has no effect on the incidence of asymptomatic parasitemia (Roberts, Harris et al. 2004). Further epidemiological evidence showed protection against severe malaria only for heterozygotes, particularly in children younger than 5 years, in Ghana (Mockenhaupt, Ehrhardt et al. 2004). In two additional studies (Williams, Wambua et al. 2005b; May, Evans et al. 2007), carriers of α^+-thalassaemia, either homozygotes or heterozygotes, had a decreased risk of severe malaria in Kenya and in Ghana respectively; however, in the latter study protection was limited to severe malarial anaemia. This finding is supported by another study from Kenya where the strongest protection from α^+-thalassaemia was against malarial anaemia, and no effect on uncomplicated malaria, parasitemia incidence or parasite density was seen. A failure of α^+-thalassaemia to protect against coma was also found in the study of Allen et al. (Allen, O'Donnell et al. 1997). The allele frequency of α^+-thalassaemia has been observed to vary along an altitudinal cline in northern Tanzania ranging from 10%-25% in high altitude villages to 45%-55% in low altitude villages, consistent with malaria transmission intensity (Enevold, Alifrangis et al. 2007); this observation is indicative of selection for α^+-thalassaemia in this area, where the prevalence of this adaptive trait is positively associated with parasite prevalence and inversely correlated with altitude within an otherwise genetically homogenous population as shown by microsatellite allele frequencies (Enevold, Alifrangis et al. 2007). Another survey in the same area showed that α^+-thalassaemia limits the decline in haemoglobin concentration associated with asymptomatic malaria, but only when malaria infection is accompanied by inflammation (Veenemans, Andang'o et al. 2008), which extends the effect of this adaptive trait to mild as well as severe malaria. However, no clear relation between this adaptive trait and sub-microscopic parasite carriage was observed in two cross sectional surveys carried out in northern Tanzania (Shekalaghe, Alifrangis et al. 2009). The molecular basis of protection remains elusive: there is no evidence of reduced rate of invasion or growth of the parasite in erythrocytes affected by this trait; however, these altered erythrocytes have been observed to bind more malaria immunoglobulin than normal erythrocytes suggesting an immune-mediated mechanism of protection (Luzzi, Merry et al. 1991; Williams, Weatherall et al. 2002). Intriguingly, α^+-thalassaemia seems to provide an effective protection against other childhood infections (Allen, O'Donnell et al. 1997; Wambua, Mwangi et al. 2006), thus reinforcing the hypothesis of an immunological basis as the mechanism of protection.

Table 1. Epidemiological studies on the haemoglobinopathies and protection against *Plasmodium falciparum* malaria infection and disease

Gene/Symbol	Genotype	Study design (N)	Age	Area/Endemicity	*In vivo*	Reference
Haemoglobin S (*HbS*)	HbAS	Cohort (237)	<8	Uganda/hyperendemic	↓UM, ↓SMA	Allison, 1954
		Case-control (619/510)	<10	West Africa/mesoendemic	↓SM	Hill et al., 1991
		Cohort (1022)	<5	Kenya/hyperendemic	↓UM	Aidoo et al., 2002
		Cohort (1054)	<10	Kenya/mesoendemic	↓SM	Williams et al., 2005a
		Case-control (2591/2048)	<10	Ghana/hyperendemic	↓SM	May et al., 2007
		Cohort (1070)	<2	Ghana/holoendemic	↓UM	Kreuels et al., 2010
		Cohort (225)	2-25	Mali/mesoendemic	↓UM	Crompton et al., 2008
	HbSS	Case-control (2305/2696)	All	Tanzania/hyperendemic	↑ SMA	Makani et al., 2010
Haemoglobin C (*HbC*)	HbAC	Cohort (299)	<10	Mali/mesoendemic	-SM	Guinet et al., 1997
		Case-control (878/2767)	<15	Mali/mesoendemic	-UM, ↓SM	Agarwal et al., 2000
		Case-control (290/580)	<10	Ghana/hyperendemic	↓SM	Mockenhaupt et al., 2004
		Cohort (256)	All	Burkina Faso/ hyperendemic	↓UM	Rihet et al., 2004
		Case-control (2591/2048)	<10	Ghana/hyperendemic	↓CM	May et al., 2007
		Cohort (1070)	<2	Ghana/holoendemic	-UM	Kreuels et al., 2010
	HbCC	Case-control (835/3513)	<15	Burkina Faso/ hyperendemic	↓SM	Modiano et al., 2001

Table 1. (Continued).

Gene/Symbol	Genotype	Study design (N)	Age	Area/Endemicity	*In vivo*	Reference
Haemoglobin E (*HbE*)	HbAE	Cohort (542)	<3	Thailand/hyperendemic	-UM	Kruatrachue et al., 1969
	HbEE	Case-control (42/175)	All	Thailand/mesoendemic	↓SM	Hutagalung et al., 1999
α⁺-thalassaemia (α⁺-*thal*)	$-\alpha/\alpha\alpha$	Case-control (290/580)	<10	Ghana/hyperendemic	↓SM	Mockenhaupt et al., 2004
	$-\alpha/-\alpha$	Case-control (249/532)	<10	PNG/hyperendemic	↓SM	Allen et al., 1997
		Case-control (655/648)	<10	Kenya/mesoendemic	↓SM , ↓FM, -UM	Williams et al., 2005b
		Case-control (2591/2048)	<10	Ghana/hyperendemic	↓SMA	May et al., 2007
		Case-control (547/280)	<5	PNG/hyperendemic	↓SMA	Fowkes et al., 2008
β⁺-thalassaemia (*β⁺-thal*)	$-\beta/\beta\beta$ $-\beta/-\beta$	Cohort (542)	<3	Thailand/hyperendemic	-UM	Kruatrachue et al., 1969

N: individuals, ↓ decrease, ↑ increase, - no effect, UM: uncomplicated malaria, SM: severe malaria, SMA: severe malarial anaemia, CM: cerebral malaria, FM: fatal malaria.

However, a recent study in Papua New Guinea provides an alternative explanation of the protection conferred by α⁺-thalassaemia in homozygosity suggesting that an increased erythrocyte count and microcytosis counterbalances the risk of anaemia during acute malaria infection (Fowkes and Day 2008). The hypothesis raised by this study is that α⁺-thalassaemic children release less haemoglobin during haemolysis compared to non-thalassaemic ones, thus reducing oxidative tissue damage, and the release of pro-inflammatory cytokines.

Taken together, these results indicate that α⁺-thalassaemia protects by limiting disease manifestations rather than decreasing parasite multiplication. The new proposed mechanism of protection recently suggested for HbS based on the ameliorating effect of HO-1 on the cascade of events leading to malaria pathogenesis (Ferreira, Marguti et al. 2011) may also be relevant for other protective haemoglobinopathies that cause chronic haemolysis, thus including α⁺-thalassaemia.

β-thalassaemia also is consistent with Haldane's malaria hypothesis due to its distribution in areas currently or previously endemic for malaria. A clear cut correlation of thalassaemia carriers in Sardinia according to altitude was demonstrated in a study by Siniscalco et al., (Siniscalco, Bernini et al. 1966), whereby the population frequency of these traits was inversely matched to the altitude cline. This correlation was consistently observed in different geographical and epidemiological contexts supporting the hypothesis of protection against malaria. The attempt to elucidate the mechanism of protection was initially based on *in vitro* studies to test erythrocyte invasion and parasite growth rates (Pasvol and Wilson 1982). Some abnormalities in invasion and growth have been observed in erythrocytes with more severe forms of β-thalassaemia without reaching conclusive evidence; no consistent evidence has been gathered for milder forms of the disease. However, subtle changes in the infected thalassaemic erythrocytes were observed, including increased surface expression of parasite derived antigen and increased binding of IgG (Luzzi, Merry et al. 1991). Enhanced phagocytosis of β-thalassaemic infected human erythrocytes was demonstrated (Ayi, Turrini et al. 2004) *in vitro*. Further observations suggested an alteration of cytoadherence and rosetting of *P. falciparum* infected erythrocytes carrying β-thalassaemia (Cholera, Brittain et al. 2008). A summary of the epidemiological studies discussed is given in Table 1.

Epistatic Interactions between Haemoglobinopathies

Epistatic interactions are anticipated due to the co-occurrence at high frequency of the haemoglobinopathies we have discussed so far. Synergistic or antagonistic interactions amongst these adaptive traits may account for their heterogenous distribution in different populations, as the relative fitness of the compound heterozygotes may differ from that of the single heterozygotes. Allison (Allison 1964) was the first to address this issue as he observed that the frequency of HbAS heterozygotes reaches 40% in some areas of East Africa, whereas it is lower in West Africa, especially in those populations where HbC occurs at relatively high frequency. One explanation proposed was that the interaction between HbC and HbS altered the equilibrium of the balanced polymorphism between HbAS heterozygote advantage and HbSS homozygote disadvantage. In fact, individuals carrying both allelic variants (HbCS) have clinical manifestations similar to sickle cell disease (Nagel, Fabry et al. 2003). This observation may help explain the restricted distribution of HbC in West Africa: the protective effect of this adaptive trait is marginal in heterozygosis (either HbAC or HbCS) differently from the balanced polymorphism of HbS. Interestingly clinical manifestations have been observed also for the compound HbCE heterozygote (Fucharoen, Fucharoen et al. 2005). Since the levels of HbF vary according to the β-globin haplotype on which HbS occurs (Labie, Pagnier et al. 1985; Nagel, Fabry et al. 1985; Oner, Dimovski et al. 1992), differences in the frequency of HbS may also depend on the specific haplotype fitness with respect to the regulation of HbF, as a longer retention of HbF may ameliorate the clinical manifestations of sickle cell disease.

A study in Kenya showed a negative epistatic interaction between the two most common haemoglobinopathies conferring protection against malaria, HbS and α-thalassaemia, despite the highly protective effect they have individually: children who are HbAS and −α/−α homozygotes show an incidence of both uncomplicated and severe malaria close to the baseline group with normal haemoglobin (Williams, Wambua et al. 2005b). A similar negative epistatic interaction was observed for HbAS and −α/αα heterozygotes in Ghana (May et al., 2007). However, the pathophysiological mechanism by which this interaction may be mediated remains unclear.

The co-inheritance of α- and β-thalassaemia results in a milder condition compared to the individual disorders (Wainscoat, Kanavakis et al. 1983) due to a lower accumulation of excess β or α globin chains; furthermore, compound α- and β-thalassaemia heterozygotes retain the malaria protection conferred by each of these adaptive traits. Therefore, the potential increased fitness of the compound α- and β-thalassaemia heterozygotes suggests that, where they coexist, their gene frequencies could be higher than in isolation and contribute to the exclusion of HbS, as observed in former malaria endemic areas such as the Mediterannean (Penman, Pybus et al. 2009).

Conclusion

The conundrum of haemoglobinopathies is still unraveled due to the patchy distribution which overlaps with malaria endemicity, but with some notable exceptions such as the absence of HbE in Africa, and conflicting evidence as to the extent and mechanisms of protection. According to population genetics theory, allelic variants of the haemoglobin which confer protection without heavy genetic load should gradually go to fixation and replace those imposing a fitness cost. However, the current distribution and frequency of the haemoglobinopathies reveals a more complex scenario. Malaria has been exerting a selective pressure on humans from the very onset of hominization (Hughes and Verra 2002), but only in recent evolutionary time, within the last 10,000 years, it has reached the high endemicity combined with a sustained host population density required for the selection of malaria resistance genes such as the haemoglobinopathies.

A better understanding of the molecular genetic basis of thalassaemia and abnormal haemoglobins due to the advances in genome wide association studies and fine mapping has made possible the precise identification of carriers with a deeper resolution compared to traditional haematological parameters, thus facilitating the screening of those at higher risk and therefore requiring prompt treatment.

In addition, recent advances in the field of immunology have led to new insights into possible pathogenic mechanisms by which the observed protection may be mediated. This knowledge may be used to identify crucial steps necessary for acquired immunity to develop and may thus be of relevance for future vaccine design.

Acknowledgements

We are grateful to all the colleagues who contributed with their work and debate to our current understanding of haemoglobinopathies. In particular, we would like to thank Pierre Buffet, Eleanor Riley, and Philip Rosenthal for their critical and constructive reviewing of the manuscript. Our deepest gratitude goes to those many participants of the studies we have described, which would have not been possible without their cooperation.

FV is currently funded by the European Community's Seventh Framework Programme (FP7/2007-2013) under grant agreement PIAP-GA_2008-218164.

Reviewed by:

dr. Pierre Buffet, MCU-PH, Service de Parasitologie Mycologie Pr. Mazier

Hôpital Pitié Salpêtrière, Paris, France, pierre.buffet@psl.aphp.fr

prof. Eleanor Riley, Department of Immunology and Infection, Faculty of Infectious and Tropical Diseases, London School of Hygiene and Tropical Medicine, London, UK, eleanor.riley@lshtm.ac.uk prof. Philip Rosenthal, Division of Infectious Diseases, Department of Medicine, University of California, San Francisco, US, prosenthal@medsfgh.ucsf.edu

References

Agarwal, A., A. Guindo, et al. (2000). "Hemoglobin C associated with protection from severe malaria in the Dogon of Mali, a West African population with a low prevalence of hemoglobin S." *Blood* 96(7): 2358-2363.

Aidoo, M., D. J. Terlouw, et al. (2002). "Protective effects of the sickle cell gene against malaria morbidity and mortality." *Lancet* 359(9314): 1311-1312.

Allen, S. J., A. O'Donnell, et al. (1997). "alpha+-Thalassemia protects children against disease caused by other infections as well as malaria." *Proc Natl Acad Sci U S A* 94(26): 14736-14741.

Allison, A. C. (1954). "Protection afforded by sickle-cell trait against subtertian malareal infection." *Br Med J* 1(4857): 290-294.

Allison, A. C. (1964). "Polymorphism and Natural Selection in Human Populations." *Cold Spring Harb Symp Quant Biol* 29: 137-149.

Aluoch, J. R. (1997). "Higher resistance to Plasmodium falciparum infection in patients with homozygous sickle cell disease in western Kenya." *Trop Med Int Health* 2(6): 568-571.

Antonarakis, S. E., S. H. Orkin, et al. (1982). "Evidence for multiple origins of the beta E-globin gene in Southeast Asia." *Proc Natl Acad Sci U S A* 79(21): 6608-6611.

Atkinson, A., M. Barbier, et al. (2011). "Evidence for epistasis between hemoglobin C and immune genes in human P. falciparum malaria: a family study in Burkina Faso." *Genes Immun.*

Ayi, K., F. Turrini, et al. (2004). "Enhanced phagocytosis of ring-parasitized mutant erythrocytes: a common mechanism that may explain protection against falciparum malaria in sickle trait and beta-thalassemia trait." *Blood* 104(10): 3364-3371.

Baruch, D. I., B. L. Pasloske, et al. (1995). "Cloning the P. falciparum gene encoding PfEMP1, a malarial variant antigen and adherence receptor on the surface of parasitized human erythrocytes." *Cell* 82(1): 77-87.

Bouharoun-Tayoun, H., P. Attanath, et al. (1990). "Antibodies that protect humans against Plasmodium falciparum blood stages do not on their own inhibit parasite growth and invasion in vitro, but act in cooperation with monocytes." *J Exp Med* 172(6): 1633-1641.

Buffet, P. A., I. Safeukui, et al. (2011). "The pathogenesis of Plasmodium falciparum malaria in humans: insights from splenic physiology." *Blood* 117(2): 381-392.

Bull, P. C., M. Kortok, et al. (2000). "Plasmodium falciparum-infected erythrocytes: agglutination by diverse Kenyan plasma is associated with severe disease and young host age." *J Infect Dis* 182(1): 252-259.

Bull, P. C., B. S. Lowe, et al. (1998). "Parasite antigens on the infected red cell surface are targets for naturally acquired immunity to malaria." *Nat Med* 4(3): 358-360.

Cabrera, G., M. Cot, et al. (2005). "The sickle cell trait is associated with enhanced immunoglobulin G antibody responses to Plasmodium falciparum variant surface antigens." *J Infect Dis* 191(10): 1631-1638.

Chakravarty, S., I. A. Cockburn, et al. (2007). "CD8+ T lymphocytes protective against malaria liver stages are primed in skin-draining lymph nodes." *Nat Med* 13(9): 1035-1041.

Chebloune, Y., J. Pagnier, et al. (1988). "Structural analysis of the 5' flanking region of the beta-globin gene in African sickle cell anemia patients: further evidence for three origins of the sickle cell mutation in Africa." *Proc Natl Acad Sci U S A* 85(12): 4431-4435.

Cholera, R., N. J. Brittain, et al. (2008). "Impaired cytoadherence of Plasmodium falciparum-infected erythrocytes containing sickle hemoglobin." *Proc Natl Acad Sci U S A* 105(3): 991-996.

Chotivanich, K., R. Udomsangpetch, et al. (2002). "Hemoglobin E: a balanced polymorphism protective against high parasitemias and thus severe P falciparum malaria." *Blood* 100(4): 1172-1176.

Chui, D. H., R. Hardison, et al. (1998). "An electronic database of human hemoglobin variants on the World Wide Web." *Blood* 91(8): 2643-2644.

Cohen, S., G. I. Mc, et al. (1961). "Gamma-globulin and acquired immunity to human malaria." *Nature* 192: 733-737.

Crompton, P. D., B. Traore, et al. (2008). "Sickle cell trait is associated with a delayed onset of malaria: implications for time-to-event analysis in clinical studies of malaria." *J Infect Dis* 198(9): 1265-1275.

Enevold, A., M. Alifrangis, et al. (2007). "Associations between alpha+-thalassemia and Plasmodium falciparum malarial infection in northeastern Tanzania." *J Infect Dis* 196(3): 451-459.

Fairhurst, R. M., D. I. Baruch, et al. (2005). "Abnormal display of PfEMP-1 on erythrocytes carrying haemoglobin C may protect against malaria." *Nature* 435(7045): 1117-1121.

Fairhurst, R. M., H. Fujioka, et al. (2003). "Aberrant development of Plasmodium falciparum in hemoglobin CC red cells: implications for the malaria protective effect of the homozygous state." *Blood* 101(8): 3309-3315.

Ferreira, A., I. Marguti, et al. (2011). "Sickle hemoglobin confers tolerance to Plasmodium infection." *Cell* 145(3): 398-409.

Flatz, G. (1967). "Hemoglobin E: distribution and population dynamics." *Humangenetik* 3(3): 189-234.

Flint, J., R. M. Harding, et al. (1993). "The population genetics of the haemoglobinopathies." *Baillieres Clin Haematol* 6(1): 215-262.

Flint, J., A. V. Hill, et al. (1986). "High frequencies of alpha-thalassaemia are the result of natural selection by malaria." *Nature* 321(6072): 744-750.

Fowkes, F. J. and K. P. Day (2008). "Alpha+ -thalassaemia and malaria in Melanesia: epidemiological perspectives." *P N G Med J* 51(3-4): 131-137.

Friedman, M. J., E. F. Roth, et al. (1979). "The role of hemoglobins C, S, and Nbalt in the inhibition of malaria parasite development in vitro." *Am J Trop Med Hyg* 28(5): 777-780.

Fucharoen, S., G. Fucharoen, et al. (2005). "Compound heterozygote states for Hb C/Hb Malay and Hb C/Hb E in pregnancy: a molecular and hematological analysis." *Blood Cells Mol Dis* 35(2): 196-200.

Galanrneau, G., Palmer C.D., Sankaran, V.G., Orkin, S.H., Hirschhorn, J.N., Lettre, G. (2010). "Fine-mapping at three loci known to affect fetal hemoglobin levels explains addtional genetic variation." *Nat Genet* 42(12): 1049-1051.

Giha, H. A., T. Staalsoe, et al. (1999). "Nine-year longitudinal study of antibodies to variant antigens on the surface of Plasmodium falciparum-infected erythrocytes." *Infect Immun* 67(8): 4092-4098.

Good, M. F. and D. L. Doolan (1999). "Immune effector mechanisms in malaria." *Curr Opin Immunol* 11(4): 412-419.

Gouagna, L. C., G. Bancone, et al. (2010). "Genetic variation in human HBB is associated with Plasmodium falciparum transmission." *Nat Genet* 42(4): 328-331.

Gray, J. C., P. H. Corran, et al. (2007). "Profiling the antibody immune response against blood stage malaria vaccine candidates." *Clin Chem* 53(7): 1244-1253.

Guerra, C. A., P. W. Gikandi, et al. (2008). "The limits and intensity of Plasmodium falciparum transmission: implications for malaria control and elimination worldwide." *PLoS Med* 5(2): e38.

Guinet, F., D. A. Diallo, et al. (1997). "A comparison of the incidence of severe malaria in Malian children with normal and C-trait hemoglobin profiles." *Acta Trop* 68(2): 175-182.

Haldane, J. B. (1949). "The rate of mutation of human genes." *Hereditas Suppl.*(35): 267-273.

Herrick, J. (1910). "Peculiar Elongated and Sickle-shaped red blood corpuscles in a case of severe anemia." *Yale Journal of Biology and Medicine* 74 (2001): 179-184

Hill, A. V., C. E. Allsopp, et al. (1991). "Common west African HLA antigens are associated with protection from severe malaria." *Nature* 352(6336): 595-600.

Hughes, A. L. and F. Verra (2002). "Extensive polymorphism and ancient origin of Plasmodium falciparum." *Trends Parasitol* 18(8): 348-351.

Hutagalung, R., P. Wilairatana, et al. (1999). "Influence of hemoglobin E trait on the severity of Falciparum malaria." *J Infect Dis* 179(1): 283-286.

Hviid, L. (2005). "Naturally acquired immunity to Plasmodium falciparum malaria in Africa." *Acta Trop* 95(3): 270-275.

Komba, A. N., J. Makani, et al. (2009). "Malaria as a cause of morbidity and mortality in children with homozygous sickle cell disease on the coast of Kenya." *Clin Infect Dis* 49(2): 216-222.

Kreuels, B., S. Ehrhardt, et al. (2009). "Sickle cell trait (HbAS) and stunting in children below two years of age in an area of high malaria transmission." *Malar J* 8: 16.

Kreuels, B., C. Kreuzberg, et al. (2010). "Differing effects of HbS and HbC traits on uncomplicated falciparum malaria, anemia, and child growth." *Blood* 115(22): 4551-4558.

Kruatrachue, M., M. Bhaibulaya, et al. (1969). "Haemoglobinopathies and malaria in Thailand." *Bull World Health Organ* 40(3): 459-463.

Labie, D., J. Pagnier, et al. (1985). "Common haplotype dependency of high G gamma-globin gene expression and high Hb F levels in beta-thalassemia and sickle cell anemia patients." *Proc Natl Acad Sci U S A* 82(7): 2111-2114.

Lang, P. A., R. S. Kasinathan, et al. (2009). "Accelerated clearance of Plasmodium-infected erythrocytes in sickle cell trait and annexin-A7 deficiency." *Cell Physiol Biochem* 24(5-6): 415-428.

Langhorne, J., F. M. Ndungu, et al. (2008). "Immunity to malaria: more questions than answers." *Nat Immunol* 9(7): 725-732.

Le Hesran, J. Y., Personne, I., Personne, P., Fievet, N., Dubois, B., Beyeme', M., Boudin, C., Cot, M., Deloron, P. (1999). "Longitudinal study of Plasmodium falciparum infection and immune responses in infants with or without the sickle cell trait." *Int J Epidemiol* 28(4): 793-798.

Lee, K. S., P. C. Divis, et al. (2011). "Plasmodium knowlesi: reservoir hosts and tracking the emergence in humans and macaques." *PLoS Pathog* 7(4): e1002015.

Liu, W., Y. Li, et al. (2010). "Origin of the human malaria parasite Plasmodium falciparum in gorillas." *Nature* 467(7314): 420-425.

Livingstone, F. (1967). *"Abnormal Hemoglobins in Human Populations: a Summary and Interpretation."*.

Luzzi, G. A., A. H. Merry, et al. (1991). "Protection by alpha-thalassaemia against Plasmodium falciparum malaria: modified surface antigen expression rather than impaired growth or cytoadherence." *Immunol Lett* 30(2): 233-240.

Mackinnon, M. J. and K. Marsh (2010). "The selection landscape of malaria parasites." *Science* 328(5980): 866-871.

Maitland, K. and K. Marsh (2004). "Pathophysiology of severe malaria in children." *Acta Trop* 90(2): 131-140.

Makani, J., A. N. Komba, et al. (2010). "Malaria in patients with sickle cell anemia: burden, risk factors, and outcome at the outpatient clinic and during hospitalization." *Blood* 115(2): 215-220.

Marsh, K., D. Forster, et al. (1995). "Indicators of life-threatening malaria in African children." *N Engl J Med* 332(21): 1399-1404.

Marsh, K. and R. J. Howard (1986). "Antigens induced on erythrocytes by P. falciparum: expression of diverse and conserved determinants." *Science* 231(4734): 150-153.

Marsh, K. and S. Kinyanjui (2006). "Immune effector mechanisms in malaria." *Parasite Immunol* 28(1-2): 51-60.

Marsh, K., L. Otoo, et al. (1989). "Antibodies to blood stage antigens of Plasmodium falciparum in rural Gambians and their relation to protection against infection." *Trans R Soc Trop Med Hyg* 83(3): 293-303.

May, J., J. A. Evans, et al. (2007). "Hemoglobin variants and disease manifestations in severe falciparum malaria." *JAMA* 297(20): 2220-2226.

Mockenhaupt, F. P., S. Ehrhardt, et al. (2004). "Hemoglobin C and resistance to severe malaria in Ghanaian children." *J Infect Dis* 190(5): 1006-1009.

Modiano, D., G. Bancone, et al. (2008). "Haemoglobin S and haemoglobin C: 'quick but costly' versus 'slow but gratis' genetic adaptations to Plasmodium falciparum malaria." *Hum Mol Genet* 17(6): 789-799.

Modiano, D., G. Luoni, et al. (2001). "Haemoglobin C protects against clinical Plasmodium falciparum malaria." *Nature* 414(6861): 305-308.

Nagel, R. L., M. E. Fabry, et al. (1985). "Hematologically and genetically distinct forms of sickle cell anemia in Africa. The Senegal type and the Benin type." *N Engl J Med* 312(14): 880-884.

Nagel, R. L., M. E. Fabry, et al. (2003). "The paradox of hemoglobin SC disease." *Blood Rev* 17(3): 167-178.

Nagel, R. L., C. Raventos-Suarez, et al. (1981). "Impairment of the growth of Plasmodium falciparum in HbEE erythrocytes." *J Clin Invest* 68(1): 303-305.

Newbold, C. I. (1999). "Antigenic variation in Plasmodium falciparum: mechanisms and consequences." *Curr Opin Microbiol* 2(4): 420-425.

Newbold, C. I., A. G. Craig, et al. (1997). "PfEMP1, polymorphism and pathogenesis." *Ann Trop Med Parasitol* 91(5): 551-557.

Nielsen, M. A., T. Staalsoe, et al. (2002). "Plasmodium falciparum variant surface antigen expression varies between isolates causing severe and nonsevere malaria and is modified by acquired immunity." *J Immunol* 168(7): 3444-3450.

Nussenzweig, V. and R. S. Nussenzweig (1989). "Rationale for the development of an engineered sporozoite malaria vaccine." *Adv Immunol* 45: 283-334.

Okuonghae, H. O., M. U. Nwankwo, et al. (1992). "Malarial parasitaemia in febrile children with sickle cell anaemia." *J Trop Pediatr* 38(2): 83-85.

Olivieri, N. F., G. M. Muraca, et al. (2008). "Studies in haemoglobin E beta-thalassaemia." *Br J Haematol* 141(3): 388-397.

Oner, C., A. J. Dimovski, et al. (1992). "Beta S haplotypes in various world populations." *Hum Genet* 89(1): 99-104.

Osier, F. H., G. Fegan, et al. (2008). "Breadth and magnitude of antibody responses to multiple Plasmodium falciparum merozoite antigens are associated with protection from clinical malaria." *Infect Immun* 76(5): 2240-2248.

Pasquetto, V., D. A. Fidock, et al. (1997). "Plasmodium falciparum sporozoite invasion is inhibited by naturally acquired or experimentally induced polyclonal antibodies to the STARP antigen." *Eur J Immunol* 27(10): 2502-2513.

Pasvol, G., D. J. Weatherall, et al. (1977). "Effects of foetal haemoglobin on susceptibility of red cells to Plasmodium falciparum." *Nature* 270(5633): 171-173.

Pasvol, G. and R. J. Wilson (1982). "The interaction of malaria parasites with red blood cells." *Br Med Bull* 38(2): 133-140.

Penman, B. S., O. G. Pybus, et al. (2009). "Epistatic interactions between genetic disorders of hemoglobin can explain why the sickle-cell gene is uncommon in the Mediterranean." *Proc Natl Acad Sci U S A* 106(50): 21242-21246.

Prugnolle, F., P. Durand, et al. (2010). "African great apes are natural hosts of multiple related malaria species, including Plasmodium falciparum." *Proc Natl Acad Sci U S A* 107(4): 1458-1463.

Rihet, P., L. Flori, et al. (2004). "Hemoglobin C is associated with reduced Plasmodium falciparum parasitemia and low risk of mild malaria attack." *Hum Mol Genet* 13(1): 1-6.

Riley, E. M., S. Wahl, et al. (2006). "Regulating immunity to malaria." *Parasite Immunol* 28(1-2): 35-49.

Ringelhann, B., M. K. Hathorn, et al. (1976). "A new look at the protection of hemoglobin AS and AC genotypes against plasmodium falciparum infection: a census tract approach." *Am J Hum Genet* 28(3): 270-279.

Roberts, D. J., Harris, T., Williams, T. (2004). "The influence of inherited traits on malaria infection." *Susceptibility to Infectious Diseases: The importance of host genetics* Edited by Bellamy R. Cambridge Univ. Press: 139-184.

Rosenthal, P. J. (2011). "Lessons from sickle cell disease in the treatment and control of malaria." *N Engl J Med* 364(26): 2549-2551.

Sambo, M. R., M. J. Trovoada, et al. (2010). "Transforming growth factor beta 2 and heme oxygenase 1 genes are risk factors for the cerebral malaria syndrome in Angolan children." *PLoS One* 5(6): e11141.

Sanchaisuriya, K., G. Fucharoen, et al. (2001). "Molecular characterization of hemoglobin C in Thailand." *Am J Hematol* 67(3): 189-193.

Santiyanont, R. and P. Wilairat (1981). "Red cells containing hemoglobin E do not inhibit malaria parasite development in vitro." *Am J Trop Med Hyg* 30(3): 541-543.

Scherf, A., R. Hernandez-Rivas, et al. (1998). "Antigenic variation in malaria: in situ switching, relaxed and mutually exclusive transcription of var genes during intra-erythrocytic development in Plasmodium falciparum." *EMBO J* 17(18): 5418-5426.

Schofield, L., J. Villaquiran, et al. (1987). "Gamma interferon, CD8+ T cells and antibodies required for immunity to malaria sporozoites." *Nature* 330(6149): 664-666.

Shekalaghe, S., M. Alifrangis, et al. (2009). "Low density parasitaemia, red blood cell polymorphisms and Plasmodium falciparum specific immune responses in a low endemic area in northern Tanzania." *BMC Infect Dis* 9: 69.

Singh, B., L. Kim Sung, et al. (2004). "A large focus of naturally acquired Plasmodium knowlesi infections in human beings." *Lancet* 363(9414): 1017-1024.

Siniscalco, M., L. Bernini, et al. (1966). "Population genetics of haemoglobin variants, thalassaemia and glucose-6-phosphate dehydrogenase deficiency, with particular reference to the malaria hypothesis." *Bull World Health Organ* 34(3): 379-393.

Snow, R. W., J. A. Omumbo, et al. (1997). "Relation between severe malaria morbidity in children and level of Plasmodium falciparum transmission in Africa." *Lancet* 349(9066): 1650-1654.

Steinberg, M. H. (2009). "Genetic etiologies for phenotypic diversity in sickle cell anemia." *ScientificWorldJournal* 9: 46-67.

Stevenson, M. M. and E. M. Riley (2004). "Innate immunity to malaria." *Nat Rev Immunol* 4(3): 169-180.

Storey, J., A. F. Fleming, et al. (1979). "Abnormal haemoglobins in the Sudan savanna of Nigeria. IV. Malaria, immunoglobulins and antimalarial antibodies in haemoglobin AC individuals." *Ann Trop Med Parasitol* 73(4): 311-315.

Su, X. Z., V. M. Heatwole, et al. (1995). "The large diverse gene family var encodes proteins involved in cytoadherence and antigenic variation of Plasmodium falciparum-infected erythrocytes." *Cell* 82(1): 89-100.

Takeda, M., M. Kikuchi, et al. (2005). "Microsatellite polymorphism in the heme oxygenase-1 gene promoter is associated with susceptibility to cerebral malaria in Myanmar." *Jpn J Infect Dis* 58(5): 268-271.

Thein, S. L. (2005). "Pathophysiology of beta thalassemia--a guide to molecular therapies." *Hematology Am Soc Hematol Educ Program*: 31-37.

Veenemans, J., P. E. Andang'o, et al. (2008). "Alpha+ -thalassemia protects against anemia associated with asymptomatic malaria: evidence from community-based surveys in Tanzania and Kenya." *J Infect Dis* 198(3): 401-408.

Verra, F., J. Simpore, et al. (2007). "Haemoglobin C and S role in acquired immunity against Plasmodium falciparum malaria." *PLoS One* 2(10): e978.

Wainscoat, J. S., E. Kanavakis, et al. (1983). "Thalassaemia intermedia in Cyprus: the interaction of alpha and beta thalassaemia." *Br J Haematol* 53(3): 411-416.

Wambua, S., T. W. Mwangi, et al. (2006). "The effect of alpha+-thalassaemia on the incidence of malaria and other diseases in children living on the coast of Kenya." *PLoS Med* 3(5): e158.

Weatherall, D. J. (1987). "Common genetic disorders of the red cell and the 'malaria hypothesis'." *Ann Trop Med Parasitol* 81(5): 539-548.

Williams, T. N., T. W. Mwangi, et al. (2005a). "An immune basis for malaria protection by the sickle cell trait." *PLoS Med* 2(5): e128.

Williams, T. N., S. Wambua, et al. (2005b). "Both heterozygous and homozygous alpha+ thalassemias protect against severe and fatal Plasmodium falciparum malaria on the coast of Kenya." *Blood* 106(1): 368-371.

Williams, T. N., D. J. Weatherall, et al. (2002). "The membrane characteristics of Plasmodium falciparum-infected and -uninfected heterozygous alpha(0)thalassaemic erythrocytes." *Br J Haematol* 118(2): 663-670.

In: Malaria: Etiology, Pathogenesis and Treatments
Editors: A. M. Peterson et al, pp. 363-379
ISBN: 978-1-62100-363-2

Chapter XV

The Role of Host Inflammatory Mediators as Biomarkers for Malaria Pathogenesis

Ivan T. Matthews and Tobili Y. Sam-Yellowe
Cleveland State University, Department of Biological, Geological and Environmental Sciences, Cleveland Ohio, U.S.A.

Abstract

Malaria pathogenesis results from a complex interplay of pro-inflammatory and anti-inflammatory mediators produced as a result of innate responses following *Plasmodium* infection. These mediators interact with host tissues and organs resulting in damage and destruction that characterizes specific syndromes associated with red blood cell destruction, vascular endothelial disturbances, microvascular obstruction, respiratory distress, retinopathy, inflammatory responses to toxins and other parasite metabolites and placental tissue destruction. The malaria syndromes define uncomplicated malaria (UM), cerebral malaria (CM), placental malaria (PM), severe malarial anemia (SA), and severe malaria (SM). Approximately 515 million cases of malaria are reported annually with 1-3 million deaths occurring in children. Five *Plasmodium* species infect humans: *P. falciparum, P. vivax P. malariae P. ovale and P. knowlesi. Plasmodium falciparum* is the agent most associated with severe and fatal malaria. Pregnant women and children make up the most vulnerable groups to develop severe pathogenesis from malaria infection. Cytokines, chemokines, vascular endothelial proteins, angiogenic factors, and other host mediators make up important mediators of pathogenesis in the host. In addition, other non-immunologic host molecules, parasite proteins, metabolites and toxins may contribute to severe pathogenesis in the host. Determining which of the mediators enhance adverse outcomes for disease progression and poor disease prognosis as well as identifying those mediators with protective effects is an area of intense investigation in malaria research. The cytokines tumor necrosis factor alpha (TNFα), interleukin (IL)-12, IL-1β, IL-10 and interferon gamma (IFNγ) are associated with the pathogenesis of cerebral malaria and severe anemia, with TNFα being strongly implicated with this form of malaria. Treatment of patients with neutralizing anti-TNFα antibodies was effective in resolving clinical symptoms. Low ratios of IL-10 to TNFα in serum correlate with severe anemia in contrast to high IL-10 to TNFα ratios seen in children with uncomplicated malaria. Levels of soluble ICAM-1, IL-1Ra, IL-2R, IL-4, IL-6, IL-6R, neopterin, angiopoeitin (ANG) 2 and TNFα are found to be highly elevated in patients with cerebral malaria, with TNFα being highly elevated in patients who died from cerebral malaria compared to patients with uncomplicated malaria. TNFα and ANG2 levels can predict poor prognosis with fatal outcomes in cases of cerebral malaria. A diagnostic test that is prognostic and capable of discriminating among the different malaria syndromes as well as distinguishing infections caused by non malaria pathogens will improve disease management of malaria and disease surveillance. A diagnostic test that incorporates host mediators of disease as well as parasite products and toxins would detect biomarkers of disease progression, diseases severity and development of cerebral malaria and will also be useful in determining the effectiveness of parasite clearance following drug treatment. In this chapter we examine studies performed to evaluate host mediators associated with malaria pathogenesis; uncomplicated malaria (UM), cerebral malaria (CM), placental malaria (PM), severe malarial anemia (SA), and severe malaria (SM) to determine the effectiveness of the mediators as biomarkers for malaria diagnosis.

Introduction

Malaria

Malaria is a prevalent parasitic disease that affects humans globally. It is the world's second biggest killer after tuberculosis (Berriman, 2010). Malaria is responsible for three-hundred to five-hundred million infections worldwide and approximately one to two million deaths annually, most of them in young children in sub-Saharan Africa (CDC, 2010). The disease is frequent in tropical and subtropical regions. Malaria is now common to 106 nations, including in Asia and Europe, threatening half the world's population (Finkel, 2007). Imported malaria remains an important challenge for public health in the United States (CDC, 2010).

Today it is not uncommon for individuals to travel from one continent to another within a twenty-four hour period. This increases the frequency for individuals to become exposed to malaria. In short, the probability of spreading the disease has heightened according to statistics and the Center of Disease Control (CDC, 2010). Malaria is caused by infection with parasites of the genus *Plasmodium*. These are single-celled organisms called protozoans. The parasites are transmitted to humans through the bite of the female *Anopheles* mosquito. Of the approximately four-hundred thirty known species of *Anopheles*, only fifty can transmit malaria in nature (CDC, 2010).

There are five *Plasmodium* species that infect humans: *P. knowlesi, P. vivax, P. ovale, P. falciparum and P. malariae* (CDC 2011). They each cause different diseases and clinical manifestations. Each species has a different host erythrocyte preference. *Plasmodium knowlesi* is found primarily in Southeast Asia and was reported in long-tailed macaques. This is currently an important human malaria species. *Plasmodium vivax* is widespread in the tropics and subtropics and extends into temperate areas uncommon in Africa. *Plasmodium ovale* is found mainly in tropical Africa, especially in Western Africa. *Plasmodium vivax and P. ovale* exhibit the hypnozoite stage in the liver and can cause relapses as well. Both species prefer to invade reticulocytes (immature erythrocytes). *Plasmodium falciparum* is widespread, but is found mostly in tropical and subtropical conditions. *Plasmodium falciparum* has a narrow host specificity and exhibits preference for all ages of the erythrocyte. *Plasmodium malariae* has a wide-range but spotty environmental distribution and prefers senescent erythrocytes. The first two species cause the most infections worldwide. *Plasmodium falciparum* is the agent of severe, potentially fatal malaria (Bayoumi *et al.*, 2009), while *P. malariae* produces long-lasting infections and if left untreated can persist asymptomatically in the human host for years, even a lifetime (CDC, 2010).

General Life Cycle of *Plasmodium*

Mosquito Stage

A female *Anopheles* mosquito ingests the infected blood of a human host containing gametocyte infected erythrocytes. The male gametocytes, (microgametocytes) will undergo exflagellation resulting in flagellated forms that will swim, find and fertilize the female gametocytes (macrogametocytes) generating zygotes. The zygotes in turn become motile ookinetes and invade the midgut wall of the mosquito where they develop into oocysts. The oocysts grow, undergo sporogony rupture, and release sporozoites. The sporozoites make their way to the mosquito's salivary glands where they become infective.

Exoerythrocytic Stage

The mosquito pierces the skin of another host and inoculates sporozoites into the human host. The sporozoites are carried by the circulatory system to the liver and invade hepatocytes (liver cells). Sporozoites undergo a process of development and multiplication known as schizogony. In the liver some of the sporozoites mature into schizonts while others enter a dormant phase known as the hypnozoite (Johnson, 2010).

These hypnozoites can reactivate and undergo schizogony at a later time, causing relapses weeks to month's even years after the initial infection. The schizonts divide and form thousands of merozoites which are released following schizont burst. The merozoites leave the liver and enter the blood stream.

Erythrocytic Stage

Merozoites invade red blood cells (erythrocytes) and undergo a trophic period during which the parasite enlarges as it ingests host cytoplasm and hemoglobin. Schizogony and gamogony take place in the blood stage. The early trophozoite is known as a ring form due to its structure. Trophozoites mature into schizonts and burst infected red blood cells, releasing more merozoites that re-enter the erythrocytes and repeat the erythrocytic cycle. This release coincides with the violent rises in temperature during the clinical manifestations of the disease. However, some merozoites instead of continuing to become schizonts, develop into gametocytes. The gametocytes are ingested by a female Anopheles mosquito during a blood meal, to continue the malaria life cycle.

Diagnosis

There are several types of procedures which have been used for malaria diagnosis for symptomatic and asymptomatic individual(s) such as microscopy, polymerase chain reaction (PCR) (Greenwood, 2002) and malaria rapid-diagnostic tests (RDTs) that identify *P. falciparum*-specific histidine-rich protein II (HRPII) (Biswas et al., 2005). Malaria is diagnosed by either a sample of venous or capillary blood (Kristiansen et al., 2001; Perlmann et al., 1997; Philippidis et al., 2004; Schaer et al., 2006) smeared on a slide and stained with Giemsa and analyzed for the presence of *Plasmodium* parasites and parasite species. Although in the hands of skilled microscopists and technichians these expensive tools through use of their specificity and sensitivity can identify malaria in the blood, unfortunately these tests are unable to differentiate individuals with symptoms of malaria infection from those with malaria disease. Identifying early signs of malaria in patients can allow for precise diagnosis and prompt therapeutic strategies (Malaguarnera *et al.*, 2002).

Treatments

Currently no vaccines are available for malaria. However, a successful phase III trial of the RTS,S vaccine shows promise with a 50 % reduction of malaria in children 5 to 17 months old (CDC, 2011). Resistance to certain drugs, particularly chloroquine has been observed contributing to elevated morbidity and mrtality in endemic areas. However, there are treatments with antimalarial drugs available such as derivatives of artemisinin (artesunate, artemether-lumefantrine), atovaquone-proguanil, quinine, doxycycline, hydroxychloroquine sulfate, and mefloquine (Parquet et al., 2010; CDC, 2011).

Pathogenesis

Malaria is a disease of the blood that is transmitted to people by infected mosquitoes. The female Anopheles mosquito can infect an individual by injecting sporozoites into the individual. The parasite gains entry into the red blood cells by binding to the erythrocyte surface receptors. The merozoite makes contact with the erythrocyte plasma membrane by the apical end. This creates an inward fold eventually forming the parasite compartment in the cytoplasm. There are numerous receptor-ligand interactions that occur during merozoite invasion (Smythe et al., 1988). Merozoite proteins such as erythrocyte binding antigen (EBA)-175, apical membrane antigen (AMA)-1 from the microneme, rhoptry neck proteins (RONs) and merozoite surface (MSP-1) protein-1, (MSP-2) protein-2, (MSP-3) protein-3, (MSP-4) protein-4 and (MSP-5) protein-5 are believed to be responsible for the initial steps of merozoite entry into the erythrocyte, including junction formation (Barnwell et al., 1998; Perkins et al., 1988; Sherman 2005; Richard et al. 2010).

The ability of the host immune system to attack host erythrocytes is significant since proteins control the time which parasitaemia rises, and the rate of direct contact to the immune system. Hyperparasitaemia is a good indicator but not always linked to predicting the severity of disease for asymptomatic children with very high parasite counts and detecting patients with very low numbers of parasites in the peripheral blood (Chitnis, 2001). Hyperparasitaemia shows differences in both adhesive proteins on merozoites and genetic differences in the host regarding red blood cell surface proteins. *Plasmodium vivax* and *P.ovale* parasites can relapse and lie dormant in the liver for several months up to five years after an individual is infected. Re-emergence of the parasites and invasion of erythrocytes causes individuals to become symptomatic. *Plasmodium knowlesi, P. falciparum, P. vivax, P.ovale* and *P. malaria* parasite density is approximately proportional with little age variation and can exist in the same area and time (Muller et al., 2009; Van den Eede et al., 2009); although, frequency of cases and nearly all deaths are caused by *Plasmodium falciparum* (Suh et al., 2004).

Symptoms of malaria comprise fever and flu-like illness, including headache, chills, tiredness and muscle aches. Vomiting, and nausea, and diarrhea may possibly arise. Malaria may cause anemia and jaundice (yellow coloring of the eyes and skin) due to the loss of red blood cells, anemia and cerebral malaria. The disease may cause seizures, kidney failure, unconsciousness, mental confusion, and death. In majority of people, symptoms start nine days to five weeks after infectivity; however some individuals experience illness as early as seven days or up to twelve months later.

Cytokines and Malaria Pathogenesis

Cytokines and chemokines are small molecular weight non-structural proteins involved in human immune responses to malaria infection or illness (Awandare et al., 2006; Beutler, 1988; Beutler et al., 1987; Cerami et al., 1988; Jason et al., 2001; Lyke et al., 2004; Nagamine et al., 2003; Schofield et al., 2005) that are manufactured by almost every cell in the body (Buechler et al., 2000; Clark, 1978; Dinarello, 2000; Sulahian et al., 2000; Vreden et al., 1992; Wong et al., 2003). Cytokines are secreted by various cells included those to fight off infections. Lymphokines are cytokines manufactured by lymphocytes however few lymphokines can be produced by non-lymphoid cells. Majority of cytokines manufactured by T-cells are identified as interleukin (IL). Interferon gamma (IFN-γ) is an essential cytokine secreted by CD8 effector T-cells that prevent replication and rid virus from an infected cell without harm. T_H1 and T_H2 cells are distinguished by specific cytokines such as IL-2, IFNγ and TNFβ for T_H1 cells and IL-4, IL-5 and IL-10 for T_H2 cells. However, both cells secrete overlapping cytokines such as IL-3 and GM-CSF. Few cytokines exert effects on distant cells while majority of cytokines exert their effects locally, and are coordinated with other membrane-bound effector molecules and can combine with receptors on target cells. Interleukin-4, IL-5 (increase the manufacturing of eosinophils) and IL-10 are produced by T_H2 cells that stimulate B cells. IFN-γ is produced by T_H1 that is the key macrophage stimulating cytokine and lymphotoxin (LT or TNF-β) that is simply cytotoxic to few cells.

Both kinds of CD4 effector T cell secrete IL-3 and GM-CSF which facilitate effector cells during an immune response by causing bone marrow cells to induce myelopoesis, manufacturing of non-specific cells in humoral and cell mediated immunity, e.g., macrophages and granulocytes. Dendritic cells are increased from bone marrow precursors stemming from IL-3 and GM-CSF stimulation.

Cytokines can by categorized by their receptors with similar genetic, structural and functional properties as follows: hematopoietins (type 1), inteferons (type 2), chemokines, immunoglobin superfamily and TNF family (majority are membrane bound) receptors. Common structural characteristics define cytokine receptor families (one subunit is shared among all family members). Cytokine receptors are usually heterodimers (more rarely heterotrimers) and can be divided into two types. The largest IL-2R family belonging to the type 1 cytokine receptors is divided into three subfamilies based on common components: IL-2Rγ, common β, and gp130. Unlike the other receptors, type 1 cytokine receptors lack protein tyrosine kinase activity and possess a Trp-Ser-X-Trp-Ser (WSXWS) motif. Following ligand (cytokine) binding, the receptor dimerizes leading to initiation of intracellular signaling pathways.

The interferon receptors (IFNR family) representative of the type 2 cytokine receptors possess characteristic conserved cysteines (CCCC) and tandem immunoglobulin-like domains localized to the extracellular domains of the subunits. In addition, type 2 cytokine receptors are able to phosphorylate tyrosine amino acid subunits (i.e. maintain their intrinsic tyrosine kinase activity).

Chemokine receptors belong to the seven-transmembrane domain receptors with domain segments connected to the GTP-binding proteins and are only expressed on select lymphocytes. The nomenclature for chemokine receptors is dependent on the family of chemokines they bind, i.e. the CC receptor (CCR) binds CC chemokines, while the CXC receptor (CXCR) binds CXC chemokines. Due to redundancy of the common receptor subunit responsible for cytokine binding and subsequent signal transduction, one receptor can frequently bind and be activated by another cytokine in the same family (Janeway *et al.*, 2007).

As a cytokine binds to a receptor, the receptor becomes activated; a secondary messenger within the cell become stimulated thus causing the cell to change its behavior. They mediate cell replication, range and the time of the immune-inflammatory response, and repair. Cytokines can bind to a receptor on each cell and can behave either in one of three ways: 1) autocrine manner -- influencing the behavior of the cell that secreted it; 2) paracrine manner-- influencing the behavior of the neighboring cells; and 3) endocrine manner-- influencing the behavior of distant cells. Each cytokine has pleiotropic effectors showing various biological activities. Cytokines are believed to behave synergistically when two or more cytokines act jointly to create a more effective end product than two cytokines functioning independently.

Interferon gamma (IFN-γ) is a cytokine that is an important regulator of immune response. Serum levels of IFN-γ were found to be significantly higher within infected patients (Wroczynska et al., 2005). Interleukin-4 is an *anti-inflammatory cytokine* that induces and regulates immune response. Interleukin-4 is believed to induce a protective T_H1 response to control infection (Robson et al., 2009). Interleukin-6 is a pro-inflammatory cytokine that is an important mediator of immune response. Interleukin 6 is also produced in significant amounts during infection (Grau et al., 1990). Tumor necrosis factor alpha (TNF-α) is a cytokine involved in regulation of immune system. Studies have observed significant levels of TNF-α in patients with severe forms of infections (Mergani *et al.*, 2010).The interleukin-1 receptor antagonist (IL-1ra) is a protein of the IL-1 cytokine family that regulates IL-1 immune responses. IL-1Ra concentrations are significant after various infectious (Keuter et al., 1994) and can be considered an efficient marker of the cytokine cascade (van Deuren et al., 1995).

Interleukin-10 (IL-10) is an anti-inflammatory *cytokine and inhibits* pro-inflammatory cytokines such as IFN-γ and TNF-α. Reports suggest IL-10 levels are increased within inflammatory infections (Kabyemela et al., 2008). Interleukin-10 is an essential anti-inflammatory cytokine, which has been shown to be an effective inhibitor of T_H1-induced cytokines, as well as IL-2 and interferon gamma (IFN-γ). Interleukin-10 is detected in malaria in general (Francischetti *et al.*, 2008) and considered to induce isotype switching (Perlmann *et al.*, 1994), from immunoglobin-M (IgM) to IgG1 and IgG3, which are believed to protect against *P. falciparum* (Tangteerawatana *et al.*, 2007; Tangteerawatana *et al.*, 2009).

Although IFN-γ has been associated with severe malaria (SM) (Deloron *et al.*, 1991; Pongponratn *et al.*, 2003), there are studies suggesting that high levels of IL-10 are directly linked with malaria (Peyron *et al.*, 1994; Sarthou *et al.*, 1997; Wenisch *et al.*, 1995). High levels of IL-10 have also been reported to exhibit a physiologic influence on immune responses (Opal *et al.*, 2000), whereas low levels of IL-10 are associated with severe anemia (SA) (Casals-Pascual *et al.*, 2006; Nussenblatt *et al.*, 2001), along with TNF-α, another specific cytokine believed to be involved in severe malaria (Clark, 2007) and has a profound impact on malaria i.e., protection and malaria pathogenesis (Gourley *et al.*, 2002; Kurtis *et al.*, 1999; Shaffer *et al.*, 1991; Singh *et al.*, 2000; Yazdani *et al.*, 2006). Studies suggest parasite sequestration occurs mostly in the brain (Eling *et al.*, 1994; Sarfo *et al.*, 2004), accompanied by high concentrations of circulating TNF-α (Clark *et al.*, 2006). Elevated levels of TNFα have been reported in the sera of cerebral malaria (CM) patients (Randall *et al.*, 2010). Findings show IL-10 as an effective regulator of inflammatory responses which can control IFN-γ and TNFα production during immunopathological processes (Taylor-Robinson *et al.*, 1999).

Combination of T_H2-induced cytokines, including IL-4, IL-10, relative to T_H1-elicited levels of IFN-γ, seems to stop the progression of malarial anemia in highly prevalent regions (Nussenblatt *et al.*, 2001). Recent studies, examining malarial infection during pregnancy (Brabin *et al.*, 1999; Buechler *et al.*, 2000; Guyatt *et al.*, 2004) have shown TNF-α to be associated with outcomes of placental malaria (PM) (Diouf *et al.*, 2007; Matteelli *et al.*, 1994; Rogerson *et al.*, 2003), as well as connection to cell-mediated inflammatory responses (Opal *et al.*, 2000) and changes in the cytokine equilibrium to facilitate T_H1 types (Eling *et al.*, 1994; Fried *et al.*, 1998; Moormann *et al.*, 1999; Rogerson *et al.*, 2003).

Decreased T_H1 proinflammatory cytokines with higher distribution levels of IFN-γ and TNF-α (Yamada-Tanaka *et al.*, 1995) together with IL-4, IL-6 and IL-10 have been evaluated in pregnant women with malaria (Raghupathy, 1997). CM and SA disease resulted in a heightened production of TNFα (Gimenez *et al.*, 2003; Grau *et al.*, 1989), which is offset by IL-10 and controlled by TNF receptors (Armah *et al.*, 2007), as observed in children with high-density parasitemia and SM (less frequently CM) (Iriemenam *et al.*, 2009). In some studies IL-6 and IL-8 have also been seen in the pathogenesis of CM and treatment with IL-1 (α or β) or IL-1receptor antagonist (IL-1ra) has produced an effect on CM and parasitemia when administered early (Eling *et al.*, 1994). Several malarial studies have reported that IL-10 (Kurtis *et al.*, 1999; Li *et al.*, 2003) may be linked with SM or can potentially act as a defense agent against the disease (Ho *et al.*, 1998; Ho *et al.*, 1995; Kurtis *et al.*, 1999; Nussenblatt *et al.*, 2001; Peyron *et al.*, 1994; Prakash *et al.*, 2006). Furthermore, the ratio between IL-10 (Jason *et al.*, 2001) and TNFα (Malaguarnera *et al.*, 2002) has been shown to determine the severity of malaria (Chaiyaroj *et al.*, 2004; Issifou *et al.*, 2003; Nussenblatt *et al.*, 2001), and malarial anemia in children (Kurtzhals *et al.*, 1998; Newton *et al.*, 1998; Othoro *et al.*, 1999).

There have been differences in chemokine, cytokine plasma concentrations and other host proteins (Malaguarnera *et al.*, 2002; Perch *et al.*, 2004; Ringwald *et al.*, 1991; Suguitan *et al.*, 2003; Sulahian *et al.*, 2000) widely reported and associated with malaria infection in adults (Kusi *et al.*, 2008; Prakash *et al.*, 2006) pregnant women and children (Cserti-Gazdewich *et al.*, 2010; Dietmann *et al.*, 2008). Several studies have been performed to examine, chemokine(s), pro-inflammatory and/or anti-inflammatory cytokine(s) with uncomplicated malaria (UM) (Dietmann *et al.*, 2009; Hesselink *et al.*, 2009), cerebral malaria (CM) (Coltel *et al.*, 2004; Curfs *et al.*, 1990; Eling *et al.*, 1994; Gosi *et al.*, 1999; John *et al.*, 2008), placental malaria (PM) (Steketee *et al.*, 2001; Steketee *et al.*, 1996; Stoiser *et al.*, 2000; Sullivan *et al.*, 1999; Tchinda *et al.*, 2007; Verhoeff *et al.*, 2001), severe malarial anemia (SA) (Matteelli *et al.*, 1994), and severe malaria (SM) (Mackintosh *et al.*, 2004; Troye-Blomberg *et al.*, 1999). Findings suggest wide conformity, both among the cellular and humoral components of the immune system, are key to elimination of *Plasmodium* from the human host (Angulo *et al.*, 2002).

Types of Cytokines, Serum Proteins and *Plasmodium* Proteins Associated with Malaria Pathogenesis

RANTES is a chemokine protein induced by cytokines. RANTES is released by cytotoxic T lymphocytes (CTL), and is a potent chemoattractant of monocytes and T cells (Appay *et al.*, 2000). Interferon gamma-induced protein (IP-10) is a protein that is secreted by several types of cells in response to IFN-γ. IP-10 has played a role in chemoattraction for monocytes, macrophages, promotion of T cell adhesion to endothelial cells, and inhibition of bone marrow colony formation (Angiolillo *et al.*, 1995).

Macrophage inflammatory proteins (MIP-1α and MIP-1β) are chemokines that cause the secretion of other pro-inflammatory cytokines such as IL-6 and TNF-α. MIP-1α and MIP-1β are chemotactic for specific types of leukocyte populations and are involved in the regulation of cell-mediated immunity (Matsukawa *et al.*, 2000). Procalcitonin (PCT) is a precursor of the hormone calcitonin. PCT has been observed to differentiate between bacterial infection and non-infectious states (Charles *et al.*, 2008). Neopterin is synthesised during an immune response upon stimulation with IFN-γ. Neopterin is associated with activation of T_H1-derived cellular immune activation and significant levels are found in infections (Murr *et al.*, 2002).

Prolactin is a protein and hormone synthesized by the anterior pituitary. Prolactin has a vital role in mediating humoral and cellular immune responses (Freeman *et al.*, 2000). Cortisol is a steroid and hormone synthesized by the adrenal gland. Significant levels of cortisol have been reported in stressful states and serious illnesses of patients (Sam *et al.*, 2004). Endoglin (sENG) is a type I membrane protein and a component of TGFβ. Elevated levels of sENG observed in humans correlate with disease and may serve as a marker for infection (Venkatesha *et al.*, 2006).

CD163 is seen in humans and belongs to the scavenger receptor cysteine family. CD163 stimulates an anti-inflammatory response and is observed during an immune response and in inflammatory diseases (Moller *et al.*, 2004). Granulocyte colony-stimulating factor (G-CSF) is a protein involved in the granulocyte formation in the bone marrow. G-CSF was discovered to be significant in patients with acute bacterial and viral infections (Pauksen *et al.*, 1994).

E-selectin is a cell adhesion molecule induced by cytokines. High levels of E-selectin are observed in various types of diseases (Mann *et al.*, 2010). Inter-cellular adhesion molecule 1 (ICAM-1) is expressed on membrane surface of cells at the sites of inflammation and infection (Rothlein *et al.*, 1988). Angiopoietins (ANG-1 and ANG-2) are proteins needed to synthesize blood vessels. ANG-2 has been associated with endothelial activation and a marker of disease severity (described in (Orfanos *et al.*, 2007)).

Monocyte chemotactic protein-1 (MCP-1) is a cytokine that belongs to the chemokine receptor family. MCP-1 is involved in migration of monocytes to an infected area and may contribute to granuloma formation during pathophysiological response (Tsuneyama *et al.*, 2001). Interleukin-8 (IL-8) is a chemokine and mediator of the inflammatory response. IL-8 is produced by a variety of cells and released during various inflammatory conditions (Bickel, 1993).

Histidine rich protein 2 (HRP2) is secreted by *Plasmodium falciparum* and is associated with infected erythrocytes and believed to be secreted by early gametocytes, as it is by trophozoites (described in (Hayward *et al.*, 2000)).

Several studies reported chemokines such as MCP–1, MIP–1α, MIP-1β, and RANTES, induce some cells to increase production of TNF-α, IP-10, MCP-1, MIP-1α, and MIP-1β, in malaria-infected patients (Suguitan *et al.*, 2003) and lower levels of RANTES in children with CM (John *et al.*, 2008). Findings suggest elevated concentrations of cortisol and decreased levels of prolactin at various ratios are an important mediator in host's immunity (Bayoumi *et al.*, 2009). Procalcitonin (PCT), a predecessor of the hormone calcitonin, has also been observed in malaria infected patients (Hesselink *et al.*, 2009), and studies indicated patients infected with SM or CM compared to patients with UM have increased serum levels of Endoglin (sENG) (Dietmann *et al.*, 2009). Prior studies have reported group B cysteine-rich scavenger membrane receptor known as sCD163 are stimulated by cytokines (e.g., IL-6 and IL-10) and were observed in significant levels in patients with UM compared to CM or SA (Kusi *et al.*, 2008). *In vivo* activation of macrophages and T cells, heighten levels of serum neopterin, was seen in children with malaria (Thuma *et al.*, 1996). Moreover, high levels of neopterin (Biemba *et al.*, 2000), procalcitonin and plasma lactate have been reported in travelers with UM or non-malaria (te Witt *et al.*, 2010). Elevations of angiopoietin-1 (ANG-1) and angiopoietin-2 (ANG-2) were also examined (Conroy *et al.*, 2009) and identified in patients with malaria.

Malaria research has indicated, all infected patients with elevated levels of ANG-2 were linked with increased lactic acid, ICAM, HRP2 and E-selectin (Yeo *et al.*, 2008). Studies also indicated that ANG-1 levels appeared to decrease as ANG-2 levels became increased in malaria infected patients (Yeo et al. 2008). ANG-1 and ANG-2 ratios were reported to be significantly different in patients without malaria (Yeo *et al.*, 2008).

Soluble ICAM-1, IL-1Ra, IL-2R, IL-4, IL-6, IL-6R, neopterin, angiopoeitin (ANG) 2 and TNFα, MIP-1α, MIP-1β,and procalcitonin may serve as prognostic indicators for the progress and outcome of malaria. A diagnostic test that combines host biomarkers with parasite proteins will improve disease management of malaria and will also serve as a useful in determinant of effectiveness parasite clearance following drug treatment.

References

Angiolillo, A. L., Sgadari, C., Taub, D. D., *et al.* (1995). Human interferon-inducible protein 10 is a potent inhibitor of angiogenesis in vivo. *J Exp Med.* 182, 155-62.

Angulo, I. and Fresno, M. (2002). Cytokines in the pathogenesis of and protection against malaria. *Clin Diagn Lab Immunol.* 9, 1145-52.

Appay, V., Dunbar, P. R., Cerundolo, V., *et al.* (2000). RANTES activates antigen-specific cytotoxic T lymphocytes in a mitogen-like manner through cell surface aggregation. *Int Immunol.* 12, 1173-82.

Armah, H. B., Wilson, N. O., Sarfo, B. Y., *et al.* (2007). Cerebrospinal fluid and serum biomarkers of cerebral malaria mortality in Ghanaian children. *Malar J.* 6, 147.

Awandare, G. A., Goka, B., Boeuf, P., *et al.* (2006). Increased levels of inflammatory mediators in children with severe *Plasmodium falciparum* malaria with respiratory distress. *J Infect Dis.* 194, 1438-46.

Barnwell, J. W. and Galinski, M. R. (1998). Malaria: parasite biology, pathogenesis, and protection. ASM Press.

Bayoumi, N. K., Elhassan, E. M., Elbashir, M. I., *et al.* (2009). Cortisol, prolactin, cytokines and the susceptibility of pregnant Sudanese women to Plasmodium falciparum malaria. *Ann Trop Med Parasitol.* 103, 111-7.

Berriman, M. (2010). *Plasmodium falciparum* genome projects. The Wellcome Trust Sanger Institute, *http://www.sanger.ac.uk/resources/downloads/protozoa/plasmodium-falciparum.html.*

Beutler, B. (1988). The presence of cachectin/tumor necrosis factor in human disease states. *Am J Med.* 85, 287-8.

Beutler, B. and Cerami, A. (1987). Cachectin--Tumour necrosis factor: a cytokine that mediates injury initiated by invasive parasites. *Parasitol Today.* 3, 345-6.

Bickel, M. (1993). The role of interleukin-8 in inflammation and mechanisms of regulation. *J Periodontol.* 64, 456-60.

Biemba, G., Gordeuk, V. R., Thuma, P., *et al.* (2000). Markers of inflammation in children with severe malarial anaemia. *Trop Med Int Health.* 5, 256-62.

Biswas, S., Tomar, D. and Rao, D. N. (2005). Investigation of the kinetics of histidine-rich protein 2 and of the antibody responses to this antigen, in a group of malaria patients from India. *Ann Trop Med Parasitol.* 99, 553-62.

Brabin, B. J., Agbaje, S. O., Ahmed, Y., *et al.* (1999). A birthweight nomogram for Africa, as a malaria-control indicator. *Ann Trop Med Parasitol.* 93 Suppl 1, S43-57.

Buechler, C., Ritter, M., Orso, E., *et al.* (2000). Regulation of scavenger receptor CD163 expression in human monocytes and macrophages by pro- and antiinflammatory stimuli. *J Leukoc Biol.* 67, 97-103.

Casals-Pascual, C. and Roberts, D. J. (2006). Severe malarial anaemia. *Curr Mol Med.* 6, 155-68.

CDC (2010). Malaria Parasites, *http://www.cdc.gov/malaria/about/biology/parasites.html.*

CDC (2011). Emerging Infectious Diseases, *http://wwwnc.cdc.gov/eid/article/16/10/10-0427_article.htm*

Cerami, A. and Beutler, B. (1988). The role of cachectin/TNF in endotoxic shock and cachexia. *Immunol Today.* 9, 28-31.

Chaiyaroj, S. C., Rutta, A. S., Muenthaisong, K., *et al.* (2004). Reduced levels of transforming growth factor-beta1, interleukin-12 and increased migration inhibitory factor are associated with severe malaria. *Acta Trop*. 89, 319-27.

Charles, P. E., Ladoire, S., Aho, S., *et al.* (2008). Serum procalcitonin elevation in critically ill patients at the onset of bacteremia caused by either Gram negative or Gram positive bacteria. *BMC Infect Dis*. 8, 38.

Chitnis, C. E. (2001). Molecular insights into receptors used by malaria parasites for erythrocyte invasion. *Curr Opin Hematol*. 8, 85-91.

Clark, I. A. (1978). Does endotoxin cause both the disease and parasite death in acute malaria and babesiosis? *Lancet*. 2, 75-7.

Clark, I. A. (2007). How TNF was recognized as a key mechanism of disease. *Cytokine Growth Factor Rev*. 18, 335-43.

Clark, I. A., Budd, A. C., Alleva, L. M., *et al.* (2006). Human malarial disease: a consequence of inflammatory cytokine release. *Malar J*. 5, 85.

Coltel, N., Combes, V., Hunt, N. H., *et al.* (2004). Cerebral malaria -- a neurovascular pathology with many riddles still to be solved. *Curr Neurovasc Res*. 1, 91-110.

Conroy, A. L., Lafferty, E. I., Lovegrove, F. E., *et al.* (2009). Whole blood angiopoietin-1 and -2 levels discriminate cerebral and severe (non-cerebral) malaria from uncomplicated malaria. *Malar J*. 8, 295.

Cserti-Gazdewich, C. M., Dzik, W. H., Erdman, L., *et al.* (2010). Combined measurement of soluble and cellular ICAM-1 among children with Plasmodium falciparum malaria in Uganda. *Malar J*. 9, 233.

Curfs, J. H., van der Meer, J. W., Sauerwein, R. W., *et al.* (1990). Low dosages of interleukin 1 protect mice against lethal cerebral malaria. *J Exp Med*. 172, 1287-91.

Deloron, P., Chougnet, C., Lepers, J. P., *et al.* (1991). Protective value of elevated levels of gamma interferon in serum against exoerythrocytic stages of Plasmodium falciparum. *J Clin Microbiol*. 29, 1757-60.

Dietmann, A., Helbok, R., Lackner, P., *et al.* (2009). Endoglin in African children with Plasmodium falciparum malaria: a novel player in severe malaria pathogenesis? *J Infect Dis*. 200, 1842-8.

Dietmann, A., Lackner, P., Helbok, R., *et al.* (2008). Opposed circulating plasma levels of endothelin-1 and C-type natriuretic peptide in children with Plasmodium falciparum malaria. *Malar J*. 7, 253.

Dinarello, C. A. (2000). Proinflammatory cytokines. *Chest*. 118, 503-8.

Diouf, I., Fievet, N., Doucoure, S., *et al.* (2007). IL-12 producing monocytes and IFN-gamma and TNF-alpha producing T-lymphocytes are increased in placentas infected by Plasmodium falciparum. *J Reprod Immunol*. 74, 152-62.

Eling, W. M. and Kremsner, P. G. (1994). Cytokines in malaria, pathology and protection. *Biotherapy*. 7, 211-21.

Finkel, M. (2007). Malaria: Stopping a global killer. *National Geographic*. 7, 32-46.

Francischetti, I. M., Seydel, K. B. and Monteiro, R. Q. (2008). Blood coagulation, inflammation, and malaria. *Microcirculation*. 15, 81-107.

Freeman, M. E., Kanyicska, B., Lerant, A., *et al.* (2000). Prolactin: structure, function, and regulation of secretion. *Physiol Rev*. 80, 1523-631.

Fried, M., Muga, R. O., Misore, A. O., *et al.* (1998). Malaria elicits type 1 cytokines in the human placenta: IFN-gamma and TNF-alpha associated with pregnancy outcomes. *J Immunol.* 160, 2523-30.

Gimenez, F., Barraud de Lagerie, S., Fernandez, C., *et al.* (2003). Tumor necrosis factor alpha in the pathogenesis of cerebral malaria. *Cell Mol Life Sci.* 60, 1623-35.

Gosi, P., Khusmith, S., Looareesuwan, S., *et al.* (1999). Complicated malaria is associated with differential elevations in serum levels of interleukins 10, 12, and 15. *Southeast Asian J Trop Med Public Health.* 30, 412-7.

Gourley, I. S., Kurtis, J. D., Kamoun, M., *et al.* (2002). Profound bias in interferon-gamma and interleukin-6 allele frequencies in western Kenya, where severe malarial anemia is common in children. *J Infect Dis.* 186, 1007-12.

Grau, G. E., Frei, K., Piguet, P. F., *et al.* (1990). Interleukin 6 production in experimental cerebral malaria: modulation by anticytokine antibodies and possible role in hypergammaglobulinemia. *J Exp Med.* 172, 1505-8.

Grau, G. E., Taylor, T. E., Molyneux, M. E., *et al.* (1989). Tumor necrosis factor and disease severity in children with falciparum malaria. *N Engl J Med.* 320, 1586-91.

Greenwood, B. (2002). The molecular epidemiology of malaria. *Trop Med Int Health.* 7, 1012-21.

Guyatt, H. L. and Snow, R. W. (2004). Impact of malaria during pregnancy on low birth weight in sub-Saharan Africa. *Clin Microbiol Rev.* 17, 760-9, table of contents.

Hayward, R. E., Sullivan, D. J. and Day, K. P. (2000). Plasmodium falciparum: histidine-rich protein II is expressed during gametocyte development. *Exp Parasitol.* 96, 139-46.

Hesselink, D. A., Burgerhart, J. S., Bosmans-Timmerarends, H., *et al.* (2009). Procalcitonin as a biomarker for severe *Plasmodium falciparum* disease: a critical appraisal of a semi-quantitative point-of-care test in a cohort of travellers with imported malaria. *Malar J.* 8, 206.

Ho, M., Schollaardt, T., Snape, S., *et al.* (1998). Endogenous interleukin-10 modulates proinflammatory response in Plasmodium falciparum malaria. *J Infect Dis.* 178, 520-5.

Ho, M., Sexton, M. M., Tongtawe, P., *et al.* (1995). Interleukin-10 inhibits tumor necrosis factor production but not antigen-specific lymphoproliferation in acute Plasmodium falciparum malaria. *J Infect Dis.* 172, 838-44.

Iriemenam, N. C., Okafor, C. M., Balogun, H. A., *et al.* (2009). Cytokine profiles and antibody responses to *Plasmodium falciparum* malaria infection in individuals living in Ibadan, southwest Nigeria. *Afr Health Sci.* 9, 66-74.

Issifou, S., Mavoungou, E., Borrmann, S., *et al.* (2003). Severe malarial anemia associated with increased soluble Fas ligand (sFasL) concentrations in Gabonese children. *Eur Cytokine Netw.* 14, 238-41.

Janeway, C. A., Travers, P., Walport, M., *et al.* (2007). Immunobiology: The Immune System in Health and Disease. 7th ed ed. Garland Pub, New York.

Jason, J., Archibald, L. K., Nwanyanwu, O. C., *et al.* (2001). Cytokines and malaria parasitemia. *Clin Immunol.* 100, 208-18.

John, C. C., Park, G. S., Sam-Agudu, N., *et al.* (2008). Elevated serum levels of IL-1ra in children with Plasmodium falciparum malaria are associated with increased severity of disease. *Cytokine.* 41, 204-8.

Johnson, J. G. (2010). The World of Biology: Chapter 26, Protozoa Life Cycle of Plasmodium - a Sporozoan, Ed.^ Eds.).

Kabyemela, E. R., Muehlenbachs, A., Fried, M., *et al.* (2008). Maternal peripheral blood level of IL-10 as a marker for inflammatory placental malaria. *Malar J.* 7, 26.

Keuter, M., Dharmana, E., Gasem, M. H., *et al.* (1994). Patterns of proinflammatory cytokines and inhibitors during typhoid fever. *J Infect Dis.* 169, 1306-11.

Kristiansen, M., Graversen, J. H., Jacobsen, C., *et al.* (2001). Identification of the haemoglobin scavenger receptor. *Nature.* 409, 198-201.

Kurtis, J. D., Lanar, D. E., Opollo, M., *et al.* (1999). Interleukin-10 responses to liver-stage antigen 1 predict human resistance to Plasmodium falciparum. *Infect Immun.* 67, 3424-9.

Kurtzhals, J. A., Adabayeri, V., Goka, B. Q., *et al.* (1998). Low plasma concentrations of interleukin 10 in severe malarial anaemia compared with cerebral and uncomplicated malaria. *Lancet.* 351, 1768-72.

Kusi, K. A., Gyan, B. A., Goka, B. Q., *et al.* (2008). Levels of soluble CD163 and severity of malaria in children in Ghana. *Clin Vaccine Immunol.* 15, 1456-60.

Li, C., Sanni, L. A., Omer, F., *et al.* (2003). Pathology of Plasmodium chabaudi chabaudi infection and mortality in interleukin-10-deficient mice are ameliorated by anti-tumor necrosis factor alpha and exacerbated by anti-transforming growth factor beta antibodies. *Infect Immun.* 71, 4850-6.

Lyke, K. E., Burges, R., Cissoko, Y., *et al.* (2004). Serum levels of the proinflammatory cytokines interleukin-1 beta (IL-1beta), IL-6, IL-8, IL-10, tumor necrosis factor alpha, and IL-12(p70) in Malian children with severe Plasmodium falciparum malaria and matched uncomplicated malaria or healthy controls. *Infect Immun.* 72, 5630-7.

Mackintosh, C. L., Beeson, J. G. and Marsh, K. (2004). Clinical features and pathogenesis of severe malaria. *Trends Parasitol.* 20, 597-603.

Malaguarnera, L., Pignatelli, S., Musumeci, M., *et al.* (2002). Plasma levels of interleukin-18 and interleukin-12 in *Plasmodium falciparum* malaria. *Parasite Immunol.* 24, 489-92.

Mann, A. P., Somasunderam, A., Nieves-Alicea, R., *et al.* (2010). Identification of thioaptamer ligand against E-selectin: potential application for inflamed vasculature targeting. *PLoS One.* 5.

Matsukawa, A., Hogaboam, C. M., Lukacs, N. W., *et al.* (2000). Chemokines and innate immunity. *Rev Immunogenet.* 2, 339-58.

Matteelli, A., Donato, F., Shein, A., *et al.* (1994). Malaria and anaemia in pregnant women in urban Zanzibar, Tanzania. *Ann Trop Med Parasitol.* 88, 475-83.

Mergani, A., Khamis, A. H., Haboor, A. B., *et al.* (2010). Lack of association between -308 tumor necrosis factor polymorphism and susceptibility to cerebral malaria among Central Sudanese children. *Int J Genet Mol Biol.* 2, 67-71.

Moller, H. J., de Fost, M., Aerts, H., *et al.* (2004). Plasma level of the macrophage-derived soluble CD163 is increased and positively correlates with severity in Gaucher's disease. *Eur J Haematol.* 72, 135-9.

Moormann, A. M., Sullivan, A. D., Rochford, R. A., *et al.* (1999). Malaria and pregnancy: placental cytokine expression and its relationship to intrauterine growth retardation. *J Infect Dis.* 180, 1987-93.

Muller, I., Genton, B., Rare, L., *et al.* (2009). Three different Plasmodium species show similar patterns of clinical tolerance of malaria infection. *Malar J.* 8, 158.

Murr, C., Widner, B., Wirleitner, B., *et al.* (2002). Neopterin as a marker for immune system activation. *Curr Drug Metab.* 3, 175-87.

Nagamine, Y., Hayano, M., Kashiwamura, S., *et al.* (2003). Involvement of interleukin-18 in severe Plasmodium falciparum malaria. *Trans R Soc Trop Med Hyg*. 97, 236-41.

Newton, C. R., Taylor, T. E. and Whitten, R. O. (1998). Pathophysiology of fatal falciparum malaria in African children. *Am J Trop Med Hyg*. 58, 673-83.

Nussenblatt, V., Mukasa, G., Metzger, A., *et al.* (2001). Anemia and interleukin-10, tumor necrosis factor alpha, and erythropoietin levels among children with acute, uncomplicated *Plasmodium falciparum* malaria. *Clin Diagn Lab Immunol*. 8, 1164-70.

Opal, S. M. and DePalo, V. A. (2000). Anti-inflammatory cytokines. *Chest*. 117, 1162-72.

Orfanos, S. E., Kotanidou, A., Glynos, C., *et al.* (2007). Angiopoietin-2 is increased in severe sepsis: correlation with inflammatory mediators. *Crit Care Med*. 35, 199-206.

Othoro, C., Lal, A. A., Nahlen, B., *et al.* (1999). A low interleukin-10 tumor necrosis factor-alpha ratio is associated with malaria anemia in children residing in a holoendemic malaria region in western Kenya. *J Infect Dis*. 179, 279-82.

Parquet, V., Henry, M., Wurtz, N., *et al.* (2010). Atorvastatin as a potential anti-malarial drug: in vitro synergy in combinational therapy with quinine against *Plasmodium falciparum*. *Malar J*. 9, 139.

Pauksen, K., Elfman, L., Ulfgren, A. K., *et al.* (1994). Serum levels of granulocyte-colony stimulating factor (G-CSF) in bacterial and viral infections, and in atypical pneumonia. *Br J Haematol*. 88, 256-60.

Perch, M., Kofoed, P., Fischer, T. K., *et al.* (2004). Serum levels of soluble urokinase plasminogen activator receptor is associated with parasitemia in children with acute *Plasmodium falciparum* malaria infection. *Parasite Immunol*. 26, 207-11.

Perkins, M. E. and Rocco, L. J. (1988). Sialic acid-dependent binding of Plasmodium falciparum merozoite surface antigen, Pf200, to human erythrocytes. *J Immunol*. 141, 3190-6.

Perlmann, H., Helmby, H., Hagstedt, M., *et al.* (1994). IgE elevation and IgE anti-malarial antibodies in *Plasmodium falciparum* malaria: association of high IgE levels with cerebral malaria. *Clin Exp Immunol*. 97, 284-92.

Perlmann, P., Perlmann, H., Flyg, B. W., *et al.* (1997). Immunoglobulin E, a pathogenic factor in *Plasmodium falciparum* malaria. *Infect Immun*. 65, 116-21.

Peyron, F., Burdin, N., Ringwald, P., *et al.* (1994). High levels of circulating IL-10 in human malaria. *Clin Exp Immunol*. 95, 300-3.

Philippidis, P., Mason, J. C., Evans, B. J., *et al.* (2004). Hemoglobin scavenger receptor CD163 mediates interleukin-10 release and heme oxygenase-1 synthesis: antiinflammatory monocyte-macrophage responses in vitro, in resolving skin blisters in vivo, and after cardiopulmonary bypass surgery. *Circ Res*. 94, 119-26.

Pongponratn, E., Turner, G. D., Day, N. P., *et al.* (2003). An ultrastructural study of the brain in fatal *Plasmodium falciparum* malaria. *Am J Trop Med Hyg*. 69, 345-59.

Prakash, D., Fesel, C., Jain, R., *et al.* (2006). Clusters of cytokines determine malaria severity in *Plasmodium falciparum*-infected patients from endemic areas of Central India. *J Infect Dis*. 194, 198-207.

Raghupathy, R. (1997). Th1-type immunity is incompatible with successful pregnancy. *Immunol Today*. 18, 478-82.

Randall, L. M. and Engwerda, C. R. (2010). TNF family members and malaria: old observations, new insights and future directions. *Exp Parasitol*. 126, 326-31.

Richard, D. MacRalid, C. A., Riglar, D. T., Chan, J. A., Foley, M., Baum, J., Ralph, S. A., Norton, R. S. and Cowman, A. F. (2010) Interaction between Plasmodium falciparum AMA-1 and the rhoptry neck protein complex defines a key step in the erythrocyte invasion process of malaria parasites. J. Biol. Chem. 285: 14815-22.

Ringwald, P., Peyron, F., Vuillez, J. P., *et al.* (1991). Levels of cytokines in plasma during *Plasmodium falciparum* malaria attacks. *J Clin Microbiol.* 29, 2076-8.

Robson, K. J. and Weatherall, D. J. (2009). Malarial anemia and STAT6. *Haematologica.* 94, 157-9.

Rogerson, S. J., Brown, H. C., Pollina, E., *et al.* (2003). Placental tumor necrosis factor alpha but not gamma interferon is associated with placental malaria and low birth weight in Malawian women. *Infect Immun.* 71, 267-70.

Rothlein, R., Czajkowski, M., O'Neill, M. M., *et al.* (1988). Induction of intercellular adhesion molecule 1 on primary and continuous cell lines by pro-inflammatory cytokines. Regulation by pharmacologic agents and neutralizing antibodies. *J Immunol.* 141, 1665-9.

Sam, S., Corbridge, T. C., Mokhlesi, B., *et al.* (2004). Cortisol levels and mortality in severe sepsis. *Clin Endocrinol (Oxf).* 60, 29-35.

Sarfo, B. Y., Singh, S., Lillard, J. W., Jr., *et al.* (2004). The cerebral-malaria-associated expression of RANTES, CCR3 and CCR5 in post-mortem tissue samples. *Ann Trop Med Parasitol.* 98, 297-303.

Sarthou, J. L., Angel, G., Aribot, G., *et al.* (1997). Prognostic value of anti-*Plasmodium falciparum*-specific immunoglobulin G3, cytokines, and their soluble receptors in West African patients with severe malaria. *Infect Immun.* 65, 3271-6.

Schaer, D. J., Schaer, C. A., Buehler, P. W., *et al.* (2006). CD163 is the macrophage scavenger receptor for native and chemically modified hemoglobins in the absence of haptoglobin. *Blood.* 107, 373-80.

Schofield, L. and Grau, G. E. (2005). Immunological processes in malaria pathogenesis. *Nat Rev Immunol.* 5, 722-35.

Sherman, I. W. Molecular Approaches to Malaria, American Soceity for Microbiology 2005

Shaffer, N., Grau, G. E., Hedberg, K., *et al.* (1991). Tumor necrosis factor and severe malaria. *J Infect Dis.* 163, 96-101.

Singh, S., Singh, N. and Handa, R. (2000). Tumor necrosis factor-alpha in patients with malaria. *Indian J Malariol.* 37, 27-33.

Smythe, J. A., Coppel, R. L., Brown, G. V., *et al.* (1988). Identification of two integral membrane proteins of *Plasmodium falciparum*. *Proc Natl Acad Sci U S A.* 85, 5195-9.

Steketee, R. W., Nahlen, B. L., Parise, M. E., *et al.* (2001). The burden of malaria in pregnancy in malaria-endemic areas. *Am J Trop Med Hyg.* 64, 28-35.

Steketee, R. W., Wirima, J. J., Hightower, A. W., *et al.* (1996). The effect of malaria and malaria prevention in pregnancy on offspring birthweight, prematurity, and intrauterine growth retardation in rural Malawi. *Am J Trop Med Hyg.* 55, 33-41.

Stoiser, B., Looareesuwan, S., Thalhammer, F., *et al.* (2000). Serum concentrations of granulocyte-colony stimulating factor in complicated Plasmodium falciparum malaria. *Eur Cytokine Netw.* 11, 75-80.

Suguitan, A. L., Jr., Leke, R. G., Fouda, G., *et al.* (2003). Changes in the levels of chemokines and cytokines in the placentas of women with Plasmodium falciparum malaria. *J Infect Dis.* 188, 1074-82.

Suh, K. N., Kain, K. C. and Keystone, J. S. (2004). Malaria. *CMAJ*. 170, 1693-702.

Sulahian, T. H., Hogger, P., Wahner, A. E., *et al.* (2000). Human monocytes express CD163, which is upregulated by IL-10 and identical to p155. *Cytokine*. 12, 1312-21.

Sullivan, A. D., Nyirenda, T., Cullinan, T., *et al.* (1999). Malaria infection during pregnancy: intrauterine growth retardation and preterm delivery in Malawi. *J Infect Dis*. 179, 1580-3.

Tangteerawatana, P., Montgomery, S. M., Perlmann, H., *et al.* (2007). Differential regulation of IgG subclasses and IgE antimalarial antibody responses in complicated and uncomplicated *Plasmodium falciparum* malaria. *Parasite Immunol*. 29, 475-83.

Tangteerawatana, P., Perlmann, H., Hayano, M., *et al.* (2009). IL4 gene polymorphism and previous malaria experiences manipulate anti-*Plasmodium falciparum* antibody isotype profiles in complicated and uncomplicated malaria. *Malar J*. 8, 286.

Taylor-Robinson, A. W. and Smith, E. C. (1999). A role for cytokines in potentiation of malaria vaccines through immunological modulation of blood stage infection. *Immunol Rev*. 171, 105-23.

Tchinda, V. H., Tadem, A. D., Tako, E. A., *et al.* (2007). Severe malaria in Cameroonian children: correlation between plasma levels of three soluble inducible adhesion molecules and TNF-alpha. *Acta Trop*. 102, 20-8.

te Witt, R., van Wolfswinkel, M. E., Petit, P. L., *et al.* (2010). Neopterin and procalcitonin are suitable biomarkers for exclusion of severe Plasmodium falciparum disease at the initial clinical assessment of travellers with imported malaria. *Malar J*. 9, 255.

Thuma, P. E., Weiss, G., Herold, M., *et al.* (1996). Serum neopterin, interleukin-4, and interleukin-6 concentrations in cerebral malaria patients and the effect of iron chelation therapy. *Am J Trop Med Hyg*. 54, 164-8.

Troye-Blomberg, M., Weidanz, W. P. and van der Heyde, H. C. (1999). The role of T cells in immunity to malaria and the pathogenesis of disease; in Wahlgren, M. Perlamnn P. (eds): *Malaria: Molecular and Clinical Aspects*. Harwood Academic, Amsterdam.

Tsuneyama, K., Harada, K., Yasoshima, M., *et al.* (2001). Monocyte chemotactic protein-1, -2, and -3 are distinctively expressed in portal tracts and granulomata in primary biliary cirrhosis: implications for pathogenesis. *J Pathol*. 193, 102-9.

Van den Eede, P., Van, H. N., Van Overmeir, C., *et al.* (2009). Human Plasmodium knowlesi infections in young children in central Vietnam. *Malar J*. 8, 249.

van Deuren, M., van der Ven-Jongekrijg, J., Bartelink, A. K., *et al.* (1995). Correlation between proinflammatory cytokines and antiinflammatory mediators and the severity of disease in meningococcal infections. *J Infect Dis*. 172, 433-9.

Venkatesha, S., Toporsian, M., Lam, C., *et al.* (2006). Soluble endoglin contributes to the pathogenesis of preeclampsia. *Nat Med*. 12, 642-9.

Verhoeff, F. H., Brabin, B. J., van Buuren, S., *et al.* (2001). An analysis of intra-uterine growth retardation in rural Malawi. *Eur J Clin Nutr*. 55, 682-9.

Vreden, S. G., van den Broek, M. F., Oettinger, M. C., *et al.* (1992). Cytokines inhibit the development of liver schizonts of the malaria parasite *Plasmodium berghei* in vivo. *Eur J Immunol*. 22, 2271-5.

Wenisch, C., Parschalk, B., Narzt, E., *et al.* (1995). Elevated serum levels of IL-10 and IFN-gamma in patients with acute Plasmodium falciparum malaria. *Clin Immunol Immunopathol*. 74, 115-7.

Wong, P. and Pamer, E. G. (2003). CD8 T cell responses to infectious pathogens. *Annu Rev Immunol*. 21, 29-70.

Wroczynska, A., Nahorski, W., Bakowska, A., *et al.* (2005). Cytokines and clinical manifestations of malaria in adults with severe and uncomplicated disease. *Int Marit Health*. 56, 103-14.

Yamada-Tanaka, M. S., Ferreira-da-Cruz, M. F., Alecrim, M. G., *et al.* (1995). Tumor necrosis factor alpha interferon gamma and macrophage stimulating factor in relation to the Severity of *Plasmodium falciparum* malaria in the Brazilian Amazon. *Trop Geogr Med*. 47, 282-5.

Yazdani, S. S., Mukherjee, P., Chauhan, V. S., *et al.* (2006). Immune responses to asexual blood-stages of malaria parasites. *Curr Mol Med*. 6, 187-203.

Yeo, T. W., Lampah, D. A., Gitawati, R., *et al.* (2008). Angiopoietin-2 is associated with decreased endothelial nitric oxide and poor clinical outcome in severe falciparum malaria. *Proc Natl Acad Sci U S A*. 105, 17097-102.

Index

A

B

C

D

E

F

G

H

J

K

L

M

N

O

P

Q

Y

Z

U

V

W

T